Textbook of Integrative
Mental Health Care

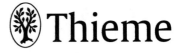

Textbook of Integrative Mental Health Care

James H. Lake, M.D.
Clinical Assistant Professor
Department of Psychiatry and Behavioral Sciences
Stanford University Hospital
Stanford, California

Thieme
New York • Stuttgart

Thieme Medical Publishers, Inc.
333 Seventh Ave.
New York, NY 10001
Associate Editor: Birgitta Brandenburg
Assistant Editor: Ivy Ip
Vice-President, Production and Electronic Publishing: Anne T. Vinnicombe
Production Editor: Becky Dille
Sales Director: Ross Lumpkin
Chief Financial Officer: Peter van Woerden
President: Brian D. Scanlan
Compositor: Compset, Inc.
Printer: Maple-Vail Book Manufacturing Group

Library of Congress Cataloging-in-Publication Data
Lake, James, 1956–
    Textbook of integrative mental health care / James H. Lake.
       p. ; cm.
    Includes bibliographical references and index.
    ISBN-13: 978-1-58890-299-3 (TMP : alk. paper)
    ISBN-10: 1-58890-299-4 (TMP : alk. paper)
    ISBN-13: 978-3-13-136671-9 (GTV : alk. paper)
    ISBN-10: 3-13-136671-0 (GTV : alk. paper)   1. Mental health services.   2. Integrated delivery
of health care.   3. Psychotherapy.   4. Psychiatry.   5. Holistic medicine.   I. Title.
    [DNLM: 1. Mental Disorders—therapy.   2. Complementary Therapies.   3. Holistic Health.
4. Mental Disorders—etiology.   WM 100 L192t 2006]
RC790.5.L35 2006
616.89'14—dc22   2006016145

Important note: Medical knowledge is ever-changing. As new research and clinical experience broaden
our knowledge, changes in treatment and drug therapy may be required. The authors and editors of the
material herein have consulted sources believed to be reliable in their efforts to provide information that
is complete and in accord with the standards accepted at the time of publication. However, in view of the
possibility of human error by the authors, editors, or publisher of the work herein or changes in medical
knowledge, neither the authors, editors, nor publisher, nor any other party who has been involved in the
preparation of this work, warrants that the information contained herein is in every respect accurate or
complete, and they are not responsible for any errors or omissions or for the results obtained from use of
such information. Readers are encouraged to confirm the information contained herein with other
sources. For example, readers are advised to check the product information sheet included in the package
of each drug they plan to administer to be certain that the information contained in this publication is
accurate and that changes have not been made in the recommended dose or in the contraindications for
administration. This recommendation is of particular importance in connection with new or infrequently
used drugs.

Some of the product names, patents, and registered designs referred to in this book are in fact registered
trademarks or proprietary names even though specific reference to this fact is not always made in the
text. Therefore, the appearance of a name without designation as proprietary is not to be construed as a
representation by the publisher that it is in the public domain.

Printed in the United States of America

5 4 3 2 1

TMP ISBN 978-1-58890-299-3
TMP ISBN 1-58890-299-4
GTV ISBN 978 3 13 136671 9
GTV ISBN 3 13 136671 0

This book is dedicated to my patients, past, present, and future, and to healers of
all traditions who are open to new ways of understanding and bringing relief to human suffering.

We shall not cease from exploration
and the end of all our exploring
will be to arrive where we started
and know the place for the first time

T. S. Eliot, "Little Gidding," *The Four Quartets*

Contents

Foreword

This volume is anchored in one of the most dramatic social shifts currently taking place in the United States: the adoption by a large proportion of the population of so-called complementary, alternative, and integrative methods of health care. As you will see, these changes have little to do with high-tech advances that make headlines, such as the decoding of the human genome, DNA manipulation, new drugs, stems cells, or organ transplantation, but instead with a fundamentally different approach to human health.

Although the profession of medicine is often regarded as a hidebound and resistant to change, if we compare it with areas such as education or the law, we can see that it is one of the most dynamic institutions in our culture. As an example of how far medicine has evolved in recent years in the area of doctor–patient relationships, consider the following account by medical ethicist Eric J. Cassell. "During the 1930s," he relates, "my grandmother saw a specialist about a melanoma on her face. During the course of the visit when she asked him a question, he slapped her face, saying, 'I'll ask the questions here. I'll do the talking.' Can you imagine such an event occurring today? Melanomas may not have changed much in the last 50 years, but the profession of medicine has" (quoted in Laine & Davidoff, 1996).

From time to time a thunderbolt descends in medicine and shakes things up, after which it is never the same. This occurred in 1993, when physician David Eisenberg and his colleagues at Harvard Medical School revealed, for the first time, the actual extent of the shift toward integrative medicine (Eisenberg, Kessler, Foster, Norlock, Calkins, & Delbanco, 1993). They found that around half of the nation's adult population visited some sort of alternative medical practitioner each year. This exceeded the number of visits made to conventionally trained doctors such as family physicians, internists, and pediatricians. Moreover, people paid for these visits almost totally out-of-pocket, because they were seldom reimbursed by insurance plans. The survey also revealed that users of nonconventional methods were not naive but were generally well-educated, affluent, white, and female. Moreover, these individuals were highly pragmatic; they did not reject conventional approaches but used nonconventional therapies in addition to them. Follow-up surveys indicate that this is not a passing fad but is gathering momentum (Eisenberg et al., 1998). In a recent survey by the National Center for Complementary and Alternative Medicine of the National Institutes of Health, up to 62% of adults in the United States use a nonconventional treatment for a variety of problems, including anxiety, depression, and other mental health problems, which are Dr. Lake's focus in this book.

When news of these trends began to sink in, the medical profession as a whole was aghast. Physicians largely responded with arrogance and condescension, portraying "alternatives" as unscientific folk medicine at best and dangerous superstitions at worst. Medical experts lamented these trends in editorials in the major professional journals, professing dismay over the fact that half the population was making "unwise" health care choices. Had educated people lost their senses? Why were people no longer content with the contributions of drugs and surgery to their lives? Why the rush to supplements, herbal products, yoga, meditation, acupuncture, "energy medicine," and homeopathy? When medical journals did address nonconventional approaches, the reports were mainly negative and focused on the side effects of specific alternative therapies or their interactions with pharmaceuticals. Some physicians implied that the providers of nonconventional care were a national menace because they lured patients away from "real" medicine; they were traitors to science because they advocated therapies that had not been sufficiently validated. Many doctors imagined that these flirtations could be educated out of patients, after which things would happily revert to normal. Seldom did physicians seriously consider that some of these therapies might actually *work*.

It was as if physicians and patients were living in parallel universes, in two different worlds. The standoff was serious. Patients, for their part, usually did not inform their physicians that they were using alternatives; when asked why, most said they did not want to be hassled by poorly informed doctors who just didn't get it. Most physicians continued to regard the emerging views as new age sophistry, and they deeply resented the growing pressure to acknowledge and engage nonconventional therapies. But it was not only physicians who were off base; many proponents of nonconventional approaches were guilty of runaway enthusiasm and wildly exaggerated claims. Both sides seemed to be falling into the situation described by linguist Alfred Korzybski: "There are two ways to slice through life: to believe everything or to doubt everything. Both ways save us from thinking."

This was not conventional medicine's finest hour. But it was nonetheless a wake-up call for many physicians—a signal that patients wanted something more, something not provided in the hospitals, clinics, and medical offices throughout the land.

What was this something more? In a landmark, nationwide survey published in 1998 in the *Journal of the American Medical Association,* Dr. John Astin (1998), then at Stanford Medical School, directly asked patients why they chose alternative health measures. Astin's survey confirmed a broad-based dissatisfaction over the quality of conventional medical care because of concerns about the questionable efficacy and safety of many established treatments, the increasing cost of medical care, and the impersonal manner of health care delivery available in health maintenance organizations and other settings. He also discovered that many individuals seek nonconventional therapies for deeply personal or spiritual reasons. They had experienced a transformational experience in their lives, Astin discovered, that deeply influenced how they viewed the world. As a result, they wanted their medical care to reflect their inner values, and they sensed in nonconventional therapies a more genuine response to these needs than is available in conventional medical care. Yet a thoroughly American pragmatism remained. Astin found that people seldom replaced conventional methods with alternative measures but used them alongside each other, as mentioned.

Integrative and *integral* are displacing the earlier adjectives *alternative* and *complementary* to describe this type of medicine. But what does integrative medicine actually integrate? By and large, it strives to attend not only to the physiological functions of the body, which is the primary focus of conventional medicine, but also to the psychological, energetic, and spiritual domains of people's lives. As Dr. Lake points out in this book, approaches used in disparate systems of medicine often rest on very different assumptions about the nature of the body, the role of consciousness in healing, and the causes or meanings of illness. Advances in conventional biomedicine in the context of complex systems theory and other emerging paradigms in Western science are making it possible for the first time to model and rigorously investigate many nonconventional therapies. The result has been steady growth in intellectual openness among both researchers and physicians to the idea of integrative medicine.

Embracing nonbiomedical approaches, and especially therapies that are based on the putative role of consciousness, "energy," or spirituality in healing, seems a grandiose or impossible project to some physicians. A surgeon colleague of mine recently vented his objections about this task. "We don't expect ministers and priests to remove an appendix," he huffed. "Why should I be expected to deal with my patients' spiritual needs?"

Others sanction the integrative approach. This includes an increasing number of our nation's 125 medical schools, the majority of which now have formal coursework in integrative medicine (Dossey, 1999).

One of the most remarkable aspects of the integral vision is attention to the role of consciousness and spiritual issues in health and illness (Dossey, 1999; Levin, 2001).[9] This has been the subject of my own research and writing for decades now. During nearly all of the 20th century, spirituality—the sense of connectedness with something beyond the individual self, however named—was completely neglected in medicine. Spirituality was considered the sole purview of ministers, priests, and rabbis, not doctors or nurses. Since 1990, however, an increasing body of evidence—over 1200 studies—has demonstrated that people who follow a spiritual path in their life (it does not seem to matter which) live significantly longer and have a lower incidence of major diseases compared with people who do not follow such a path (Helm, Hays, Fling, Koenig, Blazer, 2000; Koenig, McCullough, & Larson, 2001; McCullough, Hoy, Larson, Koenig, & Thoresen, 2000). These findings are noteworthy because mental health, Dr. Lake's concern in this book, is an area of personal health that is not only effectively addressed using a range of nonconventional and integrative biological treatments, but frequently benefits from mind–body therapies like yoga and meditation, as well as so-called energetic or spiritual approaches including Healing Touch and qigong.

Because of demonstrated correlations between spiritual beliefs and practices, health, and longevity, spirituality and basic questions about the role of consciousness and intention in health and healing become, practically by definition, the concerns of medical professionals. This does not mean physicians should begin "selling" religion or spirituality, but that they should at least inform patients about the importance of a spiritual, mind–body, or "energy" practice for health and well-being so that patients can make their own decisions about these matters. This is basically the strategy doctors follow regarding any personal behavior that is health-related, such as smoking, diet, exercise, or sexual practices. Western physicians don't have to be experts on consciousness research, energy medicine, or spirituality to perform this important service; as in any other area, they may refer to specialists such as ministers, priests, rabbis, or practitioners of the various mind–body or energy therapies if their patients request further information or advice. Some skeptics contend that people's spiritual lives are too sensitive and private for health care professionals to become involved with them. This objection was also offered a few years ago as a reason why physicians should not inquire about people's sex lives. But when the national epidemic of sexually transmitted diseases and AIDS erupted, our views about the appropriateness of medical attention to sexuality changed overnight because it was obvious that the choices people made in this area were often linked to grave health outcomes. So with choices of spiritual or mind–body practices. When we genuinely confront issues of spirituality and the role of consciousness and intention in health and healing, we physicians can respond with sensitivity and skill, as we did in the area of sexual practices.

I emphasize spirituality, mind–body practices, and "energy" medicine because these approaches illustrate the reach of the integrative perspective and how far it extends beyond conventional medicine, and also because a spiritual thread or sense of sacredness runs through a great many integrative practices, including meditation, prayer, yoga, Healing Touch, and qigong, and is a fundamental part of many established systems of medicine, including Chinese medicine and ayurveda. There are unmistakable indications that medicine is being respiritualized in the United States at the highest levels. According to one review ("Better times for Spirituality," 2001):

In a 1999 consensus report, the American College of Physicians and the American Society of Internal Medicine suggested that physician care include a review of, and attentiveness to, psychosocial, existential, or spiritual suffering of patients with serious medical illness. A year earlier, the Joint Commission on Accreditation of Healthcare Organizations (JCAHO), the body charged with evaluating and accrediting nearly 19,000 health care organizations in the United States, established Spiritual Assessment Standards as a response to the growing need for a greater understanding of how spirituality impacts patient care and service. The Association of American Colleges (AAMC) acknowledged spirituality's potential in medicine in a 1999 Medical School Objectives Project (MSOP) report. MSOP, the program that sets forth learning objectives for medical students, stated, among other criteria, that before graduation, students will have demonstrated to the satisfaction of the faculty, "the ability to elicit a spiritual history as well as an understanding that the spiritual dimension of people's lives is an avenue for compassionate care giving." (p. 12)

In 1993, only three of the nation's medical schools had coursework that examined relationships between spirituality and health; currently 84 feature coursework or lectures in this area (Fortin & Barnett, 2004).

I recently had a personal encounter with these developments that took me by surprise. I experienced a severe allergic reaction and hives, which prompted me to go to the emergency room of my local hospital. As I was being checked in, the woman who was diligently entering my insurance data into the computer said, "Now, do you have any religious or spiritual issues we should be concerned about?" For a moment I was speechless; I wanted relief from my horrific, itchy rash, not spiritual counseling. Then I remembered the JCAHO accreditation recommendations mentioned above. This clerk, an employee at an accredited health care institution, was merely doing her job and doing it well. Then I was shown to the exam room, where a nurse also asked me the same question. Their queries were sensitive and respectful, not intrusive or pushy. It was altogether a satisfying experience; my allergic reaction was treated successfully, and my spiritual needs were acknowledged. This was integrative medicine in action and a reminder of how radically the terrain is changing in health care.

Integrative medicine, as mentioned, involves the best of both conventional and nonconventional methods. It aims to achieve the optimal synthesis of biological, psychological, mind–body, energetic, and spiritual therapies addressing each patient's needs and preferences. This is illustrated in the case of Matthew Pfenninger, who developed a rapidly metastasizing brain tumor at age 18. Matthew is the son of family physician John Pfenninger, M.D., of Midland, Michigan. When the tumor defied state-of-the-art treatment at Columbia Medical Center, Dr. Pfenninger organized a "Gathering to Heal" session for his son at MidMichigan Medical Center. He was amazed when 60 of the 110 staff doctors showed up to focus on Matthew's healing through prayer or whatever way they preferred. "These were the most scientific people imaginable," Dr. Pfenninger explained, yet they were willing to come together and publicly express their love, compassion, and concern for the sick son of a respected colleague. Dr. Pfenninger was deeply touched by the event, as, apparently, was Matthew. Ten days later, follow-up scans at Columbia showed that his tumors had vanished. No one could explain what had happened. Although the tumor eventually recurred, resulting in a stormy course and a bone marrow transplant, Matthew recovered. He went on to become a straight-A engineering student and is now 27 years old (J. Pfenninger, personal communication, June 2003).

Matthew Pfenninger's brain tumor nearly killed him, and so, too, did his conventional treatments. This dilemma reveals another reason people are turning to integrative methods: the serious safety issues associated with conventional therapies. It is difficult for us physicians to acknowledge this fact, because those doctors who work in hospitals every day are understandably more focused on medicine's triumphs than its failures. We are like loving parents who see mainly the redeeming qualities of our wayward child, not the bad traits. But although modern medicine cures, it also kills, and the word is out. According to data published in 2000 in the *Journal of the American Medical Association*, nearly a quarter million persons die each year in American hospitals because of the side effects of pharmaceuticals and the errors of the health care staff (Starfield, 2000). These figures make modern hospital care the third leading cause of death in the United States, behind heart disease and cancer, and is the equivalent of a commercial passenger jet crashing every day. These statistics have been challenged, resulting in the demotion of hospital care to "only" the sixth or seventh leading cause of death. Still, in any other area this death toll would be considered a national scandal. But we have become inured to this dark side of health care, accepting it as the way things are. It gets worse. These figures are for in-hospital deaths only and do not include outpatient visits. One analysis estimates that between 4 and 18% of consecutive patients experience adverse effects in outpatient settings, resulting annually in 116 million extra physician visits, 77 million extra prescriptions, 17 million emergency department visits, 8 million hospitalizations, 3 million long-term admissions, 199,000 additional deaths, and $77 billion in extra costs (Weingart, Wilson, Gibberd, & Harrison, 2000).

It is no wonder that millions of laypersons have begun searching on their own for methods of treatment that are safer. This helps explain why the integrative health movement has been overwhelmingly a grass-roots, bottom-up, patient-driven phenomenon. Fortunately, there are also signs of internal change. The prestigious Institute of Medicine, of the National Academy of Sciences, has decried the above situation. Its 1999 report *To Err Is Human: Building a Safer Health System* was a call to arms. It declared a minimum goal of a 50% reduction of medical errors over the next 5 years. Follow-up data on the success of these efforts are awaited. Meanwhile, people continue their own explorations, as the growing integrative health care movement attests.

It is easy to criticize modern medicine for the harm it causes, but this sword cuts both ways. Safety issues are also a concern in integrative medicine and have been too little emphasized. Side effects of ingested therapies such as herbal products are becoming better known, and they also occur in the domains of energy medicine and spirituality. As our world painfully knows, spirituality and religious devotion can become twisted and used as a pretext for intolerance, terrorism, and murder. Other adverse consequences are more subtle. For example, research shows that if hospitalized patients believe their illness is due to punishment from God or that it is caused by the devil, they have a higher mortality risk following hospital discharge compared with people who do not believe such things (Pargament, Koenig, Tarakehswar, & Hahn, 2001). In this book Dr. Lake describes psychological disturbances that can sometimes occur when meditation, yoga, and qigong are practiced unskillfully or without appropriate training or supervision.

Many studies have analyzed the association of religion with prejudice and intolerance. In one review (Batson & Ventis, 1982), 34 of 44 studies found a positive relationship between traditional religious belief and practice and intolerance—in other words, the greater one's religiosity, the more intense one's prejudices often are. Only 8 of the 44 studies showed no correlation, and only 2 studies found a negative relationship, these in preadolescents and/or adolescents, suggesting that intolerance is not innate but is learned as we grow older. As a result of these findings, one team of researchers (Batson,

Schoenrade, & Pych, 1985, p. 189) came to the "very clear, if unsettling conclusion … that religion is not associated with increased love and acceptance but with increased intolerance, prejudice and bigotry."

There is also evidence that religious belief and practice often lead to destructive and cruel behavior. People with strong religious beliefs tend to advocate more punitive measures than nonreligious individuals toward several categories of criminal offenders (Kirkpatrick, 1949). Studies have found that religious people in the United States tend to be more prejudiced against African Americans (Allport & Kramer, 1946) and more intolerant of those with different political beliefs (Stouffer, 1955). In Australia, religious devotion has been found to be associated with prejudice toward those of different sexual preferences (Hong, 1984). Ethnocentrism and preference for authoritarianism have also been found to be greater among religious than nonreligious individuals (Adorno, Frenkel-Brunswick, Levinson, & Sanford, 1950).

We must be careful, however, not to make sweeping generalizations about religions. They vary enormously, and great differences exist among the followers of any given sect. Yet the briefest glance at history suggests that the above studies should be taken seriously. Holy wars, crusades, witch burnings, ethnic cleansing, and preventive or preemptive wars have all been rooted in religious zeal. This regrettable harvest led satirist Jonathan Swift to observe, "We have just enough religion to make us hate, but not enough to make us love one another."

The point is that mind–body practices, so-called energy healing, spiritual approaches, and other nonconventional therapies, do not come automatically surrounded with a celestial halo. There are unsafe integrative medical practices, just as there are toxic or lethal side effects of some conventional pharmaceuticals and surgical procedures. However, the harm done by nonconventional biological treatments as well as mind–body and and energy therapies is minuscule compared with the magnitude of suffering and loss of life that has resulted from prescribed Western medical practices.

I have dwelled on the role of religion and spirituality in health because they are a template for all the other therapies that make up the integrative portfolio, and because a spiritual element extends throughout the entire integrative perspective. The intricacies found in all spiritual, mind–body, or energetic pursuits suggest caution to anyone who is attracted to the integrative vision of human health. The stubborn fact is that *the integrative approach is not less complex than conventional medicine, but more so.* Just because a therapy is "integrative," "integral," or "holistic" does not make it effective, safe, or easy to apply.

It is difficult to define integrative medicine, but you know it when you see it. It is often displayed in the lives of great healers, such as the legendary Sir William Osler. Osler was the most influential physician in modern medicine and is known as the father of Western scientific medicine. After revolutionizing how medicine was taught and practiced in the United States and Canada, in 1905, at the peak of his fame, he was lured to England, where he became the Regius professor of medicine at Oxford University. One day he went to graduation ceremonies at Oxford, wearing his impressive academic robes. On the way he stopped by the home of his friend and colleague, Dr. Ernest Mallam. One of Mallam's young sons was seriously ill with whooping cough, a notorious killer in those preantibiotic days. The child appeared to be dying, and he

would not respond to the ministrations of his parents, physicians, or nurses. Osler loved children greatly. He had a special way with them, and they would invariably admit him into their world. When Osler appeared in his imposing ceremonial robes, the little boy was captivated. After a brief examination, Osler sat by the bedside, took a peach from a bowl, peeled it, cut and sugared it, and fed it bit by bit to the enthralled patient. Although he felt recovery was unlikely, Osler returned for the next 40 days, each time dressed in his striking robes, and personally fed the young child nourishment. Within just a few days the tide had turned, and the boy's recovery became obvious (Golden, 1999).

Osler's example is telling. He had no miracle drugs in his black bag. He worked mainly through compassion and empathy, which we used to call "bedside manner" or just plain "healing." These are the most fundamental elements in all healing traditions. Unfortunately, they became devalued during the meteoric ascent of science in the 20th century. When I was in medical school, if someone had called us "healers," we would not have known if we were being praised or damned. Integrative medicine is helping physicians reclaim the mantle of healer, and this is one of its most important contributions.

Nurses have played a monumental role in keeping alive the flame of integrative healing. No one glimpsed the integral vision more clearly than Florence Nightingale, the founder of modern secular nursing (Dossey, 2000).[8] In 1868 she wrote, "Nursing is an art; and if it is to be made an art, it requires as exclusive a devotion, as hard a preparation, as any painter's or sculptor's work; for what is the having to do with dead canvas or cold marble, compared with having to do with the living body, the temple of God's spirit? It is one of the fine arts; I had almost said, the finest of fine arts. … There is no such thing as amateur art; there is no such thing as amateur nursing" (McDonald, 2004, pp. 291–292).

Let's recall Astin's finding that people often choose alternative health care measures because of deeply held spiritual or existential beliefs. What does this mean? A key aspect of spirituality is the conviction that there are vital meanings, purposes, and directions in life; that our existence is not random; that there are underlying patterns and processes that make sense. This is one reason why people seek out therapies that are part of ancient cultures and wisdom traditions, practices such as yoga, meditation, Healing Touch, qigong, and prayer.

Meaning is an area in which modern medicine has failed the sick (Dossey, 1991). Medicine has taken its cues from biology, physics, and chemistry, and the message emanating from these areas for two centuries is that nature is meaningless. Illness, we've been assured, is caused by the deranged behaviors of the molecules and organs in our body, which follow the impersonal laws of nature, and which by definition mean nothing. If we find meaning in health and illness, it is because we insert it via our imagination, not because meaning really exists.

This view, although considered rational and even heroic by many, has run into trouble. Humans cannot live without meaning, and a sense of meaninglessness often results in despair, illness, and death. Meaning is like the air we breathe—an invisible but utterly necessary component of life—and its impact does not disappear merely because it is ignored.

A healing system that denies a place for meaning is an oxymoron, a contradiction in terms. Health-related events are seldom meaning-neutral; most people feel deeply that they reflect, symbolize, stand for, and point to specific events and processes in their lives. Even if we say that an illness was genetic in origin or was caused by an accident over which we had no control, this interpretation is rich with meaning and can convey consolation, resentment, or despair, depending on our point of view. The issue of meaning is especially important when approaching mental illness. In this book, Dr. Lake introduces the integrative practitioner to different ways of assessing, interpreting, and treating both the causes and meanings of cognitive, emotional, and behavioral symptoms, taking into account the patient's unique values and beliefs.

Aside from its concrete contributions to physical health, integrative medicine has become a reservoir of meaning and psychospiritual sustenance for millions of individuals. This is yet another reason our meaning-starved society has embraced it—and why, too, an increasing number of physicians are doing the same.

Modern medicine has evolved into one of the most spiritually malnourished professions that have ever existed. Physicians, like everyone else, have spiritual and existential needs and require meaning in their lives. But during the 20th century we learned to deny these needs because we were told that essential meanings and spirituality are incompatible with good science. This view has been deadening. It has forced physicians to renounce a defining feature of healing through the ages: its connection with the divine and its reliance on transcendent factors that go beyond the physical. Integrative medicine and the threads of spirituality and deep personal meaning that run

through it offer the possibility of helping to heal modern physicians from the affliction of meaninglessness. This is a central reason why many doctors are advocating integrative approaches, and this is especially important in the domain of mental health care.

Philosopher Ken Wilber states:

The crucial ingredient is not the integral medical bag itself—with all the conventional pills, and the orthodox surgery, and the subtle energy medicine, and the acupuncture needles—but the holder of that bag. Integrally informed health-care practitioners, the doctors and nurses and therapists, have opened themselves to an entire spectrum of consciousness—matter to body to mind to soul to spirit. . . . Body and mind and spirit are operating in self, culture, and nature, and thus health and healing, sickness and wholeness, are all bound up in a multidimensional tapestry that cannot be cut into without loss. (quoted in Schlitz, 2004, pp. 8–9)

Dr. Lake has made a significant contribution to integrative medicine in this book by helping to weave the integral tapestry around the complex issues of mental illness. In honor of his efforts to restore healing and meaning to mental health care, I bow deeply.

Larry Dossey, M.D.
Former Chief of Staff, Medical City Dallas Hospital
Former Co-Chair, Panel on Mind–Body Interventions,
National Institutes of Health

References

Adorno, T., Frenkel-Brunswick, E., Levinson, D., & Sanford, N. (1950). *The authoritarian personality.* New York: Harper.

Allport, G. W., & Kramer, B. M. (1946). Some roots of prejudice. *Journal of Psychology, 22,* 9–30.

Astin, J. A. (1998). Why patients use alternative medicine—results of a national survey. *Journal of the American Medical Association, 279*(19), 1548–1553.

Batson, C. D., Schoenrade, P. A., & Pych, V. (1985). Brother love or self concern? Behavioral consequences of religion. In L. B. Brown (Ed.), *Advances in the psychology of religion* (p. 189). New York: Pergamon Press.

Batson, C. D., & Ventis, W. L. (1982). *The religious experience: A social-psychological perspective.* New York: Oxford University Press.

Better times for spirituality and healing in medicine. (2001). *Research News and Opportunities in Science and Theology, 1*(6), 12.

Dossey, B. M. (2000). *Florence Nightingale: Mystic, visionary, healer.* Springhouse, PA: Springhouse.

Dossey, L. (1991). *Meaning and medicine.* New York: Bantam.

Dossey, L. (1993). *Healing words: The power of prayer and the practice of medicine.* San Francisco: HarperSanFrancisco.

Dossey, L. (1999). *Reinventing medicine.* San Francisco: HarperSanFrancisco.

Eisenberg, D. M., Davis, R. B., Ettner, S. L., et al. (1998). Trends in alternative medicine use in the United States, 1990–1997: Results of a follow-up national survey. *Journal of the American Medical Association, 280,* 1569–1575.

Eisenberg, D. M., Kessler, R. C., Foster, C., Norlock, F. F., Calkins, D. R., & Delbanco, T. L. (1993). Unconventional medicine in the United States: Prevalence, costs, and patterns of use. *New England Journal of Medicine, 328,* 246–252.

Fortin, A. H., & Barnett, K. G. (2004). Medical school curricula in spirituality and medicine. *Journal of the American Medical Association, 291*(23), 2883.

Golden, R. L. (1999). William Osler at 150: An overview of a life. *Journal of the American Medical Association, 282*(23), 2252–2258.

Helm, H., Hays, E., Flint, E., Koenig, H., & Blazer, D. (2000). Effects of private religious activity on mortality of elderly disabled and nondisabled adults. *Journal of Gerontological Sciences, 55A,* M400–M405.

Hong, S. M. (1984). Australian attitudes towards homosexuality: A comparison with college students. *Journal of Psychology, 117,* 89–95.

Institute of Medicine. (1999, September 1). To err is human: Building a safer health system. Available at http://www.iom.edu/report.asp?id= 5575

Kirkpatrick, C. (1949). Religion and humanitarianism: A study of institutional implications. *Psychological Monographs, 63*(304).

Koenig, H. G., McCullough, M. E., & Larson, D. B. (2001). *Handbook of religion and health.* New York: Oxford University Press.

Korzybski, A. (n.d.). Retrieved June 8, 2004, from http://www.brainyquote.com

Laine, C., & Davidoff, F. (1996). Patient-centered medicine. *Journal of the American Medical Association, 275,* 152–156.

Levin, J. (2001). *God, faith, and health.* New York: John Wiley & Sons.

McCullough, M. E., Hoyt, W. T., Larson, D. B., Koenig, H., & Thoresen, C. (2000). Religious involvement and mortality: A meta-analytic review. *Health Psychology, 19*(3), 211–222.

McDonald, L. (Ed.). (2004). *Florence Nightingale on public health care: The collected works of Florence Nightingale* (Vol. 6). Waterloo, Ontario, Canada: Wilfrid Laurier University Press.

Pargament, K., Koenig, H., Tarakehswar, N., & Hahn, J. (2001). Religious struggle as a predictor of mortality among medically ill elderly patients: A two-year longitudinal study. *Archives of Internal Medicine, 161*(15), 1881–1885.

Schlitz, M. (2004). Seeding a new model of medicine. *Shift, 3,* 8–9.

Starfield, B. (2000). Is US health really the best in the world? *Journal of the American Medical Association, 284*(4), 483–485.

Stouffer, S. A. (1955). *Communism, conformity, and civil liberties.* New York: Doubleday.

Weingart, S. N., Wilson, R. M., Gibberd, R. W., & Harrison, B. (2000). Epidemiology and medical error. *British Medical Journal, 320,* 774–777.

Available at http://nccam.nci.nih.gov/news/report.pdf

Preface: The Book in Overview

This book is about the future of medicine and the future of mental health care. It is an analysis of the ideas that are shaping the evolution of Western medicine toward new ways of thinking about the causes and meanings of illness, as well as a critical review of assessment and treatment approaches that are presently outside orthodox biomedicine. The book is about novel ways of seeing, understanding, and treating mental illness. Progress in medicine takes place when there is openness to new explanatory models of illness. When new ideas are dismissed before being critically evaluated, medicine risks becoming stagnant, politicized, and bounded by a closed set of traditions and entrenched ideologies. It risks becoming less scientific and more dogmatic. Some would contend that biomedicine as conventionally practiced has already crossed the fine divide that distinguishes science from dogma. However, many beliefs that were once accepted as facts or incontestable theories in biomedicine are now seen as crude misrepresentations, and the factual content of biomedicine is being rewritten at an ever increasing rate. Biomedicine is in a state of critical self-evaluation and rapid change. Recent progress in physics, biology, and consciousness studies has stimulated research in basic mechanisms underlying normal and abnormal states of consciousness. Entrenched theories in biomedical psychiatry are being reexamined, and novel approaches are emerging out of this dialog of self-questioning.

In North America and Europe, nonconventional assessment and treatment approaches are widely used to address a broad range of mental health problems. Some approaches rest on theories that are congruent with the prevailing Western scientific framework. Others assume the validity of paradigms that violate the core tenets of contemporary biomedicine. The increasing use of herbs or other natural substances as medicines is an example of increasingly accepted empirical approaches that do not require changes in the basic theoretical or methodological framework of Western science as it exists in the early 21st century.

Western biomedicine is at the threshold of a period of unparalleled evolution and transformation. Novel explanatory models of illness, health, and healing are being debated in leading academic institutions and in popular culture. The study of human consciousness has become an accepted field of academic research, leading to novel hypotheses about the nature of mind and mind–body in space and time. The distinction between conventional understandings of *mind* and *body* is increasingly blurred, and the role of intention in healing has

become a subject of serious inquiry. Many spiritual traditions, including yoga and Tibetan Buddhism, are providing a fertile testing ground for new models of physical reality and novel ways of understanding the causes or meanings of illness and health. The result is a dramatic shift in the kinds of questions that are regarded as legitimate to ask in conventional Western biomedical research. At present there are competing explanatory models of consciousness, but there is still no compelling evidence for a single best theory of consciousness. It follows that there can be no single theory of normal and abnormal psychological functioning, and psychiatry is obliged to remain open to novel paradigms and a variety of assessment and treatment approaches based on those paradigms.

Progress in science has been described by Kuhn in *Structure of Scientific Revolutions* as an essential evolutionary process, a kind of reciprocal and self-reinforcing transformative dialectic between the ideas and institutions of science and the beliefs, values, and skills of researchers and practitioners from many traditions. According to this criterion, conventional Western biomedicine is in a period of transformation in which established dogma is being challenged by emerging research findings and novel ways of seeing the physical, biological, energetic, and informational processes that influence health and illness. Within the first decades of the new millennium, Western-trained physicians will increasingly embrace diagnostic approaches and therapies that are currently outside orthodox medicine. Based on evidence from conventional scientific inquiry and the critical examination of emerging paradigms, including traditionally used botanicals, the roles of complex system-level phenomena in health and illness, and the putative role of "energy," information, and intentionality in healing, novel assessment and treatment approaches will gradually emerge. The result of this evolutionary process will be the establishment of integrative models of illness, health, and practical integrative approaches addressing the range of medical and mental illnesses. The continuing evolution of medicine toward a truly integrative paradigm will result in more complete understandings of fundamental biological, energetic, informational, and possibly spiritual phenomena associated with the dynamic processes that underlie disease and promote healing. The emergence of effective and *cost-effective* integrative assessment and treatment approaches in mental health care will inevitably follow from the continued evolution of Western biomedicine and other world systems of medicine. Future students of history will view the present epoch in Western medicine as a period of transition from long-held beliefs and practices embedded in 19th-century science to ideas and clinical practices that reflect the advances of 20th-century science.

The book is divided into two main parts, with appendixes. The organization of the book permits it to be read for an understanding of theory or used as a practical reference and clinical manual. The chapters of Part I discuss the conceptual foundations for integrative medicine and provide an overview of basic principles of successful integrative management. Chapter 1 presents a discussion on the evolution of integrative medicine and the issues that will shape its future. The next three chapters of Part I cover philosophical problems in medicine and integrative medicine, the relevance of emerging paradigms to the future of medicine, and general methods in integrative medicine. Specific methods for planning integrative assessment and treatment strategies addressing mental health problems are presented in Chapters 5 and 6, respectively. In my view, the first four chapters are the most important part of the book because they provide the foundations for new ways of thinking about health and illness, and they develop the underlying principles of methods for combining disparate approaches into practical integrative strategies addressing particular symptom patterns. Part II is the clinical section of the book. Conventional assessment and treatment approaches are briefly reviewed at the start of each chapter. The chapters of Part II contain detailed discussions of the evidence for nonconventional and integrative assessment and treatment approaches for many common symptom patterns.

Part I: Foundations and Methods of Integrative Mental Health Care

Chapter 1, The Evolution of Integrative Medicine and Implications for Mental Health Care, defines integrative medicine and introduces its historical background. Factors that will shape the future of integrative mental health care are discussed including research evidence supporting nonconventional approaches, unresolved efficacy and safety issues of conventional treatments, and broad social and economic trends.

Chapter 2, Philosophical Problems, develops important philosophical arguments that define the conceptual landscape of medicine in general, and integrative medicine in particular. Considerations of the nature and role of causality in medicine are discussed, and different approaches used to infer causality when assessing symptoms are reviewed. An ontological schema in the form of a truth table provides the basis for evidence tables for rating conventional or nonconventional assessment and treatment approaches developed in Chapter 4.

Chapter 3, Paradigms in Medicine, Psychiatry, and Integrative Medicine, is a review and discussion of the sources of ideas that will shape the future of medicine and eventually lead to widespread acceptance of many nonconventional or integrative approaches in general and in mental health care specifically. Evidence is reviewed for many emerging conceptual frameworks in biology, physics, and information science, and I argue for the relevance of nonorthodox ways of seeing to deeper understandings of consciousness and mental illness. It is likely that novel paradigms in Western science will help to elucidate the complex causes of mental illness, leading to fundamentally new assessment and treatment approaches that

are more effective than contemporary Western biomedical techniques. Examples of promising emerging paradigms discussed are functional medicine, new mind–body theories, complexity theory, and quantum field theory.

Chapter 4, Foundations of Clinical Methodology in Integrative Medicine, addresses two basic methodological problems: methods for planning integrative medical management and methods for obtaining reliable and pertinent information. Evidence tables are constructed showing general kinds and levels of evidence for nonconventional assessment modalities and for nonconventional treatments. The evidence tables are the initial step in systematically organizing evidence pertaining to nonconventional assessment or treatment modalities used in the management of mental or emotional symptoms. Contents of the evidence tables are simplified into three general categories: approaches that are substantiated by the available evidence, approaches that are provisional following analysis of the evidence, and approaches that are possibly effective. I argue that it is not meaningful to describe an assessment or treatment modality as substantiated or provisional in general but only with respect to a particular symptom or symptom pattern. Another important methodological problem that is addressed is the determination of degrees of compatibility between disparate kinds of medical practices that are candidates for integration. Chapter 4 also establishes methods for identifying and obtaining clinically pertinent information about assessment and treatment modalities that are being considered for combined use with other modalities.

Chapter 5, History Taking, Assessment, and Formulation in Integrative Mental Health Care, and Chapter 6, Starting and Maintaining Integrative Treatment in Mental Health Care, develop specific methods for deriving integrative assessment and treatment plans in mental health care, following the general methodological concepts developed in Chapter 4. Chapter 5 introduces methods for history taking, assessment, and formulation in the integrative management of mental or emotional symptoms. Chapter 6 develops methods for planning integrative treatment approaches in mental health care after the causes or meanings of a specified mental or emotional symptom have been assessed.

Part II: Integrative Management of Common Mental and Emotional Symptoms

Part II provides a comprehensive and critical review of the evidence supporting the use of nonconventional approaches to assess or treat common mental and emotional symptoms. Using Part II does not require familiarity with the general conceptual problems addressed in Part I. However, reading Part I first will ensure a deeper grasp of the practical methodological issues involved in integrative treatment planning when referring to the clinical chapters of the book. All nonconventional assessment and treatment approaches discussed are categorized by kind of modality on the basis of a demonstrated or putative mechanism of action, and level of evidence on the basis of an analysis of quantitative and qualitative evidence of outcomes with respect to a particular core symptom pattern. Mechanisms of action fall into four broad categories: biological; somatic/mind–body; forms of energy-information validated by Western science; and forms of energy-information not validated by Western science. The order of assessment and treatment approaches is determined on the basis of available evidence with respect to the symptom pattern being discussed. Approaches supported by compelling evidence are labeled "substantiated." Approaches for which there is significant but not compelling evidence are regarded as "provisional." Finally, those assessment or treatment approaches for which there is limited or inconsistent evidence are classified as "possibly accurate" or "possibly effective" with respect to a specified core symptom pattern. The relative strength of evidence supporting the use of a particular approach often varies considerably with respect to the symptom pattern that is being addressed. Therefore, a particular herbal that is used to treat both depressed mood and anxiety, for example, may be substantiated with respect to depressed mood, whereas it is a provisional treatment of anxiety. On the basis of criteria used in this book and available evidence at the time of writing, some conventional and nonconventional approaches are substantiated, whereas most are provisional or possibly effective with respect to a specified symptom pattern.

Chapter 7, Symptom-Focused Integrative Mental Health Care, acts as an introduction to Part II. The remaining seven chapters are organized by specific symptoms:

- Depressed mood
- Mania and cyclic mood changes
- Anxiety
- Psychosis
- Dementia and milder forms of cognitive impairment
- Symptoms related to substance abuse and dependence
- Disturbances of sleep and wakefulness

Following a brief overview of conventional biomedical approaches used to assess and treat the core symptom pattern being discussed, nonconventional assessment and treatment approaches in current use are concisely reviewed in the order of their supporting evidence. For purposes of this book, psychological treatment methods are regarded as conventional and are not addressed. The interested reader is referred to excellent current reviews of the evidence for conventional pharmacological and psychotherapy treatments, as well as the American Psychiatric Association treatment guidelines, which are available online at the APA Web site.

Evidence tables throughout Part II summarize the most important findings pertaining to the nonconventional assessment and treatment approaches discussed. Each chapter contains an algorithm addressing a primary symptom pattern. The algorithms provide the essential logic for planning integrative assessment and treatment approaches on a case-by-case basis, taking into account the patient's core symptom pattern, pertinent medical and psychiatric history in the context of treatment preferences, and realistic constraints on cost or availability. The algorithms are intended as general guides to comprehensive integrative assessment and treatment planning and do not constitute specific management programs for particular patients. Specific combinations of conventional or nonconventional treatment approaches should be recommended only when an acceptably low risk of potential contraindications has been confirmed, reviewed with the patient, and documented in the patient's chart.

General safety issues in integrative medicine and important specific safety concerns associated with particular nonconventional approaches frequently used in mental health care are discussed in Chapter 6. Potential safety issues associated with particular nonconventional or integrative approaches are summarized in the evidence tables of Part II chapters. All chapters conclude with composite case vignettes illustrating the integrative management of common symptom patterns.

Appendix A contains six tables showing integrative strategies for assessment and treatment planning, respectively, when two or more core symptom patterns are being approached at the same time. Appendix B lists published and Web-based resources pertaining to the nonconventional modalities covered in the book. The companion Web site (www.thieme.com/mentalhealth) will be updated on a regular basis and will include comments on significant new research findings, studies in progress, and emerging safety issues.

◆ My Personal Journey to Integrative Medicine

A long-standing interest in both conventional and non-Western ways of conceptualizing disease, especially the brain or mind–body, led me to the study of medicine and eventually to psychiatry, where my energy was initially divided between the neurosciences and cultural psychiatry. Since completing my residency training at Stanford University, I have prioritized learning about nonconventional approaches in mental health care for more practical reasons. In contrast to what one often hears at conferences or reads in medical journals, problems related to the effectiveness and safety of contemporary pharmacological "tools" used in Western psychiatry have been apparent to clinical psychiatrists for decades. Although medications sometimes provide dramatic relief of acute or severe symptoms, most currently used drugs have limited efficacy and effectiveness in the treatment of the major psychiatric disorders or symptom patterns discussed in this book. I have written on the assumption that many mental health professionals share my personal view that contemporary pharmacological approaches emphasize treatments of severe mental or emotional symptoms but often do not provide effective or acceptable strategies for prevention or long-term maintenance. Conventional pharmacological treatments are frequently associated with significant adverse effects or toxicities, resulting in noncompliance or early discontinuation of treatment. Many recently introduced drugs are not affordable for a growing percentage of potential users in both developed and nonindustrialized countries. For these reasons, conventional medications alone do not offer effective and realistic solutions to mental illness in most world regions. Aggressive media campaigns promoting the widespread use of conventional drugs for mental health problems have resulted in unrealistic expectations, frequent disappointment, and noncompliance. Advertisements delude patients into the naive belief that a "magic pill" will eliminate their psychological distress and rapidly restore them to "balance" and a happy life. Patients are approaching their psychiatrists or family practice physicians in increasing numbers requesting "the right pill" to restore a "chemical imbalance" they hear about in a 30-second television ad, and there is often little incentive to consider legitimate alternative approaches or to engage in the necessary and difficult work of psychotherapy. In writing this book, I have attempted to frame conventional approaches in mental health care in a realistic light while also providing accurate information about nonconventional alternatives.

Medicine is both science and intuition—healing requires skill and compassion

The fundamental commitments of any practitioner to any patient are an open mind and a compassionate heart. If the practitioner's mind is not open, new ways of "seeing" or treating illness will be overlooked, and the practitioner will have a false sense of confidence in his or her skill. In the absence of compassion, there can be no empathy, and the practitioner's understanding of the patient's suffering will be superficial and incomplete. In the absence of an open mind and a compassionate heart, the most acute intelligence or the most advanced technical skill frequently provides little relief. Technical skill cannot make up for a lack of understanding, and technology cannot replace compassion, because the relationship between practitioner and patient will be empty—without heart. The scientific practice of medicine requires objective inquiry into the nature and causes of symptoms, and a rigorous but open-minded commitment to learning new methods, sometimes in spite of the prejudices or prohibitions of the dominant paradigm or the prevailing political viewpoint. The art of medicine requires attention to intuition, often in the absence of empirical information. Competent practitioners in all systems of medicine must first master a body of information and technical skills, and continue to refine those skills while cultivating intuition and compassion (Achterberg, 1996). In my view, healing takes place when a patient experiences relief from suffering in a way that is meaningful to him or her. Healing is not merely a transient reduction in the severity of symptoms. The art of working with patients who experience mental or emotional problems rests on the skillful combination of knowledge, intuition, and compassion. When a patient benefits from the skillful implementation of an appropriate treatment, and the practitioner is guided by intuition and compassion, it can be said that healing takes place.

Authentic compassion is essential when working with any patient who is experiencing mental or emotional symptoms. Cultivating an attitude of compassion toward a patient brings relief through the patient's awareness that the practitioner is trying to stand in his or her suffering. On a more practical level, compassion engenders trust between practitioner and patient. A relationship of trust, in turn, generally leads to disclosure of personal information that provides clues to causes or meanings of symptoms that may otherwise remain obscure. The practitioner is then in a more informed position when assessing or treating a patient.

The cornerstone of competent and caring practice in all traditions of medicine is the relationship between patient and practitioner. Excellent medical care cannot take place in the absence of trust, empathy, and mutual respect. The ideas and specific integrative guidelines developed in this book certainly cannot make up for the absence of a positive and authentic relationship between a patient and a practitioner. I believe that healing takes place most deeply only when the relationship between practitioner and patient is authentic and of primary importance. In mental health care this is perhaps especially true, and in many cases the relationship between practitioner

and patient plays a more important role in health and healing than the particular methods employed. When working with patients who complain of severe mental or emotional symptoms, including depression, anxiety, or psychotic symptoms, a therapeutic relationship is premised on an empathic connection between practitioner and patient.

The dispensing of medications, increasingly the sole activity of conventionally trained psychiatrists and primary care physicians, frequently ensures the absence of meaningful contact between patient and practitioner and takes away the patient's motivation to pursue other possibly effective approaches when conventional biomedical treatments fail. This has two outcomes: The patient has the expectation that taking a medication is a sufficient way of dealing with his or her mental or emotional symptoms, and the patient is committed to a single treatment approach that may have limited efficacy or significant safety issues. This is especially concerning in view of compelling evidence for many nonconventional treatments in mental health care. Ideally, integrative medicine will personalize medical care while restoring autonomy to patients. Instead of one correct treatment, in this book I attempt to provide methods for determining many unique treatment choices in the context of a collaborative relationship between patient and practitioner where the emphasis is on maintaining wellness rather managing crises.

Integrative mental health care will enhance conventional Western psychiatry

This book is neither a critique of conventional Western biomedicine nor a defense of nonconventional medicine. I believe there are appropriate and effective roles for both established and emerging approaches in medicine, both empirically derived scientific models and intuitive ways of understanding and treating illness. Many Western biomedical treatments of mental and emotional symptoms are clearly effective, bringing relief to millions who would otherwise be unable to have relationships, work, experience pleasure, or find other sources of meaning in life. Western psychiatry rests on a coherent body of theory, research, and clinical data, and is the beneficiary of fundamental scientific advances in neurophysiology, pharmacology, molecular biology, and genetics. However, the successes of conventional biomedical assessment and treatment approaches are limited by many factors, including incomplete or erroneous understandings of the putative mechanisms of action of many drugs, the limited efficacy of many drugs in current use, significant safety problems and related compliance problems caused by toxic side effects or drug–drug interactions, and unaffordability or limited availability (because of high medication costs or poor insurance coverage) of many drugs that are regarded by Western medical practitioners as the most appropriate or effective treatments for a particular mental illness. These issues have resulted in considerable controversy over the appropriate uses of conventional biomedical treatments in mental health care, and I believe they limit the potential effectiveness of many conventional treatments. It is my strong belief that the systematic evaluation of nonconventional assessment and treatment approaches represents an informed response to the inherent limitations of contemporary biomedical approaches in mental health care.

With this goal in mind, in 2004 the board of trustees of the American Psychiatric Association (APA) established the Caucus on Complementary, Alternative, and Integrative Approaches. The caucus is the first APA-endorsed effort to evaluate non-conventional and integrative approaches in mental health care. This book partially fulfills an important objective of the caucus by providing clinical methods for integrative assessment and treatment planning in mental health care, as well as a comprehensive review of nonconventional modalities in current use.

In this book I argue for the reasonableness of establishing clinical integrative methods addressing the causes, conditions, or meanings of mental and emotional symptoms. Practical methods are suggested for combining conventional biomedical approaches and nonconventional approaches for assessing and treating mental and emotional symptoms. I have tried to embrace a neutral stance incorporating concepts and methods from conventional biomedicine and disparate nonconventional systems of medicine in order to make the book accessible to practitioners trained in all major traditions of medicine. This book is a collection of methods and clinical material that will guide the practitioner in determining when to combine disparate approaches in order to optimize assessment accuracy or treatment outcomes. My goal is to achieve a balanced synthesis of legitimate, safe conventional and nonconventional medical practices for improved outcomes in mental health care. Truly integrative clinical management can be achieved only when the practitioner's choices are informed by an objective appraisal of the evidence for the range of available conventional and nonconventional assessment and treatment approaches.

This book is intended for psychiatrists, psychologists, psychotherapists, and practitioners of non-Western systems of medicine who are open to new ways of understanding and treating mental illness. All practitioners who want to learn how to use integrative approaches to manage mental and emotional symptoms will employ this book as a practical clinical reference.

Although conventional biomedical approaches are often effective, medications alone clearly do not adequately address the complex causes and meanings of mental illness. This is especially true when the broad goal of mental health care is to provide lasting symptomatic relief while prioritizing the patient's safety and overall quality of life. Every system of medicine is constrained by inherent limitations of its theories and clinical methods, and no single assessment or treatment approach is ideally suited to all patients who report similar symptoms. Particular kinds of treatments are often ineffective or partially effective because they fail to address the complex causes, conditions, or meanings of mental and emotional symptoms. Biological treatments are beneficial in many cases but may be of limited value in cases where psychological, somatic, spiritual, or energetic causes or conditions underlie mental or emotional symptoms. Effective integrative health care addresses the disparate causes, conditions, or meanings of symptoms using multimodal approaches. Inferring the causes or meanings of a symptom pattern on the basis of empirical research or clinical observations and formulating an integrative plan that takes into account quantitative and qualitative evidence in the context of patient preferences and the availability and affordability of treatments are the essential efforts of integrative medicine. The arguments and clinical methods put forward in this book address these practical issues. The approaches discussed in this book do not replace psychological work. Psychotherapy is frequently valuable and should be

actively encouraged in patients who are motivated to work and have the capacity for insight.

◆ Why Mental Health Professionals Should Learn about Integrative Approaches

There are compelling reasons for mental health professionals and other conventionally or nonconventionally trained medical practitioners to become familiar with integrative approaches in mental health care:

◆ Many conventional assessment and treatment approaches in current use have limited efficacy.

◆ Many effective treatments have significant associated safety issues (e.g., atypical antipsychotics carry a considerable risk of diabetes; conventional antidepressants have many adverse effects).

◆ Efficacious conventional treatments are sometimes discontinued because of adverse effects or high cost. Thus, in spite of their demonstrated efficacy, they are frequently ineffective treatments for large numbers of patients who cannot tolerate their adverse effects or who cannot afford to use them for prolonged periods.

◆ Some nonconventional assessment approaches provide specific, accurate information about the causes or meanings of symptoms that may lead to more effective treatment planning.

◆ The efficacy, effectiveness, and safety of some nonconventional treatment approaches have been substantiated by compelling evidence from double-blind studies and systematic review findings.

◆ Some inexpensive nonconventional treatment approaches are as effective as established conventional treatments and may provide more cost-effective solutions to mental health problems.

◆ Individuals who experience mental and emotional symptoms frequently self-treat or receive treatment from professional nonconventionally trained practitioners at the same time they are receiving conventional biomedical therapy for the same problem, but few disclose this fact to their conventionally trained practitioner, resulting in potentially serious safety issues and poor outcomes.

◆ Because of the widespread combined uses of conventional and nonconventional approaches, mental health care in most Western countries is de facto integrative. When caring for patients who have mental health problems, it is the practitioner's responsibility to learn about appropriate, effective, and safe ways to combine disparate assessment and treatment approaches.

The majority of conventional and nonconventional treatments in current use are provisional or possibly effective because the evidence supporting their use is limited or inconsistent. As is true of nonconventional assessment and treatment approaches, conventional biomedical approaches in current use are supported by different levels of evidence. Some conventional treatments are substantiated by available research findings, whereas others are provisional or possibly effective on the basis of limited evidence or inconsistent findings. For example, many conventional drugs are not approved by the U.S. Food and Drug Administration as treatments of a particular disorder for which they are marketed. Such "off-label" treatments constitute a significant percentage of pharmacological treatments currently used in conventional mental health care. In a similar vein, many nonconventional approaches lack compelling supporting evidence, and their widespread use reflects expert consensus, social trends, or successful marketing campaigns. Considerations of safety, availability, and affordability influence patients' choices of both conventional and nonconventional approaches in mental health care.

◆ Where to Go from Here: Goals and Recommendations for the Future of Integrative Mental Health Care

The ideas and clinical material developed in this book lead to many general and specific recommendations addressing research, as well as clinical and policy issues, pertaining to nonconventional and integrative approaches in mental health care.

Research and clinical practice recommendations

The chief research and clinical practice recommendations that I propose are the following:

1. Clinical methods in integrative mental health care developed in this book should be evaluated and refined through discussions and research at centers of excellence in integrative medicine, including the program in integrative medicine at the University of Exeter, the Osher Centers (University of California, San Francisco, and Harvard University), the Stanford Center for Integrative Medicine, the Program in Integrative Medicine at the University of Arizona, and the Rosenthal Center for Integrative Medicine.

2. The National Center for Complementary and Alternative Medicine (NCCAM) of the National Institutes of Health in United States and analogous organizations in other countries (e.g., Commission E in Germany) should establish a working group of mental health professionals that will advise NCCAM as to research priorities in nonconventional and integrative assessment and treatment approaches pertaining to mental health care.

3. Research priorities at NCCAM and other government or private institutions should emphasize promising nonconventional and integrative assessment and treatment approaches that address mental health problems for which available conventional approaches are limited in effectiveness. Examples of mental health problems for which contemporary Western biomedical treatments have limited effectiveness include depression, cyclic mood changes, psychosis, and alcohol and substance abuse.

Policy recommendations

The chief policy recommendations I propose are the following:

1. The Institute of Medicine (IOM) should establish a working group within its Committee on the Use of Complementary and Alternative Medicine with the purpose of reviewing and critiquing the conceptual methods and evidence developed in this work. The working group should advise the IOM. as to policy implications for the American Medical Association, the American Psychiatric Association, and other relevant professional medical societies pertaining to research priorities and clinical practice guidelines for uses of nonconventional assessment and treatment approaches in mental health care.

2. Analysis of the cost-effectiveness of conventional, nonconventional, and integrative approaches in mental health care should be undertaken within the NCCAM, IOM, or APA, with the goal of identifying optimum integrative assessment and treatment strategies addressing the common mental health problems discussed in this book.

3. The APA recently established the Caucus on Complementary, Alternative and Integrative Approaches in Mental Health Care. The caucus should be promoted to a full Committee on Complementary, Alternative and Integrative Approaches in Mental Health Care, with the task of advising relevant committees within the APA as to legal-ethical issues, clinical practice guidelines, research priorities, and other issues pertaining to uses of nonconventional and integrative assessment and treatment approaches in mental health care.

4. The NCCAM, the APA's Committee on Complementary, Alternative and Integrative Approaches in Mental Health Care, and analogous organizations should develop professional resources for consultation on important legal and ethical issues to psychiatrists, allied mental health professionals, and nonconventional practitioners who treat patients using nonconventional or integrative approaches or refer to nonconventionally trained practitioners.

5. The DSM-V Research Agenda is currently under review within the APA, and the final version of the fifth edition of the *Diagnostic and Statistical Manual of Mental Disorders* (*DSM-V*) is due in 2012. The APA should appoint a working group within the DSM-V Research Agenda with the task of critically reviewing the evidence in favor of definitions of mental illness based on core symptom patterns and not traditional concepts of "disorder." Furthermore, the same working group should undertake a critical review of the evidence for nonconventional and integrative approaches widely used in mental health care in the United States and other Western countries, and comment on the significance and relevance of these approaches in the text of the forthcoming *DSM-V* and also in a dedicated appendix.

6. The development of an expert knowledge system incorporating the methods and clinical information contained in this book will facilitate both clinical decision making and research planning in integrative mental health care. Development of intelligent software and Web-based information tools is taking place in collaboration with faculty in the Program in Medical Informatics at Stanford University Hospital and Medical Center.

◆ This Book and How It Is Organized

This book is intended as a comprehensive and critical review of the evidence for nonconventional and integrative biological, somatic, mind–body, and energy-information methods used to assess or treat mental and emotional symptoms in adults. Special considerations are involved when working with children, and this book is not intended as a guide for mental health care in that population. A companion Web site has been created for the book (www.thieme.com/mentalhealth), and regular updates of important research findings and research in progress will be posted for the various nonconventional approaches discussed.

This book is designed to be used as a guide for physicians and other professionally trained clinicians to the integrative management of many common mental and emotional symptoms and not as a resource for self-care by patients. However, some may find it a useful resource when working together with their physician or clinician. The clinican can use the treatment-planning algorithms in Part II to develop practical integrative management strategies in consultation with the patient. The training, experience, and judgment of the clinician and the active participation and consent of the patient are necessary for safe, informed treatment choices. Patients will often benefit when the methods and clinical information discussed in this book are judiciously applied.

A comment on future revisions of the evidence tables

It is important for the reader to understand that assessment and treatment approaches discussed in this book do not have fixed or permanent rankings, because evidence supporting the use of existing nonconventional or integrative strategies will almost certainly change over time, and completely new approaches will emerge. Future research findings will result in changes in the relative rankings of many nonconventional and integrative modalities with respect to a particular core symptom pattern. For example, future negative findings may result in a shift from "provisional" to "possibly effective" for a particular treatment of chronic psychosis. By the same token, emerging positive findings may provide compelling evidence for a treatment of alcohol abuse that had previously been viewed as provisional. The same applies to conventional treatments. Some conventional approaches that are currently supported by provisional evidence may become more substantiated over time, whereas others will probably become marginalized because of future negative or inconsistent findings. Regular updates in evidence supporting particular assessment or treatment approaches, including both positive and negative findings, will be posted on the companion Web site.

This work is limited by many factors, principal among them being the incompleteness of my knowledge, understanding, and clinical experience. The ideas developed in Part I are both defined and limited by the scope of my creativity and imagination. The completeness and quality of the clinical material discussed in Part II are limited in a more concrete sense by methods developed for literature research and rating evidence. My experience as a physician and my efforts to learn about non-Western healing traditions through travel and direct experience have convinced me that many legitimate and effective approaches to treating mental illness presently are not amenable to formal Western-style research studies, nor can evidence supporting their use be found in peer-reviewed journals. Examples include highly evolved healing traditions of indigenous groups in Russia, the Americas, Africa, and Oceania. I am hopeful that future editions of this book will document theories and evidence supporting clinical techniques of these and other indigenous healing traditions as they apply to mental health care. I claim full responsibility for any omissions or factual errors in this book and invite readers to send helpful comments and information to the companion Web site.

Reference

Achterberg, J. (1996). What is medicine? *Alternative Therapies, 2*(3), 58–61.

Acknowledgments

Scholars, physicians, and healers of different traditions have provided valuable comments and criticisms to the ideas and information in this book. My mentor and friend, James Zarcone, M.D., professor of psychiatry, Stanford University Medical Center, recently emeritus, has been especially helpful and encouraging. I have been fortunate to learn from this consummate scholar and lifelong student of philosophy and medicine. Researchers, teachers, and practitioners with whom I have collaborated in efforts to build an informed dialog on integrative mental health have provided valuable comments and criticism. These include Roberta Lee, M.D., Rosenthal Center for Integrative Medicine; Michael Cohen, J.D., M.B.A., Harvard Medical School Center for Integrative Medicine; Sudha Pratikanthi, M.D., the Osher Center for Integrative Medicine University of California, San Francisco Medical School; Richard Brown, M.D., and Pat Gerbarg, M.D., at Columbia University School of Medicine; Lewis Mehl-Madrona, M.D., University of Saskatchewan; Amar Das, M.D., Ph.D., Department of Medical Informatics, Stanford Medical Center; Iris Bell, M.D., Director of Research Program in Integrative Medicine, University of Arizona School of Medicine; John Ackerman, M.D., private practice, Santa Barbara, California. Throughout I have had the pleasure of corresponding with hundreds of researchers and practitioners. These relationships continue to offer valuable insights and new findings pertaining to mind–body approaches, somatic therapies, various traditions of herbal medicine, and the uses of energy to treat mental illness.

In the fall of 2004, and again in the spring of 2006, I had the good fortune of being invited to lecture to the fellows and faculty of Dr. Andrew Weil's Program in Integrative Medicine, University of Arizona School of Medicine, Tucson. My ongoing correspondence with many graduates of that unique training program provides me with valuable insights about health and healing as well as significant research findings in integrative medicine.

Above all, I am especially indebted to my companion and wife during the years of self-absorbed research and writing that were invested in this book. While managing a busy private practice and pursuing doctorate studies in psychoanalysis, Nicole Asselborn, M.D., always found time to read sections of this book and provide fresh insights that have certainly improved both the flow and content of my writing. Finally I wish to acknowledge someone who was both a dear friend and wise teacher in the journey of ideas that led to this book. Discussions and debates with Devon Cottrell on basic philosophical questions helped to crystallize the conceptual scaffolding of this work. Devon passed away with grace and consummate skill. Her wisdom and kindness are sorely missed.

Part I

Foundations and Methods of Integrative Mental Health Care

1

The Evolution of Integrative Medicine and Implications for Mental Health Care

In contrast to conventional Western medicine, which emphasizes treating an illness, many nonconventional systems of medicine emphasize healing the whole person. The conventional model of care views the patient as the passive recipient of a psychological, physical, or somatic intervention aimed at ameliorating symptoms. Nonconventional systems of medicine regard healing as an interactive process between practitioner and patient that alleviates suffering and improves general well-being. Conventional medical treatment takes place in a directive relationship in which the patient follows medical advice. The collaborative relationship in which healing takes place emerges in the context of the intentions and attitudes of the patient and the skill, intuition, and compassion of the medical practitioner. Ideally, in integrative health care, an optimal healing environment is created within which the patient's psychological, biological, mind–body, and spiritual issues are effectively addressed in the context of an open and supportive relationship (Jonas & Chez, 2004).

For the purposes of this book, nonconventional assessment or treatments are biological, somatic, mind–body, and energy-information approaches not currently accepted in Western biomedical psychiatry. It is important to note that many nonconventional approaches are based on mainstream scientific concepts and are supported by evidence from conventional research studies. Complementary, alternative, and integrative assessment and treatment methods are different kinds of nonconventional approaches. Alternative approaches are based on concepts that are outside mainstream Western medicine. Examples include acupuncture and qigong. Complementary approaches are based on mainstream biomedical theory and supported by research evidence but are not part of the mainstream because of social, political, or ideological reasons. Herbal medicine, bright light exposure, and electroencephalogram (EEG) biofeedback are examples of complementary modalities. From the perspective of contemporary Western psychiatry, integrative approaches combine pharmacological treatments with psychotherapy. The evidence for integrative treatments that combine psychotherapy and conventional drugs is reviewed elsewhere (Sammons & Schmidt, 2003). Nonconventional approaches are seldom considered in Western psychiatry when integrative solutions are being developed. For the purposes of this book, the term *integrative* refers to combinations of conventional and nonconventional approaches. This broader definition is not restricted to prescription drugs and psychotherapy and includes the entire range of nonconventional assessment and treatment approaches.

◆ Conventional and Nonconventional Systems of Medicine Rest on Disparate Assumptions

Many nonconventional treatments, and the systems of medicine from which they originate, rest on assumptions that are fundamentally at odds with the philosophical position of Western medicine, which argues that the causes of illness are invariably reducible to physical or biological factors. Nonconventional systems of medicine rest on other assumptions, including the role of complex nonlinear processes in illness causation, the nonlocal nature of space–time, and the corollary view that consciousness has nonlocal effects on health and illness. Further, mind–body and energetic approaches argue that the role of consciousness in healing is not explainable using contemporary scientific models of brain functioning. From an integrative perspective, health and illness are manifestations of complex dynamic interactions between psychological, physical, biological, social, and spiritual factors at multiple hierarchic levels of organization in space and time (Bell et al., 2002; Reilly, 2001). To the extent that a symptom pattern is biologically determined, biological treatments will address its presumed root causes. To the extent that symptoms are manifestations of dynamic psychological issues, psychological interventions will be effective, and biological approaches sometimes serve as useful adjunctive treatments. However, in cases where dysregulation of the energetic or informational "levels" of the body–brain contributes to symptom formation, conventional assessment methods may fail to identify root causes or "meanings" of symptom patterns, and conventional biological or psychological treatments may not be effective. Biological dysregulations take place at the level of neurotransmitters, brain circuits involving several neurotransmitters, and web-like feedforward and feedback relationships between neurotransmitters (or their receptors) and other biological systems, including endocrinological and immunological factors. Functional dysregulation at a biological level can manifest as psychological symptoms, or translate into changes in energetic or informational processes in the body at one or many interrelated hierarchic levels of organization. As such, an effective biological treatment may directly or indirectly address causes, conditions, or meanings associated with a symptom pattern that are manifestations of dysregulations at biological, psychological, energetic, or informational levels. The same can be said of psychological, energetic, or informational treatments; that is, each kind of treatment can directly or indirectly affect the biological, psychological, energetic, or informational causes or conditions that manifest as a particular symptom pattern. Integrative approaches in medicine and mental health care are built on the premise that humans are complex systems of dynamically interacting biological, psychological, energetic, informational, and possibly spiritual processes. Subsequently, the goals of integrative mental health care are to characterize the causes, conditions, or meanings associated with symptom patterns and to construct appropriate treatment strategies that effectively address those factors.

Because of the number, diversity, and complexity of factors involved in health and illness, constructing a testable hypothesis regarding putative causal relationships between measurable treatment effects and presumed therapeutic benefits of many conventional and nonconventional treatments is often problematic. This issue is especially germane to studies of emerging treatments of mental illness because of difficulties inherent in measuring subjective outcomes, and basic cultural differences between concepts of "mind" and "body" and, by extension, differences in understandings of "normal" and "abnormal" emotional or mental states. In addition to its basic philosophical, scientific, and methodological foundations, the practice of biomedicine is influenced by cultural and economic factors that are difficult to quantify. These include the increasing intellectual openness of Western culture to non-Western healing approaches and the growing demand for more meaningful or more personal contact with medical practitioners, which is frequently difficult to obtain during rushed appointments in contemporary health care settings. These issues have led increasing

numbers of individuals who see a Western-trained physician to concurrently seek treatment from non–traditionally trained practitioners, including Chinese medical practitioners, herbalists, homeopathic physicians, and energy healers (Barnes, Powell-Griner, McFann, & Nahin, 2004). Increasing acceptance of nonconventional medicine in Western culture is the result of both science and social trends. Research is providing empirical evidence for many complementary and alternative approaches. Additionally, the popular appeal of nonorthodox medicine is growing because of shared cultural beliefs, including the benign role of "nature" in healing, changing attitudes toward health care, and spiritual beliefs that give patients increased feelings of empowerment and autonomy. In this broad humanistic-spiritual context, "the quest for health takes on sacred proportions, allowing the patient to discern ultimate meaning and make profound connections with the universe" (Kaptchuk & Eisenberg, 1998). Alternative medicine turns to science for legitimacy and has tried to make science "person friendly." It has been characterized as providing a vehicle for "the pathways of words, feelings, values, expectations and beliefs" that reorder and organize the disease experience involved in all traditions of medicine (Kleinman, 1973).

◆ Growing Dissatisfaction with Conventional Medical Care Is Resulting in Increased Use of Nonconventional Approaches

Broad economic issues affect the capacity of Western medicine to provide adequate health care. In the United States, these include restrictions of available treatments under managed care, Medicare, and private insurance contracts that limit reimbursement for newer, more effective drugs while promoting less expensive generics. There is growing dissatisfaction with the quality of medical care in general because of concerns over efficacy and safety of conventional treatments, complaints about the often impersonal manner of health care "delivery," and the increasing cost of medical care to the average consumer (Astin, 1998). People in the United States who use nonconventional therapies are generally more educated and twice as likely to have significant anxiety compared with those who do not. Approximately 40% of Caucasians, Hispanics, and Asians use nonconventional approaches to treat medical or mental health problems compared with over two thirds of Native Americans and less than 30% of African Americans (Astin, 1998). The same demographic groups that are critical of Western biomedicine as currently practiced are turning to nonconventional therapies for a range of medical and psychiatric problems (Eisenberg et al., 1993). This trend is based on shifting values, economic factors, renewed emphasis on healthy lifestyles, and emerging research findings supporting the use of treatments outside of orthodox Western medicine, including botanicals and mind–body practices already in widespread use in many parts of the world (Astin, 1998; Leskowitz, 1993; Rees, 2001). The growing acceptance of nonconventional medical practices reflects an increasingly consumer-driven health care environment in the context of increasing medical diversity (Kaptchuk & Eisenberg, 2001).

In the face of dissatisfaction with conventional medical care, use of nonconventional approaches is showing marked growth in the United States. Approximately 72 million U.S. adults used a nonconventional treatment in 2002, representing about one in three adults (Tindle, Davis, Phillips, & Eisenberg, 2005). If prayer is included in this analysis, almost two thirds of adults have used nonconventional therapies (Barnes et al., 2004). The overall use of the 15 most popular nonconventional treatments remained essentially unchanged between 1997 and 2002; however, use rates of some nonconventional approaches changed (Conboy et al., 2005; Tindle et al., 2005). Among those who used nonconventional approaches, 58.6% used only one modality, and 41.4% had used two or more approaches in the previous year. Visits to chiropractors declined slightly, and the number of individuals who used energy healing and biofeedback remained unchanged. Between 1997 and 2002, growth areas in nonconventional medicine included herbal medicine (12 to 18.6%) and yoga (3.7 to 5.1%). During the same 5-year period the percentage of individuals who saw a provider for herbs fell from 15.1 to 5.2%, suggesting that, although herbs are increasingly used in the general population, more people are self-treating problems without seeking professional advice. The same survey suggests that there is a trend toward increased self-treatment using homeopathic remedies and high-dose vitamins outside medical consultation. The trend toward self-treatment represents a potential safety issue in view of the uneven quality of over-the-counter natural products, the large percentage of individuals who use two or more conventional or nonconventional approaches, and the fact that almost two thirds of people who use nonconventional approaches do not disclose them to their physicians (Eisenberg et al., 2001).

Individuals who are diagnosed with a psychiatric disorder are significantly more likely to use nonconventional treatments compared with the general population (Unutzer et al., 2000). One third of individuals who report a history of generalized anxiety, mood swings, or psychotic symptoms have used nonconventional approaches to treat their symptoms (Unutzer et al., 2000). Two thirds of severely depressed or acutely anxious individuals have used both conventional and nonconventional treatments at the same time, and as many as 90% of these have seen a psychiatrist or other mental health professional (Kessler et al., 2001). The findings of two large surveys suggest that most individuals who have mental or emotional symptoms use conventional medications and nonconventional approaches at the same time (Eisenberg et al., 1998; Unutzer et al., 2000). According to one large patient survey conventional and nonconventional treatments for acute anxiety and severe depressed mood are perceived as equally effective (Kessler et al., 2001).

Changes in medical education are taking place in parallel with research advances and growing popular interest in nonconventional therapies. At the time of this writing the Consortium of Academic Health Centers for Integrative Medicine has 28 medical school members. This organization is bringing core competencies of integrative medical practice into mainstream medical education at the level of medical school and residency training programs (Kligler et al., 2004). Another significant trend that will ensure continued growth in integrative medical thinking in Western culture is increasing interest in nonconventional medicine among both conventionally trained physicians and alternative medical practitioners. According to one large physician survey, approximately half of U.S. physicians believe that acupuncture, chiropractic, and homeopathy rest on valid medical principles, and frequently refer patients to nonconventional practitioners for these therapies (Astin et al., 1998). Many Western MDs are becoming certified to

practice in one or more areas of nonconventional medicine, including massage, acupuncture, herbal medicine, and homeopathy (Astin et al., 1998; Ernst, Resch, & White, 1995). At the same time training requirements for Chinese medical practitioners and herbalists now include basic courses in human physiology and anatomy. Dual training in two or more broad systems of medicine requires enormous time, energy, and commitment and is not a realistic option for even the most idealistic and open-minded clinicians. However, increasing numbers of physicians are being introduced to a range of nonconventional modalities at intensive weekend seminars, and courses on alternative modalities are being included in the annual meetings of professional medical societies, including the American Medical Association and the American Psychiatric Association. Out of a sense of shared interest in integrative medicine conventionally and nonconventionally trained practitioners are finding ways to collaborate on patient care. The result is the gradual evolution of Western biomedicine toward truly integrative clinical methods.

◆ Efficacy and Safety Problems Limit Conventional Psychiatric Treatments

Conventional psychiatric medications are frequently effective and well tolerated. Their appropriate use permits many who would otherwise be impaired by severe cognitive, emotional, or behavioral symptoms to return to an acceptable level of functioning and restore a sense of self-empowerment, dignity, and control to their lives. Between 1.5 and 10% of the adult population of the United States and other industrialized countries take conventional psychopharmacological drugs for depressed mood, anxiety, schizophrenia, and other serious mental health problems (Ohayon & Lader, 2002). The use of pharmacological treatments in mental health care has grown steadily since the introduction of chlorpromazine, the first antipsychotic medication, in the early 1950s. Millions of individuals have benefited from important advances in neurobiology and pharmacology, resulting in novel biological treatments of mental illness. Unfortunately, the increasing use of conventional pharmacological treatments in mental health care is taking place in the context of unresolved questions about safety and efficacy. Conventional psychiatric assessment provides useful information that helps to clarify the psychological and biological meanings and causes of symptoms. However, conventional assessment approaches have limited reliability and predictive power and do not provide a complete or accurate picture of the myriad possible causes and meanings of mental illness. In spite of their successes, conventional pharmacological treatments of depression, anxiety, and other common mental health problems have limited efficacy and effectiveness, and their prolonged use is often associated with significant adverse effects (Leo, 1996; Schatzberg et al., 1997). A recent review suggests that risks associated with prescription antidepressants exceed their desired therapeutic effects (Keitner, 2004). Growing concerns over the possibility that many conventional drugs used in contemporary biomedical psychiatry have limited efficacy are complicated by increasing public alarm over safety issues and the unaffordability of many new drugs, especially among low-income patients and the elderly (Moran, 2004). This situation is made worse by shortcomings of outpatient mental health services under the constraints of managed care and health maintenance organizations, including infrequent, brief, and impersonal sessions for "medication management" only (Dubin, 2004). At the same time accumulating research findings document the benefits of nonconventional assessment and treatment approaches in mental health care.

Because of the above circumstances, increasing numbers of conventionally trained psychiatrists have moved away from strictly biomedical treatment methods and are embracing the eclectic perspectives of integrative medicine, which combines concepts and clinical methods from conventional psychiatry and disparate systems of medicine (Astin et al., 1998; Kelner & Wellman, 1997). Continued medical pluralism will probably result in increasing uses of nonconventional treatments in mental health care and eventually slow the trend in developed countries toward the widespread and frequently inappropriate uses of psychopharmacological drugs that are expensive, often have significant adverse effects, pose uncertain long-term safety risks, and in many cases have questionable efficacy (Moncrief et al., 2004). Like conventional biomedicine, nonconventional approaches are limited by ambiguous research findings, safety issues, and incomplete understandings of putative mechanisms of action. However, in view of the limitations of contemporary conventional treatments of mental illness, an important goal of future mental health research should be the systematic evaluation of promising nonconventional assessment and treatments approaches. In contrast to the generic treatment-centered approaches of biomedicine, integrative health care is patient-centered and individualized. Integrative medicine emphasizes "wellness" of the whole person and engages the patient's active participation in a process that is aimed at achieving dynamic balance rather than relief of a particular "target" symptom (Barrett et al., 2003). Through judicious combinations of conventional and nonconventional approaches, integrative medicine offers a reasonable "middle way" in mental health care.

◆ Entrenched Views of Mental Illness Bias Research Funding and Interfere with Publications of Nonconventional Research Findings

The widely shared view that mental illness is caused by pathology at the level of neurotransmitters is perpetuated by pharmaceutical industry–sponsored research and has become dogma in contemporary biomedical psychiatry. This has resulted in limited private funding for studies on most nonconventional modalities. The scientific and ideological perspectives of contemporary biological psychiatry are based on widely accepted biological theories in genetics, molecular biology, and neurobiology. Until recent decades little serious attention had been directed at evaluating nonorthodox conceptual frameworks as possible explanatory models of psychopathology. This perspective biases research funding against studies on promising nonpharmacological treatments of mental illness. A multibillion-dollar pharmaceutical industry conducts internal studies and funds most third-party research on psychopharmacological medications in the United States and other Western countries, and there is little impetus to sponsor studies on natural products much less nonpharmacological complementary or alternative treatments that are not potential sources of significant revenue. These circumstances have limited the quality and amount of data on

putative biological, mind–body, and energetic models of mental illness causation that do not rely principally on the neurotransmitter theory. The National Center for Complementary and Alternative Medicine of the National Institutes of Health is attempting to remedy this situation by sponsoring studies on different nonconventional modalities, including acupuncture, Yoga, and energy medicine. However, the status quo will likely continue as long as the pharmaceutical industry is the major funding source for research in medicine and psychiatry, and continues to invest hundreds of millions of advertising dollars annually in efforts to influence physician attitudes and popular cultural views of prescription drug use in industrialized countries.

Funding disparities between research on conventional and nonconventional treatments often translate into short, poorly designed studies involving few patients when nonconventional modalities are investigated. As a result, findings in many areas of complementary or alternative medicine research seldom fulfill criteria for methodological rigor required in Western medicine, and are subsequently regarded as inconclusive because they fail to achieve benchmarks of minimum statistical significance even in cases where outcomes are consistently positive. It is reasonable to evaluate many nonconventional treatments for which there is currently limited biomedical evidence on the basis of cumulative clinical observations over considerable time periods and consistently beneficial outcomes, and in some cases, positive findings of studies that do not follow strict Western-style research methods. The inherent biases of Western biomedicine against research in nonconventional medicine are amplified by differences in the potential statistical power of results from standard research methods or data analysis techniques used in biomedicine in contrast to typically qualitative research methods employed in much of nonconventional medical research.

Publication bias is closely tied to funding sources for medical research. The American Medical Association's Council on Scientific Affairs examined the impact of funding sources on the validity and reliability of pharmaceutical research and concluded that over half of research contracts in university- and industry-sponsored studies permitted delayed publication, more than one third allowed the drug company sponsor to delete unfavorable data prior to publication, and 30% allowed both delays in publication and selective deleting of information. Based on an analysis of 12 systematic reviews of studies on the relationship between research outcomes and pharmaceutical industry sponsorship, in 2004 the Council of Delegates of the American Medical Association issued a report confirming that studies with positive findings are more likely to be published than studies with negative findings, and that publication of negative or null findings is more likely to be delayed compared with publication of positive findings. Negative research findings of pharmaceutical company–sponsored drug studies sometimes remain classified for long periods of time. A recent analysis suggests that combining previously classified drug trials data with published findings reduces the efficacy of many widely used antidepressants to the level of placebos (Sussman, 2004). This so-called file-drawer effect has resulted in concern over the quality and objectivity of research methods used in biomedical psychiatry and the need to find ways to enforce greater public accountability of the pharmaceutical industry and the U.S. Food and Drug Administration

(FDA). The controversy over conventional pharmacological treatments in psychiatry was further increased by the FDA's decision to issue a black box warning on the use of all antidepressants in children and adolescents because of reports of significantly increased suicide risk associated with their use in this age group (Black box warning, 2004). In response to these concerns, the FDA recently directed the Institute of Medicine to critically review established FDA approaches to ensure drug safety, especially after a drug has gone to market (Mechcatie, 2005). Concerns over the reliability of pharmaceutical industry–sponsored research resulted in congressional hearings and the introduction of a bill that would require timely posting of clinical trials data in a public registry (Brewer & Colditz, 1999; Jones, 2001; Ioannidis & Lau, 2001). It is hoped that the current requirement of public disclosure of all ongoing clinical trials and outcomes will lead to closer scrutiny of industry-sponsored research (Fontanarosa, Rennie, & DeAngelis, 2004).

Publication bias has also resulted in limited numbers of citations of rigorously conducted studies on nonconventional treatments in the most widely referenced medical databases, including the largest publicly available medical database, PubMed of the National Library of Medicine (Dickerson & Min, 1993; Mancano & Bullano, 1998). Consequently, physicians and the public at large who wish to examine the research evidence pertaining to a particular nonconventional treatment face significant obstacles when searching for reliable, unbiased information. Studies on alternative treatments that are published in peer-reviewed mainstream medical journals are often framed in a cautious or negative way by journal editors. Examples include special alternative medicine issues of the *Journal of the American Medical Association* and the *Archives of General Psychiatry* (Ernst & Cassileth, 1999). In both cases negative editorial bias resulted in a distorted view of the significance of findings under discussion.

In view of the controversies over drug safety and efficacy facing the pharmaceutical industry and the FDA, it is ironic that the continuation of an almost exclusive emphasis on the development of new synthetic drugs in government- and industry-funded mental health research is probably delaying progress in the elucidation of basic mechanisms underlying the pathogenesis of psychiatric disorders. Limited funding of studies on nonconventional treatments will translate into continued slow progress in the development of novel nonconventional biological treatments, mind–body approaches, and other promising treatments in mental health care. In the absence of significant policy changes in federal research funding, there is a very real risk that the continued exclusive emphasis on psychopharmacology in mental health research will relegate future investigations of promising novel nonconventional treatments to a low priority. Subsequently, researchers and physicians will continue to ignore or a priori dismiss emerging conceptual frameworks that can potentially lead to more adequate explanatory models of mental illness. The result will be delays in the development of effective novel treatments addressing the complex biological, social, mind–body, and possibly energetic and spiritual causes and meanings of psychiatric symptoms. As noted above, the National Center for Complementary and Alternative Medicine is beginning to address this concern, but research funding of nonconventional therapies remains miniscule in comparison with billions of dollars in annual pharmaceutical industry funding of studies on conventional medications. Conceptual models that offer potentially valuable novel understandings of the biological, energetic, or "informational" mechanisms of mental illness include functional medicine, complexity theory, psychoneuroimmunology, concepts in mind–body medicine and energy medicine, and possibly also quantum field theory.

◆ Symptoms, Not Disorders, Are the Focus of Clinical Attention in Mental Health Care

In this book the primary emphasis is on symptoms rather than disorders. For practical purposes, psychiatrists, other mental health professionals, primary care physicians, and nonconventionally trained medical practitioners treat the patient's primary complaints whatever they may be, and a "disorder" is noted in the patient's chart largely for purposes of documentation requirements and insurance billing. Patients always complain of symptoms, but formal criteria for a "disorder" according to the *Diagnostic and Statistical Manual of Mental Disorders* (4th ed., *DSM-IV*) are seldom met (Krueger, 1999). Regardless of the category or name of a diagnosed "disorder," when approaching a patient the clinician focuses on the cognitive, emotional, and behavioral symptoms causing the greatest degree of impairment or distress. For example, many symptom patterns can become the focus of clinical attention when treating a patient diagnosed with bipolar disorder, including euphoric or irritable mood, disturbed sleep, depressed mood, and psychosis. Depressed mood, agitation, insomnia, and possibly impaired cognition or substance abuse often become the focus of treatment in a severely depressed patient. Patients diagnosed with an anxiety "disorder" display a broad range of symptoms that change over time and seldom conform to unambiguously worded *DSM-IV* diagnostic criteria. Symptoms evolve in unique patterns in the lifetime of every individual in relation to complex psychological, social, biological, energetic, and spiritual causes or meanings (Krueger, Caspi, Moffitt, & Silva, 1998). Because there is substantial overlap between *DSM-IV* "disorders" in terms of symptomatology, the distinctions between psychiatric "disorders" are frequently arbitrary. Thinking of mental illness in terms of *DSM-IV* diagnostic categories instead of unique evolving symptom patterns can interfere with the accurate identification, assessment, and treatment of core symptoms. Because discrete unchanging symptom patterns are seldom observed in mental illness, the concept of "disorder" in conventional psychiatry continues to change, as do the specific diagnostic criteria that correspond to most "disorders" (Shanfield, 2004; Stahl, 2003a,b). Descriptions of cognitive, emotional, and behavioral symptoms have remained relatively stable in Western culture; however, understandings of the causes or meanings of symptoms vary over time as novel paradigms and new research findings emerge. On the basis of findings from large epidemiologic studies, the validity of "disorder" as a construct has recently been called into question. Integrative approaches to health in general and mental illness in particular emphasize assessment and treatment approaches that address the unique symptoms of each patient. In some cases one primary symptom is the focus of clinical management. In other cases, the clinician must deal with two or more co-evolving symptom patterns at the same time.

◆ Progress in Integrative Medicine Has Been Slowed by the Absence of Agreement on Methods

As the global exchange of ideas and information accelerates, progress in all systems of medicine will increasingly depend on the evolution of established medical theory toward a conceptual framework capable of accommodating diverse philosophical and methodological perspectives. Integrative medicine will ideally provide a rigorously open framework that will successfully accommodate the science, intuitions, and clinical practices of disparate systems of medicine. Progress toward a truly integrative medicine has been slowed by the absence of a conceptual framework for thinking about integration from first philosophical and methodological principles. Subsequently, philosophically coherent arguments or empirically defensible methods for combining modalities from disparate systems of medicine have not been proposed. As there is presently no agreed-on conceptual framework for thinking about the basic concepts of integrative medicine, there is no professional consensus on rigorous conceptual methods for planning integrative medical management. A consequence of this fact is the absence of practical clinical guidelines for identifying assessment or treatment approaches that are most suitable for integration when managing a specified medical or mental health problem. Of equal concern, there are no guidelines for determining when to avoid combining disparate modalities because of efficacy or safety concerns.

The absence of consensus on methods in integrative medicine has led to the present state of affairs in which patients frequently self-treat complex symptoms with little or no professional guidance, and health care professionals trained in different systems of medicine combine disparate assessment or treatment approaches on the basis of little or no evidence of effectiveness or safety. The consequences of this de facto integrative approach for health care has been the absence of rigorous evidence-based methods for determining optimum treatment strategies, the continuing occurrence of unknown kinds and magnitudes of safety issues, confusion among patients about which treatments to use or avoid using for a particular problem, and controversy among both conventionally and nonconventionally trained practitioners over appropriate combinations of modalities addressing the range of medical and psychiatric symptoms. The methods and information contained in this book represent a beginning effort to address these problems.

The philosophical assumptions that are given in a system of medicine define the conceptual framework within which theorizing and practical problem solving take place. The philosophical foundations of disparate systems of medicine embody different ways of thinking about health and illness. Clearly

defining these principles is a necessary first step in constructing methods from which particular assessment and treatment approaches can then be derived. Sound methods must be based on clearly elucidated principles, and if we are to avoid ambiguity, principles must have an explicit and rigorous philosophical basis. This book discusses concepts, methods, and clinical information. In my view concepts and methods are always more important than information. A solid grounding in the concepts and methods of integrative medicine is essential for guiding understanding and competent clinical practice. The relative weight of clinical evidence supporting both conventional and nonconventional treatment approaches changes almost daily, and the evidence-based content of integrative medicine therefore evolves on a continuous basis. Conceptual methods in medicine also change but at a more gradual rate. Clinicians who have a clear understanding of the basic concepts and methods introduced in this book will be able to incorporate both established and emerging therapeutics from a range of assessment and treatment approaches with good effect.

◆ Increasing Integration Will Improve Cost-Effectiveness of Conventional Treatments in Mental Health Care

An important practical goal of integrative assessment and treatment is to reduce the use of approaches that are expensive or fail to meet acceptable requirements of cost-effectiveness, while increasing the use of less expensive or more cost-effective approaches. Methodological considerations pertaining to the selection of cost-effective approaches in integrative medicine are addressed in Chapter 4. Part II of this book reviews evidence for nonconventional approaches in mental health care, many of which are as effective as more expensive or less available conventional approaches. Effective solutions to mental health problems that are more affordable than conventional pharmacological treatments will result in reduced costs to both patients and third-party payers. The increasing use of cost-effective integrative approaches will translate into reductions in long-term costs associated with expensive conventional treatments that yield equivalent or poorer outcomes. The result will be generally improved mental health care delivery to all segments of the population and commensurate reductions in the enormous medical, social, and financial burdens of mental illness. Less tangible benefits that will accrue from integration in mental health care include increased patient autonomy, reductions in job productivity losses, and reductions in indirect costs associated with widespread and undertreated mental health problems.

References

Astin, J. (1998). Why patients use alternative medicine. *Journal of the American Medical Association, 279*(19), 1548–1553.

Astin, J., Marie, A., Pelletier, K., et al. (1998). A review of the incorporation of complementary and alternative medicine by mainstream physicians. *Archives of Internal Medicine, 158*, 2303–2310.

Barnes, P. M., Powell-Griner, E., McFann, K., & Nahin, R. (2004). Complementary and alternative medicine use among adults: United States, 2002. *Advanced Data, 343*, 1–19.

Barrett, B., Marchand, L., Scheder, J., et al. (2003). Themes of holism, empowerment, access and legitimacy define complementary, alternative and integrative medicine in relation to conventional biomedicine. *Journal of Alternative and Complementary Medicine, 9*(6), 937–947.

Bell, I., Caspi, O., Schwartz, G., et al. (2002). Integrative medicine and systemic outcomes research: Issues in the emergence of a new model for primary health care. *Archives of Internal Medicine, 162*(2), 133–140.

Black box warning on antidepressants creates concerns for clinicians. (2004). *Neuropsychiatry Review, 5*(9), 1, 25–28.

Brewer, T., & Colditz, G. A. (1999). Postmarketing surveillance and adverse drug reactions: Current perspectives and future needs. *Journal of the American Medical Association, 281*, 824–829.

Conboy, L., Patel, S., Kaptchuk, T. J., et al. (2005). Sociodemographic determinants of the utilization of specific types of complementary and alternative medicine an analysis based on a nationally representative survey sample. *Journal of Alternative and Complementary Medicine, 11*(6), 977–994.

Dickerson, K., & Min, Y. (1993). NIH clinical trials and publication bias [Electronic version]. *Journal of Current Clinical Trials,* 50.

Dubin, W. (2004, May). *Clinical practices that lead to treatment resistance* (Abstract 81D, Symposium 81). Paper presented at the annual meeting of the American Psychiatric Association, New York.

Eisenberg, D., Davis, R., Ettner, S., et al. (1998). Trends in alternative medicine use in the United States, 1990–1997: Results of a follow-up national survey. *Journal of the American Medical Association, 280*(18), 1569–1575.

Eisenberg, D. M., Kessler, R. C., Foster, C., Norlock, F. E., Colkins, D. R., & Delbanco, T. L. (1993). Unconventional medicine in the United States: Prevalence, costs, and patterns of use. *New England Journal of Medicine, 328*(4), 246–252.

Eisenberg, D., Kessler, R., Van Rompay, M., et al. (2001). Perceptions about complementary therapies relative to conventional therapies among adults who use both: Results from a national survey. *Annals of Internal Medicine, 135,* 344–351.

Ernst, E., Cassileth, B. R. (1999). How useful are unconventional cancer treatments? *European Journal of Cancer, 35*(11), 1608–1613.

Ernst, E., Resch, K., & White, A. (1995). Complementary medicine: What physicians think of it—a meta-analysis. *Archives of Internal Medicine, 155,* 2405–2408.

Fontanarosa, P. B., Rennie, D., & DeAngelis, C. D. (2004). Postmarketing surveillance—lack of vigilance, lack of trust. *Journal of the American Medical Association, 292,* 2647–2650.

Ioannidis, J. P. A., & Lau, J. (2001). Completeness of safety reporting in randomized trials: An evaluation of 7 medical areas. *Journal of the American Medical Association, 285,* 437–443.

Jonas, W., & Chez, R. (2004). Toward optimal healing environments in health care. *Journal of Alternative and Complementary Medicine, 10*(Suppl. 1), S-1–6.

Jones, T. C. (2001). Call for a new approach to the process of clinical trials and drug registration. *British Medical Journal, 322,* 920–923.

Kaptchuk, T., & Eisenberg, D. (1998). The persuasive appeal of alternative medicine. *Annals of Internal Medicine, 129*(12), 1061–1065.

Kaptchuk, T., & Eisenberg, D. (2001). Varieties of healing: 1. Medical pluralism in the United States. *Annals of Internal Medicine, 135*(3), 189–195.

Keitner, G. (2004, May). *Limits to the treatment of major depression* (Abstract No. 34). Paper presented at the annual meeting of the American Psychiatric Association, New York.

Kelner, M., & Wellman, B. (1997). Who seeks alternative health care? A profile of the users of five modes of treatment. *Journal of Alternative and Complementary Medicine, 3*(2), 127–140.

Kessler, R., Soukup, J., Davis, R., et al. (2001). The use of complementary and alternative therapies to treat anxiety and depression in the United States. *American Journal of Psychiatry, 158,* 289–294.

Kleinman, A. (1973). Toward a comparative study of medical systems: An integrated approach to the study of the relationship of medicine and culture. *Science Medicine Man, 1,* 55–65.

Kligler, B., Maizes, V., Schachter, S., et al. (2004). Core competencies in integrative medicine for medical school curricula: A proposal. *Adacemic Medicine, 79*(6), 521–531.

Krueger, R. (1999). The structure of common mental disorders. *Archives of General Psychiatry, 56,* 921–926.

Krueger, R., Caspi, A., Moffitt, T., & Silva, P. (1998). The structure and stability of common mental disorders (DSM-III-R): A longitudinal-epidemiological study. *Journal of Abnormal Psychology, 107,* 216–227.

Leo, R. J. (1996). Movement disorders associated with the serotonin selective reuptake inhibitors. *Journal of Clinical Psychiatry, 57,* 449–454.

Leskowitz, E. (1993). Spiritual healing, modern medicine, and energy. *Advances, 9*(4), 50–53.

Mancano, M., & Bullano, M. (1998). Meta-analysis: Methodology, utility, and limitations. *Journal of Pharmacological Practices, 11*(4), 239–250.

Mechcatie, E. (2005). FDA plans to strengthen drug safety program. *Clin Psychiatry News,* January, 8.

Moncrieff, J., Wessely, S., Hardy, R. (2004). Active placebos versus antidepressants for depression. *Cochrane Review.* In: The Chochrane Library, Chichester, United Kingdom: John Wiley & Sons.

Moran, M. (2004, August 20). Drug prices rise twice as fast as rate of inflation. *Psychiatric News,* p. 18.

Ohayon, M., & Lader, M. (2002). Use of psychotropic medication in the general population of France, Germany, Italy, and the United Kingdom. *Journal of Clinical Psychiatry, 63*(9), 817–825.

Rees, L. (2001). Integrated medicine: Imbues orthodox medicine with the values of complementary medicine. *British Medical Journal, 322,* 119–120.

Reilly, D. (2001). Enhancing human healing. *British Medical Journal, 322*(20), 120–121.

Sammons, M., & Schmidt, N. (Eds.). (2003). *Combined treatments for mental disorders: A guide to psychological and pharmacological interventions.* Washington, DC: American Psychological Association.

Schatzberg, A. F., Haddad, P., Kaplan, E. M., Lejoyeux, M., Rosenbaum, J. F., Young, A. H., & Zajecka, J. (1997). Serotonin reuptake inhibitor discontinuation syndrome: A hypothetical definition. *Journal of Clinical Psychiatry, 58*(Suppl. 7), 5–10.

Shanfield, S. (2004, May). *The dimensional construct in psychiatric disorders* (Abstract 12d, Symposium 12). Paper presented at the annual meeting of the American Psychiatric Association, New York.

Sparber, A., Wootton, J. C. (2002). Surveys of complementary and alternative medicine: Part V. Use of alternative and complementary therapies for psychiatric and neurologic diseases. *Journal of Alternative and Complementary Medicine, 8*(1), 93–96.

Stahl, S. (2003a). Deconstructing psychiatric disorders: 1. Genotypes, symptom phenotypes, and endophenotypes. *Journal of Clinical Psychiatry, 64*(9), 982–983.

Stahl, S. (2003b). Deconstructing psychiatric disorders: 2. An emerging neurobiologically based therapeutic strategy for the modern psychopharmacologist. *Journal of Clinical Psychiatry, 64*(10), 1145–1146.

Sussman, N. (2004). The "file-drawer" effect: Assessing efficacy and safety of antidepressants. *Primary Psychiatry,* 12.

Tindle, H. A., Davis, R. B., Phillips, R. S., & Eisenberg, D. M. (2005). Trends in use of complementary and alternative medicine by U.S. adults: 1997–2002. *Alternative Therapies in Health and Medicine, 11*(1), 42–49.

Unutzer, J., Klap, R., Sturm, R., et al. (2000). Mental disorders and the use of alternative medicine: Results from a national survey. *American Journal of Psychiatry, 157,* 1851–1857.

2

Philosophical Problems

This chapter explores important philosophical issues relevant to medicine in general and integrative medicine in particular. The discussion begins with a brief review of the disparate philosophical origins of Western medicine and non-Western systems of medicine and the significance of the resulting philosophical "gap." The context-dependent nature of methodologies that have developed within disparate systems of medicine is described. I argue that different ways of seeing illness and health phenomena are related to differences in core metaphysical assumptions. The nature and role of causality in medicine are examined, as well as established methodologies used to infer relationships between putative "causes" of symptoms. I argue that a kind of functional congruence must exist between phenomena that underlie a specified symptom pattern and phenomena operationalized as the mechanism of action of a particular assessment or treatment approach. This interphenomenal congruence explains efficacy on the basis of interactions between a defined mechanism of action and a specified symptom pattern. Disparate meanings of evidence in medicine are discussed, and unresolved philosophical problems in psychiatric classification and diagnosis are briefly reviewed. The

problem of deriving a typology of medical approaches addressing cognitive, emotional, and behavioral symptoms is discussed. The chapter concludes with an overview of philosophical issues pertaining to the development of methodologies in integrative medicine.

◆ Key Philosophical Issues

Western and Non-Western Systems of Medicine Have Disparate Philosophical Origins

The perspectives of Western medicine stand in contrast to those of other systems of medicine because of implicit assumptions about existence, causality, and time that can be traced to the cultural and philosophical roots of Western medicine. In Western culture, material existence was historically believed to be a fundamental quality of reality. According to this point of view, dynamic interactions between observable or measurable material entities (referred to as process) take place within a world ordered with respect to the presumed linear flow of time. This model reduces process to linear temporal relationships between presumed fundamental material states of existence. In Western culture assumptions about primary material categories of existence and the nature of time led to corresponding assumptions about valid ways to demonstrate the correctness of truth claims pertaining to relationships between some material states (causes) and other material states (effects). The philosophical perspective that a discoverable objective reality exists is called realism. This ancient philosophical perspective eventually led to the establishment of formal scientific methodologies based on observation and measurement, starting with Plato's Academy in Athens, and progressing to more refined methodologies with René Descartes, Francis Bacon, and, in the early 20th century, the logical positivists of Vienna and Ludwig Wittgenstein's *Tractatus Logico-Philosophicus*. Realism continued to evolve with the work of Karl Popper, who argued that a hypothesis can never be finally confirmed because only one contradictory finding is sufficient to falsify its claims. This position asserts that objective reality exists but cannot be verified or unambiguously described. Imre Lakatos extended Popper's thesis by adding the concept of heuristics and their evolutionary influence on methodologies in science. In *Against Method,* Paul Feyerabend argued that scientific method does not have a privileged position in the universe of possible approaches for investigating phenomena and should thus be viewed as no more legitimate than other methodologies. Feyerabend's anarchist position can be regarded as an extremely radical kind of relativism. Finally, in the 1960s, Thomas Kuhn put forward the idea of competing paradigms as a less extreme form of relativism in *The Structure of Scientific Revolutions* (Kuhn, 1962). According to this model, a paradigm is a conceptual framework of presuppositions that define how scientists in different traditions approach their theoretical and practical work. Like Popper and Feyerabend, Kuhn argued that ultimate "truth" is unattainable and that the acceptance or exclusion of theories in science has more to do with consensus and political affiliation than the rational demonstration of claims. Kuhn held that paradigms—which reflect shared points of view and not objective reality—evolve and are eventually overthrown as new "maps" of reality are accepted by scientists and achieve political and institutional backing. Relativism asserts that understandings of "truth" in science and in general have more to do with one's cultural and social perspective than research findings or the logical structure of a particular methodology. Most Western-trained scientists subscribe to a kind of naive realism, that is, the belief that the claimed objective reality of phenomena can be confirmed or refuted through research, in spite of the fact that this philosophical perspective was displaced by the idea of evolving paradigms decades ago.

In contrast to Western science, the primary categories of existence in Asian culture and philosophy were believed to be energy and dynamic processes involving energy. Non-Western concepts of time were not linear, and, in contrast to Western science and medicine, causality was not constrained by material processes interacting within a presumed linear ordering of time. According to this viewpoint, material states were interpreted as secondary manifestations of energy states. Implicit in these assumptions was the belief that "energy states" exist, are knowable and reportable as subjective experiences by the patient, and are observable by the skilled practitioner. Thus in many non-Western systems of medicine criteria used to establish the reality of a symptom are regarded as subjective by Western standards, and there is no perceived need in non-Western schools of

medical thought to develop a methodology that reduces phenomena to primary material causes. From the perspectives of Chinese medicine, Ayurveda, Tibetan medicine, and other non-Western systems of medicine, the truth claims of energetic conditions are asserted as factual. Analytical arguments toward the empirical basis of energetic phenomena are viewed as unnecessary because claims of "energetic" phenomena are implicit in the assumptions of Chinese medicine and other non-Western systems of medicine. For this reason, attempts to construct reductionist arguments within Chinese medicine based on a methodology borrowed from Western science and conventional biomedical criteria are frequently construed as irrelevant. From the perspectives of some nonconventional systems of medicine, the use of established empirical methodologies to investigate or confirm material causes or effects is not a productive exercise. Thus much research into efficacy claims of non-Western modalities is initiated by Western-trained scientists who use conventional biomedical criteria to investigate putative biological effects of non-Western modalities, while overlooking claims of nonmaterial kinds of causes or effects on health and illness.

There Is a Philosophical Gap between Western Medicine and Nonconventional Systems of Medicine

Francis Bacon introduced the conceptual basis of modern science at the end of the 16th century in his seminal work *Novum Organon*. Bacon's ideas rapidly evolved into what is known as *scientific method*. Scientific method is a methodology that purports to provide skilled investigators with objective or value-neutral information based on observation and analysis of the properties of natural phenomena. However, Bacon's original thesis and its modern form continue to rest on important metaphysical assumptions that often go unstated (Boss, 1994):

> Every science is ... necessarily and always based on prescientific premises. These constitute a fundamental structure that not merely sets forth in advance which inquiries are possible and which are not, but furthermore determines the very character of the science and the extent to which its results will be significant. It sets the goals for the science and establishes the procedures guaranteeing correct practical application of theory. ...

By *prescientific,* Boss means that which comes conceptually before science, delimiting what kind of thing science is, and defining its legitimate operations and core philosophical principles. Prescientific premises are, by definition, metaphysical assertions because they cannot be substantiated by objective means. All methodologies employed in science and medicine ultimately rest on prescientific metaphysical assumptions pertaining to kinds of phenomena that can have existence, properties of phenomena that are knowable, and kinds of relationships that can take place between phenomena. It follows that no particular methodology stands alone or can be completely objective or value-neutral. The methodology embodied by contemporary Western science incorporates many prescientific premises, including the tacit acceptance of Cartesian dualism, the view that human nature is reducible to a physical part and a mental part. According to the dictum, the physical and biological scaffolding and the mental qualities of human beings are dual aspects of our nature that differ in fundamental ways. Neither quality cannot be reduced to or adequately described as properties of the other kind of thing. In the broader context of dualism, contemporary Western psychiatry poses an interesting and unresolved dilemma. On one hand, proponents of biological psychiatry claim to be nondualist. They argue that normal and abnormal "states" of mental functioning are reducible to known or knowable neurobiological mechanisms. On the other hand, proponents of various schools of psychoanalysis or psychotherapy rely on metaphysical assertions about ego, id, unconscious, subconscious, or other presumed primary functions of consciousness corresponding to normal or abnormal mental states, and claim that mental functions cannot be reduced to discrete neurobiological mechanisms. Contemporary psychoanalysis and most current psychological theories therefore rest on overtly dualist models whose assumptions are generally unstated or vaguely worded. In contrast, contemporary biological psychiatry and its parent, Western biomedicine, avoid ontological and epistemological problems inherent in dualism by claiming that all normal and abnormal mental functions are reducible to knowable (i.e., if not known presently) neurobiological processes. In fact, it will be seen below that Western medicine in general and biological psychiatry in particular rest on unstated metaphysical assumptions pointing to dualist paradigms that are empirically derived or consensus-based.

The very gradual evolution of conventional Western medicine and nonconventional systems of medicine toward increasing integration is related to the fact that diverse traditions of healing are based on nonoverlapping philosophical perspectives. The philosophical gap between conventional biomedicine and nonconventional systems of medicine is a reflection of different ways of seeing in disparate paradigms. Conventional biomedicine formulates clinical practices on the assumption that causes of illness are directly related to phenomena that are observable or measurable using established empirical methods. The assumption that phenomena are measurable in ways that reflect their intrinsic properties rests on the more basic assumption that useful and accurate information about the properties of reality can validly be obtained *only* for those phenomena that are observable according to criteria (or ways or knowing) that can be made explicit. The way of seeing that is implicit in contemporary Western science and conventional biomedicine rests on philosophical propositions about the nature of "real" phenomena that cannot be independently verified. This way of seeing is called materialism, and it asserts that everything is or can be explained in terms of matter. The materialist doctrine is a metaphysical point of view that had its roots in early Greek philosophy, was adapted by Descartes to dualism, and whose specific claims have continued to change over the centuries in response to widely held scientific theories of the day. The classical concept of matter as a fundamental building block of reality was severely shaken by the advent of general relativity theory, and subsequently, quantum mechanics, in the early 20th century. Popular materialist views now conceive of objects as a kind of "lumpy energy" according to the tenets of quantum mechanics theory. However, there is no single theory of quantum mechanics but only competing interpretations that have been neither confirmed nor refuted. Recent directions in theoretical physics point to multidimensional "strings" of space–time that may comprise the fundamental fabric of the universe while providing a unifying paradigm for the divergent worldviews of general relativity theory and quantum mechanics. Presently, no consensus exists in the scientific community on whether or by what technological means divergent theories in physics can be potentially verified or refuted. The limits of contemporary scientific understanding are therefore consistent with the philosophical perspective of relativism in that, according to this view, competing theories can be neither confirmed nor refuted. Important emerging paradigms in physics and biology, and their implications for the future of medicine, are discussed in Chapter 3.

In spite of the lack of empirical evidence supporting contemporary models of physical reality, biomedicine looks exclusively to physics for reasonable constraints on its own theories. Conventional biomedicine rests on the same metaphysical assumptions about the properties of "real" phenomena that are embedded in classical materialist views of the universe. For reasons discussed above, this philosophical position (which is close to naive realism) will probably continue to evade empirical confirmation or refutation for the foreseeable future. Biomedicine borrows assumptions about reality and a methodology for verifying or refuting the existence of phenomena related to putative mechanisms of action from a naive 19th-century version of materialism that was transformed by nonclassical physics almost a century ago. The belief in biomedicine that only certain kinds of things can have existence is an *ontological* assumption. The belief that only certain prescribed empirical methodologies can yield factual information about "real" phenomena is an *epistemological* assumption. Both metaphysical assumptions comprise an argument that is the basis of contemporary methodologies in Western science and biomedicine; however, the argument is circular and philosophically unsound.

The logic implicit in conventional scientific method asserts that only "real" phenomena can function as causative agents, and it is correct to regard phenomena as real only if their existence and properties are verifiable by means of empirical methods, but empirical methods are those methods that examine properties of phenomena that are presumed to be real because they are knowable according to accepted criteria by which phenomena can be real. We are left with the circularity that putative phenomena or their properties are observable and verifiable as real using a prescribed methodology that permits verification of certain kinds of phenomena only, but the application of this methodology is a necessary test for determining whether a phenomenon is real, or by exclusion, nonexistent. The argument is in the form of an infinite regress and cannot be logically resolved. Thus philosophical assumptions embedded in scientific method reflect widely shared, unquestioned, and unverifiable metaphysical views about the nature of phenomena.

The flawed philosophical arguments of the form of thought that comprises contemporary Western science and conventional biomedicine have not impeded its widespread acceptance because of economic and political factors that ensure the dominant position of science in developed countries. The methodology of contemporary Western science has led to the creation of profitable technologies that profoundly affect human existence at many levels. Because of the economic benefits of Western science, this approach will almost certainly continue to play an important role in the world. In spite of this it is important to remark that the widespread acceptance and dominant economic position of biomedicine and Western science in general do not remedy the awkward fact that contemporary scientific method rests on shaky philosophical ground.

There is No Proof in Medicine, Only Standards of Evidence Based on Philosophical Assumptions in the Parent System of Medicine

There is no proof in medicine, only tests of verification of claimed outcomes and standards of evidence supporting those claims. By the same token, there can be no certainty of a beneficial outcome when a particular treatment approach is used, only an estimate of the likelihood that a particular outcome will occur based on statistical analysis of previous trials examining the same approach. Depending on the system of medicine, the highest level of evidence for a claimed outcome is achieved when different criteria are fulfilled. Research evidence and anecdotal reports continue to accrue for particular treatment and assessment approaches; however, claims about outcomes can only be stated probabilistically. Evidence in medicine, as in all areas of science, is inherently probabilistic and open-ended. As more data emerge, the relative strength of evidence changes in a positive or negative way. Following the same general logic, there can be no refutation of a particular treatment (or assessment approach), but only greater or lesser probability that a claimed outcome will not take place.

In biomedicine, the most substantiated treatments fulfill unambiguous criteria for specific, replicable, and clinically significant outcomes when a specified assessment or treatment approach is used and the putative mechanism of action can be adequately described and empirically verified under tightly controlled conditions that are replicable by trained investigators working independently. These criteria are held up by Western science as objective empirical indicators of both mechanism and the presumed link between mechanism and outcomes (i.e., assessment accuracy or treatment effectiveness). Many poorly substantiated treatments, according to these criteria, demonstrably fail to meet these conditions yet frequently remain in use because of ongoing claims that they are effective in some cases. Provisional treatments fulfill some but not all criteria, and may emerge as substantiated or possibly effective approaches depending on future research findings. Equivalent statements can be made with respect to substantiated versus provisional assessment approaches. This picture is complicated by the fact that in Western science and other formal systems of thought, criteria for evidence sometimes change, requiring commensurate changes in both kinds and levels of evidence referred to in support of a claimed outcome. Understandings of evidence embraced in disparate systems of medicine will probably continue to be incompatible because of differences in metaphysical assumptions about the kinds of phenomena that are believed to constitute legitimate medical evidence.

This point bears on inherent differences between the relative importance of measurement in different systems of medicine because nonphysical phenomena regarded as fundamental in many nonconventional systems of medicine are not susceptible to empirical description or measurement, and thus, according to current Western science, cannot form the basis of "scientific" evidence supporting claims of outcomes. It follows that convincing evidence for a claimed mechanism of action or outcome of a particular assessment or treatment approach is generally not forthcoming; however, empirical information or consistent subjective accounts support claims of beneficial outcomes associated with many conventional and nonconventional approaches.

The above general considerations can be translated into a practical approach to thinking about integration that can help the practitioner address actual clinical problems. Conventionally trained physicians and many nonconventional medical practitioners are trained to "see" phenomena that are believed to point to illness or health. Phenomenal indicators of illness that are observable are described as objective signs of illness, and claims of nonobservable (i.e., within a particular system of medicine) illness-related phenomena are described as symptoms. Medical practitioners learn to see the same phenomena in the same way that expert teachers see them, according to an interpretive framework that is an explicit part of training. Medical practitioners in many traditions are instructed in methods that permit them to interpret patients' subjective complaints as clinically pertinent information about the conditions or cause(s) of illness. The practitioner's interpretation of the significance of signs and symptoms in the context of a particular system of medicine defines and limits the causes of illness that are regarded as possible or legitimate, and thus defines and limits kinds of treatments that can potentially address identified or inferred causes or meanings of symptoms. In sum, different ways of seeing and assigning significance to objective signs and interpreting subjective symptoms are built into disparate systems of medicine. In the context of a particular system of medicine, a student has progressed to the point of professional competence when he or she reliably sees the same signs, elicits the same symptoms, and proficiently interprets the significance of signs and symptoms using a methodology and clinical methods endorsed by an expert clinician of the same cloth.

Different metaphors of illness embedded in disparate systems of medicine are essentially different culturally determined "ways of seeing." A problem that must be addressed is how to know when one is describing a metaphor (or "picture") for apparent signs or a claimed symptom versus actual causes or conditions associated with signs or symptoms. I am assuming that in most cases this distinction will not be clear to the practitioner, as there are seldom means for verifying that assumptions about causes or conditions associated with illness phenomena correspond to the interpretation of observed phenomena (signs) or descriptions of subjective states (symptoms). If known, it can seldom be clearly described. For example, the serotonin hypothesis can be viewed as a contemporary biological metaphor for descriptions of certain affective symptoms. It provides a simple and convenient picture that frames conventional understandings of the biological roots of symptoms but has not been demonstrated as a sufficient explanation of symptom formation (see Chapter 3 for a more detailed discussion on this point). In the same way, the idea of qi is a metaphor that is convenient for the purposes of framing symptoms according to the assumptions of Chinese medicine, but this model can neither be confirmed nor refuted. Both metaphors are higher-order descriptions of metaphysical propositions about causes of symptoms. This issue becomes relevant when the epistemological limits of methodology in medicine are being addressed. In established systems of medicine, presumed relationships exist between metaphors used to describe symptoms and the actual biological, psychological, or energetic phenomena associated with illness. In some cases, a demonstration of the specificity or accuracy of a particular assessment approach or of the effectiveness of a particular treatment suggests that there is a degree of fit between a metaphor and the symptom pattern the metaphor describes. Productive metaphors are those that consistently result in specific, accurate assessment findings or beneficial outcomes and will presumably continue in use. Metaphors that do not yield useful or reliable information about the nature of illness phenomena are less widely embraced over time and are eventually discarded.

Disparate Systems of Medicine Rest on Different Metaphysical Assumptions

Most conventional and nonconventional medical approaches lack compelling evidence supporting the existence of a putative mechanism of action. Nevertheless, they remain in widespread use because of economic, social, and political factors.

The philosophical framework of contemporary Western science and conventional biomedicine asserts that putative causes of illness or improved health that cannot be empirically verified by established conventional methods may not be included in a valid explanatory model of illness and health. However, established nonconventional systems of medicine, including Chinese medicine, Ayurveda, Tibetan medicine, and Kampo, rest on assumptions about kinds of phenomena that are causes of illness and health that radically depart from those of Western biomedicine. For example, Chinese medicine, Ayurveda, and other non-Western systems of medicine posit the existence of an elemental energetic principle present in all living and nonliving systems. Qi, in Chinese medicine, and prana, in Ayurveda, cannot be directly observed or measured using conventional empirical methods, but only inferred when illness phenomena that have significance to a skilled practitioner point to "imbalances" in this energetic principle. Concepts like qi and prana differ radically from phenomenological views endorsed by conventional biomedicine. Ways of seeing and methods for verifying the existence or characteristics of phenomena endorsed by these non-Western systems of medicine rest on metaphysical assumptions that are incongruent with the philosophical foundations of conventional biomedicine. Assumptions about the nature of phenomena associated with illness or health embedded in both conventional and nonconventional systems of medicine are philosophically equivalent to claims about phenomena that can be "real," in other words, have independent existence. The same assumptions also function as implicit propositions about phenomena that cannot be "real" or cannot have independent existence. Ways of seeing employed in disparate systems of medicine represent different ways of interpreting the significance of phenomena believed to be associated (causally or otherwise) with illness or health. Disparate ways of interpreting phenomena necessarily rest on disparate assumptions about the existence or properties of phenomena and relationships between phenomena in space and time. Different ways of seeing or assigning significance to phenomena derive from, and result in, important ontological and epistemological differences between conventional biomedicine and nonconventional systems of medicine.

A consequence of the above analysis is that a philosophical framework unifying the basic metaphysical assumptions of biomedicine and nonconventional systems of medicine cannot be constructed. Thus there can be no universal methodology shared by all systems of medicine for identifying or qualifying the properties of phenomena associated with illness (assessment), or beneficial changes (treatment), or for

verifying putative causal relationships between effects of treatments and observable outcomes (treatment validation). In the absence of a unifying philosophical framework, an empirically derived methodology for constructing integrative strategies is conceivable and has practical utility.

Assumptions embedded in any system of thought, including all systems of medicine, ultimately stand alone as unverifiable propositions that rest on metaphysical assumptions or social conventions. Different assumptions constitute the philosophical framework of disparate systems of medicine. Assumptions underlying a particular system of medicine have internal coherence and explanatory power with respect to the analysis of causes of illness or health in the context of that system of medicine. However, it will always be the case that assumptions underlying any particular system of medicine are essentially metaphysical propositions about the nature of real phenomena and kinds of relationships that can operate between phenomena, including the nature of causality in illness and health. By definition, metaphysical assumptions embedded in any particular system of medicine cannot be independently verified as more or less true, but only shown to have greater or lesser degrees of internal coherence with respect to the system of thought of which they form a part. It follows that a valid philosophical argument cannot be made in favor of claims of greater or lesser legitimacy of any particular system of medicine with respect to any other system of medicine. What remains is analysis of assumptions embedded in disparate systems of medicine with the aim of clarifying differences between core ontological or epistemological propositions. This philosophical project is a necessary precursor to developing a methodology for constructing practical integrative assessment or treatment approaches when addressing symptoms in actual clinical settings.

From the above argument, it follows that I, a Westerner trained in the tradition of Western medicine, cannot adduce an objective methodology or value-neutral way of seeing that is outside the cultural and intellectual constraints in which I live and think. Further, because I am so constrained, any methodology I construct cannot objectively identify or compare the implicit assumptions in my perspective with those of Chinese medicine or other systems of medicine. Because I cannot stand in a place that is culturally or philosophically neutral, without biases or (conscious or unconscious) assumptions that affect how I think about existence, time, and the nature of causation, I can comment on differences between disparate systems of medicine and their respective methodologies, but I cannot legitimately claim that a particular way of seeing is better, more complete, more skillful, or somehow more effective than ways of seeing employed in other systems of medicine. In other words, I cannot make the a priori claim that the methodology of Western medicine *is superior* to the methodology of Chinese medicine or other non-Western systems of medicine (or vice versa). This is an argument for the legitimacy of relativism when considering two or more disparate systems of medicine. The detailed steps of this argument are summarized below.

1. The historical-philosophical framework of a system of medicine is always given.

2. I am a Westerner embedded in Western culture and trained in contemporary Western medicine.

3. To argue for a philosophical basis for a general methodology of integrative medicine, taking into account disparate

systems of medicine, I must go outside constraints, biases, and embedded assumptions of my culture (and training).

4. I am also constrained in the way I reason and in what I know. Because I cannot see these constraints from an objective perspective, I cannot know how my constraints compare with constraints of others who think about methodology in medicine from the perspectives of other cultural-philosophical contexts.

5. Therefore, my attempts to go outside my cultural or philosophical biases to establish a "neutral" perspective will likely be unsuccessful. I will probably not be able to discern where or how I am limited (because I cannot get completely outside my cultural and intellectual traditions and forms of life), and thus I cannot accurately discern the constraints that affect my way of thinking and seeing, nor can I compare those constraints with constraints of others.

6. Propositions 1–5 are true of anyone from any cultural-philosophical perspective who is attempting to solve this problem.

7. It follows that there can be no neutral approach to constructing or "getting to" a culturally-philosophically neutral methodology in medicine.

8. I am compelled to conclude that I (*anyone from any culture*) cannot formally adduce a completely objective or "neutral" methodology. Further, I (*anyone*) cannot know the limits of the methodology I adduce with respect to other existing or conceivable methodologies. Therefore, I (*anyone*) am not in a position to objectively compare the significance of differences between methodologies in disparate systems of medicine, and can only comment on properties or characteristics of observable differences.

Some Systems of Medicine Are More Open to Integration than Others

A particular system of medicine is open to integration with another system of medicine at a conceptual level to the extent that its core ontological and epistemological assumptions accommodate assumptions of the other system of medicine, or novel assumptions in one or both systems result in philosophical congruence between the respective systems of medicine. Openness to novel assumptions about the phenomenal nature of health and illness permits novel assessment and treatment approaches based on those assumptions. The criterion of being philosophically open to integration is thus the capacity of core propositions underlying a particular system of medicine to evolve. When core assumptions that define a particular system of medicine A have a logical structure that permits the derivation of novel assumptions, other systems of medicine are potential candidates for integration with system A in cases where there is philosophical congruence between core assumptions of the respective systems of medicine. The degree of congruence between core assumptions determines the potential for integration of two or more disparate systems of medicine at a conceptual level, and kinds of issues involved when considering integrating assessment or treatment approaches on a practical clinical level. The evolution of a particular system of medicine toward greater integration with theories or clinical methods of disparate systems of medicine is determined by general social, economic, and political issues, local factors affecting access to care, and patient preferences.

These kinds of issues ultimately determine the extent to which a potentially viable methodology of integrative medicine evolves into actual integrative medical practices. The increasing dialogue between conventional biomedicine and Chinese medicine in both Asia and industrialized Western countries and the related growth in cross-referrals between conventional biomedical practitioners and Chinese medical practitioners is an example of this evolutionary process.

◆ Philosophical Problems Related to Causality in Medicine

Assumptions about causality in a particular system of medicine determine how researchers and clinicians interpret phenomena related to illness and health. These assumptions determine possible meanings of assessment and treatment in a particular system of medicine. Practical clinical methods of assessment and treatment are constrained by metaphysical assumptions about the meaning of causality and kinds of causes that are believed to operate in illness and health.

It is important to address problems related to causality in medicine because of relationships between causality and evidence in research and outcomes assessment that determine valid research or clinical methodologies in disparate systems of medicine. For example, if a particular system of medicine assumes that treatments and outcomes co-occur but in ways that cannot be adequately described in terms of linear causality, a strict empirical methodology for verifying the existence of a putative direct causal relationship between treatment and outcome is not relevant to a demonstration of efficacy. For this reason conventional empirical methodologies are frequently not used to verify claims of treatment outcomes in systems of medicine where linear causality is not assumed to operate. Analytical methodologies for inferring causality have not been put forward by many nonconventional systems of medicine because such methodologies provide relevant information only in cases where linear causality is assumed to operate.

It is convenient to conceptualize three different models of causality that are implicit in disparate ways of understanding natural phenomena, including health and illness. The most widely accepted model describes classical understandings of linear causal relationships between two or more objects or events. This model can be stated as "If *A*, then *B*"; that is, a causal relationship between an event or factor *A* and an associated outcome *B* is inferred on the basis of their observed proximity in time or space. This model is widely embraced by practitioners of Western biomedicine. Another conceptual model is useful when examining relationships between co-occurring symptoms, treatments, or outcomes that are assumed to be related but for which simple linear causal relationships do not adequately describe observed phenomena. According to this model, complex nonlinear relationships are assumed to exist between objects or events that are not related in terms of simple causes and effects. Nonlinear relationships are the domain of complexity theory (sometimes called chaos theory). Complexity theory has been applied to basic research in biology—including neurobiology, chemistry, and physics—in efforts to model complex relationships in nature. A third way of conceptualizing relationships between symptoms, treatments, or outcomes assumes the absence of both linear and complex nonlinear causality. According to this model, two or more events co-occur because of the local properties of space–time, and it is unnecessary to assume a discrete causal connection between apparently discrete phenomena. This view is consistent with quantum mechanics and quantum field theory, and is being evaluated as an explanatory model of certain therapeutic approaches currently described as "energy medicine." When a beneficial change in a specified symptom is experienced in proximity to a particular intervention, one or more of the above models can generally be invoked to explain the kinds of relationships that exist between the reported change (i.e., outcome) and the putative action or effect of the intervention. This general observation can be applied to cases where two or more symptoms are experienced at the same time, and clinical observations or assessment findings can be used to infer that dysregulation at a common biological, energetic, or informational level is associated with the formation of both symptoms. Finally, when two or more symptoms occur together, the relationship between them can shift from one of linear or nonlinear causality and possibly to acausality, depending on changes in intrinsic and extrinsic factors that affect the causes or conditions associated with the respective symptoms.

Different assumptions implicit in disparate systems of medicine about the kinds of relationships that exist between two or more co-occurring symptoms bias the practitioner's approach to assessing, classifying, and treating illness in different ways. For example, when two or more symptoms are presumed to be related in a simple linear, causal way, they are typically interpreted as a single discrete symptom pattern, or disorder. In contrast, when two or more symptoms are presumed to be only weakly or indirectly related on the basis of postulated nonlinear relationships, or when they occur together but are presumed to not be causally related, the symptoms are generally regarded as independent entities, and not as parts of a complex symptom pattern or discrete disorder. In the latter cases, the meaning of evidence of efficacy with respect to verification of treatment outcomes differs substantially from conventional biomedical understandings of evidence. In sum, different assumptions about causality in disparate systems of medicine bias models of evidence, and subsequently influence conceptual methodologies and practical clinical methods used to verify the significance of treatment outcomes.

Assumptions about causality determine how relationships between illness and health phenomena are interpreted and bias understandings of evidence in different ways in disparate systems of medicine. The kind of evidence used to support beliefs that a particular clinical approach is based on verifiable claims of mechanism of action, or is effective, is related to assumptions of causality embedded in the system of medicine from which the clinical method is derived. In other words, the classification of medical approaches according to the verifiability of a putative mechanism of action or the claimed effectiveness of a particular treatment rests on implicit assumptions about evidence, and therefore causality, that are embedded within the parent system of medicine.

When direct linear causal links are assumed to exist between phenomena believed to be related to illness or health, formal methodologies are developed to identify and analyze those links. In systems of medicine where linear causal relationships are not assumed to exist or assumed to not exist, there is no perceived need to identify or examine possible links. Thus formal methodologies are not considered relevant and are typically not adduced. In cases of the first type, assessment entails

the use of clinical methods to verify links between discrete observable phenomena. Assessment is based on empirical methods that establish evidence of the existence of putative causal relationships between two or more phenomena. Phenomena are systematically "reduced" until primary causes are established. In this reductionist approach, categories of illness are defined on the basis of inferences about similar causal patterns of origin. In cases of the second type (i.e., where linear causality is not assumed), assessment uses empirical or intuitive methods that do not rely on assigning inferred causes, and there is no agreed-on reasonable need to establish causality. In systems of medicine where linear causality is not inferred, categories of illness are frequently defined on the basis of phenomenological similarities that do not rely on classical views of causality. In this case a conceptual model is used to match information obtained through assessment with a suitable treatment.

In conventional biomedicine a treatment approach is accepted as legitimate when there is consensus on a putative mechanism of action that influences phenomena in beneficial ways that are presumably the causes of illness. In this model, there is an empirically verifiable relationship between the mechanism of a treatment and the causes of the illness being treated. In contrast, where causality is not assumed to operate, the concept of treatment has more to do with intuitive or other nonrational ways of addressing phenomena believed to be associated with illness. In cases where classical linear causality is not assumed, directing treatment interventions at discrete causes of illness is not meaningful and is seldom done. The legitimacy of a particular treatment approach and practical considerations of treatment selection follow from the intuitions and beliefs of a medical practitioner who observes or experiences the distress or manifestations of illness of each patient as a unique set of circumstances in the context of his or her training. In other words, there can be no philosophically neutral methodology that "reduces" illness to objectifiable patterns of cause and effect. Thus, in contrast to conventional biomedicine, in many non-Western systems of medicine empirical methods are not used to identify a "standard" or "best" assessment or treatment approach with respect to a particular illness.

Diverse Approaches Are Used to Infer Causation in Medicine

Induction is the principle approach used in Western medicine and some non-Western systems of medicine to establish causality on the basis of empirical observations. Causal inference in contemporary Western science rests on induction, the process of formulating a presumed law of nature on the basis of repeated observation. The fallability of this methodology was made clear by David Hume's argument that causality cannot be established through repeated observation because the observer or experimenter is limited to the observation of successive events only, and is not able to observe links between separate events. Further, any observer (or experimenter) can observe only a finite number of events under a finite number of conditions, and therefore can never observe all events that potentially bear on a particular phenomenon for which a natural law is being formulated. It follows that all natural laws are inherently probabilistic and vary in relation to local conditions where observation or experimentation is taking place. Induction continues to be accepted as the legitimate basis of contemporary scientific method, including the empirical methodology used in Western biomedicine.

Another methodology for inferring causality that is widely used in science and biomedicine is expert consensus. This approach attempts to establish causal inference on the basis of shared opinions of acknowledged experts. The National Institutes of Health, the American Psychiatric Association, and other professional medical associations use this approach to develop consensus statements about clinical methods in medicine. Inferring causality from expert consensus is inherently limited by the fact that experts are frequently self-selected and have biased views. Objective tests of the merit or validity of consensus-based conclusions are seldom performed, and history shows that different expert consensus statements during any particular time period are often at wide variance, depending on the agenda of individuals who formulate them. Furthermore, clinical methods based on expert consensus generally undergo radical revision over short periods. For these reasons arguments for causality in medicine based on expert consensus are often flawed, incomplete, and unreliable.

◆ There Are Different Meanings of Evidence in Disparate Systems of Medicine

Evidence-based medicine has become a catchphrase in contemporary Western medicine. This term reflects a widely shared skepticism among conventionally trained physicians about the validity of nonconventional medical approaches on the assumption that conventional Western medical approaches are a priori legitimate because they are "evidence-based," whereas most nonconventional medical approaches presumably lack legitimacy because of the absence of good or adequate evidence.

Questions pertaining to evidence pose important philosophical and practical problems. A discussion of models of evidence reveals disparate ideological viewpoints about ways to obtain and validate information in different systems of medicine, and it soon becomes clear that a theory-neutral methodology for designating clinical information as "evidence" for claimed outcomes is not forthcoming.

Philosophical problems pertaining to evidence in medicine are related to the general problem of deriving a methodology for determining categories of existence (ontology) and establishing criteria for assigning phenomena to classes (epistemology). The problem of evidence in medicine is related to the problem of deriving a methodology for the classification and assessment of self-reported or observed phenomena as discrete symptom patterns. Disparate systems of medicine posit the existence of illness and health phenomena on the basis of different kinds of information, ranging from conventional physiological descriptions to theorized "subtle" energies. These important distinctions are implicit in the languages and conventions of disparate systems of medicine, and there is a presumption among both conventionally and nonconventionally trained practitioners that a symptom can be accurately discerned and its clinical significance correctly interpreted by a skilled practitioner. Practitioners trained in different medical traditions are generally not aware that they are trained to "see" symptoms in ways that a priori exclude certain kinds of information while selectively reifying and giving significance to

other kinds of information believed to imply the existence of different kinds of phenomena. Findings from medical anthropology research show that clinicians from all traditions "see" information about symptoms (i.e., identify significant clinical findings) and interpret those findings according to the constraints of their unique tradition and training. There can be no objective "seeing" and no unfettered "knowing" in science and medicine. Different ways of seeing and knowing are embodied by different philosophical assumptions about kinds of phenomena that can have existence and can be observed or measured.

Assumptions about kinds of phenomena that can have existence implicitly bias beliefs about information regarded as pertinent to establishing claims of existence. Assessment is the process of making inferences about the existence of phenomena ascribed to illness. In this process the clinician is trained to see and assign significance to certain kinds of information presumably reflecting categories of phenomena that are regarded as extant in the conceptual framework of a particular system of medicine. Kinds of information that are not believed to correspond to extant phenomena are a priori dismissed or explained in terms accepted in the interpretive model. Disparate systems of medicine thus regard different kinds of information as fundamental for establishing the existence and characteristics of phenomena putatively related to illness and health. A particular medical approach is regarded as legitimate in the context of a particular system of medicine when the existence and characteristics of a putative mechanism of action or claimed outcome are confirmed by specified kinds of information that are viewed as legitimate within that system. Thus validation of clinical methods in disparate systems of medicine entails the analysis of different kinds of information in the context of different presumed phenomenal worlds.

Established systems of medicine rest on methodologies that use observation, intuition, and technological approaches to obtain information believed to be pertinent to confirming the existence of phenomena that are described as signs or symptoms. Differences in the meaning of information implicit in disparate systems of medicine have resulted in divergent conceptual models of empirical or intuitive evidence with respect to the verification of claimed treatment effects. Differences in criteria used to define the content and quality of information in disparate systems of medicine translate into divergent meanings of evidence. Disparate meanings of evidence in different systems of medicine are thus embodied in divergent understandings of information implicit in different traditions.

Contemporary Western science posits that all natural phenomena, including factors associated with health and illness, can be explained on the basis of a few categories of irreducible entities and processes. Presumed fundamental entities and processes include certain properties of matter, certain kinds of energy, and certain relationships between matter and energy (see Chapter 3 for more discussion on this point). Western science a priori excludes other kinds of putative phenomena because claims of their existence are not consistent with these assumptions of the existence and operation of certain fundamental entities and processes. Examples of excluded phenomena include consciousness as a primary kind of process, putative forms of energy or information that do not operate within normal space–time, and the direct influence of human intention on illness and health. In other words, certain putative phenomena are rejected as fictions because contemporary Western science dictates that they simply "cannot exist."

Over centuries the categories of putative phenomena that are a priori excluded by Western science have changed commensurate with ongoing evolution in research methods and emerging empirical data. Western science is a dynamic, evolving paradigm that embraces novel theoretical models when technological means permit verification of the existence of putative phenomena during any given historical era. The result is that putative phenomena become "acceptable" or "legitimate" in Western science when contemporary technologies permit confirmation of their existence by empirical means. For medicine, the result has been changing requirements of a methodology for establishing relationships between observed or subjectively reported outcomes and phenomena associated with a putative mechanism of action. Kinds of information accepted as relevant or adequate evidence of links between changes in a symptom pattern and the occurrence of a particular treatment effect have changed in commensurate ways. This has resulted in a conceptual "gap" between conventional and nonconventional systems of medicine because disparate systems of medicine rest on different ontological assumptions about phenomena that can have existence and employ different practical methods for ascertaining cause–effect relationships between putative phenomena and treatment outcomes. A circularity ensues, as phenomena that are presumed to have existence bias understandings of information that can provide valid evidence for claims of existence, whereas the kind of information that is gathered reinforces beliefs about phenomenal categories of existence. In this way, unique systems of medicine become self-reinforcing sets of assumptions about phenomena and kinds of information that are valid indicators of illness and health. There can be no universal standards of evidence for verification of the existence, causes, or characteristics of a symptom pattern or its "response" to treatment because disparate systems of medicine contain fundamentally different assumptions about the nature of phenomenal reality.

◆ Philosophical Problems in Psychiatric Classification and Diagnosis

Considerable work has been done on philosophical problems in psychiatric classification, assessment, and diagnosis (Gupta & Kay, 2002b; Radden, 1994, 1996; Sadler & Agich, 1995; Sartorius, Jablensky, Regier, Burke, & Hirschfeld, 1990). The fourth edition of the *Diagnostic and Statistical Manual of Mental Disorders* (*DSM-IV*) contains the standard nosological methodology endorsed in most Western countries. The *DSM-IV* represents the efforts of research psychiatrists to derive a theory-neutral way of classifying symptoms into discrete syndromes or disorders on the basis of empirical findings and is revised when there are changes in expert consensus on evidence for new diagnostic categories or changes in existing ones.

An important premise of Western medical diagnosis is that identification of the cause of illness is required before a formal diagnosis can be established. From a philosophical perspective, psychiatric diagnosis is especially problematic due to the complexity of presumed causes of mental or emotional symptoms, and problems inherent in identifying, measuring, or verifying relationships between putative causes and reported symptoms. Biomedical psychiatry posits both biological and social causes of mental illness, including genetically mediated or acquired dysregulation of the brain's neurotransmitters and

neural circuitry, direct or indirect effects of medical illness or substance abuse, and stressful or abusive social or family circumstances. Causal links between cognitive, emotional, and behavioral symptoms and social factors or other extrinsic stressors can often be reasonably inferred; however, it is much more difficult to identify and verify causal relationships between putative intrinsic causes (e.g., genetics, neurotransmitters, and metabolic dysregulation) and the pathogenesis or progression of a particular symptom pattern. Western psychiatric diagnosis relies on self-reported descriptions of subjective cognitive or affective symptoms obtained from the clinical interview. The goal of conventional psychiatric assessment is to correlate subjective patient reports with objective data obtained from recent medical or neurological evaluations, functional brain scans, laboratory studies, and so on. This approach is undertaken on the belief that reasonable inferences about causality in mental illness can be made on the basis of apparent temporal correlations between subjective symptoms and certain "objective" medical findings. The prevailing view is that correct inferences will lead to accurate assessment of underlying causes and appropriate, effective treatment. An inherent limitation of the methodology used in conventional Western psychiatric assessment and diagnosis is the assumption that accepted kinds of biomedical information provide a sufficient explanatory model for classifying complex symptom patterns according to discrete identifiable causes. Not only is there no convincing scientific basis for this position, but there is overwhelming evidence for the contrary view (see Chapter 6 for more discussion on this point).

Diagnosis in contemporary biomedical psychiatry is based on the assumption that self-reported subjective states provide accurate and reliable information about causes of symptoms. In fact, hypothesized causes of self-reported cognitive, affective, or behavioral symptoms are seldom identified because contemporary technologies are frequently unable to verify the existence of presumed causal factors or direct or indirect relationships between identified factors and symptoms. This problem has resulted in the absence of rigorous empirical methods for verifying putative causal relationships between subjective cognitive, affective, or behavioral symptoms and hypothesized physiological or neuropharmacological mechanisms of action. Because of incomplete knowledge about the brain and body in the context of inherent limitations of technology, contemporary biomedical psychiatry lacks a methodology for verifying claims about the causes of symptoms. By extension (at present), there is no strong methodology for verifying putative mechanisms of action of biological treatments directed at assumed biological causes of symptoms.

An analogous argument can be put forward with respect to the nonverifiability of psychodynamic and psychoanalytic models in psychiatric assessment and diagnosis. An empirical methodology has not been advanced that is capable of testing putative relationships between discrete symptoms and claims made by theoretical models in self psychology or other psychodynamic schools. Well over 100 years after Sigmund Freud announced his proposal to develop a "scientific psychology," there is still no scientific theory about putative neurobiological substrates for constructs like "ego," "id," superego," and "subconscious." Thus contemporary biomedical psychiatry rests on hypotheses that are not potentially falsifiable using available research methodology and existing technologies. Subsequently, hypothesized "causes" of psychiatric symptom patterns can be neither verified nor refuted by current Western science. By the same token, empirical verification or refutation of putative effects of biological treatments is not forthcoming.

From the above discussion it is arguable that Western psychiatry in its present form is *not* scientific because it rests on a methodology and technologies that cannot verify the theories and factual claims on which it is constructed. Western psychiatry can be understood as an eclectic worldview that incorporates diverse psychological, social, and biological explanatory models, none of which is verifiable and many of which are not even testable using existing empirical methods. In contrast to diagnosis in Western psychiatry, diagnostic categories in biomedicine are generally based on observable signs or objective empirical data that point to verifiable discrete physiological, metabolic, or infectious "causes" of subjective distress associated with particular signs. Correspondences between hypothesized causes and physical symptoms associated with medical illnesses can often be verified or refuted using available technologies, and claims of putative effects of biological treatments of many medical disorders can also be readily verified or refuted by current Western science. Thus, in contrast to biomedical psychiatry, contemporary biomedical approaches to the diagnosis and treatment of medical disorders *are* highly scientific and reliable.

The conceptual divide between biomedicine and Western psychiatry has resulted in the relatively diminished status of psychiatry in the broader context of Western medicine in general. In response, academic proponents of Western psychiatry, with strong support from the drug industry, have attempted to emulate a methodology and theories that give psychiatry a more "science-like" appearance. The overwhelming emphasis in contemporary Western psychiatry is on psychopharmacological research, genetics, and brain-imaging studies, with the goal of finding a rigorous methodology for identifying and quantifying claimed correspondences between hypothesized causes and discrete cognitive, affective, or behavioral symptoms. To date, this approach has had limited success because of incomplete understandings of basic relationships between brain structures and mechanisms and the pathogenesis of psychiatric symptoms. Progress in the debate over the causes of mental illness has been slowed in turn by slow progress in the evolution of technologies capable of falsifying competing hypotheses about neurobiological substrates of normal and abnormal brain function. An artifact of biomedical psychiatry's drive to become "science-like" to achieve greater credibility in Western scientific communities is the dismissal of nonconventional approaches before their putative mechanisms of action are rigorously evaluated or claimed outcomes are objectively appraised. This ideological bias has delayed the examination and potential integration of many nonconventional approaches in mental health care for which there is already substantial empirical evidence of both effectiveness and safety.

Through progressive and closely spaced revisions of a formal classification scheme of psychiatric "disorders" (i.e., the *DSM-IV* and its equivalent, the *International Classification of Diseases* [*ICD-10*]), biomedical psychiatry tacitly admits an incomplete understanding of the nature of mental illness, and discloses that it does not yet possess the means to accurately characterize many factors that cause or affect the course of cognitive, emotional, and behavioral symptoms. On this point it is interesting that early versions of the *DSM* put forward psychodynamic arguments for mental and emotional disorders. Subsequent versions divided symptoms along so-called functional and organic lines on the presumption that some disorders are manifestations of strictly biological processes, whereas others emerge as a consequence of extrinsic social, personality, cultural, or other factors. That approach led to considerable confusion and debate over the boundaries between functional and organic causes of mental illness. In response, the authors of the most recent version (*DSM-IV* and *DSM-IV-Text Revision* [*DSM-IV-TR*]) have eliminated the organic-functional dichotomy, claiming a neutral or "atheoretical" stance, with the goal of avoiding problems inherent in interpreting ambiguous research findings as discrete diagnostic categories of disorders. Causes are not discussed in the language of the current *DSM,* and diagnosis relies almost exclusively on self-reported history and symptoms. In other words, contemporary biomedical psychiatry addresses problems of psychiatric classification by adopting a strictly descriptive stance in an attempt to circumvent philosophical and scientific questions about causes or meanings of symptoms that are not yet resolved.

DSM diagnostic criteria claim to be valid phenomenological categories describing discrete symptom patterns; however, in its present form, the *DSM* does not adequately address the problem of delineating causal relationships between disorders and intrinsic or extrinsic factors. The result is that some *DSM* diagnostic categories probably reliably correspond to discrete symptom patterns, whereas other categories are probably mere "labels" representing ideas of patterns that do not actually exist outside the academic literature. This fact is more than a curious footnote about the current status of Western psychiatry, as the use of labels representing presumed diagnostic entities for which there is expert consensus but little reliable empirical evidence has caused a muddle in contemporary psychiatric thought. The presumption of clear understanding when there is only ambiguity and debate over important issues of methodology and theory is delaying progress in basic research, confusing clinicians, and disenfranchising millions of patients who seek more complete understandings and more effective treatments of the causes or meanings of their symptoms.

◆ Toward a Typology of Medical Approaches

Diverse approaches are used to categorize medical practices, including grouping them according to similarities in mechanisms of action, shared target symptoms addressed, kinds or levels of evidence for a putative mechanism of action or a claimed outcome, and the level of professional or public acceptance of a particular approach ("Defining and Describing Complementary and Alternative Medicine," 1997; Turner, 1998). Classification of medical practices must also take into account different ways of seeing implicit in disparate systems of medicine and the dominance of particular systems of medicine in different world regions (Cassidy, 2002). Because it is possible to categorize medical approaches in different ways, conceptual and practical boundaries between different clinical methods are frequently ambiguous. The problem of categorizing medical practices according to a formal typology can be reduced to two tasks: identifying assessment or treatment approaches that have established mechanisms of action, and identifying approaches for which there is evidence of efficacy or effectiveness with respect to a particular symptom pattern.

For the purposes of this book, assessment and treatment approaches are classified according to demonstrated or presumed underlying mechanisms of action mediating those effects and the level of evidence supporting claims of outcomes.

Five logically distinct types of clinical approaches are used in mental health care:

1. Psychological—changing symptoms through psychotherapy
2. Biological—taking a substance with the goal of changing a presumed biological substrate of a symptom
3. Somatic and mind–body—manipulating or affecting the physical body or mind–body in a prescribed manner to yield generally beneficial effects
4. Uses of forms of energy or information that have been described or validated by current Western science, with the goal of changing general functions of the brain or body in beneficial ways
5. Uses of putative forms of energy or information that have not been validated by conventional Western science, with the goal of achieving generally beneficial changes

With the exception of the last category, the above general kinds of clinical approaches apply to both conventional and nonconventional assessment and treatment methods, and are generally viewed as corresponding to levels of evidence for claims that a putative underlying mechanism of action is present or that a particular assessment or treatment method is verified or verifiable. A putative mechanism of action can be regarded as a legitimate basis of a specified treatment from the perspectives of both conventional biomedicine and the parent nonconventional system of medicine, the parent nonconventional system of medicine only, or from neither perspective. The latter case applies to some conventional and nonconventional approaches that are presently in common use but for which there is no substantial evidence supporting a claimed mechanism of action or claimed outcomes. Nevertheless, many approaches for which there is no compelling empirical evidence remain in use because research findings or clinical observations suggest that beneficial outcomes take place, or they are regarded as effective out of widely shared beliefs in spite of the absence of apparent positive outcomes.

◆ Ontological Considerations that Determine Phenomena Underlying Illness

It is important to clarify differences between core philosophical propositions contained in disparate systems of medicine, because these differences translate into divergent understandings about kinds of subjective experiences (symptoms) that *can* have existence. Phenomena associated with health and illness that are believed to have existence comprise the ontological "givens" of every system of medicine. These propositions about conditions of existence place constraints on assessment methods that are regarded as potentially valid ways to detect or measure extant phenomena. Assessment approaches regarded as valid rest on methodologies for obtaining information that is believed to accurately reflect phenomena associated with illness according to the core propositions of a particular system of medicine. What is ontologically given by propositions implicit in a given system of medicine defines and delimits understandings about symptom patterns that

can have existence and, by extension, biases how practitioners observe, measure, and interpret clinical information. The ontological givens of a particular system of medicine implicitly constrain the kinds of phenomena that are *potentially* related to changes that manifest as illness or improved health. It is assumed that when a treatment is associated with beneficial changes in reported symptoms, a putative mechanism of action operates as described within a particular system of medicine. In sum, propositions that describe what kinds of phenomena can have existence define and limit the kinds of effects or outcomes those phenomena may have on health or illness when embodied as treatments. A treatment approach that is regarded as legitimate and effective in a particular system of medicine rests on the assumption that the phenomenal basis of the treatment is verifiable as a described mechanism of action, and desirable outcomes take place when the mechanism of action operates in a beneficial way on the causes of the symptom. Depending on the conceptual framework of the system of medicine, "desirable" outcomes are observable improvements or subjectively experienced benefits to a patient who receives a particular treatment.

◆ Empirically Derived versus Consensus-Based and Intuitive Approaches

Many conventional and nonconventional medical approaches in widespread use are not substantiated by strong empirical findings. Nonsubstantiated approaches are nevertheless widely used in biomedicine and many nonconventional systems of medicine. There are two kinds of nonempirically derived medical approaches: consensus-based and intuitive. This distinction is important when developing a taxonomy of assessment and treatment approaches based on different kinds and levels of evidence. A taxonomy of disparate approaches is necessary to construct a methodology for selecting integrative medical approaches. Some nonempirically derived approaches are accepted on the basis of expert consensus on a putative mechanism of action.

Consensus-based approaches continue in widespread use due to historical, social, political, and economic influences on public policy, science, and medicine. Medical approaches based on expert consensus frequently make claims of efficacy or effectiveness that lack compelling empirical evidence and argue that a treatment is effective on the basis of a putative mechanism of action in spite of the absence of compelling evidence supporting the existence of the claimed mechanism or strong evidence of relationships between claimed outcomes and treatment effects. Examples of consensus-based treatment approaches include many drugs in current use in conventional biomedicine and many protocols for acupuncture and other kinds of nonconventional treatments.

Similar to consensus-based approaches, intuitive conventional or nonconventional approaches also lack strong empirical evidence. Intuitive medical approaches rest on shared psychological, cultural, or spiritual beliefs only, and are derived from metaphysical assumptions about illness and health that are outside contemporary scientific understandings. Practitioners of intuitive medical approaches embrace a particular belief system and make no claims that mechanisms of action underlying intuitive approaches are comprehensible by or consistent with Western scientific theories or analytical methods. Examples of

Table 2–1 Kinds of True or False Claims Pertaining to Medical Approaches in All Systems of Medicine

Mechanism of Action Is Verified or Verifiable Using Contemporary Scientific Approaches	Replicable Positive Outcomes	Replicable Negative Outcomes
Yes	Mechanism verified	Mechanism verified
	Claims true	Claims refuted
No	Mechanism not verified	Mechanism not verified
	Claims true	Claims refuted

approaches that currently fall into the domain of intuitive clinical methods include energy medicine and prayer. Intuitive approaches do not depend on empirical verification; however, in some cases conventional research designs provide evidence of their effectiveness in terms of apparent beneficial outcomes. In the same way, there is emerging evidence for the effectiveness of some consensus-based treatment approaches in conventional medicine in spite of the absence of compelling evidence verifying a putative mechanism of action or relationships between observed positive outcomes and a particular treatment. Many intuitive and consensus-based approaches used in both conventional biomedicine and nonconventional systems of medicine are associated with clinical results that are both significant and replicable. Replicable assessment findings or beneficial treatment outcomes in empirically derived, consensus-based, and intuitive medical approaches suggest that divergent assumptions embedded in biomedicine and nonconventional systems of medicine have validity. **Table 2–1** provides a framework for thinking about relationships between the verifiability of a putative mechanism of action for any medical approach and the truth of its claims.

Using contemporary research methods, the truth of a particular claim can be evaluated on the basis of two general kinds of criteria: replicable accurate assessment findings or positive outcomes with respect to a specified symptom, and the verifiability of a putative mechanism of action underlying a specified assessment or treatment approach. On this basis, it can be seen that two kinds of true claims and two kinds of false claims exist for the universe of conventional or nonconventional medical approaches. In cases where a putative mechanism of action can be confirmed to exist and verified to be correlated with desirable outcomes of a specified assessment or treatment approach, two kinds of true claims are possible: a putative mechanism of action is verified (or verifiable) and claims of assessment accuracy or treatment effectiveness are true based on replicable positive outcomes; and a putative mechanism is not verified (or verifiable), but claims are nevertheless supported by replicable positive outcomes. Likewise, two kinds of false claims are possible with respect to approaches for which a putative mechanism of action is verified (or verifiable) using conventional Western research methods: a putative mechanism is verified, but claims of assessment accuracy or treatment effectiveness are false on the basis of replicable negative outcomes; and a putative mechanism is not verified (or verifiable), and replicable negative outcomes show that the claim is false. By definition, when a putative mechanism of action is not susceptible to empirical verification, there can be no cases of particular assessment or treatment

approaches in which true or false claims rest on a verified or refuted mechanism of action, respectively.

Science evolves as changes in theory, methodology, or novel technologies permit verification of claims of mechanisms of action or effectiveness that were heretofore not susceptible to empirical verification. On this basis it is reasonable to expect that some approaches currently not regarded as verified or verifiable will be viewed as verified or verifiable in the future. Another way to express this is that some medical approaches that are currently regarded as resting on metaphysical assumptions will be verified or verifiable, whereas others will be refuted or able to be refuted based on emerging theories, novel methodologies, and future kinds of evidence.

◆ Making Judgments about Conventional and Nonconventional Medical Approaches

It is instructive to compare conventional biomedical approaches and nonconventional modalities for which claims of assessment accuracy or treatment effectiveness are true, but which rest on putative mechanisms of action that cannot be verified using the empirical methodology of current Western science. In the absence of a verifiable mechanism of action, both claims have equivalent truth value because in both cases replicable positive outcomes fulfill criteria for empirical verification that a particular approach is associated with a claimed outcome. Thus conventional and nonconventional approaches that rest on putative mechanisms of action that cannot be verified by current Western science are equivalent with respect to the kind of evidence supporting their use, assuming that claims of assessment accuracy or treatment outcomes are verified to the same degree. It is reasonable to regard conventional and nonconventional approaches for which there is an equivalent kind of evidence as equally legitimate candidates for a future integrative medicine. The claims of some conventional and nonconventional medical approaches are false because claims of effectiveness are contradicted by consistently negative outcomes, but they cannot presently be categorically refuted because a demonstration of the absence of a putative underlying mechanism of action is not forthcoming using available conventional means. The logical position of such claims can be contrasted with false claims made with respect to conventional or nonconventional clinical practices that rest on empirically verified or verifiable mechanisms of action but for which claims of effectiveness are contradicted by consistent negative outcomes. In contrast to most contemporary biomedical approaches, the assumptions on which some nonconventional approaches are based are not falsifiable using the methodology of current Western science. Because of category differences between truth claims of conventional and nonconventional medical approaches, demonstrations of the truth or falsity of claimed outcomes are necessarily undertaken in different ways.

With respect to conventional medical approaches, false claims are perspicuously false through verification of the absence of a claimed mechanism of action or a claimed outcome. In contrast, truth claims of many nonconventional approaches are not potentially verifiable using contemporary research methods are used to verify a putative mechanism of action. Because it is not possible to make judgments about the verifiability of many nonconventional approaches in Western science using contemporary research methods, the evaluation of clinical evidence supporting claims of assessment accuracy or treatment effectiveness must provide the sole basis for ascertaining the relative degree to which claims are true or false. In other words, the problem shifts from determining the kind of evidence supporting claimed outcomes to estimating relative levels of evidence corresponding to claimed outcomes of disparate assessment or treatment approaches.

From the above argument it follows that claims of empirically derived approaches can be falsified on the basis of empirical demonstrations of the absence of a putative mechanism of action or replicable negative findings of claimed outcomes. In contrast, claims of positive outcomes for intuitive approaches can be proved false, but claims that intuitive approaches work can never be categorically refuted because a demonstration of the nonexistence of a putative mechanism of action is not potentially forthcoming for intuitive practices using methodologies and technologies available in current Western science. An example of the former kind is the use of a bioassay to demonstrate that a claimed mechanism of action of an herbal medicine does not take place, thus empirically falsifying the claim. An example of the latter kind is the demonstration of the ineffectiveness of Healing Touch to treat a particular symptom pattern on the basis of consistently negative outcomes. In the latter case a claim of effectiveness of a particular clinical application of Healing Touch can be refuted empirically because of consistent negative outcomes; however, the general approach of Healing Touch cannot be refuted because current empirical means cannot potentially falsify or verify the postulated mechanism of action associated with this form of "energy" healing.

In sum, an important distinction exists between methodologies used to verify claims made for a particular conventional or nonconventional approach depending on whether the approach is empirically derived, consensus-based, or intuitive. True claims of effectiveness can be made for empirically derived and some consensus-based conventional or nonconventional approaches, and in some cases putative mechanisms of action can be empirically verified. In contrast, claims of effectiveness for intuitive approaches can be made irrespective of the absence of information about putative mechanisms of action, and refutation of these approaches is not possible using the methodologies and technologies of current Western science.

Ongoing advances in science will result in novel models of complex nonliving and living systems, including new understandings of relationships between immune functioning and mental health, and the biological and putative energetic nature of human consciousness. Continued basic research in physics and the life sciences will influence the ideas, methodology, and clinical methods of Western medicine and established systems of nonconventional medicine. Historically, significant progress in biomedicine has occurred following the emergence of new ideas in science. It is reasonable to assume that future advances in the basic sciences will continue to shape the perspectives of Western medicine in the same way. Technologies that emerge from future theories of energy, information, space, time, causality, and consciousness will result in methodologies that embody novel ways to observe and measure phenomena related to illness and health. Future methodologies in Western science will permit the empirical verification or refutation of some approaches that are currently regarded as intuitive healing methods.

Similarly, it will become possible to strongly verify certain empirically derived approaches by demonstrating the existence of a putative mechanism of action or observing claimed outcomes using novel technologies. Future technologies will permit broader understandings of biological, energetic, informational, and possibly also spiritual processes associated with both conventional and nonconventional modalities. Claims that are regarded as legitimate will change in the context of evolving theories, methodologies, and technologies, and these claims will shape the future evolution of Western science and medicine. This process will result in a continuous flux in both kinds and levels of evidence supporting uses of particular assessment or treatment approaches with respect to a specified symptom pattern. Approaches used to assess or treat a particular symptom pattern will evolve on a continuous basis in the context of changes in methodology, theory, and research methods that will translate into novel findings pertaining to claims of mechanism or effectiveness.

I have argued that important differences exist between kinds of claims that can be made in support of conventional and nonconventional medical approaches. This criterion can be used to define a basic operational difference between conventional and nonconventional approaches during any particular historical period. I have shown that conventional and nonconventional approaches are equivalent in terms of verifiability in cases where a putative mechanism of action cannot be verified but replicable positive outcomes are reported. This argument reframes the broad philosophical problem of evidence in medicine as the *problem of deriving a methodology for determining criteria that can be used to verify assessment specificity or treatment effectiveness supporting claims of outcomes associated with a particular approach.* This general statement translates into the practical problem of finding a rigorous methodology for defining kinds or levels of evidence that are sufficient to verify or refute a specific claim with respect to a particular assessment or treatment approach. The problem reduces further to establishing criteria for assigning kinds and levels of evidence to particular clinical approaches even in cases where there are no current means for verifying a putative mechanism of action. This leads back to the basic considerations of evidence addressed above. Criteria that define the "logical space" occupied by disparate clinical medical approaches provide a basis for deriving a methodology for formulating a taxonomy that includes both conventional and nonconventional approaches.

◆ From Ontology to Nosology

I have argued that the conceptual basis of integrative medicine cannot be derived from analysis of core assumptions, because disparate systems of medicine ultimately rest on irreducible metaphysical propositions about space, time, causality, and the nature of phenomenal reality. We are thus limited to certain kinds of *observable* phenomena and *measurable* outcomes associated with particular assessment and treatment approaches used in disparate systems of medicine. In view of this constraint, two basic approaches to assessment and treatment planning are possible: empirical methods are derived on the basis of observable phenomena, whereas intuitive methods are established on the basis of nonempirical means. Empirically derived methods rest on methodologies that require empirically testable observations of phenomena or empirical confirmation of putative relationships between phenomena. Disparate systems of medicine use different kinds of empirical methodologies to demonstrate claims of the accuracy or specificity of a particular assessment technique or claims of the effectiveness of a particular treatment. Empirical methodologies employed by a particular system of medicine are the basis for inferring cause-and-effect relationships between phenomena associated with illness or health in relation to the assumptions of that system. The dominant empirical methodology in Western culture is described as *scientific method*—the cornerstone of contemporary biomedicine.

The application of scientific method to the analysis of symptom patterns has led to the establishment of an explanatory theory of the causes and characteristics of illness and health that implicitly defines an ontology of symptom patterns, or a set of possible categories of pathology that can have existence according to the theory. The ontology of possible disease entities is translated into a nosology, or schema, for the classification of diagnostic categories of actual diseases, according to tenets of Western medical theory that are popular during any particular historical period. Diagnostic categories regarded as legitimate evolve in relation to changes in medical theory about possible causes and characteristics of illness. The same evolutionary process determines conceptual changes that take place in nonconventional systems of medicine according to constraints defined by the cultural contexts and intellectual traditions in which those systems of medicine originated. A review of the recent history of science illustrates that core tenets of Western scientific method are in a state of continuous evolution in response to emerging research findings and also in reaction to political, social, and economic factors. In the same way, core tenets of established nonconventional systems of medicine continue to change in response to research findings and general cultural, political, and economic factors. In biomedicine there is no constant methodology per se, but a mélange of conventions for "doing science" that are generally derived on empirical grounds but are sometimes formulated on the basis of expert consensus in the absence of compelling empirical evidence. The same is true of many nonconventional systems of medicine. The result is that understandings of legitimate categories of illness undergo continuous gradual and sometimes dramatic shifts in relation to emerging research methodologies or technologies.

Biomedicine and Western medicine in general consist of both empirically derived approaches and nonsubstantiated consensus-based approaches that are subject to continuous change in the context of fluid social and political circumstances. Certain disease entities in contemporary biomedical nosology are empirically substantiated, whereas others are based on expert consensus and largely untested assumptions about putative mechanisms of action. Disparate empirically derived or intuitive approaches comprise the corpus of medical practices in diverse cultures. This fact has led to differences in basic understandings of the causes or meanings of illness in disparate systems of medicine. The result has been that illnesses regarded as legitimate diagnostic entities within a particular system of medicine are frequently at odds with diagnostic categories that are accepted in other systems of medicine. Conventionally trained physicians regard empirically derived or intuitive approaches employed by nonconventional practitioners as nonscientific or not strictly scientific, in the sense that they do not conform to standards of contemporary Western science. This view has often led to the dismissal

of diagnostic categories in nonconventional systems of medicine before their empirical foundations are examined. Clearly some established nonconventional systems of medicine employ empirical methodologies that are comparable in internal coherence or methodological rigor to the analytic methodologies of biomedicine. On this basis there are important conceptual similarities between nosologies derived from disparate core tenets of biomedicine and established nonconventional systems of medicine. Diagnostic entities regarded as valid in Western biomedicine are not inherently more or less valid compared with nosologies of established nonconventional systems of medicine.

◆ "Optimum" Integrative Approaches

Within the limits imposed by medical technology, economics, and availability of qualified practitioners, there will presumably be an optimum integrative assessment or treatment strategy with respect to a particular symptom pattern. Assumptions that form the basis of a particular integrative approach rest on core propositions of the system of medicine in which a symptom pattern is viewed. Philosophical, technological, and cultural constraints determine the optimum "shape" of a particular integrative medical approach.

The integrative assessment or treatment approach that is optimum with respect to a particular symptom pattern depends strongly on the historical period, the geographic region, and the technological and cultural milieu. Developing an optimum integrative strategy is driven by accumulating research evidence and changing standards of evidence. When integrative medical approaches are constructed from methodologies and clinical methods used in two or more disparate systems of medicine, the size of the conceptual gap between those approaches will vary in relation to the respective parent systems of medicine in the context of economic, political, and social factors. During any given historical period, there will be an expectable gap between any two or more optimum integrative medical approaches with respect to a specified symptom pattern. Expectable "dynamic patterns" of differences between two optimum integrative approaches will emerge over long periods of time. Differences between integrative medical practices that are regarded as optimum in two or more disparate systems of medicine will thus depend on differences between the parent systems of medicine from which they are derived in the context of technological, economic, and cultural factors driving change in the systems.

Optimum integrative medical approaches will be more or less congruent with each other at the level of core propositions depending on the influences of historical, intellectual, economic, and cultural variables that shape medical practices into integrative medical approaches. Optimum integrative medical approaches evolve on a continuous basis; however, economic and cultural factors will sometimes result in widespread agreement about particular integrative approaches that become regarded as "standard" clinical methods with respect to assessment or treatment of a specified symptom pattern. For these reasons basic philosophical and scientific considerations will probably continue to play a relatively minor role in shaping the evolution of many integrative medical approaches, and variations in already established integrative approaches will probably define the future course of integrative medicine for decades to come. Two examples of change in practical integrative medical approaches that are being driven by real-world considerations include the persistence of Chinese medicine as the dominant system of medicine in most Asian cultures, and the persistence of biomedicine as the dominant system of medicine in Western Europe and North America. Both trends continue in spite of compelling technological and economic arguments in favor of using clinical methods from other systems of medicine that would probably result in increased assessment accuracy or improved outcomes if used in conjunction with established methods from either system of medicine.

A physician or other professional medical practitioner can construct an optimum integrative strategy only from the perspective of the system of medicine in which he or she is trained. Thus integrative strategies will continue to be inherently limited regardless of the conceptual framework in which they are introduced. Furthermore, it will always be true that inherent conceptual, technological, and cultural constraints on efforts to establish integrative approaches will depend on the parent system of medicine in which integration is taking place. These issues are related to the problem of defining criteria for determining practical optimum integrative medical approaches addressing a particular symptom pattern. Methodological differences predetermine criteria that are regarded as legitimate to use when practical clinical decisions are made to include or exclude a particular approach. These differences reflect different core philosophical assumptions embedded in disparate systems of medicine. Different metaphysical assumptions pertaining to the phenomenal nature of illness and health translate into different criteria for inclusion of particular assessment or treatment approaches as legitimate means for the assessment or treatment of putative causes of a particular symptom pattern. Rigorous attempts to derive integrative medical approaches in disparate systems of medicine will therefore frequently yield nonoverlapping strategies because of disparate assumptions about putative phenomena that *can* have existence and how legitimate kinds of information can be obtained about phenomena. In other words, disparate systems of medicine employ different conceptual and practical methods to verify claims of the existence of phenomena related to illness or improved health.

Measuring phenomena related to health, illness, or responses to treatment rests on assumptions about the kinds of phenomena that are knowable and how the existence of putative phenomena and their relationships with illness or health can be verified. Nonoverlapping epistemological methodologies provide the basis for assessment approaches in disparate systems of medicine. As argued above, agreement on a "final" optimum integrative approach with respect to any particular symptom pattern will not be forthcoming because of differences in assumptions embedded in disparate systems of medicine. However, it is possible to reconcile incongruent ontological or epistemological assumptions that inevitably occur when assessment or treatment approaches from disparate systems of medicine are combined. One method for doing so is to derive optimum integrative medical approaches on the basis of consensus within academic communities in different parts of the world. For example, expert practitioners in disparate systems of medicine could collaborate to develop consensus statements about "best case" integrative approaches for a particular symptom pattern. A drawback of this approach is that it is based on considerations of theory and research only, reflecting the biases of self-selected experts,

and would probably overlook or minimize the importance of practical economic and cultural considerations in integrative treatment planning. This would limit the potential utility of integrative treatment recommendations to cases in which constraints can be readily overcome. At the other extreme, technological, economic, and cultural considerations could provide the sole or chief basis for determining optimum realistic integrative approaches. In this real-world model, academic research would hold considerably less importance, and in some cases would not be considered relevant. A middle approach to developing sound realistic integrative strategies is grounded in practical, real-world considerations while acknowledging the importance of formal academic research. I believe this is the most reasonable and realistic way to think about integrative medicine, and arguments for this approach are developed in Chapter 4.

◆ Where to Go from Here: Paradigms and a Conceptual Framework for Developing a Methodology in Integrative Medicine

Asking philosophical questions about evidence, causality, and the phenomenal nature of illness ensures that a rigorous methodology will be developed to interpret relevant observations or subjective reports of symptoms. For example, can the hermeneutic methodologies of sociology or anthropology be rigorously applied to psychiatry? How relevant are the discursive approximations of hermeneutics to the verification of a claim in medicine? Do methodologies used in hermeneutics provide an accurate description of what actually takes place in medical discourse, including especially biomedical psychiatry? Biomedical psychiatry is a hybrid discipline employing empirical analysis, hermeneutics, and other science-like methodologies. Nonconventional systems of medicine rely more or less on both rational nonempirical methodologies, such as hermeneutics, and strict empirical methodologies for showing causal inference. There is no clear demarcation between the philosophical positions of the eclectic methodologies employed in biomedicine and various nonconventional systems of medicine. Both conventional biomedicine and nonconventional systems of medicine make use of similar empirical and nonempirical methodologies. There are no theory-neutral methodologies in Western medicine and nonconventional systems of medicine. Clinical approaches in biomedicine and nonconventional systems of medicine reflect shared beliefs about the utility of both rational, objective methodologies and nonrational, subjective methodologies for obtaining useful clinical information about health and illness. To different degrees all systems of medicine employ methodologies based on intuition, evidence, and expert consensus in the context of the disparate paradigms in which they operate. The practical advantages and widespread uses of both rational, objective and nonrational, subjective methodologies in medicine argue for the development of a methodology in integrative medicine that acknowledges the limitations of both approaches while incorporating their respective advantages.

Questions examined in sociology, anthropology, and other disciplines are similar to conceptual problems that must be addressed in integrative medicine in general, and integrative mental health care in particular. In this chapter I have argued that disparate systems of medicine rest on different assumptions about the nature, causes, and meanings of cognitive, emotional, and behavioral symptoms, and kinds of possible relationships between symptoms and social, cultural, biological, energetic, informational, and possibly also spiritual factors. Before addressing issues pertaining to the development of methodologies in integrative medicine, it is necessary to consider implications of divergent conceptual frameworks, or paradigms, in medicine. Paradigms constructed from coherent sets of assumptions form the basis of all systems of thought, including Western biomedicine and other established systems of medicine. Finding a suitable conceptual framework for thinking about integrative medicine will lead to a methodology for constructing practical integrative strategies. Methodologies for deriving legitimate treatment and assessment approaches in all systems of medicine are inherently limited and biased to the extent that their respective paradigms rest on assumptions about the nature of phenomena related to illness or health. Assessment and treatment approaches thus reflect core assumptions embodied in the parent system of medicine. Every system of medicine rests on assumptions about subjec-

tive experiences or observable phenomena associated with normal functioning (health) or abnormal functioning (illness). Clinical judgments about the operation of a putative mechanism of action, the accuracy of a particular assessment approach, or the effectiveness of a particular treatment are necessarily made within the paradigm in which the approach is examined. Assumptions embedded in a particular system of medicine and methodologies based on those assumptions bias judgments about practical assessment and treatment methods that are regarded as reasonable. By extension, core assumptions of integrative medicine and a methodology based on those assumptions bias judgments about legitimate combinations of disparate assessment or treatment approaches. Chapter 3 examines paradigms in science and medicine and their implications for emerging methodologies and clinical methods in a future integrative mental health care. Chapter 4 develops general methodologies in integrative medicine in the context of important philosophical and practical issues. Methodologies for planning integrative assessment strategies and integrative treatment strategies in mental health care, respectively, are developed in Chapters 4 and 5.

References

Boss, M. (1994). *Existential foundations of medicine and psychology*. Northvale, NJ: Jason Aronson.

Cassidy, C. M. (2002). Commentary on terminology and therapeutic principles: Challenges in classifying complementary and alternative medicine practices. *Journal of Alternative and Complementary Medicine, 8*(6), 893–895.

Defining and describing complementary and alternative medicine. (1997). *Alternative Therapies in Health and Medicine, 3*(2), 49–57.

Gupta, M., & Kay, R. (2002b). The impact of "phenomenology" on North American psychiatric assessment. *Journal of Philosophy, Psychiatry, and Psychology, 9*(1), 73–85.

Radden, J. (1994). Recent criticism of psychiatric nosology. *Journal of Philosophy, Psychiatry, and Psychology, 1*(3), 193–200.

Radden, J. (1996). Lumps and bumps: Kantian faculty psychology, phrenology, and twentieth-century psychiatric classification. *3*(1), 1–14.

Sadler, JZ. (1953). Epistemic value commitments in the debate over categorical vs. dimensional personality diagnosis. *Philosophy, Psychiatry, & Psychology, 3*, 203–222.

Sartorius, N., Jablensky, A., Regier, D., Burke, J., & Hirschfeld, R. (1990). *Sources and traditions of classification in psychiatry*. New York: Hogrefe & Huber.

General References

Achinstein, P. (2001). *The book of evidence*. Oxford: Oxford University Press. SR

Adler, M. (1985). *Ten philosophical mistakes: Basic errors in modern thought—how they came about, their consequences, and how to avoid them*. New York: Macmillan.

Ali, M. (2003). *The principles of integrative medicine: Vol. 2. The history and philosophy of integrative medicine*. New York: Canary Press.

Almeder, R. (1996). *Harmless naturalism: The limits of science and the nature of philosophy*. Chicago: Open Court.

Baggini, J., & Fosl, P. (2003). *The philosopher's toolkit: A compendium of philosophical concepts and methods*. Oxford: Blackwell.

Beakley, B., & Ludlow, P. (Eds.). (1992). *The philosophy of mind: Classical problems, contemporary issues*. Cambridge, MA: MIT Press.

Benesch, W. (1997). *An introduction to comparative philosophy: A travel guide to philosophical space*. New York: St. Martin's Press.

Bernstein, R. (1983). *Beyond objectivism and relativism: Science, hermeneutics, and praxis*. Philadelphia: University of Pennsylvania Press.

Beutler, L., & Malik, M. (Eds.). (2002). *Rethinking the DSM: A psychological perspective*. Washington, DC: American Psychological Association.

Bolton, D., & Hill, J. (2003). *Mind, meaning, and mental disorder: The nature of causal explanation in psychology and psychiatry* (2nd ed.). Oxford: Oxford University Press.

BonJour, L. (2002). *Epistemology, classic problems and contemporary responses*. Lanham, MD: Rowman & Littlefield.

Bunge, M. (1979). *Causality and modern science*. New York: Dover Publications.

Carnap, R. (1995). *An introduction to the philosophy of science*. New York: Dover Publications.

Clark, P., & Hawley, K. (Eds.). (2003). *Philosophy of science today*. Oxford: Clarendon Press.

Danto, A. (1997). *Connections to the world: The basic concepts of philosophy*. Berkeley: University of California Press.

Gadamer, H. (1996). *The enigma of health: The art of healing in a scientific age*. Stanford, CA: Stanford University Press.

Goldstein, M., & Goldstein, I. (1979). *How we know: An exploration of the scientific process*. New York: Da Capo Press.

Gower, B. (1997). *Scientific method: An historical and philosophical introduction*. New York: Routledge.

Gupta, M., & Kay, L. (2002a). Phenomenological methods in psychiatry: A necessary first step. *Journal of Philosophy, Psychiatry, and Psychology, 9*(1), 93–96.

Horgan, J. (1996). *The end of science: Facing the limits of knowledge in the twilight of the scientific age*. New York: Broadway Books.

Hundert, E. (1990). *Philosophy, psychiatry and neuroscience—three approaches to the mind: A synthetic analysis of the varieties of human experience*. Oxford: Clarendon Press.

Kleinman, A. (1981). *Patients and healers in the context of culture*. Berkeley: University of California Press.

Kuhn. (1962). *The Structure of scientific revolutions*. Chicago: University of Chicago Press.

Ladyman, J. (2002). *Understanding philosophy of science*. New York: Routledge.

Laudan, L. (1996). *Beyond positivism and relativism: Theory, method and evidence*. Boulder, CO: Westview Press.

Losee, J. (2001). *A historical introduction to the philosophy of science* (4th ed.). Oxford: Oxford University Press.

McGinn, C. (2000). *Logical properties: Identity, existence, predication, necessity, truth*. Oxford: Clarendon Press.

McGinn, C. (2002). *Knowledge and reality: Selected essays*. Oxford: Clarendon Press.

McHugh, P., & Slavney, P. (1998). *The perspectives of psychiatry* (2nd ed.). Baltimore: Johns Hopkins University Press.

McMillan, J. (2002). Jaspers and defining phenomenology. *Journal of Philosophy, Psychiatry, and Psychology, 9*(1), 91–92,

Meynell, H. (1998). *Redirecting philosophy: Reflections on the nature of knowledge from Plato to Lonergan.* Toronto: University of Toronto Press.

Morley, J. (2002). Phenomenological and biological psychiatry: Complementary or mutual? *Journal of Philosophy, Psychiatry, and Psychology, 9*(1), 87–90.

Murphy, E. (1997). *The logic of medicine.* Baltimore: Johns Hopkins University Press.

Radden, J. (Ed.). (2004). *The philosophy of psychiatry: A companion.* Oxford: Oxford University Press.

Rescher, N. (1999). *The limits of science.* Pittsburgh, PA: University of Pittsburgh Press.

Rosenberg, A. (2000). *Philosophy of science: A contemporary introduction.* New York: Routledge.

Rothman, K. (Ed.). (1988). *Causal inference.* Chestnut Hill, MA: Epidemiology Resources.

Rouse, J. (1996). *Engaging science: How to understand its practices philosophically.* Ithaca, NY, and London: Cornell University Press.

Rubik, B. (1996). Some limitations of the scientific epistemology and paradigm for alternative medical research. In *Life at the edge of science.* Oakland, CA: Institute for Frontier Science.

Sadler, J., & Agich, G. (1995). Diseases, functions, values, and psychiatric classification. *Journal of Philosophy, Psychiatry, and Psychology, 2*(3), 219–231.

Sadler, J., Wiggins, O., & Schwartz, M. (Eds.). *Philosophical perspectives on psychiatric diagnostic classification.* Baltimore: Johns Hopkins University Press.

Salmon, W. (1998). *Causality and explanation.* New York: Oxford University Press.

Taper, M., & Lele, S. (Eds.). (2004). *The nature of scientific evidence: Statistical, philosophical, and empirical considerations.* Chicago: University of Chicago Press.

Turner, R. N. (1998). A proposal for classifying complementary therapies. *Complementary Therapies in Medicine, 6,* 141–143.

Weinsheimer, J. (1985). *Gadamer's hermeneutics. A reading of Truth and Method.* New Haven, CT: Yale University Press.

Zachar, P. (2000). Psychological concepts and biological psychiatry: A philosophical analysis. In M. Stamenov (Ed.), *Advances in consciousness research* (Vol. 28). Philadelphia: John Benjamins.

3

Paradigms in Medicine, Psychiatry, and Integrative Medicine

There are many ways to see human beings. Some medical traditions employ ways of seeing that obtain information that can be measured and empirically verified using formal methodologies and available technologies; other traditions do not have these requirements. Conventional biomedicine and nonconventional systems of medicine rest on divergent assumptions about phenomena that can have existence and relationships between phenomena and causes or meanings of illness. These differences reflect the incommensurability of paradigms described by Thomas Kuhn in his seminal work *The Structure of Scientific Revolutions*. At this stage in the evolution of Western biomedicine, mainstream theories from physics, chemistry, and biology are accepted as a sufficient explanatory model of health and illness, including normal and abnormal brain functioning. However, there are many valid ways to conceptualize the dynamic organization of the body and brain in space and time, including social, psychological, genetic, biochemical, metabolic, biomagnetic, and "energetic" patterns of structure, process, and information. In Western medicine and some nonconventional systems of medicine, symptoms are conceptualized as subjective descriptions of effects caused by factors that can be identified and characterized in empirical terms. This explanatory model implies a deterministic correspondence between identifiable biological factors and a particular symptom pattern. Practitioners of Western biomedicine argue that nonconventional systems of medicine use different metaphors to conceptualize illness phenomena that are susceptible to empirical analysis, and that all causes of illness and mechanisms of action underlying assessment or treatment approaches rest on classical biological or physical processes that can be accurately described and sufficiently explained in the reductionist language of conventional Western science. In conventional Western psychiatry, there are competing and incommensurate theoretical viewpoints, no single adequate explanatory model, and few rigorously falsifiable hypotheses of mental illness causation. Numerous psychodynamic, genetic, endocrinologic, and neurobiological explanatory models of symptom formation reflect different ideological positions and clinical training backgrounds of mental health professionals. So far there is no unifying theory, and no single conventional model of psychopathology has been confirmed as more valid than any other.

Many nonconventional systems of medicine do not endorse the Western concept of linear causality, and their practitioners assert that illness, health, and healing can be more completely understood within conceptual frameworks that differ in fundamental ways with the tenets of Western medicine. For example, meanings of symptom patterns depend on varying subjective interpretations of the experience of illness. Alternatively, symptoms can result from interacting dynamic factors that cannot be reduced to descriptions of phenomena that are congruent with classical Western scientific theories using the language of linear causality. Nonlinear causality in the context of complexity theory or other emerging theories in physics, information science, and the life sciences may ultimately provide an adequate explanatory model of symptom formation in mental illness. Systems of medicine that do not rely on empirical observations or reproducible outcomes frequently offer beneficial clinical approaches. There is no necessary correlation between a strict requirement of empirical verification of a putative mechanism of action or measurable outcomes and the relative clinical utility of an assessment or treatment approach. Examples of this include acupuncture, massage, meditation, and mindfulness training. The disparate viewpoints of Western medicine and many nonconventional systems of medicine suggest a need to create conceptual bridges between disparate systems of medicine with the goal of differentiating misunderstandings caused by the use of different metaphors from conceptual gaps related to different ways of knowing about and interpreting phenomena.

In view of the enormous structural and functional complexity of the body and brain, and the inherent limitations of methodology and theories in current Western science, it is unlikely that the causes, conditions, or meanings of cognitive, emotional, and behavioral symptoms will be completely explained or explainable on the basis of contemporary biomedical and psychological theories. However, it is important to comment that the argument that conventional biomedicine cannot adequately explain mental illness is likewise not subject to confirmation. This problem is related to limitations of conventional biomedical models and research methods that will probably continue to yield ambiguous findings about putative biological causes of mental illness. In other words, it is likely that current Western psychiatric models of symptom formation will not be confirmed or refuted using the methodology of biomedical research and technologies available to Western science. Advances in research designs and clinical methods in conventional biomedicine will ultimately confirm some conventional models of symptom formation while refuting others. Emerging paradigms will shape future biomedical and nonconventional assessment and treatment approaches, yielding different and more complete understandings of the causes, conditions, and meanings of mental illness.

◆ Paradigms in Medicine

As defined by Kuhn (1970), a paradigm is a set of beliefs that make up a theoretical framework within which scientific theories can be critically evaluated or revised. Paradigms thus provide conceptual frameworks or "ways of knowing" that bias or filter what phenomena are believed to exist, and how observations are made and interpreted. In science, a paradigm is a way of knowing endorsed through professional consensus as a valid framework within which observations or measurements can be obtained regarding the existence and properties of phenomena using a rigorous methodology. Metaphysical naturalism is the philosophical perspective of Western science. This view asserts that all phenomena that have spatiotemporal existence are knowable using the methods of current science. A narrower perspective within metaphysical naturalism is materialism, which posits that only material entities can exist (i.e., can have the property of existence). Western science rests on materialist assumptions that are explicitly metaphysical in character. By extension , metaphysical naturalism and materialism form the implicit paradigm that underlies and defines the conceptual framework of contemporary Western medicine, although Western psychiatry is based on the shared perspectives of materialism and phenomenology. All paradigms are dynamic and changing because emerging research findings and novel ideas gradually transform ways of knowing. In reciprocal fashion, evolving paradigms permit increased openness to new findings and novel ideas such that the evolution of paradigms is self-reinforcing. Changes in the paradigmatic structure of orthodox

Western medicine have led to novel explanatory models of the causes of illness and associated practical advances in clinical methods, resulting in improvements in assessment accuracy and treatment outcomes. Because of the dynamic factors that shape the theories and clinical practice of medicine, it is likely that assessment or treatment approaches that are regarded as "optimum" in any particular system of medicine will continue to evolve, permitting different and more complete understandings of the causes or meanings of symptoms relative to the conceptual framework within which the system of medicine operates. The gradual evolution of paradigms in medicine will result in novel interpretive models that will yield alternative understandings of the causes or meanings of symptoms. New ways of understanding symptoms will in turn give legitimacy to established or emerging assessment or treatment approaches, increasing their practical clinical utility.

In any system of medicine, the value of a paradigm is related to its capacity to deepen understandings of phenomena associated with health and illness. A paradigm is practically useful if its clinical application can resolve ambiguities about the phenomenal characteristics of symptoms, resulting in a more complete and accurate assessment of causes or meanings, and subsequently, a more appropriate and effective treatment plan addressing those causes or meanings. It follows that the outcome of the clinical application of a particular assessment or treatment approach to a specified symptom reflects the capacity of the parent paradigm to sufficiently explain the causes or meanings of the symptom. Many effective though not yet established approaches in biomedicine and nonconventional systems of medicine provide important clues about the nature of the human body in space–time, and the biological, energetic, or informational properties of consciousness and phenomena associated with health and illness that may ultimately be borne out by Western science.

The clinician's conceptual framework necessarily biases his or her interpretation of causes or meanings associated with reported symptoms. Assessment and treatment approaches that are regarded as reasonable with a particular system of medicine follow from a theory of possible causes or meanings of symptoms. By extension, legitimate approaches to assessment and treatment vary significantly between disparate systems of medicine. Therefore, the paradigm within which a clinician "sees" and examines patients influences to a significant degree the phenomenal indicators of health or illness that he or she observes and legitimate interpretations of causes or meanings of signs and symptoms. In turn, interpretations of causes or meanings of signs and symptoms bias views about assessment approaches that are perceived as legitimate based on the capacity of those approaches to verify presumed causes or meanings. The adequate characterization of the properties of causes or meanings will significantly determine the relative efficacy of treatment choices selected to address the postulated causes or meanings of a particular symptom pattern. Thus, through a series of logical steps, the conceptual framework that prefigures how a clinician sees and interprets the phenomenal indicators of illness and self-reported experiences of a patient in space and time significantly influences the outcome of patient care. In Western psychiatry there is a reciprocal relationship between the analysis of symptoms and the development of an argument for the relevance of a theory of consciousness on which the analytic method is based.

Disparate theories of consciousness imply disparate explanatory models of psychopathology that rest on divergent views of causality embedded in disparate systems of medicine. The paradigm of the parent system of medicine, a derivative theory of consciousness within which normal or abnormal mental functioning is understood, and specific assessment and treatment approaches are logically related and reciprocally reinforcing concepts.

The end point of any investigation is limited by the implicit or explicit conceptual framework in which a question is asked. The kind of information that is obtained through observation or research is determined to a significant degree by the conceptual framework in which questions are asked and interpretations are made in the context of a paradigm in which the practitioner works. Contemporary biomedicine can be understood as one expression of the broad paradigm of normal science, whose dominant role in developed countries is perpetuated by widely shared cultural beliefs and pervasive economic factors, ensuring the continuation of its entrenched status in those world regions (Jobst, 1998). It is an unfortunate fact that conventional biomedical treatments have failed to adequately address medical and psychiatric illnesses in the United States and other developed countries. In the United States, 15% of the gross national product (currently approximately $1.6 trillion) is spent on health care, yet drug reactions, infections, surgical errors, or other complications of conventional medical care are among the leading causes of death and morbidity (Starfield, 2000; Zhan & Miller, 2003). The shortcomings of conventional biomedicine reflect inadequacies in normal science as an explanatory paradigm of phenomena associated with health and illness and invite serious consideration of novel ways to understand and treat physical and mental illness.

Western Biomedicine Is Based on Unexamined Materialist Assumptions

In spite of progress in the philosophy of science, contemporary understandings of illness and healing in Western biomedicine continue to reflect naive reductionist assumptions from 19th-century science pertaining to the nature of phenomenal reality and methods in science. These assumptions include the existence of simple linear relationships between identifiable, measurable effects and causes of illness, and the known or knowable nature of possible causes of illness. The assertion that all causes of illness are empirically verifiable using methods in current Western science is equivalent to the metaphysical assumption that all illness-related phenomena are reducible to described classical properties of matter and energy. Alternative models, including various schools of phenomenology and Donald Davidson's (2001) anomalous monism, have been proposed in the context of philosophical debate, but to date these ideas have had relatively little impact on Western medical thinking. The result is continued acceptance of naive metaphysical assumptions as a sufficient explanatory model of the causes of health and illness. By extension, in Western biomedicine classical ideas in biology and physics are believed to provide a sufficient explanatory model of the mechanisms underlying legitimate assessment and treatment approaches. Philosophical and ideological biases in contemporary biomedicine make it likely that naive reductionist models will continue to be regarded as sufficient and necessary explanations of health, illness, and the role of consciousness, intention, or energy in health and healing. Arbitrary limits on the propositions that define the conceptual framework of Western medicine effectively exclude consideration of a possible role of postulated nonclassical phenomena in health and illness. Nonclassical phenomena include nonlocality, intentionality, possible acausal factors in illness and health that have been proposed in relation to quantum mechanics and quantum field theory, and other theories not taken into account in explanatory models employed by contemporary Western medicine. This perspective limits contemporary understandings of health and illness and restricts legitimate methods of assessment and treatment to empirical approaches based on naive materialist assumptions. The entrenched position of naive realism in which Western biomedicine operates has delayed progress in medicine toward a more inclusive paradigm that takes into account emerging classical and nonclassical models in physics, information science, and the life sciences that would probably lead to novel and more complete understandings of the causes, conditions, and meanings of health and illness.

The viewpoint that contemporary Western scientific theories and methods provide adequate explanations of all natural phenomena is called *scientism*. Scientism rests on the implicit metaphysical assumption that all real phenomena are reducible to concepts that can be understood in terms of the theories of current science. In other words, scientism assumes that phenomena are real if and only if they are explainable on the basis of contemporary scientific theories and facts. Because this claim cannot itself be substantiated by empirical means, it is by definition a purely metaphysical assertion. Scientistic beliefs widely held in Western biomedicine have led to the rejection of calls for the rigorous scientific investigation of many nonconventional modalities on the assumption that no further light will be shed on the nature of phenomena underlying health or illness through an exploration of alternative explanatory models because Western science provides a sufficient explanation of all pertinent phenomena. Scientism therefore limits the practice of science to confirmation of theories congruent with core tenets of contemporary Western science, directing science away from unbiased inquiry into nonconventional medical practices based on claims that do not fit into the contemporary Western scientific worldview.

Historically, Western Medicine Is an Open and Evolving Paradigm

The recent history of Western biomedicine is notable for its shift away from eclectic treatment strategies incorporating plant-derived preparations toward treatments based on synthetic pharmaceuticals optimized to target specific biological markers of pathology. This shift is an evolutionary process in which a paradigm informed by indigenous healing practices grounded in disparate worldviews is being rapidly replaced with a technology-based paradigm based on naive materialism. The gradual historical paradigm shift in Western culture is reflected in a gradual transition from the use of complex mixtures of herbal ingredients to preparations of single herbs to active ingredients purified from single molecular moieties, and, finally, to synthesized analogues of isolated active molecular species engineered to achieve a specific biological effect on a target cellular receptor or other discrete molecular-level process underlying a postulated discrete, biologically unambiguous disease state. Movement away from mainstream medical use of compound herbal preparations or crude extracts

with nonspecific use indications has been accelerated by rapid advances in the understanding of biochemical, metabolic, immunologic, and other empirically verifiable biological concomitants of infectious diseases and several chronic medical disorders (Sharma, 1997). However, many of the largest pharmaceutical companies continue to invest in new-drug discovery programs dedicated to investigating naturally occurring products as candidates for molecules that will provide future treatments of physical and mental illness. The concept of "active ingredient" is now an axiom of Western pharmacology and the conventional Western medical model of biological treatment. The view that specific biological agents provide optimum treatments for discrete disease states is an oversimplification of a belief carried over from early-20th-century Western medicine, which held that purified chemical substances predictably yield desirable physiological effects on a target disease. This idea emerged from early work in the field of analytic chemistry to isolate "pure" "active ingredients" from "crude" plant abstracts based on the assumption that pure isolates would correlate with a highly selective, amplified, and therefore optimum pharmacologic effect. The concept of the active ingredient is an example of a simplistic conclusion resulting from the naive reductionism that is embedded in contemporary Western science. The active ingredient model has led to the exclusion of many traditionally used herbal formulas from rigorous scientific investigation. The result is that promising compound herbal formulas used in Chinese medicine, Ayurveda, Tibetan medicine, Japanese Kampo medicine, and other professional systems of medicine have been overlooked or not fully investigated because there is no apparent "active ingredient."

In the face of entrenched conservative views of orthodox Western biomedicine, there is increasing intellectual openness in Western culture to novel ideas about illness, health, and healing. Acupuncture and other nonconventional modalities are gradually being incorporated into Western medicine, and efforts are being made to explain their beneficial effects in the context of conventional biomedical theories. At the same time, acupuncture continues to be practiced and conceptualized according to traditional Chinese medical concepts of meridian theory. Homeopathic preparations are being evaluated in Western biomedical research studies in attempts to identify a scientifically plausible mechanism of action. Historically, the same kind of *transparadigm validation* has led to the acceptance of concepts that were originally regarded as invalid from the perspective of Western practices. Examples include the use of denatured virus particles to immunize individuals against live viruses, the use of antisepsis before and after surgery, hypnotic trance induction in the treatment of neurosis, the use of x-rays to diagnose fractures, and the use of weak electrical currents to induce seizures in the treatment of severe depression or psychosis. Each of these now mainstream approaches was at first rejected by Western medicine as spurious, ineffective, or dangerous, but was eventually accepted as reasonable and effective. Western medicine has evolved into an eclectic assemblage of disparate ideas and methods, and can accurately be described as an integrative system of medicine. The gradual acceptance of Chinese medicine by Western medical practitioners suggests that biomedicine continues to evolve toward increasing integration on both a conceptual and practical level. However, it has been argued that a truly unified paradigm that includes both Western medicine and nonconventional systems of medicine will never be achieved because nonconventional approaches are not falsifiable using current scientific methods (Federspil & Vettor, 2000).

Limitations of Conventional Western Medicine and Biomedical Psychiatry

The core propositions underlying Western phenomenological models of reality are implicit in theories of contemporary Western biomedicine. These "physicalist" assumptions limit the nature of real phenomena to kinds of physical objects or processes that can be verified or measured using contemporary scientific methods and technologies. By extension, Western biomedicine asserts that normal physiological processes and causes of pathology can be completely explained with reference to basic physical and biological phenomena, including the structural and functional characteristics of molecules, cells, and organs. Contemporary models of disease causation are thus implicitly limited to (metaphorical) descriptions of identifiable external or internal physical processes that are observable using contemporary means and that can be shown to influence biophysical processes in the body, resulting in measurable changes that are interpreted as illness or improved health. These assumptions constrain biomedicine to illnesses for which there are discrete identifiable causes; however, many symptom patterns are not adequately described using this contemporary model. Legitimate treatments of medical disorders were based on mechanisms of action that could potentially slow, interrupt, or reverse the specific organic processes that originally caused specific observable pathological changes. There were presumed correspondences between discrete causes of a particular disease state and organic factors that resulted in beneficial changes in a postulated discrete physical process underlying that disease.

Historically, in Western culture mental illness and medical illness have been regarded in fundamentally different ways. Until recent times, Western biomedicine contained an implicit assumption that a "divide" exists between the characteristics and causes of medical illness and the characteristics and causes of mental illness. A naive kind of Cartesian functional-organic dualism was a central part of Western psychiatric thought. Cognitive, affective, and behavioral symptoms were interpreted as expressions of abnormal activity in a postulated nonphysical "mind"; conversely, medical illnesses were regarded as abnormalities or pathological states of the physical body. Understandings of the phenomenal nature or causes of mental illness were based on different assumptions, namely, that functional psychological states without apparent corresponding organic causes were related to the pathogenesis of cognitive or affective symptoms. This way of thinking was based on the assumption in Western biomedicine that most mental illnesses do not have underlying physical or organic causes, and that causes of mental illness are thus necessarily nonphysical and psychological in nature: symptoms originated as maladaptive responses to internal or external stresses manifesting as abnormal or pathological states of consciousness. For example, excessive psychological stress or possibly maladaptive psychodynamic defenses, introjects, and so on, resulted in a persisting pattern of anxiety—an anxiety disorder. Personal loss often led to lasting changes in conscious states that were the psychological concomitants of depressed mood—major depressive disorder. Medical illnesses or other clearly biological factors could influence the course of

certain cognitive or affective symptoms, and there was an explicit one-to-one mapping between presumed psychological factors and hypothesized discrete psychopathological states of consciousness—psychiatric disorders. Thus, until recent decades the dynamic conceptual framework of modern psychiatry relied on metaphysical arguments and a dualist perspective that equated nonmaterial states of consciousness with assumed but empirically nonverifiable causative psychological or biological factors.

Starting in the 1960s with the discovery of neurotransmitters, contemporary biological psychiatry rapidly emerged as the dominant perspective in Western mental health care. The third edition of the *Diagnostic and Statistical Manual of Mental Disorders* (*DSM-III*, 1980) represented a concerted effort to transform the formerly dualist model into a strictly reductionist, physicalist model of mental illness causation. Successive versions of the *DSM* have become increasingly "medicalized" since the late 1970s, with the result that the implicit dualism of early understandings of mental illness has shifted to a model based largely on materialist, biological assumptions. This model assumes that complex symptom patterns can be defined as discrete disorders and classifies disorders into two major categories: those determined by genetic or other biological factors and those determined by a combination of biological and nonbiological influences, including medical, social, cultural, and family dynamic issues. Contemporary biological psychiatry claims that dysregulations at the level of specific neurotransmitters (or their receptors) correspond to, cause, and adequately explain the universe of psychiatric symptoms or disorders. This view contains the implicit physicalist assumption that specific psychiatric symptoms are caused by dysregulation in specific neurotransmitters or complex systems of neurotransmitters in ways that are strictly analogous to causation of medical disease by identifiable organic factors. This view constitutes the received doctrine of contemporary Western biomedical psychiatry in spite of the absence of compelling supporting evidence and in apparent disregard of the ongoing debate over consistently ambiguous findings of studies investigating the putative roles of neurotransmitters in the pathogenesis of mental illness. Compelling research evidence supports claims of general relationships between neurotransmitters and cognitive, affective, and behavioral symptoms. However, to date there is inconsistent and inconclusive evidence in support of specific claims that deficits, excesses, or dysregulations of particular neurotransmitters (or their receptors) correspond to or cause specific cognitive, affective, or behavioral symptom patterns or so-called psychiatric disorders. On this basis the neurotransmitter theory of mental illness has not been verified. It is of course unclear whether a sufficient explanatory model of mental illness will ultimately emerge from future refinements of the neurotransmitter theory and advances in research methods. Questions about the adequacy of the neurotransmitter theory as an explanatory model of mental illness point to ongoing concerns over research findings that suggest the limited efficacy of conventional pharmacological treatment approaches developed on the basis of this theory. These concerns are summarized in detail in Part II of this book. Research on the role of specific neurotransmitters in the pathogenesis or progression of cognitive, affective, and behavioral symptoms and clinical studies of conventional Western pharmacological treatments that address putative neurotransmitter dysregulations have yielded largely ambiguous results. Inconclusive findings pertaining to the neurotransmitter theory of mental illness include the following:

♦ Relative brain activity levels of neurotransmitters can only be indirectly and roughly estimated from cerebrospinal fluid (CSF) or urinary excretion levels of metabolites, or functional brain imaging approaches such as positron emission tomography (PET) or functional magnetic resonance imaging (fMRI), showing relative levels of regional brain neurotransmitter receptor binding activity. Existing technologies cannot provide rigorous quantitative demonstrations of putative relationships between specific neurotransmitters and particular symptom patterns.

♦ Extensive research has failed to yield clear or consistent correspondences between specific neurotransmitters, or their relative global or regional levels or activity in the brain, and the presence or absence of specific psychiatric symptoms or disorders.

♦ Research findings to date have not yielded clear or consistent correlations between changes in symptoms during psychopharmacological treatment and changes in measurable brain or CSF neurotransmitter (or metabolite) levels or activities.

♦ Many conventional psychopharmacological drugs are associated with therapeutic effects even in the absence of changes in neurotransmitters that are targeted by conventional treatments and that are the postulated causes of therapeutic effects. This observation may be consistent with a placebo effect of many conventional drugs used in mental health care.

Contemporary neuroscience provides general explanations of the anatomical and functional properties of single neurons and simple brain circuits. The putative roles of specific neurotransmitters and complex neural circuits with respect to normal and abnormal cognitive, affective, and behavioral states have not been elucidated. The claim of the serotonin hypothesis that lower brain serotonin levels correlate with relatively more depressed mood is not supported by the research data. Some depressed patients have low brain serotonin levels, but many do not. Depressed patients whose mood changes do not correlate with predicted changes in serotonin levels (i.e., with conventional drug treatment) may have dysregulations of one or more other neurotransmitter systems, or a dysregulation of other kinds of biological, energetic, or informational processes that directly or indirectly influence brain function. After decades of basic research, Western psychiatry still relies on vague descriptive models of putative biological causes of mental illness. Not only do we not understand the precise relationships between biological factors and symptom patterns, current technologies cannot potentially confirm the existence of putative relationships between specific neurotransmitters or brain circuits, and a particular cognitive, affective, or behavioral symptom pattern. Research in functional brain imaging and molecular genetics is still at a very early stage. In view of the enormous complexity of the human brain and the inherent limitations of contemporary technologies, it is unlikely that satisfactory answers to these questions will be obtained before the limits of current biomedical research methods and technologies are reached. I am arguing that the Western psychiatric model of postulated causal relationships between

neurotransmitters and receptors (and possibly genes that code for their expression) and discrete symptom patterns is a gross and misleading oversimplification of complex dynamic properties of the brain governed by neurochemical, endocrinological, immunological, biomagnetic, informational, energetic, and possibly spiritual factors that have not yet been identified, much less accurately characterized as to their possible roles in the pathogenesis or progression of cognitive, affective, or behavioral symptoms.

Complex Systems Theory Distinguishes Conventional Biomedicine from Integrative Medicine

Contemporary biomedical theory argues that a symptom pattern is attributable to one or a few causes, and that causes are ultimately biological in nature. Implicit in this reductionist materialist view is the assumption that for any symptom pattern, one or few assessment approaches will adequately characterize the underlying cause, assuming the assessment approach is prudently selected on the basis of the mechanism of action through which a specified biological cause operates to create a particular symptom. In the same vein, one or a few treatment approaches are believed to address and "correct" the specific underlying cause(s) of a symptom pattern. The complex system model stands in contrast to this linear view (Bell et al., 2002). In the framework of complexity theory, a symptom pattern is viewed as an emergent property of multiple hierarchically related causes, conditions, or meanings. According to this model, different assessment approaches may provide relevant information about causes or conditions associated with a particular symptom pattern at different levels in a dynamic system of interwoven causes and conditions. In this framework it is reasonable to consider using disparate treatment approaches addressing multiple disparate causes, conditions, or meanings of symptoms. Practical differences in assessment and treatment approaches in disparate systems of medicine reflect different assumptions in biomedicine and complex systems theory. Biomedicine assumes that linear causality operates in the dynamic interactions between natural phenomena and discrete causal relationships that exist between identifiable causal factors and disease states in a system that can be adequately characterized using current empirical methods. In contrast, the complex systems model assumes that dynamic nonlinear relationships exist between multiple hierarchically nested conditions and dynamic emergent properties of the system that are experienced and reported as symptoms (Strogatz, 2001). In some cases, for example, in the management of infectious diseases, specific symptoms are correlated with an identifiable viral or bacterial infection, and the linear biomedical model probably yields a relatively accurate description of symptom formation and is therefore an adequate basis for effective treatment planning. In other cases, for example, in mental illness, causes, conditions, or meanings associated with a symptom pattern probably vary considerably. Even in cases where conventional biomedical approaches result in reliable, clinically useful information, it is reasonable to approach complex phenomena associated with mental illness within the framework of complex systems theory and to regard biological factors as important elements of a dynamic system. In cases where it is reasonable to assume on the basis of history or assessment findings that one or two primary causes of a symptom pattern operate, a particular assessment approach will likely capture relevant information about the putative cause; however, this finding does not necessarily extend to a determination of the most effective treatment addressing the symptom pattern. Disparate treatments may adequately address an identified discrete biological cause. In fact, conventional biomedicine frequently employs many kinds of biological treatments when addressing a particular symptom pattern. By extension, it is reasonable to consider integrative approaches that address an identified cause in different, possibly synergistic ways. A corollary view is that, although a particular symptom pattern may have one or few primary causes, the patient's unique biochemical, genetic, social, psychological, and possibly energetic or spiritual constitution implies that causes vary significantly between individuals who report similar symptoms. The situation becomes more complex when one considers that in the same individual the psychological, biological, energetic, informational, and possibly spiritual causes of a symptom pattern may fluctuate over time in relation to both dynamic internal and external factors. In conventional biomedical psychiatry, it is acknowledged that persisting cognitive, affective, and behavioral symptoms in the same individual are associated with varying levels of activity in neurotransmitters and receptors, and reasons for this variability are not clear. From this observation it follows that a particular assessment or treatment approach that is appropriate for a particular symptom pattern at a particular time in the history of a particular patient may not be appropriate for another individual with a similar complaint, or the same individual reporting the same symptom pattern at a future time. Starting from the viewpoint of complex systems theory and assuming that symptoms are probably associated with multiple causes and multiple kinds of causes, combining two or more assessment approaches may more adequately capture multiple interacting causes or conditions. Subsequently, in the complex systems view, an appropriate integrative treatment plan addresses multiple causes or conditions identified through history or assessment. Different approaches to causal modeling of complex variables that are believed to operate in some nonconventional healing approaches include path analysis and the analysis of latent variables (Schuck, Chappell, & Kindness, 1997). The latter approach has been used to assess quality of life in psychotic patients (Mercier & King, 1994).

Some Nonconventional Modalities Rest on Orthodox Western Science, Whereas Others Invoke Novel Paradigms

Some nonorthodox paradigms underlying so-called nonconventional systems of medicine contain propositions that do not radically depart from assumptions embedded in orthodox Western biomedicine. For example, psychoneuroimmunology is a synthetic model that takes into account current ideas in psychiatry and biomedicine and posits that stress, immunological status, and psychiatric or neurological symptom formation are causally related. Paradigms underlying other nonconventional systems of medicine may provide more complete understandings of health and illness compared with conventional biomedicine. Clinical biomedicine has not yet incorporated concepts from emerging models in physics, biology, and information science describing structure–function relationships in complex living systems. Complexity theory and quantum mechanics (as well as quantum field theory) are

conceptual frameworks that heretofore have been overlooked as potential sources of explanatory models in medicine. These nonclassical paradigms may eventually lead to models or research methods that will clarify the characteristics of putative phenomena related to health, illness, and healing. Phenomena that are regarded as legitimate subjects of inquiry in nonorthodox paradigms but have been ignored in Western biomedical research include the role of intention in healing possibly related to coherent large-scale quantum fields associated with brain functioning; the putative beneficial role of so-called subtle energy generated by human intention or machines in immunological or neurobiological functioning (as postulated by practitioners of qigong, Healing Touch, or other forms of energy medicine); and claims of distant healing associated with postulated mechanisms through which directed human intention changes patterns of space–time, manifesting as improved subjective states of well-being.

Different Understandings of Energy and Information in Western Medicine and Nonconventional Systems of Medicine

Disparate systems of medicine postulate the existence and involvement of different forms of energy and information in health, illness, and healing. Some conventional and nonconventional assessment approaches rely on the accurate characterization of classically described energetic or informational processes that constitute the presumed causes of a particular symptom pattern. Conventional Western medicine posits that health and illness can be adequately characterized in terms of classical models of energy and information. In conventional Western psychiatry, classically accepted forms of energy provide information about brain activity associated with symptoms. Normal brain functioning is characterized by complex biomagnetic and electrical activity that can be measured using functional brain-imaging techniques, including fMRI, magneto/electroencephalography (mEEG), and quantitative EEG (qEEG). Emerging evidence suggests that there are consistent relationships between particular energetic patterns of brain function and some cognitive, affective, and behavioral symptoms; however, it is frequently difficult to determine whether energetic "abnormalities" are causes or effects of pathology. Electrical currents and pulsed electromagnetic fields are conventionally used treatments in Western psychiatry. Electrical current and focused magnetic fields probably have real-time effects on the biomagnetic properties of brain functioning, in addition to long-term effects at the level of neurochemical and biomagnetic changes in the activity of brain circuits associated with the regulation of affect and other systems.

Some nonconventional treatment approaches are based on classical forms of energy, including electromagnetic energy and sound. Examples include Western herbal medicine, functional medicine, EEG biofeedback, music and patterned binaural sounds, full-spectrum bright light exposure, microcurrent brain stimulation, and dim light exposure at selected narrow wavelengths. Treatment approaches based on classically accepted forms of energy can have both direct energetic effects and indirect informational effects on biological or energetic processes associated with health and illnesses. In contrast, treatments based on postulated nonclassical models of energy or information, including quantum mechanics, quantum information, and quantum field theory, may have both direct and subtle effects on brain functioning and physiology (Curtis & Hurtak 2004; Hankey, 2004).

Functional medicine is an important emerging paradigm that views health and illness in relationship to informational changes in complex intercellular communication processes. It rests on conventional biomedical understandings of pathophysiology in the context of assumptions of biochemical and genetic individuality (Bland, 1999). According to this model, health and illness result from interactions between the unique genetic constitution of each individual and many different internal and external factors, including infection, trauma, lifestyle, diet and, environmental influences, that can modify genetic expression and alter intercellular communication manifesting as complex physical or psychiatric symptom patterns. Disparate molecules serve as cellular mediators, including neuropeptides, steroids, inflammatory mediators, and neurotransmitters. Functional assessment approaches identify informational changes in intercellular communication associated with symptoms, and effective treatments modify the informational basis of illness, taking into account complex interactions between mediators and different cell types.

Some established and emerging nonconventional assessment approaches postulate that illness phenomena can be more completely described in terms of nonclassical forms of energy. Examples include analysis of the vascular autonomic signal (VAS), Chinese pulse diagnosis, homeopathic constitutional assessment, and gas discharge visualization (GDV). Examples of nonconventional treatment approaches based on the operation of putative nonclassical forms of energy or information include acupuncture, homeopathic remedies, Healing Touch, qigong, and Reiki. In Chinese medicine, qi is a postulated elemental energy that cannot be adequately described in the language of current Western scientific models, but may have dynamic attributes that are consistent with quantum field theory (Chen, 2004). Quantum brain dynamics (QBD) is an example of a nonclassical model that invokes quantum field theory to explain certain dynamic characteristics of brain functioning, including possibly the influences of nonclassical forms of energy or information on mental health. It has been suggested that healing intention operates through nonlocal "subtle" energetic interactions between the consciousness of the medical practitioner and the physical body or consciousness of the patient (Zahourek, 2004). In contrast, energy psychology assumes that highly developed energetic techniques, including acupuncture, acupressure, and Healing Touch, are required to affect energetic balance and health. *Mind energetics* is a recently introduced conceptual model that postulates the exchange of energy through language and intention during therapeutic encounters, and claims that energy transforms psychological defenses in beneficial ways (Pressman, 2004). Widespread interest in the role of spirituality and religion in mental health has resulted in increasing research in this area and the inclusion of a special V code in the fourth edition of the *DSM* (*DSM-IV*) for religious or spiritual problems (Turner Lukoff, Barnhouse, & Lu, 1995).

Diverse perspectives on the so-called mind–body problem exist in contemporary Western psychiatry; however, there is still no consensus on a sufficient explanatory model of mind–body interactions (Kendler, 2001). Complete understanding of mind–body interactions will probably require a convergence of classical and nonclassical paradigms (Shang, 2001). For example, light exposure therapy is known to have therapeutic effects on melatonin and neurotransmitter activity and may also interact with brain dynamics on subtle levels, possibly consistent with the postulates of quantum mechanics or quantum brain dynamics (Curtis & Hurtak, 2004). The human biofield is probably best described with respect to complex interactions between classical and nonclassical kinds of energy and information, including electrical, magnetic, acoustic, and large-scale quantum properties of living systems (Rein, 2004). Practitioners of Western medicine frequently regard energy treatments as examples of the placebo effect because of the assumption that postulated forms of energy or information on which energy treatments rest simply do not exist. Rigorous research designs investigating energy medicine are difficult to achieve, and findings on the effectiveness of directed intention and putative nonclassical energy effects on human health remain inconclusive (Abbot, 2000). Nevertheless, accumulating research evidence shows that beneficial effects of some energy treatments can be replicated under controlled conditions, suggesting that nonclassical forms of energy or information influence outcomes in some cases.

◆ Possible Future Pathways of Conventional Biomedicine

The materialist paradigm of conventional Western medicine will probably follow one of two possible future evolutionary pathways. Although it will not be necessary to go outside the established paradigm of contemporary Western medicine to develop a conceptual framework for integrative medicine, the development and validation of novel assessment and treatment approaches will require the rigorous evaluation of emerging concepts in physics, chemistry, and biology. This conservative pathway does not assume or require that violations of orthodox Western scientific models of linear causality are needed to explain illness and health, but it does assume that basic directions in future medical research will not be completely determined by entrenched economic, institutional, or intellectual biases. The conservative pathway can be described as "optimizing medicine inside the box." A more radical evolutionary pathway is possible in which an increasingly eclectic framework of Western medicine will embrace emerging ideas in physics and neuroscience as well as ideas from nonconventional systems of medicine that rest on assumptions currently outside the orthodox paradigm (Rubik, 1996). This more radical path can be described as "optimizing medicine outside the box." If the more radical pathway is followed, it is likely that Western medicine will gradually transform into a fundamentally different paradigm.

Many basic questions must be addressed to determine the relevance of a particular paradigm to medicine. These include:

◆ What kinds of entities or processes in the paradigm are believed to influence health and illness?

◆ What are the assumptions of the system of medicine in which health and illness are conceptualized?

◆ What model of space, time, and causality is assumed to operate in the system of medicine?

As discussed above and in previous chapters, the conceptual framework in which a system of medicine operates determines legitimate methods used to design research studies, identify illness phenomena, and interpret the causes or meanings of symptoms. Specific models of health and illness, and particular assessment and treatment approaches derived from those models, reflect the kinds of information believed to be relevant to understanding causes or meanings of symptoms. Factors that influence health and illness can be conceptualized as entities and processes. The kinds of entities and processes that influence health or illness, the nature and role of causality, and the attributes of a body in space and time are conceptualized in different ways in conventional biomedicine and many nonconventional systems of medicine. Implications of these differences are explored in the following sections.

Disparate Paradigms Correspond to Different Concepts of Assessment and Treatment

The conceptual framework from which a symptom is examined determines the causes or meanings ascribed to that symptom, and by extension, assessment or treatment approaches that are regarded as legitimate. Emerging nonconventional paradigms imply novel interpretive models, new understandings of causes or meanings of symptoms, and novel assessment or treatment approaches addressing those causes or meanings.

Disparate ways of explaining health and illness imply the legitimacy of different assessment and treatment approaches. Four hierarchically related paradigms embodying different assumptions about the phenomenal nature of health and illness have been proposed: the body paradigm, the mind–body paradigm, the body–energy paradigm, and the body–spirit paradigm (Tataryn, 2002). Higher order paradigms embody the assumptions of lower order paradigms and add new assumptions to them. Conventional medicine operates within the body paradigm and sometimes the mind–body paradigm. Some nonconventional systems of medicine operate within all four paradigms. Certain nonconventional approaches are based on materialist assumptions that are congruent with the body paradigm—the dominant view in orthodox Western medicine—whereas others assume the validity of dualist assumptions implicit in the remaining three paradigms. Many interventions and assessment approaches employed in both conventional and nonconventional systems of medicine fall under the body or mind–body paradigms. However, at present, only nonconventional approaches fall under the body-energy and body–spirit paradigms. Following is a summary of disparate kinds of modalities that correspond to the four paradigms.

1. *Conventional and nonconventional biological methods (**body paradigm**)* are based on biological inputs to the system that may be subtle or gross, depending on the technique employed. Subtle biological therapies include aromatherapy and essential oil massage. Herbal medicines and other natural substances, including omega-3 fatty acids, minerals, vitamins, amino acids, and amino acid precursors, provide therapeutic benefits through gross biological or pharmacological effects. The body paradigm suggests that a mechanistic overlap exists between conventional and nonconventional biological treatments. For example, S-adenosylmethionine (SAMe) and conventional antidepressants probably have similar beneficial effects on neurotransmitters associated with depressed mood.

2. *Somatic and mind–body methods (**mind-body paradigm**)* achieve therapeutic results by acting directly on the physical body or the mind–body. Beneficial physiological or psychological effects are achieved without the requirement of exogenous biological, energetic, or informational inputs. Examples of established somatic and mind–body therapies include massage, craniosacral therapy, exercise, meditation, guided imagery, yoga, and stress reduction techniques. Treatment approaches in this paradigm also operate according to biological principles described in the body paradigm.

3. *Conventional energy or information methods (**body–energy paradigm**)* employ scientifically validated forms of energy or information that are directed at the body–brain and are empirically verified (or verifiable) as causally related to a clinically useful indicator of illness or to a desired outcome. Treatment effectiveness is presumed to result from direct or indirect effects of classically accepted forms of energy or information—presumed mechanisms of action—on the biological causes of symptoms. Some energy-information modalities and some biological treatments probably share common mechanisms. For example, bright light exposure indirectly regulates brain serotonin levels in ways that are similar to the effects of some conventional and nonconventional biological treatments of depressed mood. Representative energy-information modalities that have been validated by current Western science include electroconvulsive therapy (ECT), transcranial magnetic stimulation (TMS), EEG biofeedback, other kinds of biofeedback using sound or light, vagal nerve stimulation (VNS), and bright light exposure. Assessment and treatment approaches in this paradigm operate in ways that are consistent with both the mind–body and body paradigms.

4. *Approaches based on postulated forms of energy or information (contains elements of **body–energy** and **body–spirit paradigm**)* are based on beliefs that body–mind–spirit can be described in terms of putative subtle energies that have are not verified by current Western science. The body–spirit paradigm and approaches that rely on putative nonclassical forms of energy or information raise important unresolved ontological and epistemological questions about the nature of reality, valid ways of knowing, and the phenomenal nature of the human body and consciousness in time and space. Postulated effects of subtle energies rest on presumed relationships between classically described biological functions of the body–brain and postulated energetic or spiritual attributes of human beings. Established and emerging subtle energy approaches in current use include prayer, Shamanic healing, directed intention, Reiki, qigong, and possibly also homeopathy. Putative subtle biological or energetic influences of homeopathic remedies may be related to changes in biomagnetic or quantum field dynamics. Clinical approaches within the body–spirit paradigm also operate at the levels of body–energy, mind–body, and body.

Advances in all four paradigms will permit commensurate progress in clinical approaches used to assess and treat cognitive, emotional, and behavioral problems, resulting in more complete understandings of symptoms and improved outcomes in mental health care and medicine in general. An important conceptual goal of effective integrative medical planning is to achieve a synthesis of paradigms containing interpretive models that accurately identify core causes, conditions, or meanings associated with a symptom pattern at interrelated hierarchic levels in the dynamic web of body–mind–energy–spirit. This more complete multidimensional understanding or "picture" of biological, somatic, energetic, informational, and spiritual processes will result in effective integrative treatment approaches addressing complex causes or meanings of symptoms at disparate but interrelated levels. Information from history, assessment findings, and responses to treatment will provide the clinician with useful clues, permitting more effective treatment planning. In this way, history taking, assessment,

and treatment planning are ongoing and linked in a reciprocal fashion. These ideas are the core principles of integrative medicine. A future, more integrative Western medicine will provide explanatory models of illness that address both empirical and metaphysical assumptions of contemporary Western science and nonconventional systems of medicine. **Table 3–1** summarizes the assumptions of important emerging paradigms in Western science and comments on their implications for conventional biomedicine and their relevance to nonconventional systems of medicine.

Table 3–1   Emerging Paradigms, Relevance to Nonconventional Medical Approaches, and Implications for Conventional Biomedicine

Paradigm	Relevance to Claims of Nonconventional Systems of Medicine	Implications for Western Medicine if Integrated into Orthodox Paradigm	Comments
Functional medicine	Internal and external factors affect biological mediators, including neuropeptides, neurotransmitters, and inflammatory molecules that influence the patient's unique biological constitution at level of intercellular communication	Functional medicine is an integrative model that takes into account relationships between symptoms and complex dynamic interactions at the molecular and cellular levels. This model broadens and deepens conventional Western medicine	Postulated dynamic relationships between individual genetic factors and biological mediators are consistent with psychoneuroimmunology. Putative mechanisms are difficult to confirm (using available means) for many physical, cognitive, and affective symptom patterns
Mind–body medicine	Chronic stress results in dysregulation of hormones, immunologic functioning, and neurotransmitters that manifest as cognitive, affective, and behavioral symptoms (Gilbert, 2003)	Increasing integration of mind–body practices with conventional treatments will probably result in significant improvements in patient autonomy, improved outcomes, and reduced mental health care costs	Extensive research has confirmed the medical and mental health benefits of meditation, mindfulness training, yoga, and other mind–body practices
Electromagnetic body	Normal and pathological states of complex living systems can be described in terms of electromagnetic fields (Liboff, 2004)	Interpreting aspects of health and illness in relation to interactions between electromagnetic fields (including both endogenous and external fields) and conventional molecular, genetic, and cellular processes will deepen understanding of the causes of disease	Existing conventional treatments use electromagnetic energy to disrupt ECT and rTMS brain electromagnetic activity. Emerging nonconventional therapies, including microcurrent stimulation and EEG biofeedback, operate at more subtle levels
Nonclassical forms of energy or information, including quantum mechanics (QM), quantum information, and quantum field theory (QFT)	Therapeutic benefits of acupuncture, homeopathy, and possibly energy healing may be mediated through nonclassical forms of energy or information consistent with QM, QFT, or other models (Curtis & Hurtak, 2004; Rein, 2004)	Acceptance of nonlocal influences in health and illness would fundamentally change theories and methods in contemporary Western biomedicine	Demonstrated to operate at the scale of subatomic particles Speculation about "coherent" large-scale phenomena on the scale of molecules or coordinated "groups" of cells, including neurons Impossible to design experiment that can verify or falsify claimed effects using available technology
Zero-point energy	Useful information is potentially available in space–time regions described as "empty" in Newtonian mechanics	Development of concepts and techniques to "harness" zero-point energy may be consistent with body–spirit paradigm and may provide conceptual basis for emerging assessment and treatment approaches in energy medicine	The existence of zero-point energy has not been demonstrated, and it remains purely theoretical at present. There are no existing means to verify or refute claims made by this model This model may be consistent with putative "subtle energy" modalities, including qigong, Healing Touch, homeopathy, and nonlocal effects of intention
Models of anomalous conscious states, or psi	Various models of psi argue that special states of consciousness are associated with accessing or transmitting information outside of normal space–time constraints	Validation of psi influences on complex living systems may help explain claims of energy assessment and treatment methods and the putative role of intention or prayer in healing	Poorly understood subjective variables interfere with attempts to replicate psi protocols in general, and in studies on illness or therapeutic effects in particular. Current Western research methods are unable to falsify psi models or validate specific claims of effects on illness

Table 3–1 Emerging Paradigms, Relevance to Nonconventional Medical Approaches, and Implications for Conventional Biomedicine *(Continued)*

Paradigm	Relevance to Claims of Nonconventional Systems of Medicine	Implications for Western Medicine if Integrated into Orthodox Paradigm	Comments
Holographic universe	Bohm's theory of implicate order (Bohm, 1995), later modified by Pribram in his holographic brain theory, implies that complex living structures are embedded in *N*-dimensional space–time manifolds, permitting apparent nonlocal influences between two or more brains, including possibly state changes corresponding to pathogenesis of certain illnesses or specific improvements in health	This model has been extensively discussed in the context of its implications for understanding physical-energetic-informational processes that take place in the universe. Acceptance of this paradigm by Western medicine would lead to novel models of illness causation and treatment effects in the context of contemporary theories of *N*-dimensional space–time, while avoiding metaphysical arguments of nonlocal influences	Like zero-point energy and most psi models, claims of the holographic universe model cannot be verified or refuted within contemporary science. It remains an interesting speculative model that may be congruent with emerging understandings of *N*-dimensional space–time permeating complex structures

ECT, electroconvulsive therapy; EEG, electroencephalography; rTMS, repetitive transcranial magnetic stimulation

◆ Entities, Processes, and Theories of a Body in Space–Time

Entities and Processes in Conventional and Nonconventional Medicine

Western medicine and some nonconventional systems of medicine posit the existence of entities and processes. Different meanings assigned to these terms in different systems of medicine define and limit understandings of illness and health, and, by extension, approaches to assessment and treatment, in fundamentally different ways. Disparate conceptual starting points result in different ways of seeing illness phenomena, different ways of classifying phenomena into "symptoms or disorders," and corresponding differences in treatment approaches that are regarded as "legitimate" or effective. Western biomedicine is built on foundational concepts describing dynamic patterns in linear ways. In contrast, many nonconventional systems of medicine are based on concepts that describe dynamic patterns in health or illness in nonlinear or complex ways. It is likely that all phenomena, including ordinary physical objects and energetic or informational processes, can be described as nonlinear processes, and taking this into account will clarify the dynamic interrelationships of illness phenomena.

Many nonconventional systems of medicine are process-oriented because they do not rest on presuppositions regarding primary existing physical entities. Chinese medicine, for example, posits the existence of a primary or fundamental "energetic principle," qi. Physical entities, including manifestations of health and illness, are interpreted as secondary expressions of qi. This stands in contrast to contemporary Western biomedicine, which assumes that the existence of physical entities is primary, and that energetic or informational processes are special properties of relationships between physical or biological entities. These disparate perspectives reflect fundamentally different metaphysical starting points. By definition, complex systems contain relationships between presumed entities defined by boundaries—the boundaries permit descriptions of processes or behaviors of one or more entities. When a putative process involving energy or information is viewed as primary, there is no empirical approach in contemporary Western

medicine to translate this concept into a reductionist model. This state of affairs is further complicated when one considers that both conventional biomedicine and many nonconventional systems of medicine conceptualize illness or health on the basis of process or entity metaphysical assumptions, depending on the kind of phenomenon being examined. For example, in Western medicine, models of infectious disease rest on strictly "entity" assumptions about presumed pathogens. In contrast, biological psychiatry imputes many "process" assumptions, including vaguely defined dynamic interactions between social or cultural factors and the human immune and endocrine systems, mediating stress responses, and ultimately biological events that result in mental illness.

To complicate matters more, phenomena regarded as processes by one system of medicine may be regarded as entities by another. For example, Chinese medicine views all illness phenomena as processes that manifest from postulated energetic imbalances, whereas biomedicine and many nonconventional systems of medicine construe symptom patterns as indicators of physical-biological entities resulting from pathological processes. Integrative medicine addresses this dilemma by endorsing a synthetic conceptual framework that includes both kinds of metaphysical assumptions, permitting the legitimate use of modalities based on the primary existence of energetic or informational processes and also the primary existence of physical-biological entities. On a practical level, this approach translates into viewing the same information pertaining to a symptom pattern from both a quantitative and qualitative perspective (see Chapter 4, Foundations of Clinical Methodology in Integrative Medicine, for a discussion of combined quantitative-qualitative methods). **Table 3–2** summarizes conceptual differences between contemporary biomedicine and some nonconventional systems of medicine in terms of assumptions about the roles of entities and processes in health and illness.

Disparate Paradigms Correspond to Different Understandings of Legitimate Medical Approaches

The existence and functional attributes of the body can be conceptualized in many ways, including physiological, molecular

Table 3–2   Entity and Process in Contemporary Biomedicine and Some Nonconventional Systems of Medicine

	Entity	Process
Contemporary Western biomedicine	An entity is a discrete object or thing that exists in conventional space–time.	A process is a relationship between two or more entities that takes place in classical four-dimensional space–time.
	In living systems, structures are reducible to known categories of physical entities or processes that are hierarchically related and can be described in terms of linear causality.	Certain forms of energy and information are possible and constrain all processes in all living or nonliving systems.
	Dysfunction at the level of structures ultimately manifests as symptoms that can be empirically described	No process can take place outside four-dimensional space–time.
		Processes in living systems are observable, and their characteristics are measurable, consistent, and empirically verifiable.
		Like entities, processes are related to other processes or entities in linear ways
Some nonconventional systems of medicine	There are no discrete things; there is only energy or information.	Processes describe complex nonlinear relationships between energy or information in one of many possible space–time domains.
	Four-dimensional space–time is an artificial construct.	Cognitive or affective symptoms are manifestations of nonlinear processes reflecting imbalance or dysregulation of energy or information.
	Energy and information are not constrained by the classical model of four-dimensional space–time.	Some processes in complex living systems (including the brain) are observable using conventional empirical means.
	Phenomena that are labeled entities are actually lower-order processes and manifestations of interrelationships between energy and information.	Some processes in complex living systems are not observable or measurable using conventional empirical means.
	Symptoms in illness and effects of treatments are specific examples of process entities or manifestations of relationships between structures over time	Because of inherent nonlinearity in processes affecting health and their occurrence in many possible space–time domains, consistent causes or effects of a particular symptom pattern do not occur, and there can be no standard assessment or treatment approaches

genetic, biomagnetic, and informational. Each of these viewpoints is supported by speculation and limited evidence. These disparate models reflect established or emerging paradigms about the nature and characteristics of phenomena. Some are consistent with existing classical models of physics, whereas others originate in so-called nonclassical understandings, including quantum mechanics and quantum field theory. Depending on the conceptual frameworks in which the body is imagined, fundamentally different kinds of phenomena are considered relevant to the existence and functioning of the body in space and time. By the same token, different conceptual frameworks lead to fundamentally different assumptions about kinds of phenomena that are related or not to the maintenance of health or the causes or meanings of illness. Different metaphysical assumptions contained in disparate paradigms are implicit in disparate established or emerging conventional or nonconventional modalities. The perceived legitimacy of any medical practice will ultimately be determined by the acceptance or rejection of the paradigm on which it is based. This is both a matter of future science and future consensus.

Disparate Systems of Medicine Rest on Different Assumptions of a Body in Space–Time

It is important to comment at the outset that important theoretical work is ongoing in the life sciences and consciousness studies and is taking into account complex system theory, quantum mechanics, and other nonorthodox paradigms, including the ideas of Edelman (Edelman & Mountcastle, 1978), Pribram, Penrose (1994), and others. However, this work remains highly theoretical, and until now conventional Western biomedicine has not pursued research directions into putative novel mechanisms of action suggested by emerging models of mind–brain and consciousness. In Western medicine, the assumption that only empirically verifiable entities or processes can affect living systems has led to the corollary assumption that legitimate approaches for assessing and treating presumed "causes" of symptoms can only be based on biological mechanisms. In spite of these assumptions, it has been established that, in addition to biological factors, living systems respond to many classically described forms of energy or information (which probably have indirect biological effects in some cases). In contrast to Western biomedicine, some nonconventional systems of medicine posit that "normal" and "abnormal" functional states of the body are expressions of complex relationships between structures, processes, and classically accepted or putative forms of subtle energy or information. The definition of a *subtle domain* is a field or background in which the structures or functions of brain exist or take place outside of constraints widely held to be boundary conditions in classical Newtonian space–time descriptions of existence.

Contemporary biomedicine subscribes to the materialist view that symptoms, and presumed underlying causes of illness, are reducible to knowable and measurable dysregulations or disequilibria in physiological processes that are consistent with classical Newtonian assumptions about space, time, and matter–energy relationships. Proponents of biomedicine argue that a complete understanding of normal and abnormal states of the human body is forthcoming in the context of contemporary theories in biology and physics, and that the same models can be used to explain consciousness. It is assumed that "regular" patterns of structure or function are measurable and recur in predictable ways, permitting rational inferences about empirically verifiable causes and effects in health and illness. Three important logical errors in the conceptual foundations of Western medicine limit the capacity of conventional biomedical approaches to accurately assess causes or meanings of symptoms and to effectively treat symptom patterns. These errors are implicit assumptions in Western biomedicine:

1. All phenomena affecting the properties of a complex living system are empirically measurable, and therefore empirically verifiable.
2. The system behaves in predictable linear ways, as described by classical physics and chemistry.
3. The system exists and operates in four-dimensional space–time, as described by Newtonian physics.

I am arguing that assumptions of linearity and predictability in complex biological systems, including the human brain, are naive with respect to the available research findings on normal and abnormal mental functioning and human consciousness in general. The assumption of linearity and the corollary view that discrete empirically definable cause–effect relationships exist between pathology and identifiable or empirically verifiable "factors" cannot potentially explain the dynamic relationships that characterize all but the simplest living systems. Furthermore, living systems behave in complex nonlinear ways that cannot be adequately characterized using conventional empirical methods and linear models of cause and effect. These naive assumptions are artifacts of classical models in physics that cannot accommodate complex structure–function relationships between normal or abnormal brain functional states and multiple hierarchically nested factors or processes that influence brain–body–energy.

In view of the above, it is important to consider how to modify core assumptions of Western biomedicine to permit contemporary biomedical theory to benefit from the insights of complexity theory and other emerging paradigms. Along the same lines, it is important to develop practical approaches to integrating nonconventional modalities with Western medicine in cases where putative mechanisms of action are consistent with the predictions of complexity theory and supported by emerging research findings. Examples of modalities that rely on putative nonlinear processes include EEG biofeedback, homeopathy, and energy medicine.

Physical, biological, energetic, and informational entities or processes that compose or influence the dynamic patterns of living systems probably function in both linear and nonlinear ways, and these entities or processes are hierarchically linked in space and time. This general statement can be applied to the human brain and its functions, including normal and abnormal functional patterns or states of consciousness. The multitiered biological and energetic complexity of the body and brain in space and time suggests a multitiered approach to assessment and treatment, taking into account hierarchically related bioenergetic-informational phenomena that influence normal or abnormal functioning. The dynamic multitiered complexity of the body–brain is the central premise on which the conceptual framework of integrative medicine is based.

Some assessment approaches more accurately identify states of dysregulation or "imbalance" affecting normal body–brain structures or processes that manifest as symptoms depending on the characteristics and degree of dysregulation and the relative hierarchical location of involved structures or processes. In this sense, accurate characterization of the hierarchic location of a dysregulation affecting a structure or process in the body–brain is equivalent to a determination of the causes, conditions, or meanings of the symptom pattern that is a manifestation of the dysregulation. Disparate hierarchic levels of dysregulation in the body–brain are directly or indirectly related to the manifestation of symptoms. Symptom specificity, severity, duration, and timing are related to and multiply determined by dynamic relationships between complex hierarchically interrelated factors. In this way, symptom patterns that are experienced and interpreted as illness mirror complex patterns of interrelated factors that reflect dysregulation or imbalances at various hierarchic levels in the biological, energetic, informational, and spiritual attributes of the body–brain–mind. Dysregulations or "imbalances" take place at many biological, physical, gross, or subtle bioenergetic levels. The kinds of dysregulation, their relative severity, and the complex interrelationships that exist between them will determine the severity and characteristics of observable signs or reported symptoms that are interpreted as a particular cognitive, affective, or behavioral symptom pattern.

◆ The Concept of Biochemical and Energetic Individuality and Emerging Models of a Body in Space–Time

In recent years, the concept of biochemical individuality has become increasingly accepted in Western medicine. The argument is that individual biochemical factors (and their underlying genetic basis) imply that each patient has a unique biochemical constitution and should be evaluated and treated with that fact in mind. In addition to biochemical individuality, it is possible to describe human beings as having unique biomagnetic, informational, and spiritual "constitutions."

There is growing evidence for a homeodynamic rather than homeostatic model of body–brain–energy–environment interactions at complex biological, psychological, energetic, and spiritual levels of organization of the body in space and time (Miller, 2003). *Homeodynamic efficiency* describes the extent to which complex psychophysiological factors maintain mind–body in the optimal range of functioning. This paradigm describes continuously changing dynamic factors that influence the causes and conditions of health and illness. The homeodynamic model invites consideration of assessment and treatment approaches based on psychological, biological, energy, and spiritual effects on mind–body-environment (Dossey, 1982; Jankovic, 1994; Shealy & Myss, 1993). A recently proposed paradigm called *extended network generalized entanglement theory* extends the homeodynamic mind–body model to include ideas from complexity theory, quantum mechanics, and genetics. This model suggests that the body is a dynamically self-organizing system in space and time that responds to biological, psychological, physical, and "subtle" information in the context of genetic constraints that define and limit possible patterns of self-organization (Hyland, 2003). This paradigm provides an explicit place for the operation of subtle energy therapies.

From the perspective of conventional Western medicine, patients complaining of a particular symptom are presumed to share important biologically mediated pathological signs or symptoms indicating similar or identical causes. Similar conventional biomedical treatments are administered to patients complaining of similar symptoms on the assumption that each patient is an "average case" of a specified objectively describable disorder. The impressive outcomes of many conventional treatments suggest that assumptions of average causes and average cases are correct for some illnesses, including, for example, infectious diseases, heart disease, and many kinds of cancer. However, sporadic or poor outcomes of conventional Western treatments for many disorders suggest that the average case approach to understanding pathology fails to recognize the importance of individual variability in pathogenesis. In some cases of poor outcomes, the general mechanism of a treatment may fail to address primary causes of pathology. In other cases of sporadic or poor outcomes, a treatment may be supported by a sound theory of mechanism but fail to take into account individual variability at one or more levels of biological, energetic, or informational organization. The fact that some treatments generally yield positive results in a significant percentage of patients reporting a specified symptom pattern suggests that a shared causal mechanism has been accurately identified and effectively addressed. Alternatively, consistently sporadic or poor outcomes imply significant group variation in factors that influence pathogenesis or treatment response. In view of sporadic and inconsistent outcomes of conventional Western treatments of mental illness, it is probable that cognitive, affective, and behavioral symptoms are significantly influenced by individual biochemical, energetic, informational, or other factors that are highly variable and poorly understood in current models. This view is consistent with emerging understandings of the body–brain in the context of complexity theory. Integrative assessment and treatment planning address the inherent complexity of the body in space and time by taking into account individual psychological, biological, energetic-informational, and possibly spiritual differences between individuals complaining of symptoms that are typically classified as discrete or "average" disorders in Western medicine and treated using "average" approaches, frequently yielding disappointing results.

Interpretations of "a Body" and "Embodiment" Are Different in Disparate Systems of Medicine

The problem of "a body" in space–time implies the problem of "embodiment" of structures or functions that make up a body, and the related problem of interactions between those structures or functions and phenomena outside of a body. These problems, in turn, raise questions regarding the phenomenal nature of a body, and suggest an intrinsic dualism between phenomena that can be described in material terms and phenomena that can be described using concepts of energy or information. Disparate systems of medicine are derived from disparate paradigms and embody different assumptions about the physical or energetic nature of a body and its constituent structures and functions. Questions of a body in space–time ultimately lead to

ontological and epistemological problems related to the verification of existence of phenomena presumed to play a role in the existence of a body, and their empirical characterization, respectively. Different ontological givens or epistemological perspectives implicit in disparate systems of medicine bias and limit conceptual models of a body that are regarded as legitimate within disparate systems of medicine. The concept of a "self" in various schools of psychology is related to the more general problem of a body, but it takes into account the problem of identity and the putative role of consciousness.

Concepts used to define a body in space–time are contained in categories of existence and ways of knowing that are core propositions in all systems of medicine. Those core propositions translate into overlapping or nonoverlapping schemata for identifying "normal" versus "abnormal" structural or functional states of a body, and, by extension, overlapping or nonoverlapping schemata for formulating assessment or treatment approaches addressing abnormal states. Many questions must be considered when thinking about a body in space–time:

- What kinds of phenomena (entities or processes) potentially interact with a body?
- How can correspondences between observable phenomena and a symptom pattern in a body be identified or measured?
- What kinds of correspondences between observable phenomena and symptoms can be empirically verified as causal relationships?
- What kinds of correspondences can be verified in ways that are replicable using available methods (this is the formal conventional definition of *empirical verification*)?
- What method(s) can be used to determine (kinds of) causal relationships that can be ascertained or evaluated in assessment or treatment approaches, respectively (this is the formal conventional definition of *validation of method*)?
- How do the above issues differ between disparate systems of medicine, and what is the significance of differences?

It is clear that questions of "a body" and "embodiment" introduce important conceptual issues related to choices of premises on which methods of observation, verification, and validation are based. By extension, the conceptual foundations of methodology define and limit practical approaches that are accepted as legitimate means for identifying or measuring structures or processes when examining a body and assessing treatment outcomes.

Understandings of a body are integrally dependent on the system of medicine or thought-world within which observations or measurements take place. The above questions relate indirectly to the broader problem of embodiment of consciousness, and, by extension, pathological states of consciousness that are interpreted as mental illnesses. **Table 3–3** contrasts models of a body, normal functioning (good health), and pathological functioning (symptoms) in contemporary Western medicine and a proposed model of integrative medicine that incorporates tenets of complexity theory.

Assumptions of Causality in Medicine Are Paradigm-Dependent

Many nonconventional systems of medicine invoke nondeterministic models, including Jungian synchronicity, quantum

Table 3–3 Disparate Models of "a Body" Imply Different Concepts of "Normal" and Pathological Functioning

	Contemporary Western Biomedicine	Biomedicine Incorporating Tenets of Complexity Theory
"a body"	"A body" comprises molecules, cells, and tissues. "A body" can be completely described in terms of entities (anatomy), processes (physiology), and interactions with the environment. All structures and processes exist in conventional space–time, are measurable, knowable, and therefore empirically verifiable, and can be described in conventional linear terms.	Molecular dynamics are functions of complex subatomic and molecular dynamic patterns of structure, energy, and information. Cells and their functions are functions of complex dynamics at molecular level and other hierarchic levels. Interactions between the system (i.e., "a body") and the physical, energetic, or informational environment take place in conventional space–time and at some hierarchic levels in the system (possibly also in the domain of macroscopic quantum fields). Interactions at some hierarchic levels within the system are linear; other interactions are nonlinear.
Normal functioning	Static structures and dynamic processes can be described in terms of conventional models of biological structures and processes interrelated in linear ways. Patterns of normal functioning rest on linear patterns of structure or function, and are describable and verifiable using conventional empirical methods.	There is no real distinction between "structure" and "function," which are different ways of describing complex interrelationships at different hierarchic locations in the complex system. Normal functioning can be described in general terms using basic concepts in complexity theory, but processes or structures cannot be empirically verified because they ultimately rest on chaotic, nonlinear phenomena.
Pathological functioning	Descriptions of "causes" of pathology in a biological system, including the brain, are regular, measurable, and therefore "knowable," resulting in consistently reliable assessment findings. Reliable and specific treatment principles or strategies can be derived on the basis of empirically defined biological mechanisms underlying pathology.	Nonlinear dynamics underlying pathology in complex biological systems, including the brain, are by definition not completely measurable using empirical methods, and therefore are not "knowable." Therefore, no "correct" or complete assessment finding is possible, and assessment or treatment approaches are effective when dynamic patterns associated with pathology are shifted in ways that manifest as clinical improvement.

field theory, and models of psychic functioning (psi), in efforts to explain the observed characteristics or "meanings" of symptoms outside of a limited classical model of linear causality. The debate over determinism (i.e., causality versus acausality) in nature in general, and medicine in particular, is of fundamental importance to a discussion of integrative medicine because disparate viewpoints translate into different conceptual and practical methods for verifying evidence of links between putative causes of illness and symptoms, or evidence of links between treatments and outcomes. This problem casts doubt on the appropriateness of using conventional biomedical research designs to evaluate nonconventional treatment methods based on postulated nondeterministic models of health and illness.

Philosophical issues related to the problems of "knowledge," "verification," and "causality" in conventional medicine and nonconventional systems of medicine were addressed in Chapter 2, Philosophical Problems. In brief, disparate systems of medicine rest on disparate epistemological and ontological models. Philosophical differences translate into commensurate differences in models of causality in conventional and nonconventional systems of medicine. Contemporary Western science, and by extension biomedicine, rests on the assumption of linear causality linking processes affecting health, including psychological health. Contemporary Western biomedicine asserts that some phenomena affect illness or health in ways that are observable and susceptible to empirical analysis as events that are linearly juxtaposed in time or space. Classical concepts in physics, chemistry, and biology are believed to explain sufficiently all possible causal relationships between natural phenomena, and there is no need to invoke nonclassical

theories to explain other postulated causes or meanings of phenomena or their interrelationships. Many nonconventional systems of medicine rest on the same or similar assumptions of linear causality. Examples include Western herbal medicine, chiropractic, and massage therapy.

In contrast, many nonconventional systems of medicine do not assume that symptoms are caused or related to one another in conventional linear ways, but assert that symptoms manifest in nondeterministic, possibly acausal ways. For example, in contrast to Western biomedicine, classical Chinese medicine operates according to an explicitly acausal model of the universe. The core tenets of Chinese medicine postulate that fundamental energetic states take place in the body in different ways depending on the state of balance between extrinsic and intrinsic factors. It is accepted as axiomatic in Chinese medicine that energetic states manifest as simple patterns and sometimes as complex patterns in relationship to both physical and biological causes assumed to operate in conventional biomedicine and energetic principles.

Emerging approaches in Western industrialized countries described as "energy medicine" rest on the assumption that current Western science does not provide an adequate explanatory model of the causes or conditions associated with illness and health. It is important to remark that quantum mechanics and other nonclassical paradigms in physics frame the existence of natural phenomena in the context of presumed nonlocal, acausal relationships. Observable states of entangled photons, for example, are related in exact and predictable ways, but the precise characteristics of entangled subatomic particles cannot be formally described using simple deterministic models of causality. Therefore, although entanglement between photons can be observed, the Newtonian concept of cause does not apply in the quantum domain. From this point of view (i.e., nonlocality), all that can be stated is that two separated phenomenal states are probabilistically related. A similar difficulty seems to be hindering efforts to elucidate mechanisms associated with reported beneficial outcomes in energy medicine. Correspondences have been observed between some states of human consciousness, including highly focused intention or attention, prayer, meditation, and changes in health, but empirically verifiable causes or mechanisms have not been revealed by extensive research. Energetic or informational changes that are taking place at the level of subatomic particles when entanglement is confirmed may not be the same kind of events that take place in the macroscopic world when changes in health are reported in apparent relationship to directed intention, prayer, or energy medicine. However, subjective reports of these phenomena bear interesting resemblances to one another, and nonconventional medical approaches based on assumptions of "healing energy" may ultimately provide useful conceptual models for thinking about nonlinear causation in complex living systems in general.

Prayer is widely used to treat or self-treat a range of medical and mental health problems (McCaffrey, Eisenberg, Legedza, Davis, & Phillips, 2004). There is evidence that prayer and other forms of directed intention influence biological systems on the scale of cellular activity and physiology (Astin, Harkness, & Ernst, 2000; Jonas & Crawford, 2003; Radin, Taft, & Yount, 2004). The first scientific report of an apparent nonlocal connection between sensory-isolated individuals was published in 1965 (Duane & Behrendt, 1965). EEG recordings of identical twins in separate rooms showed that when a light flashed in the eyes of one twin, increased alpha (α activity occurred in the brain of the other twin. This effect, described as *extrasensory induction*, was replicated many years afterwards by several small open trials on empathically linked individuals. Visual evoked potentials (VEPs) in one individual were correlated with above-chance brain activation in the other individual sitting inside an electromagnetically shielded room (Grinberg-Zylberbaum, Delaflor, & Goswami, 1994; Grinberg-Zylberbaum & Ramos, 1987). These early findings were subsequently confirmed by a controlled study involving 60 pairs of individuals (Standish, Johnson, Kozak, & Richards, 2001). Other studies suggest apparent nonlocal effects of intention or prayer on the basis of above-chance correlations in electrodermal activity between sensory-isolated subjects (Schlitz & Braud, 1997). Considerable controversy surrounded the publication of findings of a controlled study suggesting that VEPs in one individual correlate with above-chance activation on fMRI in the visual association cortex of an empathically linked person who is physically and electromagnetically isolated (Standish, Johnson, Kozak, & Richards, 2003). This finding has been replicated in a case study using a similar VEP paradigm and conventional EEG recording methods (Wackermann, 2003). An apparent case of macroscopic entanglement has been reported between cultured nerve cells that are electromagnetically isolated (Pizzi, 2004). Replication of this finding will offer important clues of putative nonclassical mechanisms associated with prayer and other forms of healing intention. Both classical and nonclassical paradigms have been invoked in efforts to explain apparent relationships between prayer and other forms of distant healing intention and changes in brain function measured using EEG or fMRI. From a classical perspective, extremely low frequency electromagnetic waves may explain some observed cases of apparent information transfer between two or more isolated individuals even when electromotive force shielding is used (Rubik, 2000). Observations of changes in brain activity and intention may be consistent with macroscopic quantum entanglement effects (Thaheld, 2000). It has been suggested that intention always plays a role in health care and that healing intention is thus an essential factor in both conventional and nonconventional medicine (Zahourek 2004).

Table 3–4 contrasts contemporary Western medicine in general, conventional biomedical psychiatry, and representative nonconventional systems of medicine in terms of knowledge claims used to establish evidence that a symptom or its

Table 3–4   Knowledge of Symptoms: Claims of Existence and Verification of Causes and Symptom Properties in Western Medicine, Psychiatry, and Nonconventional Medicine

	Claimed Symptom or Cause Can Exist	**Claimed Symptom or Cause Is Verified or Verifiable**	**Claimed Symptom or Cause Is Known to have X Properties**
Contemporary Western medicine	The symptom corresponds to a cause that can have material existence	The underlying cause can be observed or measured using scientifically validated empirical methods	Measurements by different researchers provide consistently reliable findings, verifying claimed characteristics of the symptom
Contemporary Western psychiatry	The cause or meaning of a cognitive or affective symptom is an established neurobiological or psychological mechanism in contemporary Western psychiatric theory	The cause or meaning of a symptom can be reasonably inferred to exist on the basis of empirical findings and is consistent with conventional models of neurobiological or psychological functioning	Patient interviews, laboratory studies, brain scans, and other biomedical assessment findings adequately characterize the putative cause(s) or meaning(s) of a symptom. Causal chains can be inferred to exist between observed or reported symptoms, and presumed neurobiological processes
Nonconventional systems of medicine	The existence of a symptom is implicit in the dynamic informational, "energetic," or spiritual state of the person who experiences it. Empirical verification of existence of a symptom is not relevant	Verification of the cause of a symptom is often impossible using conventional empirical means, but the cause can be confirmed by nonconventional "energetic" or intuitive means regarded as valid within parent system of medicine. Empirical verification of causes is not relevant	Reliable empirical data are seldom available, but the nonconventional practitioner infers or intuits properties of a symptom in the context of the parent system of medicine. Empirical verification of symptom characteristics is not relevant

cause exists, can be verified, or has certain described properties. As discussed above, differences in criteria for establishing the existence of the causes or conditions of a symptom, or verifying its properties, reflect differences in assumptions pertaining to causal versus nondeterministic models of symptom formation in disparate systems of medicine. This discussion leads into general considerations of kinds and levels of evidence in Western and other systems of medicine (see Chapter 4).

◆ Paradigms in Psychiatry

Important Advances Are Taking Place in Conventional Western Psychiatry

Recent discoveries in neuroscience and genetics suggest that orthodox models of human consciousness and mental illness are incomplete. Understandings of basic neurochemical mechanisms underlying normal brain functioning continue to evolve at a rapid rate, pointing to the limitations of the **neurotransmitter theory**. This still-current model advanced in the early 1960s characterizes neurotransmitters as substances that are invariably synthesized and released by neurons, act on postsynaptic receptors, and mediate both normal and abnormal states of consciousness in relationship to specific activity levels or dysregulations of their synthesis or receptor uptake. However, some newly identified neurotransmitters and neuropeptides are not stored in synaptic vesicles, are not released by exocytosis, and do not act at receptor sites on postsynaptic vesicles; thus they do not fulfill classical criteria for neurotransmitters. An example is D-serine, which is synthesized and stored in neuroglia. D-serine binds to *N*-methyl-D-asparate (NMDA) receptors, implicated in the pathogenesis of schizophrenia and other psychotic syndromes. Other atypical neurotransmitters that may play significant roles in the pathogenesis of psychiatric symptoms include nitric oxide, carbon monoxide, and possibly hydrogen sulfide. Nitric oxide may play an important role in learning and memory (Snyder & Ferris, 2000).

Other emerging ideas in conventional Western psychiatry promise significant advances in understanding. A recently proposed model uses nonlinear dynamics (i.e., chaos theory) to explain mood changes associated with the menstrual cycle on the basis of postulated complex influences of hormones and neurotransmitters, as well as social and psychological variables (Rasgon et al., 2003). Continued development of this model may eventually lead to effective preventive strategies addressing hormone-mediated mood disturbances. There is significant emerging evidence that complex interactions between immune functioning, neurotransmitters, and hormones play important roles in depressed mood, anxiety, and other symptom patterns (Miller, 2004). Western biomedical psychiatric research is taking into account the significance of genetic and biochemical variability in mental illness. For example, the high degree of individual variability in response to conventional drugs suggests poorly characterized differences in neurotransmitter deficiencies or imbalances associated with depressed mood, anxiety, and other symptom patterns (Delgado & Moreno, 2000). Studies on the effects of neurotransmitter depletion on mood are consistent with the view that changes in brain serotonin or norepinephrine activity levels alone do not adequately explain the causes of depression or observed differential responses to conventional antidepressants. An emerging biological treatment of mental illness called **targeted amino acid therapy** uses specific combinations of amino acids to replace or "rebalance" postulated deficiencies or imbalances in neurotransmitters while taking into account individual genetic and biochemical differences. Using this approach, the amino acid tryptophan can be administered alone or in combination with other amino acids, including L-theanine, SAMe, or others, depending on the particular neurotransmitter deficiency or imbalance that is being addressed. Tryptophan is essential for the synthesis of serotonin and can be used in the form of L-tryptophan or 5-hydroxytryptophan (5-HTP). L-theanine crosses the blood–brain barrier and is converted into γ-aminobutyric acid (GABA), the brain's principle inhibitory neurotransmitter.

Differences in response to conventional drugs are related to genetic variability (and thus ethnicity), diet, and culturally determined expectations. Genetic, cultural, and social variability translates into differences in effective dosing strategies using conventional drugs and commensurate differences in susceptibility to adverse effects (Lin, 2004). The high degree of biological variability may be especially problematic for patients of African or Asian ethnicity, potentially causing safety issues or poor outcomes (Edmond, 2004; Lawson, 2004). Advances in functional brain imaging, including positron emission tomography (PET), single photon emission computed tomography (SPECT), fMRI, and magnetic resonance spectroscopy (MRS), will permit studies on specific neurotransmitter/receptor systems implicated in the pathogenesis of mental illness, and will probably result in more specific and more effective ways to assess and treat mental illness (Nemeroff, Kilts, & Berns, 1999). Rapid progress in the understanding of genetic factors in mental illness is expected from analysis of the genetic library available in the Human Genome Project. Social, cultural, and psychological models have been advanced in efforts to more adequately explain mental illness. Nonbiological models are limited by inconsistent research findings.

The meaning of symptom causation in psychiatric illness remains obscure because of the absence of a satisfactory conceptual framework, as well as incomplete information about psychological and biological factors that putatively influence cognitive or emotional functioning. In its present form, Western psychiatry is constrained by a situation in which factors presumed to operate in symptom formation are both philosophically and scientifically ambiguous. This state of affairs stands in contrast to conventional internal medicine, in which relationships between identifiable factors and particular symptom patterns are frequently unambiguous. Resolving the problem of ambiguity will require novel research methods and technologies capable of providing consistent and reliable empirical findings in support of at least one theory of mental illness causation. Increasingly rigorous assessment and treatment approaches in conventional Western psychiatry will emerge from ongoing advances in biological psychiatry, including functional brain imaging, immunology, and genetics. Future models of mental illness causation will not depend exclusively on empirical verification of strictly biological processes and will postulate both classical biological and nonclassical kinds of phenomena to provide more adequate explanations of symptom formation and treatment response. The emerging paradigms discussed in this chapter will contribute to future theories of "normal" and "abnormal" cognitive, emotional, and behavioral functioning and will eventually lead to the development and validation of novel assessment and treatment approaches.

The Meanings of *Illness* and *Health* Are Not Clearly Defined in Western Psychiatry

The selective use of certain kinds of information as evidence of illness biases beliefs about which theories are regarded as legitimate explanations of illness and which outcomes are causally linked to a treatment addressing a specified symptom. In conventional psychiatric diagnosis, only information about putative psychodynamic states and neuropharmacological processes is considered relevant. The selective exclusion of nonpharmacological kinds of information as evidence of illness (or, conversely, evidence of the absence of pathology) biases conceptual models of psychiatric illness, permitting only certain described legitimate relationships between "therapeutic" effects and interventions. Implicit biases in the paradigm of Western biomedicine have resulted in considerable vagueness when the causes and conditions of illness and healing are examined. This becomes especially problematic when the meaning of the terms *illness* and *healing* in psychiatry is considered, as the kinds of phenomena that are believed to cause or mitigate psychiatric symptoms are intrinsically more difficult to identify, observe, and characterize than the kinds of phenomena that are believed to affect physical health in general. However, dysregulations that affect physical health frequently influence brain function in indirect ways, manifesting as specific psychiatric symptom patterns.

Western biomedical psychiatry is not a coherent body of theory and practices. Rather, it is a collection not only of different theories but also different kinds of theories about causes, conditions, and meanings associated with "abnormal" affective, cognitive, and behavioral states. This eclectic base has resulted in a wide range of views about the pathogenesis of psychiatric symptom patterns, and diverse methods of assessment and treatment based on different kinds and strengths of evidence. Using current American Psychiatric Association (APA) treatment guidelines, the same anxious patient may be approached using cognitive-behavioral techniques to "reframe" the sources of her anxious state, while being encouraged to use self-calming techniques such as guided imagery or deep breathing, and simultaneously being treated with a selective serotonin reuptake inhibitor (SSRI), addressing a presumed central neurochemical dysregulation associated with her anxious state. Cognitive-behavioral therapies rest on **behaviorism**, a theory dating to the early 20th century, which asserts that changes in cognitions result in beneficial changes in thoughts and behaviors and adaptive responses to continuing real-world stresses. This clinical approach derives from a psychological model of human functioning that was borrowed from early Pavlovian and Skinnerian concepts of classical and operant conditioning. It asserts that a causal connection exists between "thinking" or "acting" and the capacity to change abnormal or undesirable cognitive or behavioral states into normal or desirable states. These putative links have not been verified because contemporary empirical methods cannot demonstrate causal relationships between phenomena like thoughts or behaviors and the observable or self-reported phenomena of psychopathology. There are many layers of intervening or confounding factors that may account for actual changes observed in cognitive-behavioral therapy that interfere with efforts to make strong inferences about direct causal links. Although cognitive-behavioral techniques are supported by a body of evidence, they rest on a theory that cannot be falsified using

available empirical means. A neurobiological substrate has not been empirically demonstrated in support of claims for a putative biological mechanism of action underlying this treatment approach. Cognitive-behavioral therapy is thus based on outcomes studies and consensus over largely unexamined metaphysical assumptions about relationships between states of consciousness and behavioral or mental causes or effects of those states.

Accepted clinical approaches in contemporary Western psychiatry claim to be "atheoretical," in that there is no explicitly postulated conceptual model of psychopathology, and limited compelling evidence supporting what have become accepted standards of practice. As such, Western psychiatry is not a paradigm or coherent body of theories and practices. Rather, it is a strange hybrid of arbitrary conventions that have been granted the appearance of objectivity and legitimacy through expert consensus panels consisting largely of research psychiatrists in APA committee meetings who impose these views on Western psychiatry and popular culture through successive iterations of the *Diagnostic and Statistical Manual*. Therefore, although there is a presumption of rigor and objectivity in conventional psychiatric diagnosis, in many cases the process of formulating diagnostic criteria for psychiatric "disorders" is neither rigorous nor objective.

The Debate over Disorders versus Symptom Patterns in Mental Illness

Cognitive, emotional, and behavioral problems occur as complex symptom patterns that are diagnosed as discrete disorders in contemporary Western psychiatry. This approach is an artifact of the conceptual framework of biomedicine in which a particular symptom is reduced to a discrete identified or presumed underlying cause of pathological biological changes that are believed to correspond to the symptom pattern in question. Yet in mental illness there are no discrete causes, and few discrete symptom patterns recur with coherence in a predictable manner (Shanfield, 2004). In the phenomenal world of mental illness, symptom patterns are complex and change over time in relationship to different kinds of internal (biological and other) and external factors. Research studies frequently identify similar cognitive and affective symptom patterns in individuals diagnosed with *DSM-IV* disorders and normal, healthy individuals. These observations suggest that conceptualizing mental illness as a series of discrete disorders does not have construct validity. In other words, the core phenomenology of mental illness takes place at the level of symptom patterns and not coherent aggregates of symptoms that recur as discrete patterns or disorders. The definition of a "disorder" in psychiatry is based on the perceived clinical significance of symptoms in relationship to consensus-based thresholds of symptom severity or associated functional impairment below which there is no disorder, and above which a disorder is said to be present (Zimmerman, Chelminski, & Young, 2004). There is ongoing debate in academic psychiatry over the appropriate threshold values of criteria that correspond to the diagnosis of a disorder. A linear continuum of noncase, mild, moderate, serious, and severe pathology has been proposed as a model for describing the range of clinical pathology and appropriate diagnostic and treatment considerations for the psychiatric disorders currently included in the *DSM* (Regier, Narrow, & Rae, 2004). Findings from epidemiologic studies show considerable variation over time in core symptoms in individuals diagnosed with a particular psychiatric disorder, and significant interindividual variation in symptom type and severity for individuals diagnosed with the same disorder. These findings suggest that contemporary approaches in psychiatric classification are flawed, and imply that diagnostic criteria in current use do not accurately reflect the complex causes, conditions, or meanings associated with cognitive, affective, and behavioral symptoms. A more adequate descriptive model will take into account complex combinations of core symptoms in the context of dynamic internal and external factors that are highly variable over time within every patient and that are also variable between patients who report similar symptom patterns (Krueger, 1999). Factor analysis of observed patterns of psychiatric comorbidity from epidemiologic data suggests that certain core symptoms and their associated psychopathological processes underlie complex presentations of cognitive, affective, and behavioral symptoms. Prospective longitudinal studies show that symptom patterns observed in individuals diagnosed with major depressive disorder, panic disorder, social anxiety disorder, and other anxiety disorders lack stability over time (Angst 1996; Wittchen & Von Zerssen, 1987). Rather, a core symptom or symptom pattern generally changes over time along several axes. It has been suggested that core symptoms correspond to certain core psychopathological processes at one or more dynamic levels of psychological, neurobiological, informational, or possibly energetic functioning (Krueger, 1999; Krueger, Caspi, Moffitt, & Silva, 1998). The clinical chapters of this book develop the evidence for emerging nonconventional and integrative assessment and treatment approaches with respect to common patterns of cognitive, affective, and behavioral symptoms.

An emerging alternative to the *DSM* categorizes symptoms along a continuum from *normal* to *disturbed,* avoiding the need for classification of symptoms into discrete disorders that may lack construct validity (Shanfield, 2004). Genetics studies show that specific genes regulate activity in brain circuits associated with particular psychiatric symptoms, and that the neurobiological or genetic basis of a specified cognitive or affective symptom does not vary across different *DSM-IV* disorders in which the same symptom is present (Stahl, 2003a,b). This model is consistent with the observation that the same drug is often an effective treatment of similar symptoms when they occur in different disorders.

◆ Competing Perspectives in Psychiatry

At least four disparate perspectives about the nature and causes of mental illness are endorsed by contemporary Western psychiatry: disease, dimensional, behavioral, and life-story. This multiplicity of viewpoints has resulted in ongoing debate among conventionally trained psychiatrists about the treatments that are most appropriate for different symptoms (McHugh & Slavney, 1998). As discussed above, disparate perspectives of Western psychiatry rest on different implicit assumptions of the meanings or causal nature of mental and emotional symptom patterns. Each major perspective has practical implications for the use of assessment and treatment approaches. **Table 3–5** summarizes principal aspects of the four major perspectives of Western psychiatry.

The choice of a perspective from which to view human functioning largely depends on the intellectual preferences and training of the clinician. Psychiatrists are trained in the Western biomedical model and generally prefer to view psychopathology in the context of presumed underlying neurobiological abnormalities. In contrast, psychologists and other nonmedically trained mental health professionals typically prefer to approach psychopathology from more eclectic biological perspectives that take biological factors into account. Disparate perspectives are sometimes used in parallel, and their underlying assumptions are by no means mutually exclusive. Many

Table 3–5 The Perspectives of Western Psychiatry

Perspective	Implicit Assumptions	Practical Implications
Disease	Defining characteristics of mental illness are discrete abnormalities of brain structure or function.	Psychiatric diseases can be prevented or cured when underlying brain abnormalities are identified.
	Clear correspondences exist between etiology, pathological condition, and clinical entity	Treatments are pharmacologic agents that target presumed neurobiological substrates (psychopharmacology)
Dimensional	Mental illness occurs in individuals who are susceptible to distress because of their relative intellectual or emotional functioning on a quantitative scale of human psychological variation.	Causes of mental illness are the same stresses that affect all people, but result in cognitive or affective symptoms because of their relative level of intellectual or emotional functioning.
	There are no discrete mental illnesses, and patients experience different degrees or severities of symptoms depending on their relative position on the scale of variation	Distress and resulting symptoms are not "cured" but avoided.
		Treatment involves cognitive skills training to improve future coping strategies (cognitive-behavioral therapy, supportive psychotherapy)
Behavioral	Disordered behaviors result from excessive attempts to satisfy biological drives in response to cultural or social conditioning.	Mental or emotional symptoms are caused by inappropriate or excessive responses to universal physiological drives.
	Some "abnormal" behaviors result from psychiatric vulnerability in the context of anomalous early learning	Treatment entails psychological and medical approaches to prevent, improve, or interrupt abnormal behaviors (psychopharmacology and cognitive-behavioral therapy)
Life-story	Disturbing experiences result in distress and associated cognitive or affective symptoms that are subsequently incorporated into self-defeating "narratives"	Causes of mental illness are expectable responses to distressed states of mind that become fixed as narratives.
		Rescripting narratives in the context of supportive therapy will permit the patient to avoid disturbing future experiences (narrative therapy)

patients who take psychotropic meditations are concurrently in psychotherapy and regard both approaches as legitimate and effective. At present there is no consensus on a "best" perspective in Western psychiatry, but only diverse viewpoints that embody different biological or psychodynamic theories and their supporting evidence.

In more than 100 years since Sigmund Freud announced his original "project for a scientific psychology," a reliable method for verifying the neurophysiological correlates of cognitive or affective states has not been achieved. However, advances in genetics, pharmacology, and brain imaging have resulted in considerable empirical evidence supporting apparent correspondences between particular conscious or unconscious states and specific neurobiological processes or neural circuits. To date, the research evidence suggests the existence of indirect relationships between dysregulation at many complex levels of brain function or structure, and broad categories of symptoms. At this point in history, only the most basic mechanisms of brain function at the level of single neurons or systems of neurons in nonhuman animal models have been clearly explained. The enormous complexity of the brain, together with inherent constraints on the kinds of questions that can be addressed in contemporary brain research because of the limitations of available technologies and ethical constraints on research, continues to obscure efforts to elucidate basic mechanisms underlying the pathogenesis of cognitive, affective, and behavioral symptoms. Thus it is accurate to say that the goal of Freud's "project" has still not been achieved. Furthermore, it is unclear whether the broad goal of establishing causal relationships between putative discrete neurophysiological substrates and specified states of consciousness is potentially attainable or represents a productive approach to investigating the causes and characteristics of mental illness. Indeed, the question Freud originally posed more than 100 years ago, and which continues to guide contemporary research programs in psychiatry, makes an assumption that strict causal relationships exist between discrete neurophysiological substrates and specified normal mental processes and, by extension, specified cognitive, affective, and behavioral symptoms. In view of what is known about complex hierarchical relationships between cellular, synaptic, and modular components of the brain, the assumption of correspondences between discrete neurophysiological process and a specific mental state or symptom is at least naive and simplistic, and at worst irrelevant and misleading.

Different ways of thinking about brain function and the nature of consciousness have emerged since Freud's time. Perhaps the most widely embraced view at present is functionalism, one version of which postulates the existence of a corresponding specifiable brain state for any mental state. This view is essentially a contemporary restatement of Freud's idea, with the exception that correspondences are a priori assumed to exist. Functionalists would argue that the most rational, and therefore most probable, description of brain function requires the assumption that correspondences exist between discrete functional brain states and specified mental or emotional processes or experiences. In this view there is no compelling need to further verify claims of functional correspondences between brain states and mental states. Solutions to basic problems of the causes or meanings of mental illness will come from deeper understandings of human consciousness.

Cognitive Psychology and Hermeneutics Offer Alternative Explanatory Models of Mental Illness

In efforts to explain human consciousness, certain theories bypass the intrinsic limitations of empirical methods aimed at finding correspondences between presumed brain states and particular cognitive or affective states. Cognitive psychology and hermeneutics were advanced in the 20th century (Widdershoven, 1999) as methods for verifying the existence of normal or pathological states on the basis of observable behaviors or subjective reports of distress. Neither method requires the demonstration of strict correspondences between "normal" or "abnormal" brain processes and discrete mental states. Both approaches are rational in that they rely on the systematic use of logic to show meaningful relationships between phenomena, but neither approach requires verification of presumed brain states using conventional empirical means. Both methods can be used to make inferences about normal or pathological brain function, and both successfully avoid the intrinsic constraints (see discussion above) imposed by various empirical methods. It is important to briefly review the tenets of both cognitive psychology and hermeneutics to clarify differences between criteria used to show causes and effects of mental or emotional symptoms, and to consider the relevance of those differences for the structure of a conceptual framework of integrative medicine.

Cognitive Psychology as an Explanatory Model of Mental Illness

Different schools of cognitive psychology have proposed different models of normal mental states and symptom formation. A central idea of cognitive psychology is the claim that mental states or neural states can be understood as causes of actions or behaviors, and that mental and neural states that are causes cannot be reduced to each other. According to this model, irrational or pathological behavior is sometimes explained by conflicting cognitive "strategies" or incompatible behavioral rules resulting from systematic misrepresentations of percepts or situations. Stable cognitive frameworks are acquired through learning in which sensory input shapes neural circuits. Furthermore, those cognitive frameworks that are reinforced by consistent experiences will gradually become resistant to change, even when a framework results in systematic misrepresentations that are maladaptive for the individual.

On the basis of the preceding assumptions, cognitive therapy has the goal of correcting maladaptive strategies or rules, thus converting maladaptive cognitions or behaviors to more adaptive or useful strategies. According to the model, cognitive distortions, anxiety, depression, and other symptoms are manifestations of disruptive functioning due to rules that result in systematic misrepresentations. More adaptive rules are acquired through cognitive therapy, resulting in the gradual alleviation of pathological states. In this model, symptom formation is conceptualized and symptoms are treated on the basis of inferences about learned behaviors or cognitions. The cause of a symptom is a maladaptive psychodynamic process resulting in distorted beliefs or misrepresentations. Because of early learning influences, the patient makes systematic errors interpreting meanings of interactions with the environment. Empirical verification of physical causes is not relevant or necessary to an accurate understanding of psychopathology or its treatment. Therefore, there is no reference to presumed causal relationships between discrete neurobiological substrates and normal or abnormal cognitive or affective states.

Hermeneutics as an Explanatory Framework of Mental Illness

Hermeneutics was conceived by Martin Heidegger (1962) and developed by several philosophers, including Hans-Georg Gadamer (1960) and Maurice Merleau-Ponty (1962). Both hermeneutics and cognitive psychology hold that meaning is a central determinant of human beliefs and actions. However, in cognitive psychology, meaning is synonymous with cognitive representation, whereas in hermeneutics, meaning is constructed through an ongoing process of interpretation. Hermeneutics is a discursive process in which interpretation through shared dialogue transforms and clarifies meaning. This approach is used in sociology, anthropology, comparative literature, and other disciplines to demonstrate putative relationships between phenomena. Hermeneutics posits that there are no objective facts but only varying interpretations of the subjective meanings of information. The back-and-forth approach of hermeneutics results in successive levels of interpretation through the exchange of stories or narratives about different viewpoints or personal histories. The context or milieu in which a "hermeneutic circle" takes place is "pregiven" as historical tradition and shared cultural beliefs into which we are born. This milieu makes up our collective "preunderstandings." The narrative exchange of interpretations in the background of our preunderstandings eventually leads to useful interpretations of phenomena. In this process, preunderstandings, which are the premises of our worldview, also change. According to this model, progress in science takes place when novel shared meanings emerge through dialogue. Science is thus a social and political process. Hermeneutics is science-like in the sense that the process of comparing disparate interpretations of a particular phenomenon leads to reasonable shared understandings about explanations that are more meaningful or more useful in some sense. More useful explanations, in turn, have practical consequences for the carrying out of skillful actions within a particular discipline.

According to hermeneutics, pathological mental or emotional states occur when individuals fail to achieve interpretations of novel situations or information from the viewpoint of their preunderstandings. When a useful or adaptive interpretation is not successful, the individual experiences distress, which can be manifested as confusion, anxiety, depression, or other cognitive or affective symptoms. According to this view, symptoms result from distress that is experienced when an individual cannot find a way to reconcile his interpretation of a novel situation with his preunderstandings or worldview. The work of psychotherapy is to help the patient to develop a new shared dialogue (i.e., a more useful hermeneutic circle) that will eventually permit him to understand and contextualize novel situations in his existing worldview or to transform his worldview (i.e., the terms of his preunderstandings) to accommodate novel experiences.

Wide Acceptance of the Neurotransmitter Theory Has Delayed Exploration of Novel Paradigms in Western Psychiatry

Because of the absence of convincing and consistent findings, the view that there is a strict causal relationship between dysregulation of specific neurotransmitters and the pathogenesis of particular kinds of mental illness must be viewed as an interesting and crude hypothesis. It has nevertheless become widely accepted as a theory in Western medicine and popular culture in most developed countries. Many patients approach psychiatrists reporting that "my brain chemistry is out of balance.... I need a pill that can fix it...." The paucity of debate over competing conceptual explanatory models of mental illness is sustained by the view that the neurotransmitter theory is inherently correct, and provides a valid and adequate model of mental illness causation. The position of academic psychiatry is heavily influenced by the pharmaceutical industry, which has become the dominant and often sole funding source for studies on patented pharmaceutical products, while relatively few studies are done on natural products or other nonconventional treatments for which there is promising evidence.

The widely shared belief that psychopathology is caused by dysfunction at the level of neurotransmitter systems implicitly excludes consideration of other explanatory models (and treatment approaches) for which there is emerging clinical evidence. The neurotransmitter theory is essentially a self-perpetuating dogma that has been politicized by biomedical psychiatry with the support of the pharmaceutical industry as "the correct" conceptual framework within which contemporary Western psychiatry operates. For the most part, this belief restricts research to studies of only one kind of treatment (i.e., synthetic pharmaceuticals targeting a few discrete neurotransmitters or their respective receptors) based on a naive and simplistic model that remains unsubstantiated after decades of research and billions of dollars of funding at academic institutions and governmental research centers. In spite of these circumstances, the neurotransmitter theory continues to be accepted by psychiatrists and other Western-trained mental health practitioners as the dominant framework for understanding and treating mental illness.

The above factors have led to the current state of affairs in which other explanatory models of mental illness are dismissed before being seriously considered, although the strength of evidence for some alternative theories may place them on par with the neurotransmitter theory. The nonorthodox paradigms summarized in **Table 3–5** may provide future explanations of the causes of cognitive or affective symptoms, and, by extension, mechanisms of action involved when positive outcomes suggest that nonconventional treatments are effective. It is important to comment that the current dominant paradigm and many emerging alternative paradigms are not mutually exclusive. Viewing illness phenomena, especially mental illness, from a perspective that combines different paradigms may lead to deeper understandings of the causes, conditions, or meanings of symptoms, and, by extension, the mechanisms through which symptoms improve with treatment.

Advances in Basic Research Suggest Nonorthodox Paradigms Are Relevant to Psychiatry

In response to the limitations of Western medicine, in recent years alternative understandings of illness and healing have emerged in the context of nonconventional systems of medicine. Some nonconventional systems of medicine rest on metaphysical assumptions, whereas others include conventional

Table 3–6 Methods Used to Validate Nonconventional Assessment and Treatment Approaches in Mental Health Care

Method	Example	Comments
Linking evidence from emerging technologies to established biomedical technologies	Using technologies that purportedly measure the "human energy field" in conjunction with fMRI or other conventional functional imaging modalities	Consistent correlations of findings from emerging and established imaging technologies will provide clues to relationships between classical and nonclassical mechanisms in mental illness
Linking established conventional models of illness to nonconventional models of disease and healing	Analyzing outcomes from nonconventional treatments in the framework of one or more emerging paradigms (e.g., evaluating acupuncture using fMRI or other functional brain imaging); or using qEEG to monitor renormalization of brain function in relation to treatment response	Consistent correlations or predictable outcomes suggest postulated mechanism of action treatment approach is correct
Establishing objective criteria for significance of outcomes data or statistical requirements for validation of an assessment or treatment approach that is not susceptible to current science	Consensus within conventional or nonconventional medical communities over outcomes measures, trial design, and statistical power of data to conclude legitimacy of a particular "energy medicine" technique for a particular symptom pattern	This approach is frequently used to establish legitimacy for conventional medical practices for which there is incomplete empirical evidence for a putative underlying mechanism of action. The same approach can be applied to many nonconventional medical practices
Cooperative efforts between conventional and nonconventional medical practitioners to develop criteria for using nonconventional medical approaches in clinical settings when probable yields are high and probable risks are low	The NCCAM/NIH could promote development of cooperative efforts between conventionally and nonconventionally trained clinicians using nonconventional or integrative approaches in widespread practice, targeting specific mental illnesses	This approach is frequently used in conventional Western medicine in the absence of conclusive findings supporting a particular treatment. The issue here is safe, conservative practice guidelines for approaches addressing particular symptom patterns

fMRI, functional magnetic resonance imaging; NCCAM, National Center for Complementary and Alternative Medicine; NIH, National Institutes of Health; qEEG, quantitative electroencephalography

scientific assumptions about the nature of physical reality, time, space, and causality that are inherently at odds with popular beliefs about relationships between brain states and mental illness. One view argues that so-called subtle energies exist independently of the fine structure of the human central nervous system, and that irreducible energies somehow interact with physical brain structures to manifest as fundamental properties of consciousness, and therefore human experience in time and space. Metaphysical propositions underlying posited subtle energies are similar to the metaphysical concepts of some non-Western systems of medicine, including vital energies like qi and prana postulated by classical Chinese medicine and Ayurveda, respectively. Some writers interpret postulated nonphysical phenomena associated with mental functioning as ancient metaphors that describe properties of large-scale quantum field effects in complex living systems. The future validation of claimed subtle energies will require confirmation of the putative roles of both classical and nonclassical forms of energy or information discussed in previous sections.

Research in the basic sciences continues to result in the formulation of alternative explanatory models and novel understandings of the kinds of phenomena that make up the natural world. The existence of some postulated phenomena will eventually be empirically verified and shown to be related to mechanisms underlying illness and healing, and, by extension, to putative mechanisms of nonconventional assessment or treatment approaches. The existence of other postulated phenomena will eventually be refuted by a future science. Emerging paradigms in physics offer fundamentally new perspectives about the nature of space–time and causality. Novel approaches to validating claims of mechanisms of action in both conventional and nonconventional medicine will evolve from paradigms that are

currently outside of Western science. **Table 3–6** summarizes research directions that are being pursued to validate the putative mechanisms of nonconventional approaches used to assess or treat cognitive and affective symptoms.

◆ Conceptualizing Mental Illness

Overview

Contemporary biomedical psychiatry, like Western medicine in general, rests on a simplified form of Cartesian dualism that posits two fundamentally irreducible ontological categories: a physical brain and an embodied nonphysical mind. Models of consciousness whose assumptions are congruent with nonconventional medical practices diverge from the formal materialist theory of consciousness that is the basis of contemporary biomedical psychiatry. This has resulted in radical conceptual differences between the presumed role of consciousness in contemporary Western psychiatric treatments and the apparent role of consciousness in nonconventional psychiatric treatments.

Until now, Western scientific approaches have not been able to confirm or refute a theory of consciousness. Using only biological models as metaphors, contemporary scientific approaches to the study of consciousness have failed to confirm posited relationships between particular structural or functional aspects of the brain and specific states of consciousness. Indeed, different perspectives in neuroscience and artificial intelligence have led to a multiplicity of philosophical models of consciousness. Non-Western systems of medicine use nonmaterialist metaphors to frame understandings of consciousness, and have also failed to demonstrate correspondences between posited "energetic" phenomena and states of consciousness. To date, no perspective can claim a viable theory of consciousness that translates into practical methods for understanding or treating cognitive or affective symptoms. In fact, at present the problem is more basic than the refinement of research methods in hopes of identifying a postulated mechanistic basis of consciousness. Western science and non-scientific paradigms have so far come up with only vague suggestions about the kind of "thing" consciousness is, and to date there are no clear understandings, and few testable hypotheses, about putative biological, energetic, informational, or other phenomena that may somehow correspond to or cause different normal or abnormal conscious experiences.

Thinking about Mental or Emotional Symptoms Assumes a Contextual Theory of Consciousness

Implicit in any discussion of mental illness is a contextual theory of consciousness that frames understandings of cognitive or affective symptoms. Therefore, any argument on the validity or efficacy of a particular assessment or treatment approach in mental health care requires and assumes the analysis of causes or meanings of a symptom with respect to (an often implicit) theory of consciousness according to which that assessment or treatment approach is regarded as legitimate. Disparate systems of medicine incorporate disparate implicit models or metaphors of consciousness that reflect their core assumptions. The assumptions of any particular system of medicine are necessarily congruent with core assumptions of an implicit or explicit theory of consciousness, which, in turn, provides an explanatory model of the putative mechanisms of action of assessment or treatment approaches used in that system of medicine. Therefore, three factual conditions are always mutually reinforcing:

1. A particular system of medicine implies a theory of consciousness that must be congruent with that system of medicine.
2. Analysis of causes or meanings of symptoms can only take place in the context of a particular theory of consciousness.
3. Disparate theories of consciousness imply disparate explanatory models of psychopathology and, by extension, different legitimate assessment and treatment approaches.

Disparate systems of medicine use different metaphors of consciousness that define treatment outcomes in terms of desirable state changes in complex biological or "energetic" patterns that restore balance in some way, manifesting as clinical improvement. To the extent that consciousness must presumably be changed to achieve stable dynamic brain states that are therapeutic, influencing the characteristics or functions of consciousness is central to treating all cognitive or affective symptoms.

Models of Consciousness in Western Biomedicine Are Naive and Unsubstantiated

During the 20th century, models of consciousness evolved from Cartesian dualism carried over from a historically earlier period, to naive realism, to type–type and token–token identity theories, and finally to functionalist models, including most recently psychofunctionalism. The dominant model implicit in contemporary Western biomedical understandings of consciousness is a particular type of psychofunctionalism known as **computational functionalism**. This view can be described philosophically as a kind of naive identity theory, and is an unsubstantiated model that is often advanced in Western biomedicine as an explanation of the mind–body problem. According to this view, consciousness is a concept that describes "what the brain does," and the various functional properties (qualia) of consciousness are assumed to have token–token or type–type equivalence with empirically measurable neurochemical or biomagnetic events that take place at different microscopic or macroscopic levels of brain organization. In a similar fashion, naive versions of functionalism are often implicit in models of psychological or biological phenomena that attempt to explain illness and healing in the broad context of Western biomedicine. In contrast to these naive models, the **dynamic core hypothesis** of consciousness has recently emerged from the application of complexity theory to neuroscience (Tononi & Edelman, 1998). This hypothesis equates disparate conscious experiences with complex interactions among distributed groups of neurons.

The central propositions, advantages, and disadvantages of reductionist theories embedded in Western models of consciousness are listed in **Table 3–7**.

Divergent Theories of Consciousness Rest on Disparate Philosophical Assumptions

Materialist theories of consciousness are implicit in the philosophical and scientific foundations of Western biomedicine, though contemporary biomedicine does not formally develop or defend these views, which reduce mental phenomena to a presumed equivalence with entities (e.g., specific neurotransmitters and brain circuits) or physical processes (e.g., changes in activity of neurotransmitters, receptors, synapses, or neural circuits). Reductionist views of consciousness include identity theories and functionalism. These monistic theories are physicalist in viewpoint in that they posit the existence of only one fundamental kind of thing—the physical. Both functionalism and identity theories posit mental events as equivalent to identifiable physical processes in the brain. According to these views, words describing mental events are merely descriptions or "names" of processes, and there is no separate kind of corresponding mental "thing." Writers refer to different kinds of psychological or neurophysiological evidence to argue for these understandings, which are regarded in Western philosophy as mutually exclusive explanatory models of consciousness. Both direct and indirect evidence has been put forward in support of different versions of identity theory or functionalism as explanations of the relationships between consciousness and the body in health and illness. However, these models are generally not substantiated in discussions of the mind–body problem, but implicit in described mechanisms of healing and disease in the orthodox biomedical literature. The same vagueness has affected rigorous theorizing about normal and abnormal brain functioning in the domains of neuroscience and psychiatry.

In contrast to Western biomedicine, non-Western systems of medicine typically include implicit or formal views of consciousness that rest on dualist theories positing two fundamentally irreducible kinds of phenomena—the mental (or spiritual) and the physical—that interact in complex ways.

Table 3–7   Contemporary Western Theories of Consciousness Pertaining to Neurology and Psychiatry

Theory	Propositions	Advantages	Disadvantages
Type–type identity theory	*Mind* is identical with *brain*; therefore, mental phenomena are physical phenomena, and all aspects of brain function are purely physical. Each type of mental state is identical with a specific type of brain state	The mind–body problem is eliminated, as only physical states (body) are posited. Corresponds to Western psychiatric theories of mental illness and treatment resting on genetics and molecular biology, which assume type–type equivalence between brain states and mental phenomena. Current functional brain-imaging technologies are finding apparent correspondences between specific (healthy and pathological) brain states and specific mental phenomena	Requires exact verifiable correlations between specific mental states and specific brain states. This level of evidence is not possible using existing technologies. Accumulating research evidence (e.g., neural plasticity in post-stroke patients) supports the view that mental states are "multiply realized" or associated with multiple possible neurophysiological states. Cannot explain intentionality using a purely physicalist account of consciousness
Token–token identity theory	Every token or particular instance of a given type of mental state is identical with a token or particular instance of a given type of physical brain state	The mind–body problem is eliminated (see above). Neural plasticity in early development and post-CVA patients supports "multiple realized" mental states corresponding to many possible brain states. Assumes that mental states are "multiply realized"; thus repairs major weakness of type–type identity theory	Existing technologies are not able to demonstrate unvarying systematic equivalence between specific mental states and specific physical-spatial brain locations or processes. Therefore, token–token theories are inherently unverifiable. Does not avoid problem of "dualism of properties," as mental states must have corresponding mental properties. Not all brain states are identical with mental states (e.g., autonomic functions), and therefore many brain states are likely unrelated to consciousness
Metaphysical functionalism	Mind or consciousness is a function in which specific mental states can be adequately specified in formal terms of inputs, outputs, and relations to other mental states	Avoids the problem of agency in dualism. Avoids problem of verifying correspondences between mental states and brain states inherent in type–type identity theories	Does not attempt to reconcile posited brain functions with known neurophysiological processes, and is therefore not an empirical falsifiable theory
Psychofunctionalism	Materialist view that all mental functions are contained in many possible kinds of processes, including neurophysiological and cybernetic. Computational functionalism is a specific type of psychofunctionalism, which states that the mind is like a complex Turing machine in which functional elements are interrelated in complex hierarchical arrangements. Mental states are reduced to input–output functions of physical structures or states. The dynamic core hypothesis (Tononi & Edelman, 1998) is a recently proposed functionalist model that equates disparate conscious experiences with complex interactions among distributed groups of neurons	Avoids problems of dualism. Avoids paradox of behavior causality in that behaviors consist of "being in" a specified mental state (e.g., pain). Similar to token–token identity theory, in that mental states are multiply realized. Mental states are not restricted to human consciousness	Does not account for intentionality or subjectivity of many mental states, such as beliefs, attitudes, and desires (this is the problem of "absent qualia")

CVA, cerebrovascular accident

These nonphysicalist dualist models are inherently at odds with Western physicalist models and are generally regarded as a priori invalid (i.e., by Western science). On this basis, systems of medicine or particular modalities based on nonphysicalist dualist models are seldom subjected to rigorous inquiry in Western science. Dualist views introduce the problem of agency in non-Western models of consciousness. **Agency** refers to scientific and philosophical problems inherent in efforts to explain possible kinds of interactions between posited physical and nonphysical phenomena that manifest as the properties, or **qualia**, of consciousness. Contemporary Western monistic models avoid the problem of agency by positing that only physical brain processes exist, and these processes correspond to identifiable mental states. Therefore, there is no need to invoke agency in monistic models of consciousness.

Scientific Method Cannot Verify Western or Non-Western Models of Consciousness

The philosophical and scientific problem of agency according to which mental phenomena interact with physical objects or processes is avoided by monistic physicalist views like identity theories and functionalism, but remains a central problem for dualism and metaphysical monism, which postulate interactions and interrelationships between fundamentally different kinds of phenomena: the mental and the physical. Because of this basic difference, Western explanations of consciousness have historically emphasized empirical approaches to determining the behavioral or neurophysiological correlates of specific subjective or measurable experiences of consciousness (qualia). In contrast, non-Western explanations have continued to rely on metaphysical arguments postulating agency or nonphysical causation of mental or spiritual states. Neither kind of theory is potentially falsifiable using empirical means, as confirmation of the existence or absence of systematic correspondences between specified kinds of mental events and specified kinds of physical (or presumed metaphysical) processes cannot be demonstrated through measurement or observation. Attempts to do so have led to paradoxes of infinite causal chains of speculative neurobiological events (and therefore infinite regress) underlying brain processes or naive solutions such as the proposal of "super" or "sentient" neurons, which amount to neurophysiological variants of homunculus theories. Although technological approaches to studying the brain and its states (i.e., the expressions or correlates of consciousness) will continue to permit refinements in measurements of temporal, spatial, and energetic relationships between mental events and observable or experiential brain states, the complex nature of the system in time and space will continue to ensure absence of certainty as to the complete identities or properties of processes that are essential correlates of specific qualia. Therefore, neither current monistic physicalist views of Western biomedicine nor monistic metaphysical views of non-Western traditions are potentially empirically verifiable in the context of orthodox Western science.

Models of Consciousness Associated with Three Nonconventional Systems of Medicine

In contrast to Western biomedicine, non-Western systems of medicine contain implicit or formally elaborated nonreductionist no-physicalist models of consciousness. I have argued above that neither broad view of consciousness is verifiable using contemporary Western technologies in the context of scientific method, as attempts to do so lead to unsolvable problems or paradox. In spite of these philosophical and scientific issues, it is useful to consider representative professional nonconventional systems of medicine with the goal of clarifying their underlying metaphysical and empirical propositions. Core propositions underlying classical Chinese medicine, Ayurveda, and classical homeopathy are listed below.

Core Propositions of Ayurveda

◆ The physical body is a manifestation of mental tendencies carried from previous lives. The body is therefore the gross form of the mind.
◆ The body exists and allows the mind to perceive and act.
◆ The mind has a material structure—a set of observable energies and conditions.
◆ The mind is not physical matter but matter of a subtle nature—it is the most subtle form of matter.
◆ The brain is the physical organ through which the mind works.
◆ The mind is not limited to the physical apparatus of the brain.
◆ There are five levels of mind: higher self, inner consciousness, intelligence, sense mind, and ego.
◆ Chitta, the field of thought, is the level of consciousness.
◆ The human soul is the "true self," which is "pure awareness" that is linked with but not limited to the mind–body complex.
◆ There are three levels, or "primal qualities," of nature that underlie matter, life, and mind. These are Sattva (waking), Rajas (dreaming), and Tamas (deep sleep).
◆ The mind (consciousness) is the domain of Sattva.

Core Propositions of Chinese Medicine

◆ Qi is a primordial force in the universe that underlies all phenomena and determines all natural laws.
◆ Qi pervades all things manifesting as unity, continuity, and centeredness.
◆ Qi moves in a predictable patterned way, resulting in balance in nature.
◆ Qi is in balance in humans and other living and nonliving entities when it is sufficient in quantity and moves in a patterned rhythm.
◆ Many functioning constituents of qi interconnect in each entity as parts of the "cosmic whole."
◆ Body and mind are similar in kind but are different manifestations of qi.
◆ Reversible transformations of qi between body and mind manifest as disease or health, depending on the nature and direction of the transformation.
◆ Spirit (shen) is a category of qi manifested as energy on the mental plane.
◆ Imbalances of qi that affect shen can manifest in mental disturbances.

Core Propositions of Homeopathy

◆ An unseen, unified, and intelligent force organizes all natural phenomena.
◆ This fundamental force is equivalent to spirit, and is the source of life.
◆ Psychological, physiological, and cellular processes are interconnected manifestations of this unifying intelligent force.
◆ The same force manifests as health or illness, depending on its magnitude and state of balance between the environment and the body, and different internal organs.

◆ Mental and emotional attributes are manifestations of this force.

◆ Cognitive, emotional. and behavioral symptoms are manifestations of imbalances in this force.

◆ Substances that cause symptoms like those being treated (law of similars) stimulate self-healing through a "rebalancing" of this unifying intelligent force.

◆ Dilutions of substances are "succussed" to activate this force and thereby increase the potency and specificity of remedies.

Theories of Consciousness in Western and Non-Western Systems of Medicine Rest on Metaphysical Propositions

From a comparison of propositions in Western models of consciousness and major non-Western systems of medicine, it is evident that, although core propositions differ in content, they are similar in logical form. That is, core propositions in the principal world systems of medicine have in common the logical form of statements describing states of affairs or conditions of reality, and terms describing presumed relationships between these states of affairs. Neither Western nor non-Western systems of medicine contain core propositions that are empirically derived or, it has been argued, empirically verifiable. This is a significant observation with respect to the goal of determining degrees of philosophical congruence between diverse systems of medicine, and the related problem of compatibility on a theoretical and practical level when concepts or actual treatment approaches from diverse systems are combined in a single integrative treatment method.

◆ Implications of a Future Integrative Medicine for Mental Health Care

Following the above argument that the principal world systems of medicine and their derivative theories of consciousness share common metaphysical content and logical form, it is important to comment on the implications of similarities and differences between core propositions of these disparate systems for the future evolution of medicine. Congruence at the level of propositions is a measure of compatibility between disparate systems of medicine on a philosophical and possibly empirical level. Determining the types and degrees of compatibility between Western biomedicine and established non-Western systems of medicine is at the core of the debate over theoretical and practical problems in integrative medicine, which has as its major goal the development of a methodology for combining disparate approaches to optimize assessment accuracy and treatment outcomes. At present there is no rigorous methodology for achieving these goals. Relatively few integrative approaches in current use are empirically derived, much less scientifically substantiated. Therefore, a practical value of this work is elaboration of the philosophical and scientific constraints of a system of thought (i.e., propositions and their relationships) from which the methodology of a rigorous integrative medicine can be derived. Below I review arguments developed in Chapters 2 and 4 toward a truly integrative medicine that may eventually result in a synthesis of the underlying philosophical propositions of disparate systems of medicine.

Congruence between Disparate Systems of Medicine

◆ Western biomedicine rests on propositions that describe consciousness as reductionist and physicalist, whereas non-Western systems of medicine rest on propositions that describe relationships between a "universal force" and manifestations of this force as matter, consciousness, or other "natural" phenomena.

◆ Propositions underlying Western biomedicine contain metaphysical assumptions about correspondences between physical brain states and conscious (i.e., nonphysical) experience.

◆ Propositions underlying Ayurveda, Chinese medicine, and homeopathy contain metaphysical assumptions about "forces" or "energies" that manifest as physical and nonphysical phenomena, including consciousness.

◆ The propositions underlying Western biomedicine and non-Western systems of medicine are different in content but similar in logical form, in that all contain metaphysical statements of assumed states of affairs.

◆ The core propositions of models of consciousness implicit in Western biomedicine are therefore nonverifiable by scientific method using contemporary technologies.

◆ The core propositions of implicit models of consciousness in non-Western systems of medicine are similarly nonverifiable (i.e., using empirical means).

◆ Western biomedicine and non-Western systems of medicine are philosophically compatible systems of thought, as both rest on propositions that share the same kind of logical form, and both rest on metaphysical assumptions about the nature of consciousness and relationships between consciousness and physical states of affairs.

◆ Therefore, a basic kind of logical and philosophical congruence exists between Western biomedicine and non-Western systems of medicine with respect to shared metaphysical approaches in deriving models of consciousness and the nature of conscious states.

◆ Philosophical congruence of systems of medical thought that are divergent at the levels of theory and practical methods suggests compatibility between Western biomedicine and non-Western systems of medicine on a conceptual and possibly a methodological level.

◆ It is therefore philosophically defensible to consider practical empirical ways of integrating Western biomedicine and non-Western systems of medicine with the goal of establishing a broad, systematic logicophilosophical framework that will permit understanding conscious experiences in new ways, providing novel approaches to the assessment and treatment of "abnormal" conscious states (i.e., cognitive and affective symptoms).

A future integrative medicine will result from a synthesis of paradigms containing disparate interpretive models of the causes or meanings of symptoms. Different and more complete understandings of complex dynamic relationships between biological, somatic, energetic, informational, and possibly spiritual processes associated with symptom formation will lead to more effective integrative assessment and treatment approaches addressing causes or meanings of symptoms at multiple interrelated hierarchic levels. A future, more integrative perspective of Western medicine will lead to explanatory models of illness and healing that more adequately address both empirical and metaphysical assumptions implicit in contemporary Western science and non-Western systems of medicine. Increasing intellectual openness to nonconventional systems of medicine in Western cultures will result in the continuing evolution of conventional Western biomedicine toward a truly integrative medicine incorporating established reductionist and emerging nonreductionist understandings of relationships between consciousness, illness, and health. Research into nonconventional treatments that use intentionality, meditation, or prayer will elucidate the putative role of consciousness in health and healing. The future integrative clinician will judiciously use information from the patient's history, assessment findings, and outcomes to plan "multilevel" assessment and treatment strategies. New findings will lead to novel treatment approaches, and the ongoing biological, energetic, or informational assessment of outcomes will lead to progressively more accurate understandings of hierarchically related causes or meanings of a symptom pattern.

A general methodology for integrative medicine is developed in the following chapter. Methodologies for deriving integrative assessment and treatment approaches in mental health care are described in Chapters 5 and 6, respectively.

References

Abbot, N. C. (2000). Healing as a therapy for human disease: A systematic review. *Journal of Alternative and Complementary Medicine, 6*(2), 159–169.

American Psychiatric Association. (1980). *Diagnostic and statistical manual of mental disorders* (3rd ed.). Washington, DC: Author.

Angst, J. (1996). Comorbidity of mood disorders: A longitudinal prospective study. *British Journal of Psychiatry Supplementum, 30,* 31–37.

Astin, J., Harkness, E., Ernst, E. (2000). The efficacy of "Distant Healing": A systematic review of randomized trials. *Annals of Internal Medicine, 13*(11), 903–910.

Bell, I., Caspi, O., Schwartz, G., et al. (2002). Integrative medicine and systemic outcomes research. *Archives of Internal Medicine, 162,* 133–140.

Bland, J. (1999). New functional medicine paradigm: Dysfunctional intercellular communication. *International Journal of Integrative Medicine, 1*(4), 11–16.

Bohm, D. (1995). *Wholeness and the implicate order.* New York: Routledge.

Chen, K. W. (2004). An analytic review of studies on measuring effects of external QI in China: Review article. *Alternative Therapies in Health Medicine, 10*(4), 38–50.

Curtis, B., & Hurtak, J. (2004). Consciousness and quantum information processing: Uncovering the foundation for a medicine of light. *Journal of Alternative Complementary Medicine, 10*(1), 27–39.

Delgado, P. L., & Moreno, F. A. (2000). Role of norepinephrine in depression. *Journal of Clinical Psychiatry, 61*(Suppl. 1), 5–12.

Davidson, D. (2001). *Subjective, intersubjective, objective.* Oxford: Clarendon Press.

Dossey, L. (1982). *Space, time and medicine.* Boston: Shambala.

Duane, T. D., & Behrendt, T. (1965). Extrasensory electroencephalographic induction between identical twins. *Science, 150*(694), 367.

Edelman, G., & Mountcastle, V. (1978). *The mindful brain: Cortical organization and the group-selective theory of higher brain function.* Cambridge, MA: MIT Press.

Edmond, H. (2004, May). *Ethnicity, culture and psychopharmacology, Asian perspectives, Symposium 44: Culture, ethnicity, race and psychopharmacology—new research perspectives.* Paper presented at the annual meeting of the American Psychiatric Association, New York.

Federspil, G., & Vettor, R. (2000). Can scientific medicine incorporate alternative medicine? *Journal of Alternative Complementary Medicine, 6*(3), 241–244.

Gadamer, H. G. (1960). *Wahrheit und Methode: Grundzuge einer philosophischen Hermeneutik.* Tubingen: Mohr.

Gilbert, M. (2003). Weaving medicine back together: Mind–body medicine in the twenty-first century. *Journal of Alternative Complementary Medicine, 9*(4), 563–570.

Grinberg-Zylberbaum, J., Delaflor, M., & Goswami, A. (1994). The Einstein/Podolsky/Rosen paradox in the brain: The transferred potential. *Physics Essays, 7*(4), 422–428.

Grinberg-Zylberbaum, J., & Ramos, J. (1987). Patterns of interhemispheric correlation during human communication. *International Journal of Neuroscience, 36,* 41–53.

Hankey, A. (2004). Are we close to a theory of energy medicine? *Journal of Alternative and Complementary Medicine, 10,* 83–86.

Heidegger, M. (1962). *Being and time.* San Francisco: Harper.

Hyland, M. (2003). Extended network generalized entanglement theory: Therapeutic mechanisms, empirical predictions, and investigations. *Journal of Alternative Complementary Medicine, 9*(6), 919–936.

Jankovic, B. (1994). *Neuroimmodulation: The state of the art.* New York: New York Academy of Sciences.

Jobst, K. (1998). Toward integrated healthcare: Practical and philosophical issues at the heart of the integration of biomedical, complementary and alternative medicines [Editorial]. *Journal of Alternative and Complementary Medicine, 4*(2), 123–126.

Jonas, W., & Crawford, C. (Eds.). (2003). *Healing, intention and energy medicine: Science, research methods and clinical implications.* New York: Churchill Livingstone.

Kendler, K. (2001). A psychiatric dialogue on the mind–body problem. *American Journal of Psychiatry, 158*(7), 989–1000.

Krueger, R. (1999). The structure of common mental disorders. *Archives of General Psychiatry, 56,* 921–926.

Krueger, R., Caspi, A., Moffitt, T., & Silva, P. (1998). The structure and stability of common mental disorders (DSM-III-R): A longitudinal-epidemiological study. *Journal of Abnormal Psychology, 107,* 216–227.

Kuhn, T. (1970). *The structure of scientific revolutions* (2nd ed.). Chicago: University of Chicago Press.

Lawson, W. (2004, May). *Pharmacotherapy in African Americans, Symposium 44: Culture, ethnicity, race and psychopharmacology—new research perspectives.* Paper presented at the annual meeting of the American Psychiatric Association, New York.

Liboff, A. (2004). Toward an electromagnetic paradigm for biology and medicine. *Journal of Alternative and Complementary Medicine, 10*(1), 41–47.

Lin, K. (2004). *Ethnicity, pharmacogenetics and psychopharmacotherapy, Symposium 44: Culture, ethnicity, race and psychopharmacology—new research perspectives.* Paper presented at the annual meeting of the American Psychiatric Association, New York.

McCaffrey, A., Eisenberg, D., Legedza, A., Davis, R., & Phillips, R. (2004). Prayer for health concerns: Results of a national survey on prevalence and patterns of use. *Archives of International Medicine, 164,* 858–862.

McHugh, P. R. & Slavney, P. R. (1998). *The perspectives of psychiatry.* Baltimore: Johns Hopkins University Press.

Mercier, C., & King, S. (1994). A latent variable causal model of the quality of life and community tenure of psychotic patients. *Acta Psychiatrica Scandinavia, 89,* 72–77.

Merleau-Ponty, M. (1962). *Phenomenology of perception.* London: Routledge & Kegan Paul.

Miller, A. (2004, May). *Advances in psychopharmacology: Immune system pathology in psychiatric disease.* Paper presented at the annual meeting of the American Psychiatric Association, New York.

Miller, D. W. (2003). Homeodynamics in consciousness. *Advances in Mind–Body Medicne, 19*(3–4), 35–46.

Nemeroff, C., Kilts, C., & Berns, G. (1999). Functional brain imaging: Twenty-first century phrenology or psychobiological advance for the millennium? *American Journal of Psychiatry, 156*(5), 671–673.

Penrose, R. (1994). *Shadows of the mind: A search for the missing science of consciousness.* Oxford: Oxford University Press.

Pizzi, R. (2004, April). *Non-local correlation between human neural networks on printed circuit board.* Paper presented at the Tucson Conference on Consciousness, Tucson, AZ.

Pressman, M. (2004). Mind energetics: evolution and arrival. *Seminars in Integrative Medicine, 2,* 36–47.

Radin, D., Taft, R., & Yount, G. (2004). Effects of healing intention on cultured cells and truly random events. *Journal of Alternative and Complementary Medicine, 10*(1), 103–112.

Rasgon, N., Pumphrey, L., Prolo, P., et al. (2003). Emergent oscillations in mathematical model of the human menstrual cycle. *CNS Spectrums, 8*(11), 805–814.

Regier, D. A., Narrow, W. E., & Rae, D. S. (2004). For DSM-V, it's the "disorder threshold," stupid [Letter to the Editor]. *Archives of General Psychiatry, 61,* 1051.

Rein, G. (2004). Bioinformation within the biofield: Beyond bioelectromagnetics. *Journal of Alternative and Complementary Medicine, 10*(1), 59–68.

Rubik, B. (1996). Toward an emerging paradigm for biology and medicine. In *Life at the Edge of Science.* Oakland, CA: Institute for Frontier Science.

Rubik, B. (2000, July). *Electromagnetic and other subtle energies in Psi research.* Paper presented at the Esalen Invitational Conference, Big Sur, CA.

Schlitz, M., & Braud, W. (1997). Distant intentionality and healing: Assessing the evidence. *Alternative Therapies in Health and Medicine, 3*(6), 62–73.

Schuck, J. R., Chappell, L. T., & Kindness, G. (1997). Causal modeling and alternative medicine. *Alternative Therapies in Health and Medicine, 3*(2), 40–47.

Shanfield, S. (2004). *The dimensional construct in psychiatric disorders, Symposium 12: Behavioral dimensions of psychiatric disorders.* Paper presented at the annual meeting of the American Psychiatric Association, New York.

Shang, C. (2001). Emerging paradigms in mind–body medicine. *Journal of Alternative and Complementary Medicine, 7*(1), 83–91.

Sharma, H. (1997, May/June). Phytochemical synergism: Beyond the active ingredient model. *Alternative Therapies in Clinical Practice,* 91–96.

Shealy, C., & Myss, C. (1993). *The creation of health: The emotional, psychological, and spiritual responses that promote health and healing.* Walpole, NH: Stillpoint Publishing.

Snyder, S., & Ferris, C. (2000). Novel neurotransmitters and their neuropsychiatric relevance. *American Journal of Psychiatry, 157,* 1738–1751.

Stahl, S. (2003a). Deconstructing psychiatric disorders: Part I. Genotypes, symptom phenotypes, and endophenotypes. *Journal of Clinical Psychiatry, 64*(9), 982–983.

Stahl, S. (2003b). Deconstructing psychiatric disorders: Part 2. An emerging neurobiologically based therapeutic strategy for the modern psychopharmacologist. *Journal of Clinical Psychiatry, 64*(10), 1145–1146.

Standish, L. J., Johnson, L. C., Kozak, L., & Richards, T. (2001). *Neural energy transfer between human subjects at a distance.* Paper presented at Bridging Worlds and Filling Gaps in the Science of Healing, Kona, HI.

Standish, L. J., Johnson, L. C., Kozak, L., & Richards, T. (2003). Evidence of correlated functional magnetic resonance imaging signals between distant human brains. *Alternative Therapies in Health and Medicine, 9*(1), 122–125, 128.

Starfield, B. (2000). Is U.S. health really the best in the world? *Journal of the American Medical Association, 284*(4), 483–485.

Strogatz, S. (2001). Exploring complex networks. *Nature, 410,* 268–276.

Tataryn, D. (2002). Paradigms of health and disease: A framework for classifying and understanding complementary and alternative medicine. *Journal of Alternative and Complementary Medicine, 8*(6), 877–892.

Thaheld, F. (2000). Proposed experiment to determine if there are EPR nonlocal correlations between two neuron transistors. *Apeiron, 7,* 3–4, 202–205.

Tononi, G., & Edelman, G. (1998). Consciousness and complexity. *Science, 282,* 1846–1851.

Turner, R. P., Lukoff, D., Barnhouse, R. T., & Lu, F. G. (1995). Religious or spiritual problem: A culturally sensitive diagnostic category in the DSM-IV. *Journal of Nervous and Mental Disease, 183*(7), 435–444.

Wackermann, J. (2003). Dyadic correlations between brain functional states: Present facts and future perspectives. *Mind and Matter, 2*(1), 105–122.

Widdershoven, G. (1999). Cognitive psychology and hermeneutics: Two approaches to meaning and mental disorder. *Journal of Philosophy, Psychiatry, & Psychology, 6*(4), 245–253.

Wittchen, H., & Von Zerssen, D. (1987). *Verlaufe behandelter und unbehandelter Depressionen und Angst-storungen: eine klinisch-psychiatrische und epidemiologische verlaufsuntersuchung.* Berlin: Springer-Verlag.

Zahourek, R. P. (2004). Intentionality forms the matrix of healing: A theory. *Alternative Therapies in Health and Medicine, 10*(6), 40–49.

Zhan, C., & Miller, M. (2003). Excess length of stay, charges, and mortality attributable to medical injuries during hospitalization. *Journal of the American Medical Asscociation, 290,* 1868–1874.

Zimmerman, M., Chelminski, I., & Young, D. (2004). On the threshold of disorder: A study of the impact of the DSM-IV clinical significance criterion on diagnosing depressive and anxiety disorders in clinical practice. *Journal of Clinical Psychiatry, 65,* 1400–1405.

General References

Achinstein, P. (2001). *The book of evidence.* Oxford: Oxford University Press.

Albert, D. (1994). *Quantum mechanics and experience.* Cambridge, MA: Harvard University Press.

Ashton, H. (1992). *Brain function and psychotropic drugs.* Oxford: Oxford University Press.

Auyang, S. (1998). *Foundations of complex-system theories in economics, evolutionary biology, and statistical physics.* Cambridge: Cambridge University Press.

Beakley, B., & Ludlow, P. (Eds.). (1992). *The philosophy of mind: Classical problems, contemporary issues.* Cambridge, MA: MIT Press.

Bohm, D., & Peat, D. (2000). *Science, order and creativity* (2nd ed.). New York: Routledge.

Bolton, D., & Hill, J. (2003). *Mind, meaning, and mental disorder: The nature of causal explanation in psychology and psychiatry* (2nd ed.). Oxford: Oxford University Press.

Boss, M. (1994). *Existential foundations of medicine and psychology.* Northvale, NJ: Jason Aronson.

Brown, H., & Harre, R. (Eds.) (2001). *Philosophical foundations of quantum field theory.* Oxford: Clarendon Press.

Cartwright, N. (1999). *The dappled world: A study of the boundaries of science.* Cambridge: Cambridge University Press.

Casti, J. (1990). *Paradigms lost: Tackling the unanswered mysteries of modern science.* New York: Avon Books.

Conrad, L., Neve, M., Nutton, V., Porter, R., & Wear, A. (1995). *The Western medical tradition: 800 BC to AD 1800.* Cambridge: Cambridge University Press.

Dalal, A. (Ed.). (2001). *A greater psychology: An introduction to the psychological thought of Sri Aurobindo.* New York: Tarcher/Putnam.

Dethlefsen, T., & Dahlke, R. (1990). *The healing power of illness: The meaning of symptoms and how to interpret them.* Dorset, England: Element Books.

Dossey, L. (1991). *Meaning and medicine: Lessons from a doctor's tales of breakthrough and healing.* New York: Bantam Books.

Dossey, L. (1999). *Reinventing medicine: Beyond mind–body to a new era of healing.* San Francisco: Harper San Francisco.

Elitzur, A., Dolev, S., & Kolenda, N. (Eds.). (2005). *Quo vadis quantum mechanics?* New York and Berlin: Springer.

Fabrega, H. (1997). *Evolution of sickness and healing.* Berkeley: University of California Press.

Gallagheer, S., & Shear, J. (Eds.). (1999). *Models of the self.* San Diego: Imprint Academic.

Goldstein, M., & Goldstein, I. (1979). *How we know: An exploration of the scientific process.* New York: Da Capo Press.

Good, B. (1994*). Medicine, rationality, and experience: An anthropological perspective.* Cambridge: Cambridge University Press.

Griffin, D. (1997). *Parapsychology, philosophy, and spirituality: A post-modern exploration.* Albany: State University of New York Press.

Grof, S. (1985). *Beyond the brain: Birth, death and transcendence in psychotherapy.* Albany: State University of New York Press.

Hahn, R. (1995). *Sickness and healing: An anthropological perspective.* New Have, CT: Yale University Press.

Hart, T., Nelson, P., & Phuakka, K. (Eds.). (2000). *Transpersonal knowing: Exploring the horizon of consciousness.* Albany: State University of New York Press.

Healy, D. (2002). *The creation of psychopharmacology.* Cambridge, MA: Harvard University Press.

Heisenberg, W. (1999). *Physics and philosophy: The revolution in modern science.* Amherst, NY: Prometheus Books.

Holland, J. (1998). *Emergence: From chaos to order.* Cambridge, MA: Perseus Books.

Horgan, J. (1996). *The end of science: Facing the limits of knowledge in the twilight of the scientific age.* New York: Broadway Books.

Hundert, E. (1990). *Philosophy, psychiatry and neuroscience—three approaches to the mind: A synthetic analysis of the varieties of human experience.* Oxford: Clarendon Press.

Jibu, M., & Yasue, K. (1995). Quantum brain dynamics and consciousness: An introduction. In M. Stamenov & G. Globus (Eds.), *Advances in consciousness research* (Vol. 3). Philadelphia: John Benjamin.

Kaku, M. (1997). *Visions: How science will revolutionize the 21st century.* New York: Anchor Books Doubleday.

Kass, L. *Beyond Therapy: Biotechnology and the pursuit of happiness, a report by the President's Council on Bioethics.* (2003). New York: Regan Books.

Kiev, A. (Ed.). (1996). *Magic, faith, and healing.* Northvale, NJ: Jason Aronson.

Kleinman, A. (1988). *Rethinking psychiatry: From cultural category to personal experience.* New York: The Free Press.

Kuhn, T. (1977). *The essential tension: Selected studies in scientific tradition and change.* Chicago: University of Chicago Press.

Kuriyama, S. (1999). *The expressiveness of the body and the divergence of Greek and Chinese medicine.* New York: Zone Books.

Lewontin, R., Rose, S., & Kamin, L. (1984). *Not in our genes: Biology, ideology, and human nature.* New York: Pantheon Books.

Lloyd, G. (1996). *Adversaries and authorities: Investigations into ancient Greek and Chinese science.* Cambridge: Cambridge University Press.

Lockwood, M. (1989). *Mind, brain & the quantum: The compound "I."* Cambridge, MA: Blackwell Publishers.

Lorimer, D. (2004). *Science, consciousness and ultimate reality*. Exeter, England: Imprint Academic.

Margolis, H. (1993). *Paradigms and barriers: How habits of mind govern scientific beliefs*. Chicago: University of Chicago Press.

McEvilley, T. (2002). *The shape of ancient thought: Comparative studies in Greek and Indian philosophies*. New York: Allworth Press.

McHugh, P., & Slavney, P. (1998). *The perspectives of psychiatry* (2nd ed.). Baltimore: Johns Hopkins University Press.

Micale, M. (Ed.). (1993). *Beyond the unconscious: Essays of Henri F. Ellenberger in the history of psychiatry*. Princeton, NJ: Princeton University Press.

Morowitz, H., & Singer, J. (Eds.). (1995). The mind, the brain, and complex adaptive systems. In *Proceedings of the Santa Fe Institute studies in the sciences of complexity* (Vol. 22). Menlo Park, CA: Addison-Wesley.

Nadeau, R., & Kafatos, M. (1999). *The non-local universe: The new physics and matters of the mind*. Oxford: Oxford University Press.

Petitot, J., Varela, F., Pachoud, B., & Roy, J. (Eds.). (1999). *Naturalizing phenomenology: Issues in contemporary phenomenology and cognitive science*. Stanford, CA: Stanford University Press.

Pickering, A. (1995). *The mangle of practice: Time, agency, and science*. Chicago: University of Chicago Press.

Pico, R. (2002). *Consciousness in four dimensions: Biological relativity and the origins of thought*. New York: McGraw-Hill.

Rescher, N. (1999). *The limits of science*. Pittsburgh, PA: University of Pittsburgh Press.

Rosenthal, D. (1991). *The nature of mind*. Oxford: Oxford University Press.

Rubik, B. (Ed.). (1989). *The interrelationship between mind and matter*. Paper presented at a conference hosted by the Center for Frontier Sciences, Philadelphia.

Rubik, B. (1996). *Life at the edge of science: An anthology of papers by Beverly Rubik*. Oakland, CA: Institute for Frontier Sciences.

Salthe, S. (1985). *Evolving hierarchical systems: Their structure and representation*. New York: Columbia University Press.

Schwartz, G., & Russek, L. (1999). *The living energy universe: A fundamental discovery that transforms science and medicine*. Charlottesville, VA: Hampton Roads.

Stapp, H. (1993). *Mind, matter, and quantum mechanics*. Berlin: Springer-Verlag.

Stone, M. (1997). *Healing the mind: A history of psychiatry from antiquity to the present*. New York: W. W. Norton.

Talbot, M. (1999). *The holographic universe*. New York: HarperCollins.

Thagard, P. (1992). *Conceptual revolutions*. Princeton, NJ: Princeton University Press.

Tiller, W. (1997). *Science and human transformation: Subtle energies, intentionality and consciousness*. Walnut Creek, CA: Pavior Publishing.

Tseng, W., & Streltzer, J. (Eds.). (1997). *Culture and psychopathology: A guide to clinical assessment*. New York: Brunner-Mazel.

Valle, R., & von Eckartsberg, R. (Eds.). (1989). *Metaphors of consciousness*. New York: Plenum Press.

Van Loocke, P. (Ed.). (2000). The physical nature of consciousness. In M. Stamenov (Ed.), *Advances in consciousness research* (Vol. 29). Philadelphia: John Benjamin.

Velmans, M. (2000). *Understanding consciousness*. Philadelphia: Routledge.

Wallace, B. (2003). *Choosing reality: A Buddhist view of physics and the mind*. Ithaca, NY: Snow Lion Publications.

Wallace, B. (Ed.). (2003). *Buddhism and science: Breaking new ground*. New York: Columbia University Press.

Welton, D. (Ed.). (1999). *The body: Classic and contemporary readings*. Oxford: Blackwell.

Wider, K. (1997). *The bodily nature of consciousness: Sartre and contemporary philosophy of mind*. Ithaca, NY: Cornell University Press.

Wilber, K. (2000). *Integral psychology: Consciousness, spirit, psychology, therapy*. Boston: Shambhala.

Wilber, K. (2001). *Quantum questions: Mystical writings of the world's greatest physicists*. Boston: Shambala.

Williams, R. (1998). *Biochemical individuality: The basis for the genetotrophic concept*. New Canaan, CT: Keats Publishing.

Wright, J., & Potter, P. (2003). *Psyche and soma: Physicians and metaphysicians on the mind–body problem from antiquity to enlightenment*. Oxford: Clarendon Press.

Yasue, K., Jibu, M., & Senta, T. (2001). No matter, never mind: Proceedings of Toward a Science of Consciousness—fundamental approaches. In *Advances in consciousness research* (Vol. 13). Philadelphia: John Benjamins.

4

Foundations of Clinical Methodology in Integrative Medicine

Ideally, a conceptual framework for integrative medicine will provide a new language for describing illness and health in a more complete way, taking into account phenomena that are not adequately addressed in the languages and paradigms of many established systems of medicine. This framework will result in a new methodology for planning integrative assessment and treatment strategies addressing psychological, cultural, biological, energy-informational, and possibly spiritual causes or meanings of medical and psychiatric symptoms. To be of practical value, a conceptual framework underlying a methodology for integrative medicine must translate into accurate statements about the validity of theoretical claims and the effectiveness of clinical approaches. The methodology will permit the elaboration of clinical methods for combining particular assessment or treatment approaches into integrative strategies that effectively address a specified symptom pattern.

The premises underlying methodologies in medicine addressed in this book are generally implicit in philosophical assumptions embedded in the cultural background. Assumptions underlying methodologies in disparate systems of medicine reflect ways of seeing that are a priori accepted in disparate cultures or intellectual traditions. Because of their divergent cultural origins and disparate premises, methodologies embody implicit truth claims pertaining to the efficacy of clinical approaches used in the parent system of medicine. In other words, beliefs about the efficacy of a particular modality necessarily follow from core assumptions implicit in a particular system of medicine. Thus disparate clinical approaches cannot be evaluated using objective means alone, and many systems of medicine regard the formal validation of assumptions underlying methods as irrelevant or unnecessary. Consequently, many systems of medicine do not have strict requirements for empirical methods (or other "objective" approaches) that demonstrate the existence of a putative mechanism of action or verify claimed outcomes of a modality because the truth of a claim that a mechanism of action is present or that an outcome takes place is implicit within the conceptual framework that embodies the system of medicine. The conceptual frameworks of many systems of medicine, including, for example, Chinese medicine, Tibetan medicine, and Ayurveda, lead to unquestioned acceptance of truth claims pertaining to assessment and treatment approaches among professionally trained practitioners in those systems of medicine. These issues must be taken into account when practical integrative methods incorporate non-Western systems of medicine.

The principal work of this chapter is the establishment of a methodology for deriving practical clinical methods in integrative medicine. Methodologies for constructing specific integrative assessment and treatment plans addressing common cognitive, affective, and behavioral symptoms are developed in Chapter 5, History Taking, Assessment, and Formulation in Integrative Mental Health Care. The initial problem that must be addressed is the development of a methodology and elaboration of criteria for verifying the existence and operation of a putative mechanism of action and confirming claims that a particular assessment or treatment modality has beneficial outcomes with respect to a specified symptom. I argue in this chapter that current research methodologies employed by Western biomedicine are not appropriate tools for examining putative mechanisms of action underlying some nonconventional modalities. In other words, the truth claims of some nonconventional modalities cannot potentially be falsified or verified by current Western science (Dossey, 1995). It is interesting that the same argument applies to certain clinical approaches in widespread use in conventional Western medicine. Mechanisms of action underlying many contemporary Western medical treatments have not been verified by empirical means, yet these approaches continue in widespread use through professional consensus. An example is the use of certain antiseizure medications to treat cyclic mood changes associated with bipolar disorder in spite of the absence of compelling evidence and the lack of approval by the U.S. Food and Drug Administration for these clinical uses. In view of such cases, it is arguable that Western medicine does not always substantiate modalities in current use on the basis of its own "gold standards" of evidence.

In the practice of medicine, there are no universal criteria for verifying that a putative mechanism of action exists or that a treatment is effective with respect to a specified symptom. Blinding and the use of placebos to determine whether outcomes are related to treatment effects are relatively recent innovations, and rest on different assumptions when used in biomedicine and many nonconventional systems of medicine (Ernst & Resch, 1996). Beliefs about the effectiveness of a particular clinical approach in medicine have as much to do with professional consensus and economic factors as with rigorous methodologies for assessing empirical evidence of efficacy or effectiveness. Considerable interest has recently focused on "evidence-based medicine" in response to the ambiguous status of "evidence" in conventional Western medicine.

◆ Overview

The development of a sound methodology for integrating biomedical and nonconventional modalities requires the solution of both conceptual and practical problems. Basic philosophical issues and paradigms in medicine were addressed in Chapters 2, Philosophical Problems, and 3, Paradigms in Medicine, Psychiatry, and Integrative Medicine. An ontology of phenomena associated with illness or health and a typology of legitimate medical practices, that is, practices for which empirically testable truth claims can be made, were established. Different understandings of the meaning and role of evidence in verifying claims of a putative mechanism of action or a reported outcome were reviewed. A framework for a hierarchy of evidence was established for comparing disparate modalities on the basis of empirical and subjective criteria. The hierarchy of evidence provides a framework for developing practical integrative strategies in the symptom-focused chapters of Part II. Planning integrative health care involves making clinical decisions on the basis of the highest level of both quantitative and qualitative evidence, keeping in mind patient preferences, values, available medical resources, and other practical constraints. All methodologies used to rank information as evidence assume that certain ways of knowing are more valid than others. As discussed in Chapter 2, the validity of a particular epistemological approach rests on assumptions about kinds of phenomena that can have existence. This is always and necessarily true because assumptions about extant phenomena implicitly bias methodologies used to ascertain existence. In other words, methodologies used to verify claims of outcomes rest on mutually reinforcing epistemological and ontological assumptions. Because of this, a particular methodology of evidence ranking will continue in use when underlying epistemological and ontological assumptions are mutually reinforcing systems of thought.

In sum, there can be no single methodology for assessing evidence obtained within any system of medicine, and there can be no value-neutral way to ascertain a best or most valid methodology. There are only different methodologies that continue to evolve and provide different ways of seeing for practitioners trained in disparate systems of medicine. It is instructive to characterize evidence-ranking methodologies with respect to the theoretical or practical goals of assessing or using evidence, and differences between kinds of information regarded as evidence. With these concepts in mind, a methodology is adduced with the goal of constructing evidence tables for practical use in planning clinical integrative methods in mental health care.

This chapter is organized into two main parts. In the first, a conceptual framework is established for the integration of conventional and nonconventional medical practices. Considerations of kinds and levels of evidence for determining when to include disparate modalities are addressed. The methodology derived is based on the general logical-philosophical framework adduced in Chapter 2 for categorizing conventional and nonconventional modalities according to differences in the verifiability of the existence of putative mechanisms of action or the truth of claims of effectiveness. The resulting truth table provides the schema for a hierarchy of levels and kinds of evidence for both conventional and nonconventional modalities while avoiding biases inherent in evidence-based medicine (EBM) that a priori exclude many nonconventional modalities. Measures of rigor and relevance are used to assess quantitative and qualitative evidence supporting claims of outcomes when nonconventional modalities are used. Using this approach, disparate nonconventional modalities can be mapped onto a general hierarchy of evidence. Constructing the evidence tables is a necessary first step in systematically organizing evidence pertaining to nonconventional assessment or treatment modalities used in the management of cognitive, affective, or behavioral symptoms.

In Part II of this book, contents of the evidence tables are simplified into three general categories: approaches that are substantiated, approaches that are provisional, and approaches that are possibly effective. (Note: Although some nonconventional modalities have been refuted on the basis of compelling negative evidence, such approaches are generally not in current use and are therefore not discussed in Part II.) I argue that it is not useful to describe a particular assessment or treatment modality as substantiated or provisional in general, but only with respect to a specified symptom pattern. This is necessarily true because a particular modality may be demonstrably effective as a treatment of a specified symptom but have questionable efficacy with respect to a different symptom pattern. Substantiated modalities are those assessment or treatment approaches for which there is compelling evidence that use of the approach reliably enhances the accuracy or specificity of assessment findings, or improves treatment outcomes with respect to a specified cognitive, affective, or behavioral symptom. Substantiated modalities rest on compelling positive evidence from rigorously controlled studies, provisional modalities are based on strong evidence from research and clinical observations, and modalities designated as possibly effective rest on limited or inconsistent research and clinical evidence. Criteria used to designate a particular modality as substantiated, provisional, or possibly effective with respect to a specified symptom are determined by both quantitative and qualitative approaches used to evaluate claims of outcomes. Conventional and nonconventional modalities fall into three general classes: empirically derived, consensus-based, and intuitive. By definition, the evaluation of empirically derived modalities requires the assessment of empirical evidence. In contrast, the validation of modalities that are perpetuated through professional consensus or are based on intuition does not rely on rigorous demonstrations of empirical evidence. In other words, modalities that are maintained through consensus, which comprise the majority of conventional and nonconventional assessment and treatment

approaches in current use, are frequently endorsed by a professional medical society in the absence of compelling empirical evidence. Most consensus-based clinical methods will probably eventually qualify as provisional, some will likely become substantiated by compelling evidence, and others will be viewed as possibly effective because of inconsistent findings. By definition, intuitive clinical medical approaches are not susceptible to analysis or verification using available empirical methods. At the present time in the history of medicine, representative intuitive approaches are Healing Touch, Reiki, qigong, and other so-called energy medicine techniques. Analogous to the evolution of consensus-based approaches, some intuitive modalities will probably eventually be designated as substantiated or provisional on the basis of future advances in basic science or medical theory that will make it possible to verify the existence of putative "energetic" mechanisms of action in empirical terms. Emerging technologies may also permit the future verification of claimed beneficial "energetic" effects of prayer or healing intention on human physiology or consciousness.

The evidence tables provide a conceptual framework for thinking about reasonable choices in integrative medical management. Following considerations of levels of evidence, the next methodological problem is the determination of degrees of compatibility between disparate kinds of clinical approaches that are candidates for integration. A multifactorial approach is developed that takes into account evidence of compatibility or synergy between disparate approaches as well as safety, economic issues, availability, and patient preferences. The problem of determining when to use a clinical approach for which there is little or no compelling evidence of effectiveness is addressed. The first part of this chapter concludes with a general discussion of the concept of algorithms for planning integrative health care using the above methodology. Algorithms provide the logical framework for planning optimum integrative medical care with respect to identified core symptoms. The chapters in Part II of this book use the basic methodology developed in this chapter to construct symptom-focused integrative medical strategies targeting common cognitive, affective and behavioral symptoms.

In the second part of this chapter, a methodology is established for identifying and obtaining clinically pertinent information about assessment and treatment modalities that are candidates for integrative management plans. A methodology is put forward for identifying and extracting information from reliable resources including medical databases, nonindexed journals, conference proceedings, professional association guidelines, and expert interviews. Information obtained using this methodology provides the clinical content for the evidence tables used in Part II. Limitations of methodology are identified and suggestions are offered for future improvements in literature research methods.

◆ Methodology in Integrative Medicine

The term **methodology** can refer to two kinds of conceptual operations. In its broadest sense, *methodology* refers to a general kind of analytical approach to solving problems based on the application of rules. In a narrow sense, a methodology is a specified set of rules addressing a defined problem. A rule is a proposition that defines what kinds of things exist and how extant things can be verified or categorized. Rules are ultimately determined through consensus on ontological categories of phenomena and epistemological approaches to verifying the existence or characteristics of those phenomena. Opinions that contribute to consensus agreements about rules generally come from scholars who have expertise in a particular discipline, for example, a particular system of medicine. Therefore, methodology is often determined through expert consensus to the extent that it is rule-governed. The rules of a particular methodological approach in medicine or any other system of thought can be rational, nonrational, or both rational and nonrational. Rational rules include analytical tests that verify the existence of putative phenomena or characterize relationships between phenomena. The parameters and goals of analytical tests are expressions of premises about phenomenal reality embedded in disparate systems of medicine. The result is that tests considered analytical and based on rational analysis in one system of medicine are sometimes viewed as subjective and nonrational by practitioners of a disparate system of medicine. Nonrational rules include propositions that define subjective criteria incorporated in a specified methodology used to establish the existence or properties of phenomena. This state of affairs is further complicated by the fact that the same medical practice can be interpreted as rational or nonrational, analytic or subjective, depending on the perspective from which it is viewed. For example, conventionally trained Western physicians view pulse taking in Chinese medicine as completely subjective, whereas Chinese medical practitioners assert that they are following a prescribed systematic methodology that permits identification of objective energetic imbalances. The Western physician claims to measure and identify phenomena in themselves. In contrast, the Chinese medical practitioner claims to measure and identify phenomena with respect to his or her subjective energetic state. Western biomedicine asserts the validity of strictly analytical methodologies for obtaining objective data using empirical means, whereas Chinese medicine and other nonconventional systems of medicine claim validity of a methodology that combines analytical and intuitive means to obtain both objective and subjective information about a patient in relation to the practitioner.

Clearly, the meanings of **rational** and **intuitive** are defined relative to the conceptual framework of the system of medicine from which a particular medical approach is evaluated. Historically, in Western philosophy reality was assumed to be material, and "process" was derivative of phenomena that were reducible to certain fundamental material states of existence. Therefore, assumptions about primary categories of existence led to assumptions about ways to show the truth of claims about relationships between material states (effects) and other (dynamic) material states (causes). This eventually led to scientific method, which was already implicit in assumptions of Western philosophy. In contrast, in Asian philosophical systems, including Taoism and Buddhism, the primary categories of existence were believed to be energy and dynamic processes involving energy. In this philosophical model, material existence is interpreted as a particular manifestation of energetic processes or their interactions. Implicit in these assumptions was the assertion that energy states exist, are knowable, and can be accurately reported by patients or observed by clinicians. Therefore, in Asian systems of medicine, criteria used to establish the reality of a symptom were entirely subjective, and there was no requirement or possibility for developing a reductionist methodology that could trace phenomena back to presumed primary material causes. According to this view, the truth of

claims of energetic conditions is given, and there is no need to (indeed, it would be construed as irrelevant or nonsensical) to construct philosophical or empirical arguments about energetic phenomena as these are factual states of affairs implicit in the assumptions of Asian philosophy. Thus questions pertaining to empirical methods for verifying a putative mechanism or a claimed outcome are not relevant. The assumptions underlying any methodology are implicit in the philosophical structure of the system of medicine from which the methodology originates. For this reason there is no perceived need to "defend" a methodology, that is, when the assumptions of a particular system of medicine are accepted as a priori true, the assumptions underlying its methodology will also be regarded as a priori true, and the methodology will be accepted as valid.

In sum, distinctions between rational/analytical and nonrational/intuitive methodologies cannot be made with respect to disparate systems of medicine for the reason that a methodology that is regarded as rational and analytical in one system of medicine may be regarded as nonrational and intuitive in another. Comparative remarks about analytical versus intuitive or rational versus nonrational methodologies can therefore be made only from the relative perspective of a particular system of medicine. It is necessary to conclude that any methodology cannot be categorically described as rational or nonrational. This will always be true because any particular clinical approach can only be described as rational or nonrational, analytical or intuitive with respect to criteria employed in a particular system of medicine for validating a methodology or verifying outcomes according to that methodology.

The Absence of a Methodology in Integrative Medicine: Causes and Consequences

The term **integrative medicine** has been in widespread use for many years. However, until now, there has been no coherent theory of integration, nor has a practical clinical methodology for combining disparate approaches been advanced. Most writing on integrative medicine emphasizes research on mechanisms of action underlying nonconventional medical modalities as examined from the viewpoint of contemporary biomedicine. To date, rigorous attempts have not been made to establish a theory- or value-neutral methodology for appraising disparate systems of medicine starting from a philosophical analysis of core assumptions. A consequence has been the increasingly critical regard or outright dismissal of nonconventional systems of medicine or specific nonconventional medical approaches by Western biomedicine in the name of science. In spite of the fact that these opinions frequently lack empirical evidence, orthodox Western medicine remains strongly biased against the majority of nonconventional medical theories and approaches. A consequence has been the absence of a systematic program to examine nonconventional theories of health and illness in contexts where investigators are not inherently biased against those theories. In recent years research sponsored by the National Center for Complementary and Alternative Medicine (NCCAM) of the National Institutes of Health (NIH) has been conducted in many areas of nonconventional medicine. However, most NIH-sponsored studies are conducted in academic medical centers, follow conventional biomedical methodologies to examine nonconventional approaches, and have the stated goal of abstracting the active ingredient or identifying a central therapeutic mechanism of action.

The methodology used in conventional biomedical research to evaluate nonconventional modalities fails to address conceptual problems posed by fundamental differences between core assumptions of particular nonconventional systems of medicine and contemporary biomedicine. In other words, no consideration is given to the problem of how to objectively validate research methods, and there is a presumption that contemporary biomedicine provides valid and adequate ways to evaluate putative mechanisms of action and test efficacy claims of any particular nonconventional medical approach. Therefore, many NCCAM-sponsored studies represent efforts to evaluate nonconventional medical theories and clinical approaches in the context of contemporary theories and traditions of Western biomedicine that are implicitly at odds with the claims of a putative mechanism of action or efficacy of many nonconventional assessment and treatment approaches. When a biomedical research methodology is used, some nonconventional medical approaches are found to work, and others are judged ineffective. Those approaches that are phenomenologically close to contemporary biomedicine in terms of similarities between putative mechanisms, and for which current biomedical techniques can measure claimed effects, are verified by biomedical research methods and found to be effective. In contrast, those nonconventional medical approaches resting on (phenomenologically) disparate kinds of claimed mechanisms, and for which current biomedical technologies cannot measure claimed effects are refuted, are designated as ineffective. Conventional biomedical investigations of nonconventional medical approaches serve to ensure that those theories or approaches that are like contemporary biomedicine will be validated or verified, and those theories or approaches that are unlike contemporary biomedicine will be proven invalid or refuted. This approach is analogous to examining contemporary biomedical approaches from the viewpoint of Chinese medicine, Ayurveda, or another established nonconventional system of medicine, and making judgments about the validity of claimed mechanisms of action or the effectiveness of particular biomedical approaches solely on the basis of the evaluative methods or philosophical assumptions of those disparate systems of medicine. Attempts to understand biomedicine in this way would probably be received as arbitrary and absurd by Western researchers and physicians, yet an equivalent approach is the unquestioned cornerstone of the biomedical research methodology used to evaluate approaches used in nonconventional medicine.

In spite of the obvious logical and methodological flaws that limit contemporary biomedicine's efforts to elucidate nonconventional medical approaches, there is reason for optimism. The ongoing evolution of scientific theories and commensurate advances in technology will provide future biomedical researchers with the means to validate methodologies used in certain nonconventional systems of medicine, and to verify claims of efficacy of particular nonconventional medical approaches that are rejected by current Western science. The steady conceptual and technological evolution of medicine has transformed the paradigms and clinical practices of Western medicine and other world systems of medicine from earliest historical periods. As this evolutionary process continues, Western medicine and so-called nonconventional systems of medicine (i.e., that are open to evolution) will embrace assumptions pertaining to novel kinds of phenomena related to health or illness. Some claims that are now rejected as spurious will be verified, while conversely, some claims of mechanism

or efficacy that are presently accepted in Western medicine will be dismissed. However, at present Western biomedicine generally rejects the legitimacy of nonconventional systems of medicine prior to evaluating putative mechanisms of action or efficacy claims of particular treatments. This view is perpetuated by contemporary standards of medical education, the financial interests of the pharmaceutical industry, insurance companies, and regulatory bodies that define "legitimate" medical practices in Western countries.

The absence of a conceptual framework for combining assessment or treatment approaches from disparate systems of medicine has resulted from a perceived fundamental "gap" between worldviews due to nonoverlapping and sometimes mutually exclusive ontological and epistemological assumptions embedded in disparate systems of medicine (see Chapter 2). This gap constrains efforts to develop conceptual models of illness and health that are regarded as valid by practitioners of disparate systems of medicine. Different philosophical starting positions have ensured broad differences in practical methodological approaches in assessment and treatment, leading to a widespread perception of an inherent incompatibility between disparate systems of medicine. The absence of practical integrative methods for assessing patterns of illness and formulating suitable medical approaches has perpetuated scientific and ideological disputes over presumed fundamental mechanisms of action in illness and healing. This state of affairs makes it difficult to determine when it is appropriate to consider combining nonconventional or conventional assessment or treatment methods in patient management.

Planning Integrative Approaches Requires a Balance of Rigor and Relevance

Regardless of differences between the paradigms from which disparate conventional or nonconventional modalities originate, similar methodologies can be used to establish the effectiveness of a modality with respect to a specified symptom. This is true because determinations of effectiveness rest on observations of outcomes only—there is no epistemological requirement of a proof of a putative mechanism of action. Criteria used to characterize and measure outcomes provide a legitimate means for determining the effectiveness of a particular modality in both conventional biomedicine and nonconventional systems of medicine. When addressing cognitive or affective symptoms, outcomes often reflect subjective reports of the presence or absence of distress that do not correspond to objectively measurable changes in brain function or physiology that are difficult or impossible to describe empirically. This applies both to assessment tools used in Western psychiatry and outcomes measures of nonconventional assessment approaches. Many possible sources of bias result in nonspecific effects of treatments on reported outcomes (Gray, 2004):

- *Hawthorne effect:* Subjects do better solely because they are being studied.
- *Pygmalion effect:* Expectations of experimenter influence outcomes.
- *Placebo effect:* Subject's expectation of improvement and "nonspecific" psychotherapeutic effects leads to improvement above chance.

Because of the intrinsically subjective nature of cognitive and affective symptoms, as well as the limitations of study designs, the placebo response rates of most psychiatric disorders to conventional treatments are consistently high (Gray, 2004). Outcomes in Western psychiatry are generally defined as "significant" when there is a 50% or greater reduction in the target symptom. Thus a combination of high placebo response rates and other sources of bias frequently confound efforts to determine the efficacy of conventional psychiatric treatments. A consistently large placebo effect and other sources of bias inherent in conventional biomedical research designs is complicated by the fact that many nonconventional modalities are not susceptible to quantitative methods of analysis using available technological means. Examples include all mind–body practices, healing practices popularly described as "energy medicine," the majority of compound herbal formulas used in nonconventional systems of medicine, and homeopathy. Considerable efforts have been made to develop qualitative tools that will permit empirical evaluation of assessment or treatment approaches that are not susceptible to quantitative analysis.

To make informed judgments about differences in effectiveness when considering which conventional or nonconventional approaches to include in an integrative management plan, it is first necessary to find ways to compare disparate modalities. A comparison of modalities requires clarification of characteristics that are regarded as significant, and therefore a method for assigning relative degrees of significance to observed similarities or differences. In other words, a comparison of two or more disparate modalities assumes the existence of a classification system, or typology, of modalities ("Defining and Describing Complementary and Alternative Medicine," 1997; Turner, 1998). (Conceptual problems involved in the classification of approaches in medicine are addressed in chapter 2.) Statistical comparisons of clinician-observed outcomes are often of questionable reliability because they reflect differences in self-reported subjective experiences. This is especially true when evaluating treatments of mental illness. Both conventional and nonconventional treatments of cognitive or affective symptoms face intrinsic limits because of the subjective nature of symptoms being treated. In view of the inherent unreliability of quantitative methods for comparing outcomes of two or more approaches used to obtain or compare subjective patient reports, it is reasonable to introduce measures of rigor and relevance (Richardson, 2002). **Rigor** refers to the strength of evidence used to establish claims that a specified modality actually works, and **relevance** refers to the appropriateness of a specified modality with respect to the needs and preferences of a particular patient. The evaluation of rigor in outcomes data provides an objective measure of the quality of evidence supporting disparate modalities. In assessing the effectiveness and appropriateness of assessment and treatment approaches, the clinician must find a balance between rigor and relevance that adequately addresses the presenting complaint and is acceptable to the patient.

When an acceptable balance of rigor and relevance has been achieved, the problem of compatibility between disparate modalities is addressed. A methodology is introduced for determining degrees of compatibility when treatments are candidates for combined use. Incompatible modalities are those that are contraindicated in combination; treatments that are neutral, additive, or synergistic with respect to each other are compatible and desirable in combination.

The next methodological problem addressed in this chapter is the choice of parallel versus sequential assessment or treatment approaches in the context of current symptoms, patient history, practical constraints, and preferences. Examples of both approaches are provided to illustrate important differences between parallel and sequential approaches in integrative medical management. A particular integrative plan must be selected after quantitative and qualitative approaches have been used to determine rigor, compatibility, and mode (i.e., parallel vs. sequential) of implementation. After viable choices have been identified, the clinician and patient work together to decide on the suitability or relevance of a particular combination of assessment and treatment approaches with respect to the health problems, preferences, and circumstances of the patient. In this sense, relevance is broadly determined by reviewing the history of treatments for a similar problem while taking into account the patient's preferences, availability, and affordability of professional conventional and nonconventional medical services, along with the judgment of the supervising clinician. The thoughtful consideration of rigor and relevance is fundamental to determinations of appropriate integrative medical strategies. This general discussion of practical concepts in integrative health care concludes with a methodology for addressing ongoing changes in symptoms, ambiguity in assessment findings, poor or absent treatment responses, or research findings suggesting the relevance of novel assessment or treatment approaches.

What to Consider When Planning Integrative Medical Management

When formulating a practical integrative management strategy, the clinician must address five basic issues:

♦ The symptom pattern that is the focus of clinical attention
♦ The patient's history of response to previous treatments for similar symptom(s)
♦ Particular assessment or treatment methods to consider
♦ Practical issues of cost, availability, patient preferences, and values that will determine the "shape" of a realistic and acceptable integrative strategy
♦ How to assess outcomes

In addition to these basic considerations, a rigorous methodology for combining disparate modalities in an integrative strategy that is safe, effective, and realistic should take into account the following questions on a case-by-case basis with respect to a particular symptom pattern:

♦ Can the clinician identify treatments that enhance outcomes and shorten response times?
♦ Can the clinician identify assessment approaches that enhance the accuracy or predictive power of findings?
♦ Will combining the specified assessment or treatment approaches optimize assessment accuracy or treatment outcomes?
♦ How can two or more specified treatments be combined to ensure the highest degree of compatibility or synergy?
♦ What are reasonable criteria for determining when it is appropriate to combine assessment or treatment modalities in parallel or sequentially with respect to a specified symptom pattern?
♦ What are reasonable criteria for determining when it is appropriate to combine specified assessment and treatment modalities when addressing complex symptom patterns?

◆ What are reasonable criteria for combining specified treatments to improve compliance or enhance patient satisfaction with ongoing care?

◆ What is a practical methodology for measuring outcomes? In other words, what are reasonable criteria for obtaining useful information about outcomes in assessment accuracy or treatment effectiveness?

Conceptual Problems When Considering the Integration of Empirically Derived, Intuitive, and Mixed Approaches

Relatively few integrative strategies in current use are based on systematic reviews of randomized controlled trials (RCTs) demonstrating the effectiveness or safety of particular treatment combinations with respect to a specified symptom pattern. Therefore, at present most clinical integrative approaches incorporate treatments that are presumed to be compatible on the basis of unsubstantiated reports of outcomes, or consensus-based standards of practice. The same is arguably true for the majority of biomedical interventions in current use (Bloom, Retbi, Dahan, & Jonsson, 2000; Smith, 1991). Most contemporary biomedical or nonconventional modalities and most integrative medical practices in current use rest on expert consensus and have not been verified by replicable positive findings from controlled studies. However, as discussed above, expert consensus guidelines frequently rest on inconsistent evidence and are seldom formulated using a validated methodology.

Many systems of medicine use assessment and treatment approaches that are empirically derived from experimental or observational evidence of a mechanism of action, outcomes, or both. Some systems of medicine incorporate approaches that rest on core assumptions about a putative mechanism of action that cannot be verified by empirical evidence either because the mechanism of action is described in metaphysical terms or the technological means required for verification are currently unavailable. By definition, assessment and treatment approaches based on assumptions that are not potentially verifiable using current science are intuitive. Qigong is an example of an intuitive approach. In this ancient energetic healing tradition, a qigong master "projects" qi into the patient with the intention of "rebalancing" postulated energetic principles to achieve improved health and well-being. A mechanism of action for qigong has not been verified by Western science; however, studies have demonstrated that the regular practice of qigong is associated with measurable changes in heat, low-frequency sound, or electromagnetic energy at the practitioner's fingertips (Lake, 2001). Patients who receive qigong treatments frequently experience physiological changes that may be associated with the claimed effects of qigong, for example, "energy" flowing from a qigong master resulting in beneficial changes in autonomic activity. Qigong is an intuitive approach for which empirical evidence of a putative mechanism of action will probably not be forthcoming for many decades, if ever. However, accumulating evidence supports claims of consistent beneficial physiological effects. Finally, some systems of medicine incorporate both empirically derived and intuitive approaches. Examples include Chinese medicine, Ayurveda, and Tibetan medicine. **Table 4–1**

Table 4–1   Conceptual Problems in the Integration of Approaches from Empirically Based, Intuitive, and Mixed Systems of Medicine

Category	Representative System of Medicine or Clinical Approach	Important Characteristics	Comments Regarding Integration
Empirically derived only	Naturopathic medicine Biomedicine Western herbal medicine	Claims of mechanism of action and/or outcomes are verified or verifiable (definition). Assumes classical model of space–time, matter–energy, and linear causality	Modality can be integrated with other empirically based approaches if certain criteria are met (see below). Modality can be integrated with intuitive approaches when research or anecdotal evidence suggests effectiveness and safety
Intuitive only	Healing Touch Other forms of energy medicine, including Reiki and qigong	Claims of mechanism are not empirically verifiable (definition). Claims of outcomes are verified or verifiable. Criteria for demonstrating effectiveness usually ambiguous. Practitioner's intention or consciousness presumed necessary for effectiveness. Combined use with empirically based approaches sometimes recommended, but generally viewed as unnecessary	No empirically verifiable basis for integration with other systems of medicine because of absence of congruent core propositions (definition). Can be integrated with other empirically based or intuitive approaches when there is sufficient research or anecdotal evidence to support efficacy and safety claims
Mixed systems (incorporate empirically based and intuitive approaches)	Chinese medicine Ayurveda Tibetan medicine	Measures of efficacy and effectiveness frequently ambiguous. Practitioner's intention or consciousness important to outcomes when both empirical and intuitive approaches are used. Combinations of empirically based and intuitive approaches often prescribed as standard of medical practice	Combines empirically based and intuitive assessment and treatment approaches in holistic framework. "Mixed" systems of medicine are highly synthetic collections of disparate theories and clinical methods

summarizes conceptual issues that must be addressed when considering integrating empirically based or intuitive modalities.

Empirically based methods from disparate systems of medicine can be compared on the basis of degrees of similarity between mechanisms of action. Intuitive approaches, conversely, cannot be compared in this way because their core assumptions are metaphysical propositions and, by definition, cannot be verified using empirical means (see discussion above). This difference translates into an important distinction between a methodology for integrating empirically based approaches with other empirically based approaches and a methodology for integrating intuitive approaches with other intuitive or empirically based approaches. Empirically derived approaches are verified when evidence for a mechanism of action or claims of effectiveness is obtained from research or anecdotal reports. It is possible to compare the mechanisms of action or degrees of effectiveness of two or more empirically based approaches with respect to a specified symptom pattern.

Different Methodologies Are Used in Disparate Systems of Medicine

There is ongoing debate and controversy over research methodologies in nonconventional medicine. Whereas some argue that the same conventional research standards should be applied to investigations of nonconventional modalities, others argue that the methodology used in current biomedical research cannot adequately characterize the mechanisms of action underlying many approaches. Examples include homeopathy and qigong (Bengston, 2004; Zhang, 2004). Contemporary biomedicine claims that legitimate medical practices rest on valid claims of mechanism. By definition, valid claims are reducible to verifiable mechanistic descriptions of natural processes familiar to Western science. The phenomenological nature of presumed underlying processes determines whether or not a particular modality may be regarded as legitimate. Once the existence of a putative mechanism of action is established, empirical means must be used to verify causal relationships between phenomena that constitute the mechanism of action and observable effects or outcomes of a treatment based on an empirical description of the mechanism. Empirically verifiable causal relationships between a putative mechanism of action and expected outcomes are essential properties of the system and must be shown to be consistently present such that the mechanism of action operates in the claimed way. A modality rests on valid assumptions when available measurement techniques reliably demonstrate the existence of strict causal relationships between observable effects of that medical approach and expected observable outcomes when the modality is applied in a specified way. The assumptions underlying a modality are regarded as nonvalid when claims of outcomes cannot be linked to a putative mechanism of action using conventional empirical methods of measurement or observation (Murphy, 1997). According to this view, many nonconventional modalities rest on inherently nonvalid assumptions because empirical demonstrations of correspondences between putative mechanisms and claimed effects are not forthcoming using conventional techniques. Nonconventional practitioners nevertheless claim that their approaches are based on valid assumptions and have good efficacy on the basis of principles foreign to contemporary Western science and biomedicine. For example, practitioners of Chinese medicine claim that inserting and rotating fine needles in certain points on the skin causes changes in the distribution and balance of qi in a complex network of "meridians," ultimately manifesting as desirable and expected improvements in an "energetic imbalance." At present there is no Western technology capable of verifying (or refuting) the existence of qi, or characterizing putative relationships between the skillful insertion of acupuncture needles and desirable changes in a target symptom. However, recent brain-imaging studies are providing indirect biomedical evidence in support o some claims of Chinese medical acupuncture. Specific examples of emerging nonconventional assessment approaches used to evaluate putative energetic properties of qi related to particular symptom patterns are discussed in Part II of this book.

It is important to remark that the same factors that constrain verification of a putative mechanism of action underlying treatments in Chinese medicine also constrain available empirical means for verifying the existence and operation of mechanisms of action that are assumed to correspond to beneficial effects of psychopharmacological agents used in Western medicine. For example, the mechanisms of action associated with some antidepressants in common use are poorly understood, and contemporary neuroscience lacks methods capable of verifying causal relationships between putative neuropharmacological effects of antidepressants in the brain and observed beneficial outcomes in patients who take these drugs. A well-known example is the antidepressant bupropion (Wellbutrin), for which a mechanism of action has not yet been clearly described following extensive basic and clinical research. In spite of the failure of contemporary biomedical research methodology to verify putative mechanisms of action underlying many established treatments, consistent positive outcomes are observed for both acupuncture and conventional antidepressants. Both treatment approaches remain in widespread use on the basis of consistent positive outcomes even in the absence of empirical verification of a putative underlying mechanism of action.

Evidence-Based Medicine Places Limits on Western Biomedicine and Often Excludes Complementary, Alternative, and Integrative Approaches

Sound research in conventional biomedicine relies on the validity of trial design, outcomes measures, and statistical analysis methods. Applying the results of a clinical trial to a particular patient involves making an inference about the applicability of general findings to a specific case. Interpreting the results of a clinical trial is largely a matter of determining the validity of the trial design. **Construct validity** refers to the adequacy of the research design selected to test a hypothesis. Outcomes measures are determined on the basis of construct validity. Statistical methods used to test hypotheses in conventional psychiatric research are frequently limited by the absence of outcomes data that are required for rigorous evaluation, and alternative approaches are being explored (Lieberman, 2001). **Internal validity** is a measure of how effectively a research protocol controls for confounding variables. Randomization and double-blinding are methods to achieve internal validity in conventional Western biomedical research. The **external validity** of a study is the degree to which the findings of the study can be used to infer the general applicability of study findings to a population with a similar illness. For example, poor compliance with a treatment that has demonstrated efficacy for a particular illness can reduce the external validity of findings because it will interfere with expected outcomes based on the findings of a study in which compliance is rigorously controlled. Finally, ***statistical validity*** refers to the appropriateness of statistical tools used to analyze the significance of outcomes (Docherty, 2001). The above "levels" of validity define constraints on information attainable using a conventional research methodology and limit biomedical research to phenomena that are susceptible to the kinds of empirical analysis that necessarily follow from the application of these concepts. Thus investigations of illness phenomena or putative mechanisms of action that are not easily described in terms of discrete entities generally result in inconclusive or negative findings.

In recent years Western biomedicine has embraced ***evidence-based medicine,*** which uses a hierarchy of evidence approach to assess the significance of findings with respect to the parameters of a study design, together with systematic reviews and meta-analyses supporting clinical practices. EBM had its origins in the early 1980s and has developed a large following in academic medicine. It relies heavily on systematic reviews of the conventional medical research literature to "guide the judicious use of current best evidence in making decisions about the care of individual patients" (Sackett et al., 1996). Specific clinical decisions are made on a case-by-case basis following a review of "best evidence" in the context of the physician's expertise and the patient's preferences. Current EBM methods are available at http://medicine.ucsf.edu/resources/guidelines. Other sources include the center for evidence-based medicine at Oxford (www.cebm.net/index.asp), the center for evidence-based medicine at Toronto (http://cebm.toronto.ca), and the center for evidence-based mental health (http://cebmh.com).

Students of Western medicine are taught that evidence-based medicine employs a rigorous methodology for identifying best evidence and undergo training in that methodology to better learn clinical decision making in patient care. According to the tenets of EBM, the highest or most reliable level of evidence of efficacy for any treatment modality is obtained through a systematic review of rigorously conducted randomized controlled trials. Progressively lower levels of evidence include individual RCTs with narrow confidence intervals, all-or-none case series, systematic reviews of cohort studies, individual cohort studies, and RCTs with less than 80% follow-up. EBM places evidence obtained from cohort studies, case series, and expert opinion at the low end of the evidence hierarchy. Proponents argue that information obtained from these study designs is inherently less reliable because it is less susceptible to rigorous controls or quantitative analysis when compared with randomized controlled trials.

Prior to the introduction of evidence-based medicine, standards of practice in conventional Western biomedicine were based largely on expert consensus, which EBM explicitly relegates to one of the lowest levels in the hierarchy of evidence. Most biomedical treatments in current use do not yet adhere to the highest standards of EBM (Dalen, 1998). Western physicians are taught that EBM embodies the ideal standard of good treatment planning; however, relatively few Western physicians actually practice EBM because they are not familiar with its methodology or lack the time and resources to do so. In spite of the benefits of EBM in treatment planning, most conventionally trained physicians continue to make treatment recommendations on the basis of their own clinical experience and intuitions, and sometimes defer to the opinions of local experts. Relatively few physicians rely on a rigorous analysis of findings in the medical literature in clinical decision making. EBM methodology clearly brings a new level of rigor to the analysis of diverse findings and is a valuable tool in clinical treatment planning. Recent studies suggest that EBM can be validly applied to both nonconventional medicine and Western biomedicine (Wilson, Mills, Ross, & Guyatt, 2002), and that rigorous treatment planning in nonconventional medicine must endorse the same standards of evidence used in biomedicine (Fontanarosa & Lundberg, 1998; Haynes, 1999). In response to these challenges, the evidence-based Complementary and Alternative Medicine (CAM) working group was formed (Wilson & Mills, 2002), with the goal of finding ways to apply the rigorous empirical methodology of EBM to the evaluation of putative mechanisms of action and effectiveness of nonconventional modalities.

Efforts to adapt nonconventional medical research to biomedical research standards are ongoing, and significant progress is being made in many areas. However, such efforts may prove to be inherently self-limiting. EBM methodology, for example, excludes some kinds of potentially relevant research and clinical information, or assigns such information to lower levels of significance in a hierarchy of evidence that is implicitly biased in favor of the kinds of study designs traditionally used in Western biomedical research. Criteria for relative levels of evidence in EBM reflect implicit assumptions in Western medicine about kinds of information that correspond to legitimate evidence. For example, EBM assumes that clinically useful information is forthcoming only from study designs based on certain statistical measures of significance. The statistical measures used describe putative correlations of causes and outcomes that can be directly observed and isolated (i.e., controlled for) from all other possible interfering or confounding variables. Furthermore, only those causes or outcomes that are observable or measurable using available technologies belong to categories of phenomena for which legitimate claims of existence can be made (see Chapter 2). Evidence-based medicine assumes that if a treatment is legitimate, a discrete mechanism of action has been identified or is at least identifiable, and that a predictable, deterministic causal relationship exists between treatment effects, the putative mechanism of action, and statistical measures of outcomes obtained using available technological means. EBM equates postulated causes and effects with discrete biological mechanisms. In contrast to Western biomedical treatments, many nonconventional approaches cannot be adequately explained in this reductionist framework. EBM does not acknowledge the relevance of emerging paradigms in health and illness (Richardson, 2002). EBM asserts that study findings may be interpreted as rigorous only after sequential series of significant outcomes have been obtained from identical study designs using identical statistical methods. Finally, EBM assumes that averaged results of systematic reviews or meta-analyses of several studies can be validly applied to individuals, providing clinically pertinent guidance in treatment planning (Churchill, 1999).

EBM assumptions about the requirements of a valid methodology for obtaining medical information contain implicit biases against the methodologies of many nonconventional systems of medicine as well as many particular nonconventional assessment and treatment modalities (Vickers,

1999). A consequence has been the relegation of many nonconventional modalities to the lowest levels of the EBM evidence hierarchy in spite of robust findings consistent with the claims and worldviews of nonconventional medical systems of medicine.

In Western medical circles, many nonconventional modalities are dismissed as spurious treatment choices before evidence for them is rigorously appraised. This situation is complicated by the growth and practice of EBM in Western biomedicine and requirements of cost containment in health maintenance organizations (HMOs) and managed care, which often stipulate as a requirement for reimbursement that physicians use the lowest-cost treatments available in spite of compelling evidence in favor of other, often more effective, biomedical treatments. In the face of rigorous standards of biomedical evidence using EBM methodology, important economic and social constraints define the broad context of mental health care in the United States and other Western industrialized countries, resulting in the continued use of approaches that are arguably not evidence-based (i.e., by EBM criteria) in ~40% of clinical decisions by psychiatrists or other Western physicians who treat mental health problems (Drake et al., 2001; Geddes et al., 1996). Psychiatrists are increasingly aware of EBM; however, few base clinical practice decisions exclusively on its principles, out of the concern that EBM does not take into account many conventional treatments in widespread use, including off-label pharmacological treatments and innovative psychotherapy approaches (Borenstein, 2004).

New Approaches to Thinking about Evidence and Algorithms in Integrative Medicine

Algorithms for medical decision making in conventional Western biomedicine are limited by inconclusive biomedical research evidence, heavy reliance on expert opinion, and lack of awareness of the rigorous standards of evidence-based practices in the general medical community (Stein, 2004). Expert consensus is frequently the basis of clinical decisions in nonconventional medicine. Historically, standards of medical practice have incorporated guidelines based on expert consensus more often than adhering to strictly scientific requirements of "evidence" popularly subscribed to during a particular historical period or in a particular cultural setting. Expert consensus guidelines are generally defended as "authoritative" on the basis of interpretations of outcomes that purport to show consistent therapeutic effects of medical practices not yet subjected to rigorous scrutiny. Authoritative interpretations are generally made by clinicians or researchers who have political influence through academic or institutional affiliations. Consensus-based practices in both conventional and nonconventional medicine are essentially self-reinforcing beliefs that selectively exclude kinds of evidence or modes of investigation that are not congruent with the premises of the parent system of medicine in which they originate. This state of affairs has led to the mutual disregard of relevant and potentially valuable evidence by conventional biomedicine and many nonconventional systems of medicine. In sum, treatment planning in conventional medicine generally excludes evidence supporting nonconventional approaches, and by the same token treatment planning in nonconventional medicine often excludes evidence for conventional approaches. Integrative algorithms address this problem by taking into account the evidence for both biomedical and nonconventional assessment and treatment approaches.

Below, I propose a novel kind of evidence hierarchy based on a synthesis of core tenets from contemporary Western evidence-based medicine and models of evidence used to evaluate nonconventional modalities that are outside of current Western biomedical thinking. The resulting integrative model of evidence permits the derivation of a hierarchy of quantitative and qualitative evidence while acknowledging important differences in the quality and kind of information available from the evaluation of both conventional and nonconventional modalities. Diverse kinds of information supporting claims of efficacy for a particular nonconventional approach are considered from the conceptual frameworks of both biomedicine and the nonconventional system of medicine from which the modality is derived. Steps are taken to avoid ideological or methodological constraints or biases inherent in biomedicine or disparate nonconventional systems of medicine. This synthetic approach for constructing hierarchies of evidence leads to strategies incorporating best evidence from a broad range of sources in response to well-formulated clinical questions following a critical appraisal of the quality of information supporting the use of both conventional and nonconventional modalities with respect to a specified symptom. The resulting integrative methodology provides physicians and nonconventionally trained practitioners with a comprehensive range of clinical choices in contrast to the inherent limitations of a strictly biomedical EBM methodology or other, more narrowly defined ways of constructing evidence hierarchies used by nonbiomedical systems of medicine. Integrative treatment planning takes into consideration both quantitative and qualitative evidence pertaining to all potentially beneficial psychological, somatic, mind–body, "energy information," and possibly spiritual approaches in addition to established conventional biomedical approaches. The goal of this synthetic methodology is to enhance the quality of medical care and improve outcomes.

Disparate Systems of Medicine Use Different Criteria for Determining the Validity or Efficacy of Assessment or Treatment Approaches

Based on cumulative research data, the collective experiences of physicians and other professionally trained medical practitioners, along with the reports of patients, it is reasonable to conclude that many established conventional biomedical modalities are probably efficacious and effective in spite of the absence of unequivocal proof according to the criteria of EBM. By the same token, it is reasonable to argue that many established nonconventional modalities are efficacious and effective in spite of the absence of compelling biomedical evidence. The historical evolution of medicine is characterized by the entrenchment of medical practices regarded as efficacious on the basis of consistent positive outcomes, as well as the gradual abandonment of practices believed to lack efficacy. The present historical period is a case in point, in that relatively few conventional or nonconventional medical practices in current use are substantiated by strong evidence of a putative underlying mechanism, yet many modalities in all traditions of medicine remain in widespread use because of consistent positive outcomes, expert consensus on presumed efficacy in spite of the absence of conclusive data, or social and economic factors influencing popular views of medical practices. In the absence of compelling empirical evidence, true claims about possible underlying mechanisms of action associated with conventional or nonconventional medical practices cannot be made on the basis of formal biomedical criteria. However, as will be discussed below, contemporary empirical methods used to establish the validity or effectiveness of conventional medical approaches are not necessarily appropriate or sufficient for establishing the effectiveness of some nonconventional modalities. The verification of a specified assessment or treatment approach requires the demonstration that a putative mechanism of action exists and is correlated with a claimed outcome. As I have previously explained (see Chapter 2), arguments for verification in medicine are intrinsically circular in that the existence of certain kinds of phenomena is implicit in the methodology used to verify their existence. Objective or neutral views of health or illness are not possible from the perspectives of biomedicine or disparate nonconventional systems of medicine. There is no objective point of view. Thus different interpretations of the causes, characteristics, or meanings of symptoms cannot be shown to be more or less true than other interpretations from the perspective of an objective perspective. Although it is meaningful to assert that competing perspectives of medicine exist, it is spurious to argue that a perspective embodied within a particular system of medicine is somehow more complete or "better" than any other perspective. This problem becomes especially germane to a discussion of integrative medicine when interpreting the clinical significance of the highly subjective illness phenomena of concern to psychiatry.

Recently, efforts have been made to establish methodologies for evaluating the efficacy of nonconventional modalities on the basis of criteria that are not strictly biomedical. This approach emphasizes measures of outcomes over evidence of causation. It has been argued, for example, that a nonconventional modality is based on valid assumptions (i.e., about the characteristics of phenomena underlying illness) if the prescribed implementation of that modality is associated with consistent reports of outcomes reasonably expected to occur if the claimed effect of the modality takes place. It is important to note that this criterion does not require empirical verification of a presumed underlying mechanism of action using standard biomedical tests, nor does it include a requirement that claimed effects operate according to contemporary biomedical theory. The only requirement is that a correspondence is consistently observed to take place between the "skillful" implementation of an assessment or treatment approach and a desirable outcome that is expected in the conceptual framework of the parent system of medicine. Outcomes of some nonconventional treatments are measurable using accepted biomedical measures. For example, reduction in hepatic enzymes is expected following the administration of milk thistle (*Silymarin* spp.) extract in patients diagnosed with hepatitis. Outcomes of other nonconventional treatments are difficult or impossible to objectively assess on the basis of quantitative biomedical criteria. In these cases, outcomes necessarily rely on patient reports of changes in subjective symptoms, and there are generally no empirically measurable "signs" corresponding to beneficial changes. For example, anxious patients who self-treat their symptoms using regular qigong practices frequently report significant reductions in anxiety levels that cannot be objectively verified to take place or to be related to qigong. There is an ongoing

Table 4–2 Quantitative and Qualitative Measures of Outcomes Following Medical Treatment

♦ Observable response to a clinical problem that had not improved with previous kinds of treatment

♦ Alleviation or reduction of chronic physical or psychological effects of ill health

♦ Improved overall feelings of health and well-being following treatment

♦ Reduction in the frequency or intensity in relapsing ill health or return of a specified symptom or symptom pattern that is the focus of treatment

♦ Improved general level of comfort, including the reduction or alleviation of distress or symptoms causing distress

♦ Enhanced social, psychological, relationship, or employment functioning

♦ Reduction or alleviation of the patient's sense of suffering

♦ Enhanced capacity for insight or ability to manage one's own medical or psychological health

♦ Enhanced capacity to influence external factors that directly or indirectly undermine a patient's state of medical or psychological health

♦ Improved patient satisfaction with the kind or quality of care

debate over the meaning of *outcome* in nonconventional medical research. As is also true of Western medicine, three kinds of outcomes or effects can take place in the context of medical treatment (Long, 2002):

♦ Effects related to the general philosophy or principles of a system of medicine

♦ Effects arising from the relationship between a patient and a healer

♦ Effects resulting from the application of a particular technique

Of course, these three kinds of effects operate in conventional Western biomedicine, but are frequently overlooked in research designs and clinical practice. Because of the different kinds of effects in both Western medicine and nonconventional systems of medicine, many quantitative and qualitative methods are useful when assessing outcomes. **Table 4–2** lists outcome measures used to determine whether a desired effect has been achieved following treatment (Coates & Jobst, 1998).

It is clear from the above discussion that desirable outcomes of conventional and nonconventional treatments of both medical and psychiatric symptoms are reportable or observable but seldom quantifiable. The problem of verification of reported changes in subjective states during or following treatment is germane to the validation of both conventional and nonconventional approaches in medicine and psychiatry. Though important conceptual differences exist between biomedicine and nonconventional modalities, for practical purposes the "gap" between conventional and nonconventional treatments may not be very wide when assessing the effectiveness of treatments in mental health care because in both instances outcomes data are based on the analysis of reports of subjective symptoms that cannot be quantified or empirically verified as causally related to an intervention. Again, this is necessarily true because there are presently no reliable means to objectively confirm putative correlations between a treatment and a beneficial outcome when treating cognitive or affective symptoms. Assessment methods examine correspondences between "causes" of dysfunction and observable clinical signs or reportable symptoms. Repeated findings of similar correspondences suggest causal correlations between putative causes and observable changes in specific signs or symptoms. In psychiatry, functional brain-imaging research suggests possible correlations between "dysfunction" at certain levels of metabolic or neuropharmacological brain activity and depressed mood, anxiety, or schizophrenia. However, due to the structural and functional complexity of the brain and inherent limitations of contemporary technologies, biological psychiatry presently lacks a strong empirical methodology for verifying strict relationships between specific putative causes of presumed central nervous system (CNS) dysfunction and specific cognitive or affective symptoms. It is likely that this ambiguous state of affairs will continue for the foreseeable future. Because of this, it is unclear when or whether Western psychiatry will become an exact science. Because of the inherent vagueness of cognitive, emotional, and behavioral symptoms, and intrinsic methodological constraints on the problem of verifying causal relationships between treatments and outcomes in mental health care, subjective indicators of treatment outcomes will continue to play a central role in assessing the effectiveness of both conventional and nonconventional treatments.

Methodologies for Verifying Effectiveness in Biomedicine and Nonconventional Medicine Use Similar Criteria

Disparate criteria used to validate putative mechanisms of action in conventional and nonconventional medical approaches reflect differences between the perspectives of the parent systems of medicine. In contrast, similar, and in some cases identical, criteria are used to establish the clinical effectiveness of particular conventional and nonconventional approaches. The reasons for this go back to differences between requirements of a methodology used to confirm the existence of a putative mechanism of action, as well as requirements of a methodology used to verify the effectiveness of a particular clinical approach. In Western science the validity of a medical practice can be established only through verification that a putative underlying mechanism of action is the basis of that medical practice and operates in the claimed manner. Validation thus requires two kinds of proof: verification of the existence and characteristics of phenomena that are the putative basis of a mechanism of action, and verification of presumed causal relationships between those phenomena and the claimed effects (outcome) of a particular modality. Although this process appears to call for objective means for establishing the existence of a thing and verifying causal relationships between it and other phenomena, the means for doing so are in fact self-referential and therefore not objective.

The following example will help to clarify this point. Using the empirical criteria of contemporary biomedicine, the existence and characteristics of a putative mechanism of action can be established only when the phenomenal basis for that purported mechanism is verifiable according to the kinds of empirical criteria required in the methodology of contemporary Western science. On examination it becomes clear that criteria required for verification in Western science rest on assumptions that are implicit in the philosophical framework of Western science and, by extension, biomedicine, about kinds of phenomena that can have existence. According to the dictum, only those phenomena that can be observed or measured using contemporary technologies can have existence. Using conventional biomedical logic, putative phenomena associated with a claimed treatment effect that are not susceptible to verification through observation or measurement using contemporary Western empirical means are a priori rejected as nonexistent. This point goes to the heart of the philosophical and conceptual gap between conventional and nonconventional systems of medicine (see Chapter 2). Criteria for evidence supporting claims of existence of a putative mechanism of action reflect assumptions in disparate systems of medicine about the kind and quality of information necessary to verify the existence of a mechanism of action and confirm claims of efficacy. The argument is circular, because the empirical methodology employed in biomedicine to verify the existence of a putative mechanism of action or its efficacy in terms of outcomes measures, predetermines "good" or "adequate" approaches to both experimentation and clinical practice. The researcher or clinical practitioner therefore "sees" what is permitted within the conceptual framework of conventional biomedicine, and there is no place for claims of treatment mechanisms or outcomes that depart from assumptions built into many nonconventional systems of medicine because such claims are regarded as a priori lacking legitimacy.

The current gold standard biomedical research design is the randomized controlled trial in which all variables that potentially affect outcomes are assumed to be knowable and possess characteristics that can be accurately described. The validity of an RCT design is based on the assumption that all variables potentially affecting outcomes are subject to known constraints (i.e., controls) imposed by the researcher in the experimental design. In the ideal case, there is double blinding: Neither experimenters nor patients are aware of which patients are enrolled in either the "active" or "placebo" arm of the study. Conventional RCT research designs are based on the assumption that effectiveness rests on the demonstration of efficacy against a suitable placebo. Although this is probably a legitimate way to characterize conventional pharmacological treatments, it does not adequately describe many nonconventional or integrative treatments that operate at multiple synergistic levels and are therefore not verifiable using simple empirical measurements of discrete biological effects. RCT research designs frequently employ measures of "effect size" that are statistically underpowered with respect to the intervention being studied, fail to take into account possible nonspecific beneficial effects, or ascribe such effects to placebo when they occur. The result is that conventional RCT studies of many nonconventional modalities, including acupuncture, homeopathy, and Healing Touch, conclude that they are ineffective (Walach, 2001). The RCT design reinforces the closed, self-referential character of contemporary biomedical research because of the assumption that all variables potentially affecting outcomes are identifiable and subject to control. In this context, *control* implies that the experimenter can identify and modify the relative strengths (dosing) or timings of phenomena that directly or indirectly affect outcomes. The same constraints apply to investigations of the validity or effectiveness of assessment approaches because of the assumption that phenomena affecting the accuracy of assessment findings are able to be verified and in some way "controlled." The Western-style research methodology used to evaluate the efficacy of conventional medical approaches is designed to identify and examine only phenomena that are believed to exist and to be relevant to illness according to contemporary Western biomedical theory. Only phenomena assumed to have existence according to orthodox Western science are regarded as suitable for biomedical research. Therefore, biomedical research methodology is in effect "closed" to the investigation of putative mechanisms of action resting on phenomena that potentially affect health or illness but are not reducible to categories of existence described in contemporary Western science. Furthermore, RCT research designs measure only statistical correspondences between a described treatment and a measured outcome effect.

RCT designs are not able to provide information about possible mechanisms of action or subjective aspects of treatment from the patient's perspective. Finally, RCT studies are often poorly designed, and because of their short duration or limited numbers of enrolled subjects, their findings often lack the requisite statistical power to establish significant correspondences between treatments and outcomes. This issue is especially problematic for biomedical research on mental illness where brief premarketing trials sometimes fail to adequately characterize effect sizes or side effect risks of new drugs. Because of these inherent constraints, RCT and other quantitative research designs are more suited to investigations of biological treatments, including conventional psychopharmacology and herbal medicines. In contrast, qualitative research methods are more suitable for the investigation of mind–body, energy, or spiritual approaches. Other factors that often interfere with or limit biomedical research studies of nonconventional modalities include the following (Verhoef, Casebeer, & Hilsdew, 2002; Walach, 2001):

◆ Nonconventional interventions are often complex, incorporating multiple modalities and making quantitative analysis of underlying mechanisms or cause–effect relationships between treatments and outcomes very difficult.

◆ Many nonconventional modalities are not standardized, but individualized and flexible in adaptation to the history, needs, and circumstances of each patient.

◆ Many nonconventional modalities are used to assess or treat nonspecific or multifactorial conditions.

◆ Nonconventional treatments are typically used to restore balance rather than remove a putative cause of a specified symptom or symptom pattern.

◆ Because the mechanisms of action of many nonconventional modalities are difficult or impossible to quantify, it is often impossible to identify an appropriate placebo response in nonconventional medical research, making outcomes studies very difficult or impossible.

◆ RCT study designs have the express goal of minimizing the impact of the patient–provider relationship, which is a desirable or necessary aspect of many nonconventional modalities.

The above issues have practical implications that limit investigations of many nonconventional modalities within the context of Western biomedical theory and biomedical research methodologies. For example, whereas some nonconventional modalities rest on mechanisms of action that are congruent with core assumptions of contemporary biomedicine (e.g., Western herbal medicine), many nonconventional approaches rest on putative mechanisms that are not reducible to categories of phenomena accepted in Western science (e.g., acupuncture). For the reasons cited above, relying

on the same standards of experimental evidence to verify a putative mechanism of action will invariably lead to refutation of certain nonconventional modalities because current Western science is not able to "capture" or adequately characterize their underlying mechanisms. Even though putative mechanisms of action underlying many nonconventional modalities cannot be verified using conventional means, some nonconventional modalities are supported by compelling evidence of efficacy or effectiveness on the basis of controlled studies or consistently positive observations. It is therefore inappropriate and unreasonable to use conventional research designs, including the RCT or other standardized methods in biomedical research methodology, to determine the legitimacy of certain nonconventional modalities resting on putative mechanisms that are not susceptible to verification using this methodology. Western medicine employs RCT study designs to obtain aggregate data about frequencies of response and strengths of association between particular treatments and outcomes.

The tension between quantitative and qualitative research methodologies mirrors the ideological conflict between EBM and patient-centered care. Both are useful and relevant, and methodologies that combine them take advantage of the useful features of both (Verhoef et al., 2002). A methodology that combines qualitative approaches and established quantitative methods will result in valuable information about the personal, individualized experiences of illness and healing. In cases where the outcome of an RCT study shows no treatment effect, it is possible that the nonconventional modality worked in ways other than expected, or specific individuals benefited from the intervention in subjective ways or in observable ways that were not assessed as outcomes. Reliance on RCT study designs to validate nonconventional modalities will not only fail to confirm a putative mechanism of action in many cases, but will also lead to the rejection of potentially legitimate assessment and treatment approaches that are not susceptible to verification using the current methodology of biomedical research (Richardson, 2000). It is, of course, reasonable to conduct RCT studies on nonconventional modalities that are susceptible to quantitative investigation. However, even in cases where it is conceptually possible to design an adequate RCT protocol to investigate a particular nonconventional approach, it is seldom practical to implement RCT studies outside of Western medical institutions because of the high cost of most RCT studies, as well as the frequent absence of private or public funding (Linde, 2000). These practical constraints have led to the widespread use of observational studies in the investigation of many nonconventional modalities. In sum, continued reliance on RCT studies and other standardized biomedical research designs will probably delay or confound efforts to investigate putative mechanisms of action and verify outcomes for many established and emerging nonconventional approaches (Long, 2002).

What can be done in the face of the above dilemma, and is it possible to rigorously evaluate nonconventional modalities while not a priori rejecting their premises? Can this be achieved using a biomedical research methodology founded on premises that are inherently biased against many nonconventional approaches? These questions raise the general issue of quantitative versus qualitative methods in the investigation of natural phenomena, including health and illness. Theory building in Western science has evolved from strict reliance on positivism, to realism, and most recently to relativism; however, the practical work of biomedical research and clinical practice continues to be grounded in a positivist epistemology. According to this view, the question of the validity of a particular assessment or treatment approach is equivalent to the capacity for empirical verification of the existence of a putative mechanism of action or claimed outcomes associated with that approach. This view gives primacy to information obtained using quantitative means. Because of its historical origins and philosophical bias, Western science asserts that qualitative methods necessarily yield unreliable information on the basis of the assumption that rigorous means for verifying causal relationships between treatments and outcomes or for accurately measuring effect sizes are not possible in the absence of quantitative empirical methods (see Chapter 3). The philosophical position of Western science is thus inherently biased against many nonconventional systems of medicine whose clinical approaches are not (presently) susceptible to rigorous quantitative investigation or verification. Many non-Western-trained medical practitioners work with narratives of health and illness that cannot be reduced to a positivist way of knowing.

Emerging Research Methodologies in Nonconventional Medicine—Single-Case Studies, Case Series, ATI, Design-Adaptive Allocations, and Participant-Centered Analysis

In response to the above concerns, researchers and practitioners of nonconventional medicine have proposed novel methodologies and clinical approaches that take into account the comparative strengths and weaknesses of established quantitative and qualitative research methodologies (Richardson, 2002). Considerable thought has been put into the development of rigorous qualitative and combined quantitative-qualitative methodologies appropriate for the investigation of nonconventional modalities. A practical outcome of this effort has been renewed discussion of research methodologies that are not inherently limited by the conceptual and technological constraints of Western biomedicine. The use of fixed-response quantitative research methods to gather clinical patient data frequently excludes important subjective outcomes and fails to capture patients' beliefs about the "meanings" of health and illness. Qualitative methodologies have been found useful for gathering outcomes data relevant to the experiences and clinical outcomes of a particular patient in response to a range of medical interventions. Qualitative criteria include ratings of consistency of training, duration of training, the historical duration of use of a particular nonconventional modality, how well established the use of a particular modality is for a specified cognitive or emotional symptom, the level of concern (if any) over potential safety issues when a nonconventional modality is administered by a professional practitioner, and the existence of a coherent body of theory supporting specific uses of a particular approach. Combined quantitative and qualitative methodologies are used to study complex systems in general, including the analysis of economic and social trends. Combining quantitative and qualitative methodologies in medicine permits researchers to more adequately address the complex factors that contribute to health and illness (Vuckovic, 2002). Anecdotal reports often suggest that a particular nonconventional assessment or treatment approach is appropriate or beneficial for a specific problem. However, limited evidence from formal research studies substantiates the

treatment in question. The probability that studies on nonconventional modalities will yield useful information about mechanisms of action or outcomes is increased when conventional RCT research designs are complemented by other research methods, including observational studies, case series analysis, double-blinding, design-adaptive allocations, participant-centered research, and "N of 1" trials (Linde, 2000).

Different qualitative and combined quantitative-qualitative research methodologies used to investigate nonconventional approaches have been elaborated, and novel criteria for research designs for evaluating nonconventional approaches have been proposed.

The issue of blinding in conventional research designs remains controversial. For many conventional and nonconventional treatments, it is difficult or impossible to "blind" both patient and researcher to the intervention. For example, a surgeon is necessarily aware of the surgical procedure being used, and a Chinese medical practitioner is aware that he or she is administering a protocol that is believed to be beneficial or a protocol that is believed to be ineffective. The absence of double-blinding can potentially bias analysis of research findings. A proposed solution is the use of a "dual-blind" research design, in which the patient is blinded, the researcher administering the treatment is not blinded, but a second investigator who evaluates outcomes is blinded. It has been suggested that this approach can improve the integrity of research in both conventional and nonconventional medicine by bypassing problems related to nonblinded experimenters (Caspi, Millen, & Sechrest, 2000). When a particular approach is potentially beneficial for the patient's symptoms but has little supporting evidence, the single-case ($N = 1$) study may provide a valid way to determine whether the approach is actually beneficial and safe (Johnston & Mills, 2004). A **single-case study** is a prospective trial on one individual in which the treatment being investigated is administered and withheld in alternating fashion while an agreed-on outcome is measured. Depending on the specific research question that is being asked, a single-case study can be performed in a single- or double-blind fashion, can be randomized or nonrandomized, and may or may not include a placebo–control arm. Single-case studies can follow a crossover design or a continuous treatment protocol. In contrast to conventional research designs that define treatment outcomes in terms of probabilities, single-case studies result in definitive, individualized outcomes for each patient. This approach also has drawbacks and limitations, including the impossibility of generalizing findings to other patients, and the fact that findings may not be applicable to illnesses that are "unstable" over time (i.e., because long-term changes in baseline symptoms in the patient on which a single-case study is performed cannot be taken into account in treatment planning using this method; Ernst, 1998a,b).

Case series are sometimes used to estimate the possible benefits of a particular medical treatment for a given population. Case series are accumulated reports of uncontrolled findings from one or more individuals. Although case series sometimes point clinicians and researchers in useful directions, they are limited because they cannot account for placebo effects or other nonspecific treatment effects. Participant-centered analysis is a variant of the case series in which multiple measures of a single variable are taken for each individual in a sample. This methodology permits statistical analysis of complex relationships between treatments and outcomes at the individual level and makes up for some of the disadvantages of typical case series (Aickin, 2003). In integrative mental health care, single-case studies and case series analysis are methodologies that can help clarify the potential benefits of treatments that are currently ranked as possibly effective, but for which substantiated or consistent research findings are currently lacking. ***Aptitude × treatment interaction*** (ATI) is a recently suggested conceptual framework for analysis of outcomes in integrative medicine research. This approach assumes that outcomes depend on the match or mismatch between patient characteristics, or aptitudes, including biological, psychological, and cultural factors that affect treatment response, and the specific treatment received. The model regards outcomes as manifestations of dynamic interactions in a complex system and argues that effective treatment planning must take these factors into account (Caspi & Bell, 2004). A method called design-adaptive allocations has been suggested as an alternative to the conventional randomization used in RCT studies (Aickin, 2002). This method may permit a better balance between treatment groups and more accurate measurement of factors affecting outcomes, and may be especially useful for analyzing findings in small studies that would generally be viewed as statistically "underpowered" in Western medicine. Increasing global interest in nonconventional medicine at the World Health Organization (WHO) has led to the establishment of a program aimed at developing universal tools to assess quality of life changes in response to medical interventions from the perspective of any system of medicine (Liverani, 2000). The goal of the WHO universal valuation system is to develop effective qualitative and quantitative methodologies for assessing treatment effectiveness at biological, individual, and social levels of functioning. This program will help to determine the cost-effectiveness of various nonconventional modalities compared with more expensive conventional treatments for the range of medical and mental health problems. Research methodologies in energy medicine pose special problems, including the identification of placebo or "sham" treatments, the determination of controlled conditions, and the choice of appropriate statistical and qualitative methods for outcomes analysis (Jonas & Chez, 2004).

I have argued that the kinds of distinctions between particular modalities based on tests of verification of putative mechanisms of action will change as the conceptual framework of science evolves and novel technologies arise. Some approaches that are currently regarded as validated only within a particular nonconventional system of medicine will be regarded as validated by a future biomedicine. It is likely that some medical practices in current use that have not been validated by either biomedicine or nonconventional systems of medicine (i.e., consensus-based or intuitive modalities) will become validated by emerging research methodologies in a future form of biomedicine or a future nonconventional system of medicine. The converse is also to be expected, in that some assessment and treatment approaches that are now accepted as valid or substantiated within biomedicine or a particular system of nonconventional medicine will probably be empirically refuted by emerging methodologies or future technologies capable of demonstrating the absence of a postulated mechanism of action. The research methodology and theories of Western science have undergone continuous change since their invention, resulting in commensurate shifts in the perspectives of medicine (see Chapter 3). It is reasonable to expect that the continuing evolution of science and technology will result in changes in the kinds and strengths of evidence associated with

particular conventional and nonconventional approaches. We can anticipate that ongoing evolution in the methodologies, theories, and technologies of conventional and nonconventional systems of medicine will lead to shifts in verifiable truth claims for particular approaches, and to commensurate changes in their relative positions in a hierarchy of evidence. For example, certain modalities that are now provisionally accepted clinical methods based on nonvalidated claims of beneficial "effects" of energy or information will likely become validated by a future science capable of demonstrating their putative underlying mechanisms of action.

Typologies of contemporary medical practices generally make distinctions between biological, somatic, mind–body, and spiritual techniques. Assigning disparate assessment tools and treatment modalities to categories does not differentiate them on the basis of the quality of evidence for claims of a mechanism of action or efficacy with respect to a specified symptom. Because of this, conventional typologies of medical practices are of limited value in identifying assessment or treatment approaches that are more or less valid according to biomedical or nonconventional criteria, or more or less efficacious with respect to a particular medical or psychiatric symptom pattern. This problem can be addressed by assigning assessment or treatment practices to logically possible categories of kinds and levels of evidence. With respect to a specified symptom, a particular modality is assigned to a level of evidence and kind of evidence on the basis of criteria used to determine the current status of truth claims of a putative mechanism of action or, or on the basis of criteria used to verify claims of effectiveness (see Chapter 2). Using this approach, any particular modality is based on implicit or explicit propositions that correspond to particular truth claims of a putative mechanism or observed efficacy. With respect to contemporary Western science and available technologies, any conventional or nonconventional modality has an exact location in an evidence hierarchy in which there are many possible levels and kinds of evidence.

Efficacy versus Effectiveness, and Considerations of Cost-Effectiveness Analysis, Cost-Utility Analysis, and Cost-Benefit Analysis in Integrative Management

Treatment efficacy refers to measured results of a treatment in a randomized clinical trial under ideal controlled conditions, including a homogeneous patient population, specially trained therapists, and monitored outcomes. Treatments that are efficacious under ideal conditions may not be effective in the real world because of differences between patients, the absence of ideal conditions, and the unmonitored application of the treatment. ***Treatment effectiveness*** deals with outcomes measures in real-world clinical settings. Limitations of conventional psychiatric treatment in this regard include differences in diagnostic skills of practitioners, diverse skill levels in psychotherapy and psychopharmacology, poorly documented differences in dosing and drugs used for particular disorders or symptoms, and uncontrolled differences between patients, such as poor compliance and differences in self-motivation or the concurrent use of undisclosed treatments. Some treatments have good efficacy and effectiveness but are very expensive to implement. The result is that less effective but inexpensive treatments are sometimes more cost-effective compared with more effective, expensive treatments. The efficacy and effectiveness of some nonconventional treatments are comparable to existing conventional treatments but are safer and significantly less expensive. Many physicians believe that an "efficacy gap" exists with respect to depression because available treatments are not regarded as fully effective, yet efficacious and cost-effective alternatives are frequently not available through conventional health care delivery systems (Fisher, van Haselen, Hardy, Berkovitz, & McCarney, 2004). When these factors are considered together with increasing prices and limited insurance coverage for many new drugs, nonconventional treatments become practical, cost-effective solutions for increasing numbers of patients. Conventional mental health services are seldom delivered in ways that are cost-effective. In the United States, the current economic crisis at the state level has led to cuts in Medicaid budgets, resulting in more restrictions on care for chronically mentally ill individuals. This has resulted in limited access to medications and less individualized care. HMOs are also attempting to cut costs on a continuous basis by restricting access to drugs. Restricting access to conventional medications results in higher costs related to increased patient acuity associated with increased visits to doctors' offices and emergency rooms, as well as increased hospitalizations. It has been argued that cost-containment measures are thus resulting in increased expenditures from doctor visits and hospitalizations that are exceeding savings on drug costs (Horn et al., 1996).

Cost-effectiveness refers to the cost of achieving a given outcome. Cost-effectiveness analyses of conventional and nonconventional approaches are difficult to perform and rely on accurate measurements of both effectiveness and cost. Outcomes measures are based on appraisals of treatment effectiveness using both quantitative and qualitative criteria. Some outcomes measures are objective (e.g., changes in blood pressure), whereas others are highly subjective (e.g., changes in mood). The subjective outcomes expected for many nonconventional treatments, together with the subjective measures used to assess changes in cognitive or affective symptoms, limit the value of comparisons of outcomes from disparate approaches used in mental health care. Treatment costs can be measured in direct and indirect terms. Direct costs include the cost (if any) of the intervention itself, practitioner fees, the cost of medicines (natural or synthetic), and administrative costs. Indirect costs include the cost of time off work necessary to obtain treatment, as well as the intangible costs of distress when treatment is not successful. If two treatment approaches have similar outcomes, the less expensive approach is sometimes more cost-effective, depending on the balance of direct and indirect costs between the two treatment modalities. This will vary depending on the unique mix of symptoms, symptom severity, and complex needs and circumstances of each patient. In other words, because of the very individualized nature of integrative health care, generic indices of cost-effectiveness for different integrative strategies are seldom forthcoming. One treatment (or treatment combination) may be more effective, whereas a very different conventional or nonconventional treatment (or treatment combination) may be significantly more cost-effective. For example, in some cases moderately effective interventions that cost little to implement, including regular exercise, changes in diet, stress reduction, and bright light exposure, provide cost-effective solutions when used alone or in conjunction with conventional approaches. Clinical decisions to recommend effective versus cost-effective treatments depend on a complex analysis of local resources and symptom severity in the context of the particular patient's preferences and financial resources. Cost offsets alone should never be the sole basis for treatment decisions, though in real-world clinical decision making, they almost always play a significant role.

Cost-utility analysis is a form of cost-effectiveness analysis that is based on measures of distress and life quality. Cost-utility analysis measures the desirability of outcomes to the patient. By definition, this approach is highly subjective and relative to the cultural context in which treatment takes place. In contrast to cost-utility analysis, ***cost-benefit analysis*** compares the financial cost of treatment to the financial benefits of treatment, and subjective factors are not considered. On this basis, some approaches that have high cost-benefit ratios may have low or unacceptable cost-utility, depending on the preferences and perspectives of the individual patient (White, Resch, & Ernst, 1996). It follows that a nonconventional intervention perceived by a patient as enhancing the quality of his or her life will probably be more sought after than some conventional treatments that result in equivalent or better objective outcomes that may have superior cost-benefit ratios but are not perceived as enhancing the quality of life. This issue, in the context of increasing concerns about the efficacy and safety of many conventional drug treatments used in mental health care, explains why nonconventional treatments that are perceived as "life quality enhancing" and are available to patients at little or no cost (e.g., physical exercise, mind–body practices, and dietary changes) are being pursued at increasing rates.

Considerations of Effectiveness versus Cost-Effectiveness in Integrative Treatment Planning

In cases where a patient who is initially treated with conventional drugs does well on reduced doses of medications when using a nonconventional treatment concurrently, the integrative approach has equal or better effectiveness and equal or better cost-effectiveness compared with the conventional treatment alone. The argument for equivalent effectiveness and improved cost-effectiveness is stronger in cases where a patient who has previously responded to a conventional drug does well when taking a nonconventional treatment only. Cases in which symptoms improve when an integrative treatment replaces a conventional treatment that has previously failed provide the strongest evidence for nonconventional medicine. Differences in cost-effectiveness depend on comparative costs of conventional versus nonconventional approaches in the context of the patient's circumstances and preferences. In cases where integrative treatments are equally or more effective or cost-effective compared with available conventional treatments, eliminating or lowering the dose of a conventional medication frequently translates into fewer safety issues, improved treatment compliance, generally improved outcomes and reduced relapse rates, and reduced long-term costs to the patient in terms of lost productivity and direct treatment costs.

The skillful practice of integrative medicine can improve cost-effectiveness through the judicious use of compatible treatments that enhance outcomes while preserving or reducing treatment costs. Increased cost-effectiveness can be achieved by improving outcomes at the same cost or obtaining similar outcomes at reduced cost. The comparative cost-effectiveness of conventional versus integrative treatments addressing a specified symptom pattern will depend on actual costs and local availability of different treatment choices. It is obvious that cost-effectiveness is not improved in cases where a nonconventional or integrative treatment has comparable efficacy but is more expensive or more difficult to obtain compared with a conventional treatment approach. The same applies to considerations of conventional treatments when nonconventional treatments are equally or more effective, more affordable, or more accessible. Effective conventional or integrative treatments are more or less cost effective depending on the unique circumstances of every patient, and evaluations of cost-effectiveness must be made on a case-by-case basis.

Establishing a Hierarchy of Levels and Kinds of Evidence for Claims of Validity or Efficacy

Arguments for the use of a particular methodology to evaluate the efficacy of a specified conventional or nonconventional modality can be characterized as valid (Murphy, 1997) so long as it is possible to verify that the methodology can ascertain whether a putative mechanism of action is present and is the basis for claims of efficacy of the modality. In other words, a claim that a particular medical approach is an appropriate treatment of a specified symptom is a valid claim if the existence of a putative mechanism of action can be verified using a defined methodology. In contrast, a particular modality is an effective assessment or treatment approach with respect to a specified symptom if consistent positive outcomes can be empirically demonstrated using a defined methodology when that modality is applied regardless of the absence of compelling evidence for a postulated mechanism of action. Thus a methodology used to evaluate a specified modality can be determined to be valid or nonvalid irrespective of symptoms for which the modality is intended, but a particular modality can be characterized as more or less effective only with respect to a particular target symptom pattern. The problem of establishing the validity of a methodology rests on determining what criteria are sufficient to establish the existence and operation of a claimed mechanism of action associated with a specified modality. By convention, validated modalities are those for which an accepted methodology has been used to establish a high level of evidence for a putative mechanism of action that is believed to be necessary in order for the specified treatment to have the claimed effect. In Western medicine findings from laboratory studies comprise the highest level of evidence in support of the validity of a methodology used to demonstrate a claimed mechanism of action. Conversely, effective medical practices are those for which a putative mechanism of action might or might not be established, and for which substantial evidence supports claims of beneficial outcomes with respect to a specific symptom pattern. One or more kinds of evidence are generally accepted as providing verification of claims that a specified modality has a beneficial outcome with respect to a particular symptom pattern. Kinds of evidence used to substantiate efficacy or effectiveness include reliable clinical observations, replicated findings from randomized controlled trials, and, to a lesser extent, consistent anecdotal reports or expert opinion.

The distinction between a sufficient proof of validity (i.e., of a methodology used to evaluate a clinical method) and a sufficient proof of efficacy or effectiveness of a specified clinical method is central to an understanding of differences between empirically derived, consensus-based, and intuitive medical approaches. For example, it is possible to establish the validity, effectiveness, or both validity and effectiveness of any specified empirically based approach. In contrast, by definition, only the effectiveness of consensus-based and intuitive modalities has been established. This is a significant fact when one realizes that most conventional and nonconventional approaches in current use do not fulfill criteria required for the empirical verification of a putative mechanism of action, and are therefore maintained either through expert consensus or shared intuitions, values, and so on. Criteria used to verify a putative mechanism or claimed outcome of an empirically derived modality are different than criteria for determining the effectiveness of intuitive practices. However, in both cases, assumptions about mechanisms of action underlying effective modalities are necessarily congruent with assumptions about relationships between phenomena that "cause" (or are interpreted as) illness, and relationships between phenomena that "cause" (or are interpreted as) improved health. Conventional biomedical modalities and nonconventional empirically based modalities that can potentially be validated by the research methodology of contemporary Western biomedicine must rest on phenomena that are explainable on the basis of conceptual models describing the nature of physical objects and certain conventionally accepted kinds of bioenergetic processes that characterize the potential interactions of those objects or processes. In contrast, intuitive modalities do not depend on empirically derived models of causality, and therefore do not require the existence of conventionally agreed-on categories of phenomena. However, some intuitive modalities may ultimately be shown to rely on mechanisms that are congruent with the assumptions of Western science.

In sum, conceptual approaches for appraising the legitimacy of a specified modality from the viewpoint of a particular system of medicine are essentially criteria sets used to determine the validity of a methodology used to demonstrate a putative mechanism of action of the specified modality relative to phenomena that are ontologically legitimate categories of existence from the perspective of the parent system of medicine. It follows that empirically based modalities regarded as validated from the perspective of one system of medicine are often regarded as nonvalid from the viewpoints of other systems of medicine whose methodologies are based on disparate ontological assumptions. However, a specified intuitive modality may be regarded as effective from the perspective of a particular system of medicine that a priori excludes some empirically based modalities because of putative mechanisms of action that do not fulfill specific ontological criteria required by that system of medicine. An example of this is the growing acceptance of Healing Touch in conventional Western hospitals and clinics in the United States and Western Europe. In fact, this often turns out to be the case because it is not possible to formulate analytical descriptions of claimed mechanisms underlying intuitive medical practices. Therefore, using a formal empirical methodology, the phenomenological bases of disparate intuitive modalities cannot be empirically described or compared with one another or with consensus-based or empirically derived modalities. For these reasons, there can be no "science" of intuitive modalities in the same sense that there is a science of empirically derived modalities. It follows that intuitive modalities cannot be a priori excluded as lacking legitimacy because the limited methodology used in conventional biomedical research and the limitations of technology cannot demonstrate with certainty that their putative mechanisms of action do not exist and operate in the way that is claimed. In other words, the methodology supporting a particular intuitive modality cannot be invalidated by current Western science or any other empirical methodology, nor can claims of a putative mechanism underlying a particular intuitive approach be falsified or verified using conventional empirical means. This is always and necessarily true because, by definition, intuitive modalities can be evaluated and compared with other empirically derived, consensus-based, or intuitive approaches only on the basis of measures of efficacy or effectiveness, and never on the basis of empirical demonstrations of a putative mechanism of action (for reasons discussed above). Therefore, a methodology for establishing effectiveness, but not a methodology used to establish the existence of a putative mechanism of action, necessarily provides the sole basis for identifying intuitive approaches that are appropriate to consider for inclusion in integrative management strategies.

Considerable variation often exists in the strength of available evidence for a putative mechanism of action or the claimed effectiveness of a specified conventional or nonconventional modality with respect to a specified symptom pattern. This fact is due to diverse study designs, the range in the size of studies examining a particular modality, and commensurate differences in the quality and significance of findings with respect to the target symptom pattern. A general hierarchy of levels and kinds of evidence therefore provides only a crude conceptual model, and it is necessary to construct separate tables showing the levels and kinds of evidence for any particular modality with respect to a specified symptom pattern. Our subject is mental health, and our central task is to develop tables showing kinds and levels of evidence for particular assessment and treatment modalities with respect to specified cognitive, affective and behavioral symptoms. The common symptom patterns covered in Part II of this book are

◆ Depressed mood
◆ Mania and cyclic mood changes
◆ Anxiety
◆ Psychosis
◆ Disturbances of memory and cognition
◆ Symptoms related to substance abuse and dependence
◆ Disturbances of sleep and wakefulness

Many nonconventional modalities in current use to assess or treat cognitive and affective symptoms are based on limited evidence from clinical studies, have been examined in studies that are small or methodologically flawed (i.e., by Western scientific standards), or have a record of inconsistent results. Like the majority of established conventional approaches, most nonconventional modalities used as treatments of specific symptom patterns have not been empirically validated using the methodology of Western medicine or the parent nonconventional system of medicine. In the methodology developed below, both quantitative and qualitative criteria are used to assess kinds and level" of evidence supporting nonconventional modalities. The use of both kinds of criteria to evaluate evidence relates directly to the practical work of integrative medicine, because both empirically obtained quantitative information and qualitative or self-reported subjective information are needed to ensure an accurate and complete understanding of most conventional and nonconventional modalities. Quantitative criteria include

Table 4–3 Quantitative and Qualitative Criteria Used to Assess Evidence for Nonconventional Assessment and Treatment Modalities

Quantitative Criteria

◆ Numbers of studies done, kinds of studies (basic research and clinical investigations, randomized controlled trials, cohort studies, case series, etc.) and significance of findings

◆ Systematic reviews or narrative reviews and significance of findings

◆ Studies in progress, objectives, and preliminary findings (if any)

◆ Specificity of findings by major cognitive, affective, or behavioral symptom (i.e., how the specified assessment or treatment modality enhances diagnostic accuracy or improves treatment outcomes)

Qualitative Criteria

◆ Unresolved research issues influencing study design

◆ Other unresolved issues (e.g., safety, availability, cost, and insurance coverage)

◆ Described uses of specified modality in conjunction with other conventional or nonconventional modalities with respect to a specified cognitive, affective, or behavioral symptom

◆ Best resources for further information for patients or clinicians

◆ Patient preferences and attitudes toward recommended modality

statistical measures describing the quality, numbers, and types of biomedical studies pertinent to a particular nonconventional modality. Qualitative criteria include information pertaining to unresolved research issues, preliminary findings of ongoing trials, clinician and patient perceptions and preferences, cost, and availability. Quantitative criteria are the basis of evidence-ranking methods in Western medicine. In contrast, subjective, qualitative information that is typically excluded from biomedical evidence is often the cornerstone of evidence-ranking methods in nonconventional systems of medicine. **Table 4–3** includes both quantitative and qualitative criteria that are useful means of evaluating the relative merits and weaknesses of a particular nonconventional modality with respect to a specified symptom pattern.

Constructing Hierarchies of Quantitative Medical Evidence

Philosophical arguments for the conceptual basis of evidence hierarchies are presented in Chapter 2. Different approaches are appropriate when evaluating quantitative versus qualitative medical evidence. **Table 4–4** lists relevant criteria for an evidence hierarchy used to evaluate quantitative information about kinds and levels of evidence with respect to a putative mechanism of action or a claimed outcome for particular conventional or nonconventional assessment or treatment approaches that are susceptible to empirical verification. This is also the basis for the methodology used to evaluate quantitative evidence for clinical approaches discussed in the chapters of Part II. According to this schema, there are seven general kinds and five general levels of evidence.

With respect to the first four kinds of evidence, empirical information is available and permits judgments about both the existence of a putative mechanism of action (i.e., within the context of current Western science) and the claimed efficacy or

Table 4–4   Kinds and Levels of Evidence for Developing Evidence Hierarchies

---

Kinds of Quantitative Evidence

Efficacy is verified, and putative mechanism of action is verified.

Efficacy is verified, and putative mechanism of action is not verified.

Efficacy is verified, and putative mechanism of action is refuted.

Efficacy is refuted, and putative mechanism of action also is refuted.

Efficacy is verified, and putative mechanism of action is unverifiable.

Efficacy is unverified, and putative mechanism of action is unverifiable.

Efficacy is refuted, and putative mechanism of action is unverifiable.

Levels of Quantitative Evidence

"*N* of 1" trials or systematic reviews of randomized controlled studies

Randomized controlled studies where follow-up is greater than 80%

Cohort studies

Case control studies or observational studies

Expert opinion

---

effectiveness of an approach. In contrast, for the last three kinds of evidence, empirical verification of claims of effectiveness is possible, but for reasons discussed above it is not possible to make judgments about the existence of a putative mechanism of action. The last three kinds of evidence—efficacy verified, efficacy unverified, and efficacy refuted—are relevant when evaluating intuitive modalities for which there are sometimes data on effectiveness but for which, by definition, there is no reliable information about a putative mechanism of action. In the three last cases, a putative mechanism of action is unverifiable using contemporary Western scientific means. Recall that this is the defining criterion for all intuitive modalities. The above levels of evidence are present in widely used methodologies for the evaluation of both biomedical and nonconventional assessment and treatment approaches. It is interesting to note that evidence-based medicine assigns "expert opinion" to the lowest level of quantitative biomedical evidence because strong correspondences between expert opinions and research evidence are frequently not present (Gray, 2004). It is significant that many established clinical practice guidelines in conventional biomedicine rely on expert opinion in the absence of higher levels of evidence according to the principles of EBM.

I have argued elsewhere that the overall strength of evidence for use of a particular modality with respect to a specified symptom pattern can be expressed as a factor of the level and kind of evidence while taking into account a measure of the relative significance of findings for a specified kind of evidence and cumulative results at a given level of evidence. To be of practical clinical value, all evidence hierarchies must provide accurate and relevant evidence pertaining to particular assessment or treatment modalities with respect to a specified symptom. It is meaningful, therefore, to talk about levels or kinds of evidence for a particular modality only with respect to a specified symptom pattern. A putative mechanism of action and beneficial outcomes associated with a particular modality can be verified by compelling research findings with respect to a specified symptom pattern. Another modality that is being considered with respect to the same symptom pattern may be supported by moderately strong evidence from open studies or case reports. In such cases the optimum treatment

for the specified symptom pattern should include the modality for which the strongest kind and highest level of evidence are present. However, in some instances the patient may have already tried what is arguably the optimum treatment (i.e., on the basis of the evidence hierarchy) but failed to respond, a qualified local provider of that treatment may not be available, or the patient may refuse the recommended approach because of cultural preferences or financial constraints. In any of these cases, to develop an integrative treatment plan that is both supported by evidence and acceptable to the patient, it is often necessary to consider treatments for which there are supporting data but not always compelling evidence. The clinician and patient ideally should work together to select potentially beneficial treatments that represent realistic choices in view of patient preferences and extenuating circumstances. In sum, the evidence hierarchies should be used as a general guide to planning reasonable assessment or treatment approaches in the broad context of realistic constraints and patient preferences. A methodology for evaluating both quantitative and qualitative evidence for purposes of planning integrative health care is developed in the following section.

Evaluating Both Quantitative and Qualitative Evidence

There are four general levels of evidence based on possible combinations of different kinds of quantitative and qualitative evidence supporting the use of a particular assessment or treatment modality with respect to a specified symptom pattern. In some cases, high-quality studies will have been conducted but not yet analyzed in a systematic review. In other cases, studies may be ongoing or recently concluded but not yet published, or published in specialty journals but not yet subjected to a critical peer-review process. The combined quantitative-qualitative model used here takes these considerations into account in an effort to provide a balanced methodology for weighing the evidence supporting uses of both conventional and nonconventional assessment and treatment approaches when different levels and kinds of evidence are available for disparate approaches that are being considered for possible inclusion in an integrative management plan. An assessment or treatment approach is substantiated with respect to a specified symptom when there is a consistent and high level of supporting evidence, the approach is in established clinical use, and it is widely accepted by a relevant community of professional practitioners. Provisional approaches are supported by significant but less compelling evidence, although they are often in widespread clinical use and are often endorsed by conventional or nonconventional medical practitioners or a relevant professional association. For purposes of this book, a particular assessment or treatment approach is regarded as possibly effective when limited or inconsistent research findings support its use with respect to a specified symptom pattern, and if endorsed by a relevant professional group its use is limited or controversial. A modality is refuted (with respect to a specified symptom pattern) when consistent negative findings of well-conducted studies or at least one systematic review confirm negative findings. If the approach is still used, it is not endorsed by a relevant professional association and remains highly controversial. For obvious reasons very few conventional or nonconventional modalities in current use have been refuted by compelling negative findings. Most assessment and treatment approaches in current

Table 4–5   Criteria for Determining the Level of Evidence for Assessment and Treatment Approaches

1. Substantiated (in current use and effective)

Systematic review findings are compelling or strongly support claims that a particular assessment modality provides accurate information about the causes or meanings of a symptom pattern or that a particular treatment approach results in consistent positive outcomes with respect to a specified symptom pattern, *or* three or more rigorously conducted double-blind randomized controlled trials (cohort studies for assessment approaches) support claims of outcomes when the modality is employed to assess or treat a specified symptom pattern. The modality is in current use for the assessment or treatment of a specified symptom pattern, *and* the use of the modality with respect to a specified symptom pattern is endorsed by a relevant association of professional practitioners.

2. Provisional (in current use and probably effective)

Systematic review findings are highly suggestive but not compelling, or have not been conducted because of insufficient numbers of studies or uneven quality of completed studies, *or* three or more rigorously conducted double-blind randomized controlled trials (cohort studies for assessment approaches) yield findings that are suggestive but not compelling, and the approach is in current use for the assessment or treatment of a specified symptom pattern. The use of the modality with respect to a specified symptom pattern may be endorsed by a relevant association of professional practitioners.

3. Possibly effective (in current use and possibly effective)

Fewer than three well-designed studies or three or more poorly designed studies have been done to determine whether a particular assessment modality provides accurate information about causes or meanings of a specified symptom pattern or to determine whether a particular treatment modality results in consistent positive outcomes with respect to a specified symptom pattern. Research findings or anecdotal reports are limited or inconsistent, *and* there are insufficient quality studies on which to base a systematic review or meta-analysis. The modality is in current use but remains controversial and may be endorsed by a relevant association of professional practitioners.

4. Refuted (may be in current use but refuted by evidence)

For a particular assessment modality, findings of three or more rigorously conducted studies or at least one systematic review consistently show that the approach does not provide accurate information about causes or meanings of a specified symptom pattern.

For a particular treatment modality, findings of three or more rigorously conducted studies or at least one systematic review consistently show that the modality does not result in beneficial outcomes with respect to a specified symptom pattern. Refuted approaches are generally not in current use, are not endorsed by a relevant society of professional practitioners, and if used, are highly controversial.

It is important to recall that the double-blind, randomized, controlled trial is the current gold standard in biomedical research used to verify efficacy claims of treatments; however, the cohort study is the gold standard used to verify outcomes of assessment approaches. Substantiated modalities are those conventional or nonconventional assessment or treatment approaches in current use for which claims of assessment accuracy or treatment efficacy have been verified either by findings of a systematic review or by consistent positive outcomes from at least three well-designed outcomes studies, and the approach is endorsed as the standard of practice by a relevant association of professional medical practitioners. Using the same criteria, there is provisional evidence for a modality with respect to a specified symptom when the findings of a systematic review or at least three outcomes studies provide suggestive but not compelling evidence, the approach is in current use with respect to a specified symptom, and the approach is endorsed by a relevant professional body. By definition, provisional approaches are supported by good evidence; however, the continued widespread use and endorsement of many provisional approaches with respect to a specified symptom pattern strongly suggests that claims of assessment accuracy or treatment efficacy have merit even when those claims have not yet been corroborated by large numbers of well-designed outcomes studies or systematic review findings. A modality is possibly effective when the evidence supporting its use for a specified symptom pattern is uneven because of a limited number or quality of outcomes studies or inconsistent findings. Possibly effective approaches are sometimes endorsed by a relevant professional group. It is reasonable to regard a modality as refuted with respect to a specified symptom pattern when consistently negative research findings do not support claims of assessment accuracy or treatment efficacy, and the modality is not endorsed by a relevant professional group. In some cases a particular approach is endorsed by a professional group of conventional or nonconventional medical practitioners, but outcomes studies yield consistently negative findings. I am taking the conservative viewpoint that such approaches should be regarded as refuted for all reasonable intents and purposes. It is conceivable that certain modalities that are presently regarded as refuted according to the above criteria will emerge as provisional modalities with future positive findings. Most biomedical and nonconventional approaches that are currently refuted will likely continue to be regarded as refuted. In the same vein, some approaches that are currently designated as provisional with respect to evidence supporting their use for a specified symptom pattern will probably become substantiated or refuted on the basis of future research findings or systematic reviews.

Clearly, the evidence base supporting uses of conventional or nonconventional assessment or treatment modalities is constantly changing. There are two basic reasons for changes in the relative strength of evidence for any particular assessment or treatment approach with respect to a specified symptom pattern: emerging research findings suggest that a particular approach is more or less likely to result in beneficial outcomes, and new methodologies for assessing the kinds and levels of evidence are endorsed, resulting in system-level changes in criteria for evaluating claims of mechanism of action or efficacy. Ongoing revisions of the evidence tables in the companion Web site www.thieme.com/mentalhealth take both of these factors into account.

use are supported by at least some objective evidence of beneficial outcomes and are endorsed by a professional group of nonconventional practitioners. **Table 4–5** lists criteria for determining whether a particular modality is substantiated, provisional, or possibly effective.

This evidence-ranking methodology employs combined quantitative and qualitative criteria to determine whether a particular approach is substantiated, provisional, possibly effective, or refuted in terms of the evidence supporting its use for the assessment or treatment of a specified symptom pattern. This approach can be applied equally to any conventional or nonconventional assessment or treatment approach.

Kinds and Levels of Evidence in Medicine Will Continue to Change

Future research findings will verify claims of putative mechanisms of action or efficacy for certain nonconventional modalities that now qualify as provisional while refuting others. Novel assessment and treatment approaches will continue to emerge in biomedicine and nonconventional systems of medicine, and many of these will become viable modalities in a future integrative medicine. Depending on the kind and quality of available evidence, future approaches will become regarded as substantiated, provisional, or possibly effective with respect to future standards of evidence. It is important to note that determinations of levels of evidence are closely related to the category to which a particular modality belongs. Basic differences between criteria used to determine the pertinent evidence base, or to establish the relevance of empirically derived, consensus-based, or intuitive modalities translate into commensurate differences in criteria used to determine whether modalities belonging to disparate classes are regarded as substantiated, provisional, possibly effective, or refuted with respect to a specified symptom pattern. Thus the criteria used to determine whether a particular modality is substantiated or provisional are determined, first, in relation to the class of the modality (i.e., empirically derived, consensus-based, or intuitive), and second, in relation to the level of evidence supporting the use of the modality with respect to a specified symptom. The definition of a particular modality as empirically derived, consensus-based, or intuitive is a function of whether requirements for certain kinds or levels of qualitative or quantitative evidence are fulfilled. Qualitative information is potentially available for each of the three classes of modalities, but quantitative information is potentially available for only empirically derived and consensus-based approaches. Recall that, by definition, intuitive modalities remain in use in spite of the absence of empirical evidence, and their claims are not verifiable using (current) empirical methods. In contrast, consensus-based modalities remain in use in spite of negative evidence or in the absence of compelling positive findings in spite of the fact that their claims are susceptible to empirical verification. The class of a particular modality is determined by the quantitative or qualitative criteria that are fulfilled for efficacy claims of that modality with respect to a specified symptom. Four logically possible cases of combined evidence spaces of qualitative and quantitative information are possible for any particular conventional or nonconventional modality. **Table 4–6** shows possible evidence spaces corresponding to empirically derived, consensus-based, and intuitive modalities.

The level and kind of evidence for a particular modality with respect to a specified symptom pattern determine whether a particular modality is substantiated, provisional, possibly effective, or refuted. This composite factor can be described in terms of evidence space. For empirically derived modalities, substantial evidence exists with respect to a specified symptom when compelling quantitative and qualitative evidence exists (A) for a claimed outcome. A particular empirically derived modality is provisional with respect to a specified symptom pattern when the evidence space contains suggestive findings because of different levels of qualitative and quantitative evidence (B or C). Finally, an empirically derived modality is refuted with respect to a specified symptom when both quantitative and qualitative findings are negative or highly inconsistent (D). By definition, consensus-based modalities are not supported by compelling empirical evidence, but continue in practice in the face of ongoing debate over the significance of inconsistent or limited quantitative and qualitative evidence (B and C). Evaluating the evidence for intuitive modalities presents a dilemma because intuitive modalities are not (presently) subject to verification using conventional empirical methods. In such cases, supporting, inconsistent, or negative evidence is not relevant to clinicians' judgments about the acceptability or appropriateness of a particular intuitive modality with respect to a specified symptom. Intuitive approaches nevertheless remain in use because both clinicians and patients believe they are effective outside of considerations of quantitative or qualitative evidence. The efficacy of intuitive modalities cannot be verified or refuted by Western science using contemporary methods or technologies. However, shared interpretations of qualitative evidence, including consistent reports of improved health, frequently support the continued use of intuitive modalities. Intuitive modalities are sometimes supported by qualitative but not quantitative evidence, and often have no supporting evidence whatsoever. Future scientific theories will accommodate the assumptions of some nonconventional intuitive modalities, and in some cases novel technologies will permit the verification of a putative mechanism of action or a claimed beneficial effect, and those intuitive approaches will subsequently become redefined as consensus-based or empirically derived assessment and treatment methods in conventional medicine.

Recall that the kind and quality of evidence for any particular conventional or nonconventional modality will vary, often considerably, depending on the symptom pattern that is being addressed. The evidence tables in Part II of this book rate assessment and treatment modalities used to treat a specified symptom pattern as substantiated, provisional, or possibly effective (possibly accurate for assessment approaches) with respect to that particular target symptom. This method takes into account cases where discrepancies exist between the strength of quantitative and qualitative evidence, and permits the practitioner to evaluate the merits of evidence supporting the use of a range of nonconventional assessment or treatment approaches for different primary symptoms and on a case-by-case basis. For example, if clinical data supporting the use of a particular aromatherapy protocol in anxiety are

Table 4–6 Potential Evidence Spaces for Empirically Derived, Consensus-Based, and Intuitive Modalities

Kind of Evidence	Level of Evidence			
	A	B	C	D
Quantitative	Compelling evidence	Compelling evidence	Negative or inconsistent evidence	Negative or inconsistent evidence
Qualitative	Compelling evidence	Negative or inconsistent evidence	Compelling evidence	Negative or inconsistent evidence

cited in only one specialized database, are not mentioned in the peer-reviewed professional literature on aromatherapy, and are excluded from review articles or omitted from systematic reviews of studies of aromatherapy in mental health, or are not included in a treatment protocol endorsed by a relevant professional association of aromatherapy practitioners, it is reasonable to doubt the credibility of the source. In this case, the particular aromatherapy treatment in question would be designated as a "possibly effective" treatment of anxiety, and more substantiated treatments would be considered when formulating a suitable integrative treatment plan. At present few nonconventional assessment approaches have been strongly substantiated. The majority of nonconventional approaches in current use to assess the causes or meanings of cognitive, affective, and behavioral symptoms are provisional or possibly accurate because of limited available quantitative or qualitative evidence from cohort studies or clinical observations.

The same comment can be made for the majority of conventional biomedical assessment approaches used in conventional mental health care. Serological analysis, urine analysis, and structural or functional brain-imaging studies frequently provide useful diagnostic information pertaining to multiple factors related to mental illness, but the extent to which they provide a definitive picture of the primary causes of cognitive or affective symptoms remains unclear. In contrast to the many established, effective conventional and nonconventional treatment approaches, the paucity of substantiated assessment methods in Western biomedical psychiatry has significantly delayed progress in the evolution of mental health care. This problem is discussed in more detail in Chapter 5.

Empirically derived modalities that are not presently substantiated can be potentially confirmed or refuted by future evidence, but the level of evidence supporting their use may remain relatively unchanged following additional studies. Consensus-based modalities can become empirically substantiated, refuted, or remain unsubstantiated but often continue in widespread use. The efficacy of some intuitive modalities will probably be empirically verified by future technologies, and they will fulfill criteria for provisional or substantiated modalities. Some intuitive approaches will be refuted by future research, whereas others will probably continue in use regardless of considerations of evidence because of their popular appeal to patients or clinicians. **Table 4–7** shows possible

evolutionary pathways of empirically derived, consensus-based, and intuitive modalities.

The above criteria provide useful guidelines for identifying assessment or treatment choices that are most substantiated with respect to a specific symptom pattern. Provisional modalities are sometimes reasonable choices in integrative management when more substantiated approaches have proven ineffective or unsafe, or when more substantiated approaches are not realistic choices because of practical constraints or personal preferences. The evidence tables given in this book will be updated regularly (refer to the companion Web site www.thieme.com/mentalhealth for such updates), and the relative position of a particular modality in evidence space will change as significant new supporting or disconfirming evidence emerges with respect to a specified symptom pattern. The relative strength of evidence supporting the use of a particular modality for the assessment or treatment of a specified symptom will probably vary over time depending on the emerging evidence for that modality in relationship to changes in the evidence spaces of other modalities used to treat the same symptom pattern. In this way, the comparative "weights" of evidence for all modalities relevant to the management of a specified symptom will be revised on an ongoing basis. Ultimately, the clinician's choice of particular assessment or treatment modalities will be based on an evaluation of evidence in favor of disparate modalities at any given time, taking into account a particular patient's history of responses to previous treatments, patient preferences, financial or availability constraints, and the practitioner's training and clinical experience.

Sequential versus Parallel Interventions and Comments on Order of Precedence in Integrative Treatment Planning

The integrative practitioner must take into account many factors in addition to considerations of evidence ranking to decide whether to recommend two or more treatments in parallel versus sequential treatments. Similar considerations apply to the selection of assessment approaches when evaluating the causes or meanings of symptoms. When the evidence suggests that two or more disparate treatments have equivalent efficacy, the selection of a treatment or treatments, as

Table 4–7 Possible Evolutionary Pathways of Empirically Derived, Consensus-Based, and Intuitive Modalities

Category of Modality	Empirical Data Support Use*	Future Methods, Theories, or Technologies Permit Substantiation	Future Methods, Theories, or Technologies Yield Inconsistent Results
Empirically derived	Always (S) Sometimes (P) Rarely (PE)	The modality continues in use and is supported by increasing evidence	The modality is refuted or continues in use at lower level of evidence
Consensus-based	Sometimes (S, P, or PE)	The modality becomes accepted as empirically derived (level of evidence varies)	The modality is refuted or continues in use as intuitive modality
Intuitive	Never (criteria for S, P, and PE cannot be evaluated and so do not apply)	The modality becomes accepted as empirically derived	The modality continues in use as an intuitive approach: empirical evidence is not relevant to clinical acceptance

*An empirically derived or consensus-based modality is substantiated (S), provisional (P), or possibly effective (PE) with respect to the level of empirical evidence that supports claims of a putative mechanism of action or beneficial outcomes. Intuitive modalities sometimes remain in use regardless of the absence of substantiating evidence or the presence of contradictory evidence.

well as the order in which treatments are recommended, should be determined on the basis of the following criteria:

♦ A (conventional or nonconventional) treatment that was effective and well tolerated when previously used by the patient for similar symptoms should be strongly recommended.

♦ A (conventional or nonconventional) treatment that was previously effective for similar symptoms but was not well tolerated should be recommended following a trial on a treatment that probably has equivalent effectiveness but may be better tolerated.

♦ When the evidence suggests that a (conventional or nonconventional) treatment approach is probably effective for a specified symptom pattern, but the treatment requires a highly skilled practitioner to administer, the approach should be recommended only when a qualified local practitioner is available, and in cases where the approach is both affordable and acceptable to the patient.

♦ When two or more (conventional or nonconventional) treatments have equal efficacy and there is similar risk of adverse effects, cost should be an important deciding criterion.

♦ When the patient has tried all substantiated (conventional or nonconventional) treatments that are affordable, available, and acceptable (to the patient) without benefit, it is reasonable to consider provisional approaches.

♦ Criteria for determining the order of precedence of provisional approaches are the same as those used for substantiated approaches.

♦ Depending on the evidence, patient preferences, cost, and availability of qualified practitioners, combining a provisional approach with a substantiated approach may provide synergistic benefits.

♦ As new approaches are tried, previously tried unsuccessful (conventional or nonconventional) approaches should be discontinued unless there is evidence that they have synergistic effects when used with the new approach.

♦ Possibly effective treatments should be considered only after substantiated or provisional approaches (i.e., for the specified symptom pattern) have been tried without benefit or in cases where evidence supports the use of a possibly effective approach together with a particular substantiated or provisional approach.

♦ In cases where all substantiated and provisional approaches have been tried without benefit, or are unavailable, unaffordable, or unacceptable to the patient, it is sometimes reasonable to try a possibly effective approach if there is a qualified local practitioner, the patient provides informed consent to receive the treatment, and the patient is motivated to try that approach. In such cases, the $N = 1$ method can be used to evaluate the efficacy of a particular treatment for a specific patient even in the absence of compelling evidence. Using the $N = 1$ approach will help the clinician to determine whether a possibly effective treatment is potentially beneficial for the patient and can sometimes lead to an effective individualized treatment plan.

The evidence tables in Part II of this book facilitate the identification of particular assessment or treatment practices that fulfill criteria for different levels or kinds of evidence and that can be combined in compatible or synergistic ways. Reviewing the evidence tables is an essential step in planning clinical management addressing cognitive, affective, and behavioral symptoms.

Algorithms given in Part II provide a logical framework for thinking about reasonable sequences of assessment and treatment approaches addressing a particular patient and his or her unique symptoms. The clinician's task is to select modalities that are effective, appropriate for the patient, and locally available. The practical steps in this process are discussed in Chapters 5 and 6.

♦ Literature Research Methodology and Constructing the Evidence Tables

In this section, a methodology is developed for constructing a series of tables for planning integrative management strategies addressing common cognitive, affective, and behavioral symptoms covered in Part II of this book. Criteria for selecting primary and secondary sources of data are suggested, the general plan for constructing the tables is presented, and search strategies for obtaining reliable information are described. A methodology for identifying ancillary information sources is briefly reviewed. Primary sources include mainstream databases on Western biomedicine or nonconventional medicine. Secondary sources include newsletters (both circulating and electronic), expert interviews, unpublished data, and personal communications where relevant. A plan is described for periodically reviewing and updating contents, and optimizing the general logical structure and search parameters of queries used to construct the tables to enhance their utility as tools for planning the integrative management of mental health problems. Evidence tables are constructed to illustrate levels of evidence and degrees of compatibility for disparate conventional and nonconventional modalities. Finally, the basic concept and uses of the Web site that accompanies this book (www.thieme.com/mentalhealth) are presented.

The essential purpose and central value of the evidence tables is to facilitate decision making in planning integrative medical management. The tables must contain information that is useful for solving practical problems in the day-to-day management of patient care. They must provide accurate, unbiased coverage of disparate nonconventional and integrative modalities relevant to the assessment or treatment of common mental health problems. The tables show relative levels of evidence or compatibility, and must have an open structure, permitting repositioning of assessment or treatment modalities when new findings emerge. Using this approach, the tables afford a flexible integrative treatment-planning tool incorporating the most relevant modalities based on the best available evidence at any given time.

In constructing the tables, information about mechanisms of action, efficacy, and safety was obtained for both assessment and treatment approaches. A computerized literature search was used to identify citations of systematic reviews or meta-analyses of randomized controlled studies, individual RCTs, and case reports pertaining to nonconventional medical approaches for the common cognitive, affective, and behavioral symptoms examined in this book. A manual literature search of published and unpublished papers and conference proceedings supplemented the computerized search. In addition to completed studies, preliminary findings pertaining to ongoing research or clinical trials were obtained from several sources, including the Cochrane database of clinical trials (www.cochrane.org/reviews) and the NIH–NCCAM database of ongoing clinical trials (http://nccam.nih.gov.clinicaltrials) in alternative medicine. Preliminary findings from these resources were used to identify promising research areas and significant emerging trends in clinical applications of the range of nonconventional and integrative approaches used in mental health care.

Rationale for Search Methodology Used to Construct the Evidence Tables

Three basic kinds of information can be obtained from the literature about nonconventional modalities: studies on efficacy of a particular modality, studies on the efficacy of a particular combination of biomedical or nonconventional modalities, and studies on the safety of a particular combination of biomedical or nonconventional modalities. There are many ways to search for medical information. For purposes of constructing the evidence tables used in Part II of this book, a search strategy was employed that used several different approaches in parallel. This approach takes into account the fact that any particular search strategy is inherently self-limiting or biased against certain kinds of medical information. Search strategies typically used to obtain medical evidence rank the significance of findings on the basis of the presumed validity of the study design. Western biomedicine assigns different degrees of validity to different study designs (Gray, 2004). The randomized controlled trial is regarded as the most rigorous conventional study design, and the most reliable medical information is generally assigned to conclusions of a systematic review of several RCTs designed in exactly the same way. Evidence-based medicine compares the findings of systematic reviews or meta-analyses of RCTs to determine the relative merits of evidence pertaining to different kinds of treatments for a particular symptom pattern. However, systematic reviews and meta-analyses are inherently limited in many ways, and often provide unreliable or biased information (Jadad & Gagliardi, 1998). For example, the value and validity of systematic review findings are often affected by reporting bias. Many studies are excluded from the review process for reasons other than study quality or size (Gray, 2004), including

◆ Significant findings are more likely to be published than nonsignificant findings.
◆ Studies with significant findings are more likely to be published in journals that are indexed in a medical database.
◆ Significant findings are more likely to be published in English-language journals, and nonsignificant findings are more likely to be published in non-English-language journals.
◆ Studies with significant findings are more likely to be cited compared with studies with nonsignificant findings.

For these reasons, the conclusions of different systematic reviews of the same studies sometimes differ. A meta-analysis increases the statistical power of a study, or the capacity of the study design to detect significant differences between two or more treatments that are being compared. Different sources of bias affect meta-analysis findings, including biases in publication, reference selection, methods of data extraction, and outcomes caused by improper blinding, incomplete randomization, or the use of certain kinds of inclusion or exclusion criteria (Mancano & Bullano, 1998). An example of publication bias is the observation that a meta-analysis based on published data only is more likely to show beneficial effects of a treatment compared with a meta-analysis that takes into account unpublished data, because published results are more likely to be positive than negative (Dickerson & Min, 1993).

At the level of individual RCTs, there are limited data for many nonconventional modalities, which have therefore largely been investigated using cohort studies or case control studies. There are many reasons for this fact, including limited funding for large prospective trials of most kinds of nonconventional modalities and intrinsic problems designing RCTs that can examine putative mechanisms of action underlying many nonconventional modalities. Because of these constraints, RCTs examining many nonconventional modalities and systematic reviews of such RCTs will probably continue to be relatively infrequent compared with the number of RCTs and systematic reviews of conventional medical approaches. Therefore, relying on information from systematic reviews or meta-analyses of published RCTs or analysis of individual RCTs for determinations of the efficacy of nonconventional treatments will inherently bias search results against many nonconventional modalities (Mancano & Bullano, 1998). In view of the above, a reasonable compromise approach to determining accurate and clinically useful information about nonconventional modalities is to combine different kinds of search strategies. For example, where limited or no data are available from systematic reviews of RCTs or individual RCTs investigating a particular nonconventional assessment or treatment modality for a specified mental health problem, the results of cohort studies or case series can provide useful information. Where necessary, basic research data on the efficacy or effectiveness of nonconventional modalities were supplemented by expert interviews or professional practice guidelines published by associations representing particular nonconventional modalities. In all cases, clinical decisions ultimately rest on the clinician's judgment in the context of relevant medical literature.

Conceptual Steps for Obtaining Information for the Evidence Tables

Valuable data sources are those that provide current, reliable information that is useful for clinical problem solving. At present, most medical databases emphasize conventional biomedicine over nonconventional medical practices. However, growing interest in nonconventional medicine among both physicians and patients has resulted in the inclusion of citations on many nonconventional modalities in Medline (www.pubmedcentral.nih.gov) and other mainstream medical databases. Several medical databases covering numerous nonconventional modalities have been designed for use by medical practitioners and patients. At the same time, specialized databases have been created with the goal of providing information about focused areas of nonconventional medicine, for example, Chinese medicine, Western herbal medicine, and homeopathy.

In this section I will discuss the design of the evidence tables that provide essential information for integrative treatment planning, as described above. The evidence tables include claims of efficacy for specified nonconventional assessment or treatment modalities corresponding to citations obtained through Web-based or manual searches of primary or secondary sources, expert opinion, or my own clinical experience. Citations examined during the initial literature research phase included meta-analyses or systematic reviews of randomized controlled trials, individual randomized controlled trials, cohort studies, case control studies, and other study designs investigating uses of nonconventional assessment or treatment modalities in mental health care. For purposes of constructing the evidence tables, searches of systematic reviews or individual studies pertaining to strictly conventional biomedical psychiatry were not made. Statements describing uses of modalities in conventional Western psychiatry included in Part II chapters are based on general practice guidelines and current review articles, and not based on an exhaustive review of the literature. As such, general statements pertaining to the efficacy or effectiveness of a particular biomedical assessment or treatment approach for a specified mental health problem are described in overview in the introductory sections of Part II chapters but are not included in the evidence tables. For purposes of constructing evidence tables for use in planning integrative mental health care, it is assumed that claims of efficacy for conventional biomedical modalities can be reliably substantiated by existing practice guidelines endorsed by the American Psychiatric Association (APA) or other guidelines describing standards of psychopharmacological treatment of cognitive, affective, and behavioral symptoms (e.g., the Texas Medication Algorithms). The National Guideline Clearinghouse (www.guideline.gov) indexes most established guidelines for conventional biomedical treatments and some nonconventional modalities. Existing guidelines supporting conventional biomedical approaches in mental health care are based on expert consensus following comprehensive reviews of the peer-reviewed biomedical literature. It is important to recall that not all clinical practice guidelines are based on best evidence, according to the standards of evidence-based medicine (Browman, 2001). Clinical practice guidelines reflect the biases and professional experiences of their authors. Conventional practice guidelines therefore reflect expert consensus on biomedical approaches regarded as legitimate and evidence-based in the context of contemporary Western medicine. Contemporary biomedical practice guidelines typically do not take into consideration evidence pertaining to most nonconventional modalities. For example, the literature review process on which APA-endorsed guidelines or other mainstream practice guidelines are based largely ignores citations of studies on nonconventional modalities (Beckner & Berman, 2003; Dickerson & Min, 1993). Cases of negative peer review bias against publications on nonconventional medicine suggest that this is a significant problem interfering with accurate reporting of research findings. Negative reviews of nonconventional medical research studies sometimes rely on misrepresentations of findings, misleading statements, failure to refer to the relevant research literature, selective use of certain published papers reporting negative findings, and inaccurate reporting of contents of published papers (Morley, Rosner, & Redwood, 2001; Resch, Ernst, & Garrow, 2000). The concept underlying the integrative evidence tables used in this book takes into account exclusion biases in conventional biomedical databases. Treatment-planning tables are constructed from critically reviewed claims of efficacy or effectiveness in citations obtained from reliable resources on nonconventional approaches.

Selecting Resources to Search When Constructing Evidence Tables for Integrative Management of Cognitive, Affective, and Behavioral Symptoms

Formulating a question that can be answered by searching the literature is the essential first step in obtaining clinically pertinent information (Gray, 2004). A clearly phrased question is the basis for any literature search. If the question is ambiguous, the literature search will be unfocused, important resources will be overlooked, and relevant information will be missed. According to the logic of evidence-based medicine, questions about the efficacy of a particular assessment or treatment modality with respect to a specified illness are best answered with reference to certain kinds of evidence obtained from studies based on certain kinds of research designs, or even better, statistical analyses of several high-quality studies on the same question. Questions about treatment efficacy, for instance, are best answered by randomized controlled trials, and the reliability or specificity of an assessment approach is best determined by cross-sectional studies (Guyatt & Rennie, 2002). However, the situation is complicated by the fact that there are many levels of RCTs, and important differences exist between the significance of findings of different RCTs, depending on study design, size of trial, follow-up, and so on. Evidence-based medicine is rapidly gaining acceptance among Western-trained physicians as a legitimate method for critically appraising the evidence in support of any conventional or nonconventional modality. Recently published textbooks on complementary and alternative medicine have embraced EBM as an appropriate paradigm from which to objectively assess evidence of efficacy and safety. The methods of EBM are inherently limited by implicit materialistic assumptions that have resulted in the a priori exclusion of many nonconventional modalities as spurious or irrelevant.

Considerations of levels of evidence in planning integrative medical management are addressed earlier in this chapter. In general, it is important to keep in mind that the kind of evidence sought, that is, whether it is evidence of safety, treatment efficacy or effectiveness, or assessment accuracy or specificity, and the particular modality being studied, will determine the resources that will most likely yield clinically useful information, and will subsequently define the most efficient search strategy with which to obtain relevant information (Jadad & Gagliardi, 1998).

Some databases include only citations of studies that meet strict research biomedical criteria, including RCT design, tests for statistical significance, and peer review. In contrast, specialized databases on particular nonconventional systems of medicine may include citations of all publications in which abstracts contain certain key words, making it difficult to discriminate between speculative essays, commentary, and peer-reviewed research when scanning content (Allais, Voghera, DeLorenzo, Mana, & Benedetto, 2000). This is complicated by the fact that many mainstream medical databases as well as resources of nonconventional modalities use different approaches and terminology to describe or index studies on nonconventional treatments. For example, in PubMed, Best Evidence, and EMBASE, citations of studies on nonconventional modalities are not completely indexed, making it difficult to locate pertinent citations (Beckner & Berman, 2003). Fewer than half of known clinical trials on any given nonconventional modality are included in PubMed. Therefore, exclusive reliance on PubMed will result in serious omissions of relevant hits pertaining to nonconventional modalities. Disparate criteria for peer review in conventional and nonconventional systems of medicine, combined with the selective exclusion of citations on topics outside of a defined area of interest, and different approaches to indexing, reflect the biases and beliefs of medical practitioners or administrators who design medical databases. This fact has resulted in the limited usefulness of any particular medical database for the purposes of performing a comprehensive review of the literature pertaining to both conventional and nonconventional approaches relevant to a specified medical or mental health problem. Because many mainstream medical databases do not index publications on nonconventional modalities, and many research studies on nonconventional modalities are unpublished or published in journals that are not peer-reviewed, a comprehensive search strategy must cover nonindexed publications, including conference proceedings and newsletters. Non-English-language articles must also be obtained and reviewed because of the likelihood that English-language studies are biased in favor of conventional modalities. In sum, there is no unbiased or methodologically neutral approach for selecting citations in general or using specialized conventional or nonconventional medical databases. Practical consequences of this fact include the following:

◆ No single medical database is a comprehensive source of reliable information about both conventional and nonconventional medical practices.

◆ Combining citations from disparate databases will result in a spectrum of data reflecting the biases and beliefs implicit in the source databases.

◆ There are no objective criteria for determining on what basis to include or exclude databases as sources. This problem applies equally to considerations of including or excluding other (i.e., nondatabase) sources of information pertaining to a particular system of medicine or modality.

◆ The coverage areas and specific content of medical databases will almost certainly overlap, resulting in redundant entries when evidence tables are constructed from them. A methodology for interpreting the significance of overlapping or redundant entries is therefore important when developing clinically useful evidence tables.

Practical Considerations When Identifying Resources and Selecting Primary and Secondary Sources

This section briefly reviews the methodology used to fill in the evidence tables in Part II of this book. As noted above, I am assuming that APA practice guidelines and other mainstream practice guidelines are legitimate primary sources of information on contemporary Western biomedical practices in mental health care.

A practical first step in developing evidence tables for planning integrative mental health care is to review efforts that have already been made to gather reliable sources of accurate, up-to-date information about conventional and nonconventional medical practices pertaining to the assessment and treatment of mental health problems. This has been done independently by at least two large private organizations: the Rosenthal Center for Integrative Medicine, at Columbia University, and the Cochrane Collaboration, based at Johns Hopkins School of Medicine. The Cochrane databases provide valuable prefiltered resources. These include the complementary medicine field in the Cochrane registry of systematic reviews (www.update-software.com/abstracts/mainindex.htm). The registry includes reviews conducted by Cochrane reviewers and others who are not affiliated with the Cochrane Collaboration. Cochrane systematic reviews are superior to narrative reviews because they are required to specify both inclusion and

exclusion criteria, and make explicit remarks about studies that are included or excluded from a review. Because of the stringent criteria used to select studies for review and rigorous standards applied to the analysis of research designs and outcomes, the findings of Cochrane reviews are frequently negative or inconclusive. In addition to the Cochrane database of systematic reviews, the Cochrane Collaboration puts out the Database of Abstracts of Reviews of Effectiveness (DARE), which provides citations of both Cochrane and non-Cochrane reviews for comparison (http://nhscrd.york.ac.uk/darehp.htm). The Cochrane Collaborative Review Groups (CRGs) are another valuable resource for researchers (www.cochrane.org/reviews/index.htm). CRGs are formed around professional reviewers who systematically examine published and unpublished studies pertaining to specific medical or psychiatric illnesses. Cochrane CRGs collect information on emerging evidence for treatments of depression, anxiety, dementia, cognitive impairment, and schizophrenia. The Cochrane resources also include a database containing economic evaluations and health technology assessments from which it is possible to estimate cost-effectiveness of specific nonconventional modalities with respect to a specified mental health problem. This information can be important when determining whether a particular nonconventional intervention is affordable or cost-effective.

In contrast to the Cochrane methodology, which relies exclusively on RCT research designs, evidence mapping examines the quality and relevance of many research methodologies (Katz et al., 2003). Evidence mapping also differs from the Cochrane methodology by not excluding studies that are a priori regarded as methodologically flawed. This approach begins with identification of individuals who have expertise in a specific area of medicine. A "region of medical evidence" is subsequently mapped, and a search for the relevant evidence "terrain" is conducted. An evidence map is constructed from the terrain, and the process concludes with an overview of the "lay of the land." Evidence mapping differs in significant ways from other methodologies used to synthesize evidence in medicine. For example, unlike the Cochrane field approach, evidence mapping does not a priori exclude studies that are considered to be methodologically "weak" for various reasons. Furthermore, in contrast to the Cochrane databases and other resources of prefiltered medical information, studies other than RCTs are included in the terrain of evidence mapping. Evidence mapping ensures that nonconventional medical modalities that have not been examined in RCTs are included in the evidence base that is considered in medical decision making. Problems associated with the evaluation of evidence in nonconventional and integrative medicine are more amenable to evidence mapping compared with the Cochrane field approach and other, more established methodologies. This book uses aspects of the Cochrane field approach and evidence mapping to identify and evaluate medical evidence.

U.S. government agencies, including the National Center for Complementary and Alternative Medicine of the National Institutes of Health, and the Department of Agriculture (http://agricola.nal.usda.gov/), have developed Web sites and Web-searchable databases covering a broad range of modalities after systematically reviewing information sources pertaining to both conventional and nonconventional medicine. Government databases are probably the best sources for safety information pertaining to nonconventional modalities, though negative bias and exclusion bias should be taken into account when reviewing citations. Useful sources of safety information include

◆ U.S. Food and Drug Administration (www.fda.gov)
◆ Healthfinder (www.healthfinder.gov)
◆ American Botanical Council (www.herbalgram.org)

Citations included in governmental or academic databases reflect standardized Western biomedical criteria for determining the rigor of study design, appropriate data analysis, and significance level of results. These criteria reflect the intellectual perspectives and needs of clinicians and researchers more than the interests or needs of patients seeking practical information about a specified conventional or nonconventional assessment or treatment approach. The NCCAM and Rosenthal Center Web sites include links to other web-based resources on nonconventional medical practices that are considered by their developers to be sources of reliable citations (i.e., on the basis of criteria used by those organizations). The Rosenthal Center Web site (www.rosenthal.hs.columbia.edu/) was developed in consultation with the Alternative Medicine Foundation (AMF), which also hosts its own Web site (www.amfoundation.org/) covering a range of nonconventional modalities. Citations that are included in academic or government-sponsored Web sites are frequently excluded from more patient-oriented Web sites. In addition to links to related Web-based resources, many nonaffiliated Web sites on nonconventional medicine include chat rooms and newsletters summarizing interesting emerging findings that have not yet been published or, in some cases, will not be published in mainstream medical journals.

Defining Search Parameters and Establishing Search Strategies

Basic Considerations

A great deal of thought has been put into developing search strategies for obtaining reliable information pertaining to uses of nonconventional modalities. Searching Web-based resources on nonconventional medicine entails four basic steps (Beckner & Berman, 2003):

1. Defining a question in a clear and unambiguous way
2. Selecting appropriate resources, search tools, and a methodology to answer the question
3. Conducting searches and refining search methodology
4. Correctly interpreting findings for research or clinical use

Many online resources include built-in search engines. Others are searchable using a variety of search engines. All search engines have advantages and disadvantages that should be considered when designing a search strategy. For purposes of researching this book, directory search tools, directory with search engine, and multiengine search tools were employed at different times depending on the resources being searched. In addition to considerations of search tools, other specific issues addressed when developing the search methodology and information resources included

◆ Selecting terms describing the cognitive, affective, and behavioral symptoms covered in Part II of this book
◆ Selecting terms describing different kinds of studies (e.g., RCT, case control study, and cohort study) when

investigating claims of mechanism of action, efficacy, or effectiveness

◆ Using key words such as *safety, contraindications,* and *adverse effects* when querying Web-based resources for safety information
◆ Identifying the most appropriate search engines to use when searching particular databases
◆ Selecting primary Web-based databases (including prefiltered and nonfiltered databases)
◆ Selecting secondary Web-based or other data sources, including newsletters and Web-based chat rooms
◆ Identifying suitable software for condensing or abstracting results of Web-based searches into searchable summaries
◆ Choosing Boolean strings of search terms defining unambiguous research or clinical questions pertaining to particular assessment or treatment approaches used for specified symptoms
◆ Determining appropriate "cut-off" periods limiting citation publication dates when searching different resources
◆ Setting limits on numbers of citations selected for use in the evidence tables in general, and in each cell of the evidence tables

◆ **Searches use both symptom labels and *DSM-IV* nomenclature**
Cognitive, affective, and behavioral symptom patterns but not disorders define the framework in which both conventional and nonconventional modalities are examined in this book. Reasons for this are discussed in Chapters 2 and 3 and will not be repeated here. Key words describing symptoms are the preferred search method for finding relevant citations of studies on nonconventional modalities pertaining to mental health problems. However, to ensure the broadest possible coverage, synonym lists were constructed including symptom labels of common symptoms and the nomenclature of common psychiatric disorders as given in the fourth edition of the *Diagnostic and Statistical Manual of Mental Disorders–Text Revision* (*DSM-IV-TR*) and the 10th edition of the *International Classification of Diseases* (*ICD-10*). Key words used to search for pertinent citations were obtained from thesauri of both prefiltered and primary databases. Sample searches using only conventional biomedical nomenclature for psychiatric disorders as defined, for example, in the *DSM-IV-TR* and the *ICD-10* biased results in favor of citations on conventional modalities, and there were few relevant "hits" pertaining to nonconventional modalities in mental health care. To capture the greatest number of relevant citations from the medical and anthropological literature, descriptors of major categories of cognitive, affective, and behavioral symptoms used in both biomedicine and nonconventional systems of medicine were used as key word search terms. *Sadness* and *depressed mood,* for example, were used instead of *major depressive disorder. Anxiety* and *fear* were used instead of *generalized anxiety disorder* or *panic disorder.* Specialized lexicons were developed using modality-specific key words to improve yields of searches for citations on nonconventional modalities.

Limitations of EBM Literature Research Methods

Evidence-based medicine experts recommend the use of prefiltered resources to streamline searches of what they describe as "foreground questions" pertaining to a specific patient, and browsing in authoritative textbooks on specialty areas of medicine to obtain relevant information on "background questions" pertaining to general issues about the efficacy or effectiveness of a particular treatment (Guyatt & Rennie, 2002). However, unlike Western biomedicine, nonconventional medicine is not a single entity based on a coherent set of principles or assumptions. At present, nonconventional modalities are informed by diverse theories and opinions about the causes or meanings of illness from the perspectives of disparate systems of medicine. For example, different textbooks on nonconventional medicine often use the same information in support of very different recommendations, and there is no "average" point of view representing the philosophies or clinical methods of nonconventional medicine because it is not clinically useful to condense the divergent perspectives of many nonconventional modalities into a single averaged framework. Because there are no authoritative textbooks covering all areas of nonconventional medicine, we are left with two primary sources of information: database searches and expert consultations. Going back to basic principles of EBM, Web-based searching using prefiltered resources was considered a reasonable and efficient initial approach.

The EBM Working Group has developed the "4S" approach in an effort to achieve the most efficient literature research methodology for obtaining clinically relevant information pertaining to any medical question. **Table 4–8** summarizes the basic logic of the 4S approach, including unresolved issues in each step of the search process as formulated in evidence-based medicine.

◆ **A modified 4S approach will improve results of searches on nonconventional modalities**   As noted above, the 4S approach is intrinsically biased in favor of citations of conventional modalities and does not adequately reflect important basic research or clinical studies on many nonconventional modalities. The results of an initial literature review obtained using the 4S method can be balanced by examining guidelines of professional associations representing nonconventional systems of medicine (Gray, 2002). Using this approach, inquiries pertaining to the efficacy of an assessment modality are most reliably addressed in cross-sectional studies, whereas questions about efficacy and effectiveness are most reliably addressed by RCTs or reviews of RCTs, and accurate information about safety issues is available in cohort or case control studies (Gray, 2002).

In view of the identified limitations of the 4S methodology, I have developed a "modified" 4S approach that takes advantage of the strengths of the established EBM methodology while supplementing it with other search methods to ensure adequate coverage of the nonconventional medical literature. My goal was to develop the most efficient methodology for obtaining the best available evidence pertaining to nonconventional modalities in mental health care. The modified 4S approach includes a combined initial search and a secondary search, which has the purpose of supplementing omissions and correcting for other biases in findings of the initial search. There are three basic stages of the proposed search methodology. In the initial search, selected sources of prefiltered or primary medical data were queried. These included the Cochrane databases, the TRIP database (www.tripdatabase.com), the set of CAM citations available through the British Library (AMED, www.ovid.com/site/catalog/DataBase/12.jsp?top=2& mid=3&bottom=7&subsection=10), and Bandolier (www.jr2. ox.ac.uk/bandolier/kb.html), among others. Prefiltered databases were searched by key word, and some were searched

Table 4–8   The "4S" Methodology of Literature Research in Evidence-Based Medicine

Systems

Querying high-quality prefiltered sources of frequently updated reliable data, especially systematic reviews. System-level databases include Clinical Evidence, the National Electronic Library for Mental Health (NELMH), and clinical practice guidelines, including those published by the American Psychiatric Association, the National Guideline Clearinghouse, and the Canadian Medical Association. Some prefiltered sources are more established than others, inclusion criteria differ for different prefiltered sources, and some are more comprehensive sources of information about certain mental health problems.

Synopses

If clinically relevant citations are not obtained from searches of prefiltered databases, a logical next step is to query databases of structured abstracts of high-quality systematic reviews or individual studies. *Evidence-based mental health* is an example of a synopsis of conventional biomedical data on treatments in mental health care. Synopses have been appraised for quality, but many relevant studies that do not meet strict biomedical inclusion criteria are excluded.

Syntheses

If relevant information is not obtained from a search of systems or synopses, the architects of evidence-based medicine (EBM) suggest finding syntheses, or high-quality systematic reviews. The Cochrane Database of Systematic Reviews, the Database of Abstracts of Reviews of Effectiveness (DARE), and the Health Technology Assessment Database are regarded as excellent sources of systematic reviews. Other sources of high-quality systematic reviews include the Agency for Healthcare Research and Quality (AHRQ) and the National Health Service Centre for Reviews and Dissemination.

Studies

EBM guidelines suggest that searching Medline or other databases for single studies should be pursued only when relevant information is not obtained from searches of systematic reviews, structured abstracts of systematic reviews, or prefiltered sources of systematic reviews or guidelines. Although this approach will yield relevant citations that may not be included in published systematic reviews or prefiltered sources, Medline searches typically yield a large number of irrelevant or marginally relevant citations that take considerable time to review. For this reason, in most cases searches of non-prefiltered databases like Medline are not practical or productive approaches for obtaining useful clinical information for the busy clinician.

using a multiengine approach. Peer-reviewed special reports summarizing research or clinical uses of various nonconventional modalities were also examined in the initial search.

The initial search yielded the majority of useful citations for established and provisional nonconventional assessment and treatment modalities. Relevant citations from the initial search were constructed into two general evidence tables: (1) nonconventional assessment approaches in mental health care and (2) nonconventional treatment approaches in mental health care. The secondary search methodology obtained information from textbooks, peer-reviewed journals that are not indexed in online resources, and interviews with expert nonconventional medical practitioners or Western physicians who use nonconventional approaches in the treatment of mental health problems. Online database directories were used to identify specific databases containing relevant citations. Useful directories of online resources on nonconventional medicine included the Rosenthal Center for Integrative Medicine,

Table 4–9 Obtaining Information on Nonconventional Approaches in Mental Health Care

Initial search

1. Cochrane Collaboration—complementary medicine field
2. Cochrane Database of Systematic Reviews
3. Cochrane Database of Abstracts of Reviews of Effectiveness (DARE)
4. Cochrane registry of clinical trials
5. Bandolier evidence-based summaries
6. British Library AMED database
7. Evidence-based online resources in medicine and nonconventional medicine
8. Other prefiltered databases, including www.Clinicalevidence.com and TRIP

Secondary Search

1. Textbooks on alternative medicine and integrative medicine
2. Online resources pertinent to psychology or psychiatry that include citations on nonconventional medical research (e.g., PsychInfo)
3. OMNI (Organizing Medical Networked Information), Biomed Central, Combined Health Information Database (CHID)
4. Online news sites and newsletters covering nonconventional medicine
5. Peer-reviewed journals of nonconventional medicine
6. Expert interviews by major nonconventional modality
7. Professional nonconventional medical association guidelines
8. PubMed searches of principal authors that came up frequently in the prefiltered searches
9. Manual searches of unpublished journals and conference proceedings identified in initial literature research or expert interviews

Shoring Up Leads

1. Obtain key studies or unpublished information provided by expert practitioners.
2. Optimize key word searches using high-yielding databases and search engines.

McMaster University Alternative Medicine Resources, and Healthfinder. Professional associations of nonconventional medical practitioners also provided valuable advice regarding useful online resources for particular nonconventional modalities. The third and final stage of research was intended to "shore up" results obtained in the first two stages. It consisted of returning to the most useful resources to ensure that all relevant citations had been identified and examining leads provided by experts, online newsletters, or unpublished sources. **Table 4–9** summarizes the three stages used to obtain information for use in the evidence tables.

Constructing the Evidence Tables

Phase 1: Identifying Nonconventional Assessment and Treatment Modalities

Searches were conducted in several phases. The first phase was performed automatically once primary and secondary sources were established and access to identified primary Web-based databases was obtained. At this stage, abstracts and biblio-

graphic information were pulled from the databases, but not full-length articles. Results of the initial automated search yielded two general sets of citations pertaining to nonconventional assessment and treatment approaches, respectively. Results were sorted into predefined cells of the phase 1 evidence tables by major symptom and categories of treatment or assessment modalities. Redundant citations were eliminated. Citations supporting use of one assessment or treatment modality for more than one symptom, or more than one nonconventional modality for a specified symptom, qualified for two or more cells in the phase 1 evidence table, and were not considered to be redundant citations. Therefore, in cases where these conditions are met, the same citation is included more than once in the evidence tables, depending on the relative strength of evidence supporting its use. For example, many citations commented on evidence supporting the use of a particular modality for more than one core symptom. Such citations were included in all cells in the phase 1 evidence table for which there was an indication of a specific clinical application. At this stage, the evidence table was manually checked for errors, including redundant entries, completeness of abstracts, and completeness of bibliographic information.

Comments pertaining to safety and compatibility are included in the evidence tables where information is available. Combining modalities that are known to be compatible or synergistic is often reasonable, whereas combining modalities where safety issues are documented or can be inferred can result in significant risk to patients and should always be avoided. In cases where the absence of compelling research or clinical data does not permit a determination of compatibility between two or more modalities being considered for inclusion in an integrative management strategy, the clinician should take the most conservative approach available to minimize patient risk. These practical issues are discussed in Chapters 5 and 6.

Phase 2: Sorting Information by Kinds and Levels of Evidence

In this stage, the assessment and treatment datasets from phase 1 were further divided according to levels and kinds of evidence supporting empirically derived, consensus-based, or intuitive modalities. This required a manual sorting of the information developed in phase 1. A semiquantitative approach was used to rate modalities according to findings reported in citations as "substantiated," "provisional," "possibly effective," or "refuted" using the criteria developed in the first part of this chapter.

Phase 3: Resolving Discrepancies between Findings

In several cases, both "substantiated" findings and "provisional" findings pertaining to the same nonconventional modality were reported in equally reliable sources. For example, peer-reviewed papers on rigorously conducted studies on St. John's wort in depressed mood report inconsistent findings, resulting in an ongoing debate within the Western psychiatric community about the efficacy of this herbal product. In cases where discrepancies were identified following a thorough review of the literature, the position of a particular modality in the evidence tables was determined on a case-by-case basis through analysis of the available literature in the context of the author's clinical experience and professional judgment or in consultation with an expert in the clinical use of that particular modality. Systematic reviews or meta-analyses were used, when available, to resolve conflicts when significant discrepancies existed between reliable information sources pertaining to the efficacy or safety of a particular nonconventional modality in the treatment of a specified symptom pattern. However, conclusions of systematic reviews or meta-analyses were not the final or sole basis for designating a modality as "substantiated," "provisional," or "possibly effective." In cases where evidence remained ambiguous following the above review process, a particular modality was included in the lower of two levels of evidence pending results of future quantitative and qualitative studies.

◆ **The evidence tables will be updated on a continuous basis**   It is important to note at this juncture that progress in the management of cognitive, affective, and behavioral symptoms using nonconventional approaches is uneven. Whereas a great deal of reliable information exists for some nonconventional modalities when applied to a particular core symptom, there are relatively few reliable reports supporting the use of many nonconventional approaches for which the quality of data is uneven or consistently poor. This fact does not necessarily translate into the automatic exclusion of such nonconventional modalities from consideration in integrative treatment planning. For example, the modality in question may be in widespread use by professionally trained nonconventional practitioners who report consistently positive outcomes; or preliminary findings of ongoing studies may point to efficacy and safety for a particular modality that presently lacks substantial supporting evidence on the basis of formal studies by Western medical researchers or investigators examining the modality from the perspective of the parent system of medicine. Conversely, preliminary findings may suggest that the approach lacks efficacy or is associated with unresolved safety problems. In all cases the judicious clinician should recommend a particular modality, or refer a patient for a particular treatment, only after carefully evaluating the available evidence and becoming familiar with preliminary findings or potential safety issues. Before recommending a particular assessment or treatment plan, the clinician is encouraged to consult the companion Web site (www.thieme.com/mentalhealth) to ensure that the most current information has been taken into account.

Using the Evidence Tables Together with the Integrative Planning Algorithms

All chapters in Part II conclude with algorithms for planning integrative management of a specified core symptom. The algorithms show the logical steps used in integrative management and are intended to be used with the evidence tables. All Part II chapters conclude with composite vignettes illustrating the integrative management of the symptom patterns discussed in this book.

Future Literature Research Methods

Available information for many nonconventional assessment and treatment approaches is limited in both quantity and quality. The result is a gap between most conventional and nonconventional approaches with respect to both the kind and level of supporting evidence. Future revisions of the algorithms will be implemented in the form of knowledge systems linking primary data sources to the evidence tables in seamless fashion. Advances in online searching will soon provide conventional and nonconventional medical practitioners with decision support tools offering almost real-time updates and critical new findings pertaining to the safety, efficacy, and compatibility of a broad range of assessment or treatment modalities.

As envisioned, a future "modality-specific" literature research methodology will combine the most appropriate search tools with the most relevant information sources and the most efficient search strategies. The resulting optimized search methodology will eventually be available as an online tool in the companion Web site to this book. Regular updates will incorporate ongoing advances in methodology and Web-based resources into a future modality-specific search methodology. Continuous automated or manually programmed updates using Web-based or unpublished resources will result in content revisions of the evidence tables, and commensurate changes in the relative weights of evidence supporting assessment or treatment modalities with respect to a specified symptom pattern for any choice point in the integrative planning algorithms. Using voice recognition software and simple graphics tools, practitioners evaluating patients will soon have the capability to input historical patient data, including detailed treatment response history, patient preferences, comments on local availability, and cost of particular modalities, and instantly obtain a series of contingent integrative management approaches optimized with respect to defined parameters of patient data, preferences, availability, and cost. Advances in information technology will permit clinicians from all backgrounds to rapidly and accurately determine optimum integrative management strategies addressing the unique complaints and preferences of each patient.

References

Aickin, M. (2002). Beyond randomization. *Journal of Alternative and Complementary Medicine, 8*(6), 765–772.

Aickin, M. (2003). Participant-centered analysis in complementary and alternative medicine comparative trials. *Journal of Alternative and Complementary Medicine, 9*(6), 949–957.

Allais, G., Voghera, D., DeLorenzo, C., Mana, O., & Benedetto, C. (2000). Access to databases in complementary medicine. *Journal of Alternative and Complementary Medicine, 6*(3), 265–274.

Beckner, W., & Berman, B. (2003). *Complementary therapies on the Internet.* St. Louis, MO: Churchill Livingstone.

Bengston, W. (2004). Methodological difficulties involving control groups in healing research: Parallels between laying on of hands for the treatment of induced mammary cancers in mice to research in homeopathy. *Journal of Alternative and Complementary Medicine, 10*(2), 227–228.

Bloom, B. S., Retbi, A., Dahan, S., & Jonsson, E. (2000). Evaluation of randomized controlled trials on complementary and alternative medicine. *International Journal of Technology Assessment in Health Care, 16*(1), 13–21.

Borenstein, D. (2004, May 4). Evidence: psychiatry. *Psychiatric News,* p. 3.

Browman, G. (2001). Development and aftercare of clinical guidelines: The balance between rigor and pragmatism. *Journal of the American Medical Association, 286,* 1509–1511.

Caspi, O., & Bell, I. (2004). One size does not fit all: Aptitude x treatment interaction (ATI) as a conceptual framework for complementary and alternative medicine outcome research. Part II: Research designs and their applications. *Journal of Alternative and Complementary Medicine, 10*(4), 698–705.

Caspi, O., Millen, C., & Sechrest, L. (2000). Integrity and research: Introducing the concept of dual blindness. How blind are double-blind clinical trials in alternative medicine? *Journal of Alternative and Complementary Medicine, 6*(6), 493–498.

Churchill, W. (1999). Implications of evidence based medicine for complementary and alternative medicine. *Journal of Chinese Medicine, 59,* 32–35.

Coates, J. R., & Jobst, K. A. (1998). Integrated Healthcare: A way forward for the next five years? A discussion document from the Prince of Wales's Initiative on Integrated Medicine. *Journal of Alternative and Complementary Medicine, 4*(2), 209–247.

Dalen, J. (1998). Conventional and "unconventional" medicine: Can they be integrated? [Editorial]. *Archives of Internal Medicine, 158,* 2179–2181.

Defining and describing complementary and alternative medicine. (1997). *Alternative Therapies in Health and Medicine, 3*(2), 49–57.

Dickerson, K., & Min, Y. (1993). NIH clinical trials and publication bias (Doc No. 50). *Online Journal of Current Clinical Trials.*

Docherty, J. (2001). Interpretations and conclusions in the clinical trial. *Journal of Clinical Psychiatry, 62*(9), 40–43.

Dossey, L. (1995). How should alternative therapies be evaluated? *Alternative Therapies, 1*(2), 76–85.

Drake, R., Goldman, H., Leff, H., et al. (2001). Implementing evidence-based practices in routine mental health service settings. *Psychiatric Services, 52,* 179–182.

Ernst, E. (1998a). Establishing efficacy in chronic stable conditions: Are "*N* = 1 study" designs or case series useful? *Forschende Komplementarmedizin, 5*(1), 128–130.

Ernst, E. (1998b) Single-case studies in complementary/alternative medicine research. *Complementary Therapies in Medicine, 6,* 75–78.

Fisher, P., van Haselen, R., Hardy, K., Berkovitz, S., & McCarney, R. (2004). Effectiveness gaps: A new concept for evaluating health service and research needs applied to complementary and alternative medicine. *Journal of Alternative and Complementary Medicine, 10*(4), 627–632.

Fontanarosa, P., & Lundberg, G. (1998). Alternative medicine meets science. *Journal of the American Medical Association, 280,* 1618–1619.

Geddes, J., Game, D., Jenkins, N., et al. (1996). What proportion of primary psychiatric interventions are based on evidence from randomized controlled trials? *Quality in Health Care, 5,* 215–217.

Gray, G. (2004). *Concise guide to evidence-based psychiatry.* Washington, DC: American Psychiatric Publishing.

Gray, G. E. (2002). Evidence-based medicine: An introduction for psychiatrists. *Journal of Psychiatric Practice, 8,* 5–13.

Guyatt, G., & Rennie, D. (Eds.). (2002). *Users' guide to the medical literature: Essentials of evidence-based clinical practice.* Chicago: AMA Press.

Haynes, B. (1999). A warning to complementary medicine practitioners: Get empirical or else. *British Medical Journal, 319,* 1629–1632.

Horn, S., Sharkey, P., Tracy, D., et al. (1996). Intended and unintended consequences of HMO cost-containment strategies: Results from the Managed Care Outcomes Project. *American Journal of Managed Care, 2,* 253–264.

Jadad, A., & Gagliardi, A. (1998). Rating health information on the Internet: Navigating to knowledge or to Babel? *Journal of the American Medical Association, 279,* 611–614.

Jonas, W., & Chez, R. (2004). Recommendations regarding definitions and standards in healing research. *Journal of Alternative and Complementary Medicine, 10(1),* 171–181.

Johnston, B. C., & Mills, E. (2004). N-of-1 randomized controlled trials: An opportunity for complementary and alternative medicine evaluation. *Journal of Alternative and Complementary Medicine, 10*(6), 979–984.

Katz, D. L., Williams, A. L., Girard, C., et al. (2003). The evidence base for complementary and alternative medicine: Methods of evidence mapping with applications to CAM. *Alternative Therapies in Health and Medicine, 9*(4), 22–30.

Lake, J. (2001). Qigong. In: Shannon, S. *Complementary and alternative medicine in psychiatry.* New York: Academic Press.

Lieberman, J. (2001). Hypothesis and hypothesis testing in the clinical trial. *Journal of Clinical Psychiatry, 9,* 5–8.

Linde, K. (2000). How to evaluate the effectiveness of complementary therapies. *Journal of Alternative and Complementary Medicine, 6*(3), 253–256.

Liverani, A. (2000). Subjective scales for the evaluation of therapeutic effects and their use in complementary medicine. *Journal of Alternative and Complementary Medicine, 6*(3), 257–264.

Long, A. (2002). Outcome measurement in CAM: Unpicking the effects. *Journal of Alternative and Complementary Medicine, 8*(6), 777–786.

Mancano, M., & Bullano, M. (1998). Meta-analysis: Methodology, utility, and limitations. *Journal of Pharmacy Practice, 11*(4), 239–250.

Morley, J., Rosner, A. L., & Redwood, D. (2001). A case study of misrepresentation of the scientific literature: Recent reviews of chiropractic. *Journal of Alternative and Complementary Medicine, 7*(1), 65–78.

Murphy, E. (1997). *The logic of medicine.* Baltimore, MD: Johns Hopkins University Press.

Resch, K., Ernst, E., & Garrow, J. (2000). A randomized controlled study of reviewer bias against an unconventional therapy. *Journal of the Royal Society of Medicine, 93*(4), 164–167.

Richardson, J. (2000). The use of randomized controlled trials on complementary therapy: Exploring the methodological issues. *Journal of Advanced Nursing, 32*(2), 398–406.

Richardson, J. (2002). Evidence-based complementary medicine: Rigor, relevance and the swampy lowlands. *Journal of Alternative and Complementary Medicine, 8*(3), 221–223.

Sackett, D. L., Rosenberg, W. M., Gray, J. A., et al. (1996). Evidence-based medicine: What it is and what it isn't. *British Medical Journal, 312,* 71–72.

Smith, R. (1991). Where is the wisdom? *British Medical Journal, 303*(6806), 798–799.

Stein, D. (2004) Algorithms for primary care: An evidence-based approach to the pharmacotherapy of depression and anxiety disorders. *Primary Psychiatry, 11*(6), 55–78.

Turner, R. (1998). A proposal for classifying complementary therapies. *Complementary Therapies in Medicine, 6,* 141–143.

Verhoef, M., Casebeer, A., & Hilsdew, R. (2002). Assessing efficacy of complementary medicine: Adding qualitative research methods to the "gold standard." *Journal of Alternative and Complementary Medicine, 3,* 275–281.

Vickers, A. (1999). Evidence-based medicine and complementary medicine. *ACP Journal Club, 130,* A13–A14.

Vuckovic, N. (2002). Integrating qualitative methods in RCTs: The experience of the Oregon Center for CAM. *Journal of Alternative and Complementary Medicine, 8*(3), 225–227.

Walach, H. (2001). The efficacy paradox in randomized controlled trials of CAM and elsewhere: Beware of the placebo trap. *Journal of Alternative and Complementary Medicine, 7*(3), 213–218.

White, A., Resch, K., & Ernst, E. (1996). Methods of economic evaluation in complementary medicine. *Forschende Komplementarmedizin, 3,* 196–203.

Wilson, K., & Mills, E. J. (2002). Evidence-Based Complementary and Alternative Medicine Working Group. Introducing evidence-based complementary and alternative medicine: Answering the challenge. *Journal of Alternative and Complementary Medicine, 8*(2), 103–105.

Wilson, K., Mills, E. J., Ross, C., & Guyatt, G. (2002). Teaching evidence-based complementary and alternative medicine: 4. Appraising the evidence for papers on therapy. *Journal of Alternative and Complementary Medicine, 8*(5), 673–679.

Zhang, H. L. (2004). Qigong commentary. *Journal of Alternative and Complementary Medicine, 10*(2), 228–230.

5

History Taking, Assessment, and Formulation in Integrative Mental Health Care

I have argued in earlier chapters that the concept of "disorder" in mental health is not supported by available epidemiologic evidence, and that a more valid and clinically useful construct is a continuum of symptom patterns that can be inferred on the basis of subjective reports of the quality and severity of emotional, behavioral, or cognitive symptoms. An integrative approach to history taking can be used to gather pertinent information about the patient's social, psychological, and medical history, in addition to his or her cultural framework and any pertinent spiritual beliefs and experiences.

In this chapter, contemporary approaches in Western psychiatric assessment are critiqued. Ethical and liability considerations pertaining to establishing a contract with a new patient, providing ongoing integrative care, and making referrals to other practitioners are reviewed from the perspective of integrative medicine. Established and emerging nonconventional assessment methods are briefly reviewed. The logic for using single versus multiple assessment approaches is discussed. The concept of a multitiered formulation of causes or meanings associated with a symptom pattern is introduced as the cornerstone of effective integrative treatment planning. The reader is referred to Part II for detailed presentations of the evidence for specific approaches used to assess the common symptom patterns discussed in this book.

For all practical purposes, there are no compelling safety reasons for avoiding the use of any assessment method or any combination of methods because almost all assessment approaches involve the passive monitoring of biological, biomagnetic, somatic, or "energetic" functioning.

◆ Overview

Every human being is unique at the level of social, cultural, psychological, biological, and possibly "energetic" functioning, and the complex causes or meanings of cognitive, emotional, and behavioral symptoms are likewise unique. Individuality limits the validity of generalizations about health and illness and precludes exclusive reliance on systematic reviews or meta-analyses of strictly quantitative assessment findings. The individual variability and complexity of possible causes or meanings of symptoms suggest that case reports provide valuable information when evaluating the relevance of assessment approaches. Integrative assessment approaches in mental health care will result in more productive and cost-effective approaches in integrative treatment planning, combining the most effective conventional biomedical and nonconventional treatments targeting a specific symptom pattern. Within the next decades, physicians will increasingly use assessment approaches that are now outside the domain of orthodox biomedicine. Methods in integrative medicine will permit the individualized assessment of mental and emotional symptom patterns addressing the unique symptom patterns and circumstances of every patient. The evolution of biomedicine toward a truly integrative paradigm will result in deeper understandings of fundamental biological, "energetic," informational, and spiritual causes and meanings associated with mental illness.

◆ The Limitations of History Taking and Assessment in Western Psychiatry

Contemporary Understandings of Biological and Environmental Causes of Mental Illness Are Incomplete

Western psychiatry endorses the general view in biomedicine that mental illness results from complex interactions between genetic and environmental factors, yet current gene–environment models do not explain the majority of mental illnesses. The belief that internal and external factors "cause" mental illness and that there are genetic predispositions to

maladies mentales dates to Freud (1909/1955). Early twin studies had their origin in Sir Francis Galton's work in the late 19th century (Galton, 1876; Rosanoff et al., 1934). Research findings suggesting a strong role of heredity in mental retardation, criminal behavior, and alcohol abuse became the basis of a form of eugenics called the "racial hygiene" doctrine, which was used by Hitler to justify the mass extermination of the mentally ill and handicapped (Meyer-Lindenberg, 1991). In current genetic epidemiology studies, genetic-marker strategies, which take into account gene–environment interactions, have largely replaced family and twin studies (Risch, 1997). Important current concepts in medical genetics include susceptibility genes and polygenic disorders. Genetic epidemiology has been largely replaced by molecular genetics, and the recently completed Human Genome Project has provided researchers with a complete human genetic map. In molecular genetics research, gene mapping (genomics) is combined with proteomics, which has the goal of creating a database of correspondences between complex polygenic interactions and effects on protein synthesis that may manifest as medical or psychiatric illness (Anthony, 2001). This monumental undertaking has been called the Human Proteome Initiative. Current research in molecular genetics uses gene mapping of polygenic markers possibly associated with increased susceptibility to a particular mental illness. A related step is gene cloning to determine whether an identified gene is associated with changes in protein synthesis that affect neurotransmitter or receptor structure or function in ways that can be expected to produce psychiatric symptoms. The almost exclusive emphasis on molecular genetics research in biomedical psychiatry has led to concerns that the research agenda embraced by Western psychiatry has become too narrow in scope (Lippman, 1992). To date genetic studies in psychiatry have resulted in largely inconclusive findings, possibly because simple correlations do not exist between discrete mental illnesses and discrete mutations of single genes (Merikangas & Swendsen, 1997). Advances in the understanding of the biological basis of mental illness using gene mapping and other molecular genetics techniques have been limited by poorly defined, complex interactions between multiple genes and gene–environment interactions (Owen, Cardno, & O'Donovan, 2000; Owen, Holmans, & McGuffin, 1997). With the exception of the association between the APO E-4 allele and a subset of individuals with early-onset Alzheimer's disease, it has not been possible to identify discrete relationships between specific genetic problems and the phenotypes of specific psychiatric disorders. There is also evidence of genetic factors in some cases of bipolar disorder, depressive or anxiety symptoms, schizophrenia, and alcoholism (Cutrona et al., 1994; Kendler, 1995; Kendler et al., 1987; Reiss et al., 1995; Wahlberg et al., 1997).

The absence of compelling findings from genetics research is complicated by the inherently subjective nature of cognitive, emotional, and behavioral symptoms and the paucity of knowledge about specific effects of complex environmental factors on genes, human physiology, and brain function, including molecular regulatory processes that cause changes in neurotransmitters or receptors associated with mental illness (Plomin, 1994). Because of the polygenic and environmental factors that influence the formation and progression of cognitive, emotional, and behavioral symptoms, it is unlikely that existing techniques in molecular genetics will adequately characterize their complex causes. The continuing focus on molecular genetics as the "holy grail" of psychiatric research has diminished the relative importance of studies on social and cultural factors, including poverty, unemployment, and ethnic conflicts, and biological but nongenetic concomitants of mental illness (Thomas, Romme, & Hamelijnck, 1996). In response to the perceived "narrowing" of Western psychiatry to molecular genetics, a multiaxial framework that takes into account complex levels of possible causes or influences of mental illness has been proposed (McDowall, 1987). According to this model, environmental factors potentially affecting mental illness include the natural chemical environment, the "synthetic" chemical environment, and the macrosocial and microsocial environment of each person.

Methods in Conventional Psychiatric Assessment and Diagnosis Are Limited and Continue to Evolve

Conventional methods used to assess and diagnose medical illnesses are based on the systematic observation of objective "signs" of structural or physiological abnormalities related to symptoms of illness. In contrast, conventional methods used in Western psychiatric diagnosis rely on the use of inference to determine the presence of pathology on the basis of self-reported subjective states and the use of standardized interview instruments, most commonly the Mini-Mental State Examination (MMSE). Few empirically verifiable physiological, biochemical, or genetic signs are used in psychiatric assessment. Instead, the clinician gathers subjective symptoms of distress whose causes are seldom verifiable using objective empirical means. The essential logic of contemporary Western biomedicine is the identification of significant symptom patterns, and the subsequent determination of reasonable treatments based on identified or inferred causes of symptoms. The implicit assumption is that a biological or other functional cause is not present if it cannot be empirically verified. In cases where there is a physical complaint but no empirical evidence of a corresponding cause on the basis of contemporary biomedical assessment methods, the complaint has no basis—it is not "real," and is therefore branded psychosomatic. Some nonconventional systems of medicine relate symptoms to fundamentally different biological, social, energetic, or spiritual events or processes. In other words, disparate systems of medicine rest on different ontological and epistemological assumptions. Subsequently, clinicians trained in different traditions "see" illness phenomena and infer their causes or meanings in ways that are congruent with the ontological and epistemological assumptions implicit in their parent system of medicine. Disparate sets of assumptions correspond to different understandings of "evidence" in medicine. Novel ways of seeing or constructing illness phenomena derive from or lead to novel paradigms. Basic philosophical issues that are important for an understanding of the conceptual basis of integrative medicine are discussed in Chapter 2, Philosophical Problems. Chapter 3, Paradigms in Medicine, Psychiatry, and Integrative Medicine, discusses the relevance of established or emerging paradigms to integrative medicine.

Conventional psychiatric assessment is based almost exclusively on structured interviews and a brief mental state examination in conjunction with a review of pertinent medical or psychiatric records. The biopsychosocial model stipulates the use of a tiered approach for obtaining information about possible associations between the patient's biological, psychological, and social history and reported mental or emotional symptoms. Methods of assessment and observation used in Western psychiatry have changed little since the late 19th century, have not been validated through rigorous empirical testing, and continue to rely on statistical or narrative interpretations of patient reports of highly subjective phenomenological experiences (Berrios & Markova, 2002). There is a schism between the proposed "atheoretical" empirically based descriptive methods of contemporary psychiatry and the subjective information obtained from interviews that are frequently the sole basis for diagnosing an individual with a psychiatric disorder. Structured clinical interviews are used infrequently in actual clinical settings. Conventional structured interviews have improved over time; however, their validity in terms of interrater reliability continues to be questioned (Regier et al., 1998). Thus, for practical purposes, Western psychiatric assessment seldom uses its own "gold standard" assessment methods, which are of questionable validity when they are used. This problem is made worse by the fact that the means to validate psychiatric diagnoses using objective clinical or biological criteria are not practically available in most cases (Wittchen, Hofler, & Merikangas, 1999). In addition to the structured interview, laboratory studies are ordered in cases where the physician suspects an underlying medical cause of mental or emotional symptoms. Frequently ordered tests include thyroid studies, complete blood count (CBC), urinalysis, serum iron levels, and assays of liver enzymes and kidney function. Conventionally trained psychiatrists sometimes refer patients who complain of possible neurological symptoms to a neurologist for a formal evaluation, including electroencephalography (EEG) and brain scans, to obtain detailed structural or functional information about the brain to rule out primary diseases of the central nervous system. Functional neuroimaging, including functional magnetic resonance imaging (fMRI), quantitative electroencephalography (qEEG), and positron emission tomography (PET), will play an increasingly important role in future conventional psychiatric assessment (Gordon, 2002). Information obtained from structured interviews and laboratory and neuroimaging studies provides the clinician with a broad diagnostic picture of possible social, psychological, or biological causes of symptoms, and points to social, psychological, or biological treatments that can reasonably be expected to address identified causes or meanings of symptoms.

Debate is ongoing over the validity of diagnostic criteria in the fourth edition of the *Diagnostic and Statistical Manual of Mental Disorders* (*DSM-IV*), and diagnostic principles used in the *DSM* continue to evolve in response to new research findings and the work of expert committees. Since the first edition of the *DSM* in 1952, the number of defined disorders has increased from 106 to 365. Important advances in scientific understandings of the causes of mental illness certainly occurred during the first 40 years of the *DSM*; however, they do not provide a sufficient explanation of the 300% expansion in the number of discrete categories, or labels, of psychopathology during this period. Inconclusive and limited data pertaining to putative psychodynamic or biological causes or meanings are available for the majority of disorders, and reliable histories confirming these causes or meanings are generally difficult or impossible to obtain (Beutler & Malik, 2002). At the time of writing, 10 diagnostic research meetings have been planned to stimulate the discussion and debate that will shape the fifth edition of the *DSM* (*DSM-V*), which is currently planned for release in 2010 (Sirovatka, 2004). The research agenda for *DSM-V* outlines issues that are being addressed by psychiatrists who are revising the concepts and language of the current version. An important goal of this effort is to improve the overall validity of psychiatric diagnosis by shifting criteria from "syndromal" to "etiologic." The research agenda addresses basic issues of nomenclature, including attempts to formulate a more adequate definition of the term *mental disorder*. Six working groups were established at a *DSM* research planning conference in 1999. These groups are focusing on advances in developmental science, cultural issues in psychiatric diagnosis, difficulties in the diagnosis of personality disorders, issues pertaining to nomenclature, new findings from neuroscience and genetics, and disability and impairment (First, 2002). Although the *DSM-V* research agenda will probably result in improvements in construct validity of *DSM* diagnostic categories, at the time of writing a working group has not been tasked with systematically reviewing the literature on assessment methods used to evaluate cognitive, emotional, and behavioral symptoms in nonconventional systems of medicine. In the absence of such considerations, the *DSM-V* will probably continue to be biased in favor of existing conventional biomedical or psychodynamic models of mental illness.

In conventional biomedicine, assessment is a process of confirming correspondences between a described symptom pattern and putative underlying causes. Two assumptions are implicit in this process: (1) available technological means have the capacity to identify all pertinent information regarding possible causes of symptoms, and (2) the concept of (linear) causality that has been historically applied to the understanding of natural processes is sufficient to explain the origins, characteristics, or causes of medical or psychiatric symptoms. Evidence-based medicine (EBM) claims to base diagnostic conclusions and choices in treatment planning on a rigorous evaluation of pertinent empirical information accepted as valid indices of illness or health. However, the approach to history taking used in EBM relies on narrowly formulated questions, ensuring that potentially relevant information is a priori excluded when formulating an integrative assessment and treatment plan. The skillful integrative clinician uses "open" questions suggesting multiple ways of seeing symptoms and interpreting their possible causes, meanings, or interrelationships. This open approach to history taking naturally leads to a more open approach to assessment and formulation, resulting in an integrative treatment plan that addresses multiple possible levels of causation or meaning.

Limitations and Safety Concerns Must Be Taken into Account When Considering Nonconventional Assessment Approaches

Before recommending or using any conventional or nonconventional approach to assess a mental or emotional symptom pattern, the clinician should always review the evidence with respect to a specified mental or emotional symptom pattern. Compared with the relatively robust findings supporting many nonconventional treatment approaches in mental health care, there are limited data for most nonconventional assessment methods. Furthermore, most nonconventional assessment approaches that have been carefully evaluated using Western-style

research designs generally do not result in findings that are reproducible, sensitive, or specific (Ernst & Hentschel, 1995). Examples of the latter include iridology, hair analysis, kinesiology, radionics, clairsentient diagnosis, and electroacupuncture. The use of consensus-based or intuitive nonconventional assessment approaches for which there is limited supporting evidence may result in avoidance of more substantiated conventional or nonconventional approaches that can more reliably and more accurately identify the causes of symptoms. In such cases, misdiagnoses or missed diagnoses may potentially harm the patient by delaying appropriate care. This concern goes back to the ethical and liability issues discussed above. Research evidence for the range of conventional and nonconventional assessment approaches is accumulating at a rapid rate. The position of integrative mental health care is that both conventional and nonconventional assessment approaches should be considered when evaluating cognitive, emotional, and behavioral symptoms, and that the selection of clinical methods should depend foremost on the strength of evidence, while taking into account the clinician's experience, cost, and availability issues (if any), and the patient's preferences. The reader is encouraged to consult the companion Web site to this book (www.thieme.com/mentalhealth) to ensure that recommendations are based on the most current and reliable information available.

Symptoms—Not Disorders—of Mental Functioning or Emotional Distress

I have argued that the concept of disorder in Western medicine is a construct, and that the historical origins of classification and diagnosis in Western psychiatry are artifacts of 18th-century metaphysics. Below, I review arguments for this position and suggest that cognitive, emotional, and behavioral symptoms are reports of unique subjective experiences associated with distress or impairment. I am arguing that making reasonable inferences about the psychological, biological, energetic, informational, or spiritual causes or meanings of symptoms is fundamental to the derivation of adequate and effective treatment plans. In the context of the historical roots of contemporary Western psychiatry and in view of the absence of strong empirical methods capable of identifying putative biological causes of mental or emotional symptoms, most psychiatric disorders can be regarded as convenient and arbitrary constructs. As discussed above, current ideas in psychiatric nosology simplify the complex and subtle phenomenology of mental or emotional symptoms into discrete categories of pathology that seldom match observed symptom patterns. *DSM* criteria used to define disorders in Western psychiatry do not provide explanations of how symptoms originate or "hang together" in patterns that are reported by patients. Thus contemporary models of disorders in psychiatry not only fail to improve understandings of symptoms, but frequently result in increased confusion over their causes or meanings. The end result of contemporary Western psychiatric diagnosis is a label of a "disorder" that has limited validity and little relevance to an accurate understanding of the characteristics, causes, or meanings of reported mental or emotional symptoms. In other words, *DSM* criteria do not provide an accurate, complete, or clinically useful picture of mental or emotional symptom patterns. Instead of working within the constraints and biases of Western psychiatric nosology, I am proposing that increased emphasis should be placed on obtaining more complete information about multiple possible causes or meanings of symptom patterns to better understand what approaches might reasonably be expected to alleviate distress or impairment associated with symptoms.

The characterization of particular symptom patterns as discrete disorders rests on the assumption that disparate symptoms are related to one another in complex ways that reliably form dynamic patterns. Furthermore, contemporary Western psychiatry asserts that symptom patterns composing a disorder are stable over time or recur according to a described temporal pattern, and that the symptom pattern can be verified by qualified, independent observers. Using these criteria, a psychiatric disorder can be understood as a pattern of a pattern, or a "meta-pattern" of emotional or mental symptoms that are stable over time. Categories of experiences that are regarded as symptoms are determined by the framework within which subjective experiences are reported and examined. The choice of framework (i.e., the system of medicine in which a particular symptom pattern is examined) therefore biases interpretations of particular symptom patterns as disorders. For example, the text revision of *DSM-IV* (*DSM-IV-TR*) contains implicit assumptions about kinds of subjective experiences that are regarded as significant or interrelated. In Western psychiatry certain patterns of subjective experiences are regarded as disorders, whereas other patterns are regarded as normal variants of affect, cognition, or behavior. Classification schemes used in other systems of medicine rest on different assumptions about the meanings and relative significance of particular symptom patterns in the context of empirical methods, or "rules," for identifying a symptom and assessing its effect on or meaning to the patient. In sum, objective criteria regarded as valid across disparate systems of medicine have not been put forward, and there is no agreed on method for verifying the existence of subjective mental or emotional experiences, their putative causes or meanings, or claims of consistent patterns of relationships between them.

There can be no empirically verifiable understanding of a disorder as it pertains to mental health in the context of any particular system of medicine or between disparate systems of medicine because current empirical tests do not reliably verify psychological, biological, energetic, or other putative causes of symptoms. By extension, there are no empirical means for verifying presumed relationships between symptoms to determine whether symptom patterns correspond to criteria used to define a disorder in disparate systems of medicine. Because empirically verifiable or objective knowledge of relationships between subjective experiences is not available or verifiable, accurate statements about differences between disorders of mood or cognition as they are defined in disparate systems of medicine cannot be made. In view of these limitations, it is legitimate to comment on reports of subjective mental or emotional experiences, and to characterize certain experiences as "symptoms" or signatures of distress or impairment reflecting "abnormal" or "maladaptive" mental or emotional functioning with respect to an assumed "normal" range of experiences. However, it is not legitimate to describe unique symptom patterns as instances of disorders. The ongoing debate over disorders versus symptom patterns in Western psychiatry is reviewed in Chapter 3. To develop valid and clinically useful diagnostic concepts, the architects of future versions of the *DSM* must address the above conceptual and methodological problems in current diagnostic methods.

Integrative Assessment Methods Incorporate and Broaden Conventional Approaches

Contemporary biomedical approaches in history taking and medical assessment yield valuable information that helps to clarify biological, psychological, and social factors related to cognitive, emotional, and behavioral symptoms. However, assessment methods used in Western medicine and psychiatry are inherently limited because their principles are based on implicit assumptions that place restrictions on the phenomena that can potentially explain the causes or meanings of symptoms. Biomedical psychiatry assumes that discrete causes of symptoms are biological processes manifesting as distressing emotions, impaired cognitive functioning, and so on. Indirect causes of symptoms include acute or chronic social, cultural, or other stresses that lead to biological (including neurobiological and endocrinological) changes manifesting as symptoms. In Western psychiatry, meanings of symptoms are psychodynamic interpretations of distress or impaired functioning resulting from maladaptive responses to internal or external stresses. An integrative perspective acknowledges these conventional concepts as legitimate but insufficient to explain the spectrum of causes or meanings of emotional or mental symptoms. In addition to classical neurophysiology, integrative medicine conceptualizes causes as dynamic energetic or informational processes affecting the body or brain at numerous hierarchic levels, including neuroimmunological functioning, interacting biomagnetic fields, and possibly also nonclassical energy-information processes, including large-scale coherent quantum states or other "subtle" energetic or informational phenomena associated with consciousness. From the perspectives of integrative medicine possible meanings of symptoms include conventional psychodynamic interpretations in addition to cultural, spiritual, and anomalous aspects of consciousness that are a priori dismissed by current science. Disparate ways of "seeing" causes or meanings of symptoms have profound implications for the practice of medicine. When possible causes or meanings of a symptom are not evaluated, there will be limited insight into the most appropriate or most effective treatments addressing that symptom. Integrative assessment methods deepen conventional models of mental illness by clarifying and expanding appropriate treatment options to more fully address the range of causes or meanings of symptoms.

In cases where significant empirical data support putative causes of a mental or emotional symptom pattern, postulated relationships between measurable biological factors and subjective complaints are seldom confirmed because of the complexity of intervening hierarchical relationships between causes and presumed corresponding symptoms. Assessment approaches used in contemporary Western psychiatry, including urine assays of neurotransmitter metabolites, serum endocrinological assays, and structural and functional brain-imaging technologies (e.g., computed tomography, MRI, qEEG, fMRI, single photon emission computed tomography, and PET) yield largely nonspecific information about the patient's general state of health, or general brain structure and function. Therefore, the kind and quality of information available from contemporary Western psychiatric assessment generally do not permit reliable inferences about specific relationships between mental or emotional symptoms and their postulated causes at the level of molecules, neurons, or brain circuits. The ambiguous state of affairs of Western

Table 5–1   Verifying Causation When Assessing Physical versus Mental/Emotional Symptoms

Criterion	Physical Symptoms	Mental/Emotional Symptoms
Putative causal factors of symptom are identified or identifiable using available scientific means	Yes	No—indirect inferences only
Putative causal factors are verified or verifiable as causes of symptom	Often	No—the brain is too complex to permit empirical verification of the most basic postulated relationships between symptoms and putative causes using available scientific means
Treatment addressing unambiguous causal factors is specific, and effectiveness is empirically verifiable	Sometimes	No—absence of unambiguous information about possible causes and the absence of a falsifiable model of pathogenesis have resulted in general treatments that presumably affect putative causes of symptoms

psychiatric assessment has resulted in numerous models but few falsifiable hypotheses linking mental or emotional symptoms to putative underlying causes of brain dysfunction. **Table 5–1** compares criteria used in Western medicine to verify causes of physical symptoms versus cognitive, emotional, and behavioral symptoms.

To summarize, the construct validity of the idea of a psychiatric disorder rests on the assumption that symptom patterns recur in highly organized ways, and that self-reported subjective states provide accurate and reliable information about the quality and severity of symptoms. With few exceptions, the existence of psychiatric disorders can be neither verified nor falsified because contemporary technologies lack the capacity to correlate unambiguous information pertaining to mental or emotional symptoms with empirically verifiable neurobiological structures or processes—there are no reliable markers for psychiatric disorders. Exceptions to this include the severe form of bipolar disorder (bipolar I), severe psychotic syndromes, and some dementias. In both cases, identified genetic or neurobiological factors probably play important roles in the progression of illness, and there is considerable overlap in the characteristics and severity of symptoms between individuals diagnosed with the same disorder.

Integrative Assessment May Improve Accuracy and Cost-Effectiveness of Mental Health Care

Conventionally trained physicians frequently consider using or recommending nonconventional assessment or treatment approaches only after mainstream approaches have failed. From the perspective of Western medicine, this is regarded as a "conservative" approach, because it gives precedence to conventional medical approaches over nonconventional methods (Eisenberg, 1997). However, some nonconventional approaches are substantiated by compelling research evidence, whereas some conventional approaches in current use have limited or inconsistent supporting evidence. In other cases, clearly effective conventional assessment or treatment approaches may not represent realistic options because of expense, limited availability, or patient preferences. In integrative medicine the order of precedence of assessment or treatment recommendations is related to evidence in the context of realistic constraints and patient preferences. Thus mainstream biomedical approaches do not necessarily constitute the most expedient, most effective, most cost-effective, or most preferred initial management plan. The use of well-substantiated nonconventional assessment approaches together with conventional biomedical approaches will

permit future clinicians to obtain more accurate and specific information about the causes, conditions, or meanings of cognitive, emotional, and behavioral symptoms. This will result in improved reliability of findings compared with current methods, and a more complete picture of biological, energetic, or informational causes or psychological or spiritual meanings associated with mental or emotional symptoms. Improved accuracy and reliability of findings will enhance the cost-effectiveness of presently used assessment methods. The integration of biomedical and nonconventional assessment approaches will prove useful in cases where conventional medical-psychiatric assessment approaches, including brain scans, serologic studies, and neuropsychological inventories, result in ambiguous findings. The benefits of integrative approaches in psychiatric assessment include the following:

◆ An integrative assessment approach will help clarify the medical and psychiatric differential diagnosis when conventional assessment methods have failed to identify the causes or conditions associated with a symptom pattern, or the patient's medical or psychiatric history is vague or complex.

◆ Combining conventional assessment methods with nonconventional biological assessment approaches based on current medical theory, including qEEG and urinary or serologic studies of neurotransmitter metabolites and immunologic or endocrinological factors, will result in increased specificity and accuracy when ruling out possible biological causes or markers of mental or emotional symptoms.

◆ Combining conventional assessment methods with emerging approaches that are currently outside of biomedicine will clarify the role of possible energetic or informational causes of mental or emotional symptoms.

◆ The derivation of integrative assessment approaches and their use in algorithms will address the neurobiological, somatic, mind–body, energetic, or informational causes or conditions underlying mental or emotional symptoms.

Emerging Paradigms Are Yielding New Tools for Psychiatric Assessment

Alternative conceptual frameworks, or paradigms, in science and medicine are resulting in novel explanatory models of illness. Chapter 3 discusses the implications of emerging paradigms for our understanding of the nature and causes of physical and mental illness. New ways of thinking about complex living systems, space–time, causality, consciousness, energy, and information are resulting in novel methods for assessing putative causes of symptoms. The conceptual framework in which a symptom pattern is evaluated determines interpretations of causes or meanings that are regarded as legitimate. Subsequently, treatment choices addressing the causes or meanings of a symptom are selected in the context of the system of medicine in which the symptom is evaluated. Disparate conceptual frameworks define different interpretive models used in medicine, resulting in different inferences about causes or meanings of the same symptom. Many nonconventional assessment approaches result in findings that may permit novel explanations of illness phenomena currently explained in strictly psychodynamic or biomedical terms. Identified causes or meanings of a symptom pattern translate into treatment choices regarded as legitimate in relation to the system of medicine in which the symptom is evaluated. Treatment choices recommended on the basis of findings from different assessment approaches will expectably result in different outcomes. In integrative mental health care, the key to selecting assessment approaches is to identify the paradigm or blend of paradigms that contain interpretive models of illness that may provide more accurate or more complete information about different causes or meanings of a particular symptom pattern. The most productive assessment strategy results in a picture of complex causes and meanings of a symptom pattern that is more accurate or complete than available using other strategies. The findings of integrative assessment provide the basis for a treatment plan that adequately addresses disparate causes and meanings of a symptom pattern.

◆ Nonconventional Assessment Methods in the Evaluation of Mental or Emotional Symptoms

Future Integrative Methods Will Assess Biological, Somatic, and Energy-Information Causes and Meanings of Mental Illness

Novel clinician-centered assessment approaches (e.g., kinesiology and Healing Touch) and emerging technologies will permit future clinicians to capture information that is unattainable using contemporary biomedical approaches. The result will be a more complete understanding of neurobiological, somatic, and energetic factors associated with psychiatric symptom patterns. Assessment approaches based on emerging scientific paradigms or non-Western conceptual frameworks are frequently rejected by Western physicians because these approaches have not been adequately examined to determine the validity of claims of a putative underlying mechanism of action, or their specificity or reliability with respect to a particular symptom (Ernst & Hentschel, 1995). Important philosophical and methodological issues pertaining to the determination of causes of a mental or emotional symptom are discussed in Chapters 2 and 4, respectively.

Nonconventional assessment approaches can be divided into four categories with respect to the conceptual framework or paradigm in which they originate: assays of biological structure or function, measures of bodily structure or function on a gross level (somatic), measuring forms of energy or information that have been validated by Western science, and measuring forms of energy or information that are not validated by Western science. Significant advances in the

biological assessment of cognitive, emotional, and behavioral symptoms are taking place in functional medicine. Emerging technologies including qEEG and heart rate variability (HRV) are providing useful clinical information about functional dysregulations of the brain and heart that are related to mental illness. Assessment approaches that purport to detect forms of energy or information that are not (yet) validated by Western science are also being used to assess mental health problems. These include applied kinesiology, pulse diagnosis in Chinese, Ayurvedic, and Tibetan medicine, analysis of the vascular autonomic signal (VAS) and gas discharge visualization (GDV).

Emerging Assessment Methods in Functional Medicine Will Add Significantly to Current Understandings of Mental Illness

At present, biological assessment methods are more widely accepted compared with other approaches. Functional medicine uses both emerging and conventional quantitative analysis methods to assess relationships between nutritional status, neurotransmitters, endocrine and immune function, and mental or emotional symptoms. Widely used tests include serum and urinary assays of neurotransmitters and their metabolites, vitamins, minerals, amino acids and their metabolites, hormones, fatty acids, proinflammatory cytokines (e.g., interleukin [IL]-6, IL-8, and IL-1b), and immunologic factors, as well as blood chemistries. Relationships between immunity and psychiatric symptoms are complex, and the same immunologic dysregulation is often found in patients with different major symptom patterns. At present there are no specific or sensitive immunologic markers of particular mental or emotional symptoms (Dantzer, Wollman, Vitkovic, & Yirmiya, 1999). For example, chronic depressed mood is associated with suppression of some immunologic factors (e.g., lower natural killer cell activity and decreased lymphocyte) and excess activity of others (e.g., increased neutrophils and increased haptoglobin levels), but these relationships are inconsistent. Elevated IL-6 is often present in schizophrenia and mania and in individuals who have been severely traumatized.

Horrobin (1996, 1998) has proposed a ***membrane phospholipid*** model of schizophrenia, which argues that abnormal metabolism of phospholipids resulting from genetic and environmental factors manifests as a chronic severe symptom pattern classified as schizophrenia in Western psychiatry. The finding of deficient levels of certain essential fatty acids in the red blood cells of schizophrenics is consistent with Horrobin's hypothesis (Vaddadi et al., 1996). The membrane phospholipid hypothesis may provide a unifying conceptual framework for understanding not only schizophrenia, but also bipolar disorder, and possibly dyslexia, schizotypal personality disorder, other schizophrenia-like syndromes, and other psychiatric disorders. The hypothesis suggests that a spectrum of psychiatric disorders is associated with abnormalities at the level of the neuronal membranes, and that the nature and severity of symptoms are related to the magnitude and type of metabolic errors leading to abnormal phospholipid metabolism. Severe psychiatric syndromes like schizophrenia develop when genetic errors of metabolism resulting in chronic brain deficiencies of dietary fatty acids are combined with other metabolic abnormalities that result in errors of fatty acid incorporation in phospholipid membranes or abnormally high rates of removal of fatty acids from nerve cell membranes by phospholipases. Evidence in support of the membrane phospholipid model in the pathogenesis of psychotic syndromes includes the following (Horrobin, 1998):

◆ MRI brain-imaging studies show relatively increased rates of phospholipid breakdown in the brains of never-medicated schizophrenics.

◆ Reduced electroretinogram (ERG) response is found in schizophrenics, an indicator of reduced retinal docosahexaenoic acid (DHA).

◆ Clozapine has been shown to increase red blood cell phospholipid amino acid and DHA levels, suggesting that this may be a mechanism of action for clozapine, or other atypical antipsychotic drugs, in addition to its dopamine-blocking effects.

◆ Clozapine is known to act like a prostaglandin E analogue, which may relate to its antipsychotic mechanism of action in regulating neuron membrane lipid metabolism.

Findings from neurotransmitter depletion studies suggest that both norepinephrine and serotonin have important but indirect roles in depressed mood. There are no clear or consistent correlations between particular symptom patterns and dysregulation of specific neurotransmitter or receptor systems, as there is considerable variation between patients with similar histories and symptoms. The artificially induced depletion of normal brain levels of norepinephrine or serotonin does not result in symptomatic worsening of depressed patients, suggesting that other neurotransmitters, including the monoamines, and possibly endocrinologic or immunologic factors are also involved in the pathogenesis of depressed mood or other symptom patterns (Delgado & Moreno, 2000). Central nervous system (CNS) levels, and therefore serum or urine metabolite levels, of some neurotransmitters follow a diurnal pattern of variation, including norepinephrine, epinephrine, and phenylethylamine (PEA). A possible CNS deficiency state of a specific neurotransmitter that follows a circadian pattern can best be determined by performing an assay when levels are expected to be high. In contrast, a possible CNS excess of a specific neurotransmitter can best be determined by taking measurements when levels are expected to be low according to the normal diurnal variation of the neurotransmitter. The use and timing of conventional medications or nonconventional treatments, diet, stress, and activity level can influence neurotransmitter levels. Urine specimens collected in the early morning are less likely to be affected by these factors, and therefore will more likely show a baseline deficiency or excess of a specific neurotransmitter. Calculating ratios of neurotransmitters to creatinine in the urine compensates for urinary dilution and may provide more accurate indicators of CNS levels of specific neurotransmitters compared with measurements of neurotransmitters alone. Unpublished findings from a large case series suggest that reduced attention in both children and adults is associated with relatively lower CNS serotonin and higher epinephrine levels, while anxiety is associated with relatively lower levels of glutamate (personal communication, Gottfried Kellerman, PhD, December 2004). The chapters in Part II review the research evidence for specific assays as biological markers of mental or emotional symptom patterns or predictors of treatment response. Emerging methods will permit clinicians to develop treatments that address unique intracellular nutritional and antioxidant factors associated with the patient's mental health problem (Boerner, 2001).

Quantitative EEG Studies and HRV Analysis Will Become Standard Assessment Approaches in Mental Health Care

Methods used to assess mental or emotional symptoms based on monitoring electromagnetic or biomagnetic fields include HRV monitoring of fluctuations in electrical heart rhythms, and qEEG for measuring dynamic patterns of brain electrical activity. The scientific basis of both HRV and qEEG has been validated by extensive research findings. However, neither approach is in current widespread use for the assessment of mental or emotional symptoms. It is likely that advanced qEEG brain-mapping techniques will become standard tools for the assessment of treatment-resistant depression, problems of inattention, traumatic brain injury, and many other mental health problems.

Assessment Approaches That Measure Putative Forms of Energy or Information Not Validated by Western Science Will Probably Enhance Current Approaches

The increasing use of energetic assessment approaches will aid clinicians' efforts in making inferences about possible energetic or informational causes or meanings of cognitive, emotional, and behavioral symptoms patterns. Intuitive approaches used by "energy healers" and machines that purportedly measure dysregulations in "subtle energy fields," including GDV, have emerged from beliefs or observations about correspondences between putative energy phenomena or information fields and emotional or psychological states. Empirical verification or refutation of approaches that claim to measure subtle energy phenomena will probably require many more decades of research. However, accumulating evidence supporting the use of Chinese pulse diagnosis as a technique in both medical and psychiatric assessment will rapidly increase popular and professional acceptance of this and other energetic methods.

Ancient techniques and technology-based methods are being used to assess responses to acupuncture and qigong. Traditional Chinese medical diagnosis employs four basic approaches: inspection, listening and smelling, inquiring, and palpation. Using these methods, the skilled practitioner obtains both empirical and intuitive information about the energetic balance between yin and yang, the two fundamental forms of qi (vital energy) that influence health and illness. Biomedical research on the validity of assessment approaches in Chinese, Ayurvedic, and Tibetan medicine has been slowed by the absence of objective measurements of postulated fundamental energetic principles. Measuring changes in skin electrical resistance has been used to assess qi energy and the effects of acupuncture treatment (Zhang & Chang-Lin, 2002). Brain-imaging research using fMRI has recently validated claims of predicted therapeutic effects when specific acupuncture points are stimulated (Zhang et al., 2004). Machines have been developed that purport to measure indicators of qi in meridians (Borg, 2003). The measurement of electrodermal potentials at acupoints following qigong treatment may provide accurate information about changes in electrical activity associated with beneficial effects of qi (Syldona & Rein, 1999). Research findings suggest that Chinese medical practitioners can be trained to quantify measures of yin and yang in a reliable manner, permitting standardized assessments of postulated energetic changes before or after treatment (Langevin et al., 2004). Subjective responses to Chinese medical treatments are also useful indicators of outcomes. Beneficial changes following acupuncture frequently include improved attitude toward health and positive lifestyle changes (Gould & MacPherson, 2001).

Analysis of the pulse is a fundamental approach in the assessment of physical and mental illness in four major world systems of medicine: Western biomedicine, Chinese medicine, Ayurveda, and Tibetan medicine. The methods used to detect and interpret the subtle characteristics of the human pulse have been refined over millennia of clinical experience. The skillful use of pulse diagnosis requires years of training under the guidance of an expert teacher. A specialized lexicon is used to describe dozens of pulse qualities that continue to elude description in conventional biological terms. Empirical findings support the use of information obtained from the pulse in the assessment of medical illnesses. However, at the time of writing, no formal studies have been done to determine the specificity of pulse diagnosis in the assessment of particular mental and emotional symptom patterns. Anecdotal reports and case histories suggest that certain characteristics of the pulse as described in Chinese, Ayurvedic, or Tibetan medical assessment correspond to particular energetic imbalances manifesting as mental or emotional symptoms. Based on his own extensive research and clinical experience, Hammer (2001) has suggested that pulse characteristics in Chinese medical assessment reflect three levels of severity of psychological symptoms. Mild to moderate symptoms, including general feelings of anxiety, transient depressed mood, and irritability, are often associated with a "tight" or rapid rate when taking the pulse at the pericardium position and "smooth vibration" over the entire pulse at all depths. More severe psychological symptoms are often associated with a pulse that is felt as a "rough vibration" over the entire pulse, and "slipperiness" in some aspects of the pulse. The most severe kinds of mental or emotional symptoms are frequently associated with the most abnormal energetic qualities of the pulse, resulting in a "pulse picture" that is "overwhelmed" by "chaos" in the circulation (Hammer, 2001).

Assessment Methods from Ayurveda and Tibetan Medicine May Help to Clarify Energetic Causes of Cognitive, Emotional, and Behavioral Symptoms

Ayurveda and Tibetan medicine are highly evolved systems of medicine that approach physical and mental illness in a truly integrative way using a range of physical, psychological, and spiritual methods. Tibetan medicine and Indian Ayurvedic medicine are related historically and share many basic concepts and methods in healing, although they also diverge in important ways (Bodeker, 2001; Clifford, 1990). Both systems of medicine posit the existence of three "humors" (in Sanskrit *dosha,* and in Tibetan, *nyes-pa*), or fundamental energetic elements, that combine in subtle ways to influence health and illness. Interactions between the three humors are invoked to explain different mental and

emotional functions and their afflictions, including thinking, feeling, reacting, and remembering. The three doshas of Ayurveda are Vata, Pitta, and Kapha. The corresponding humors of Tibetan medicine are called rlung, mKhris-pa, and bad-kan. Psychological, physical, and spiritual approaches are used to assess energetic imbalances that manifest as cognitive, emotional, and behavioral symptoms in Ayurvedic and Tibetan medicine. The identification of external and internal influences that contribute to energetic imbalances provides the clinician with an accurate understanding of complex causes or conditions underlying medical and mental illness. Assessment begins with a detailed history of physical, psychological, and spiritual functioning, including sleep patterns, dietary habits, and emotional and behavioral patterns. The physical examination includes analysis of the urine, careful examination of the tongue and eyes, and palpation of the pulses in several places. The patient's unique energetic constitution and any significant recent changes in health or activity are determined from history and assessment findings. A suitable integrative treatment plan consisting of psychological, physical, and spiritual interventions is constructed to address identified energetic imbalances associated with the patient's complaints. Common mental and emotional symptom patterns are frequently associated with excesses in a particular humor. More complex symptom patterns manifest when there are concurrent excesses or imbalances in two or more humors.

Analysis of the VAS May Help to Substantiate Traditional Energetic Assessment Methods

An emerging approach that is adding to assessment methods used in Chinese medicine and energy medicine is analysis of the vascular autonomic signal. The VAS is a postulated reflex that is triggered by different biophysical or energetic stimuli inside or outside the human body. Proponents of this model argue that the VAS reflex maintains the body's principal systems, including the endocrine, immune, and central nervous system, in homeodynamic balance, and that optimum energetic balance is disrupted by both external and internal stresses. For several decades acupuncturists have used the VAS reflex to assess the energetic conditions underlying both medical and psychiatric symptom patterns. Recent studies suggest that the VAS reflex can be reliably captured using Doppler monitoring of arterial wall movement (Ackerman, 2001). Research findings suggest that that subtle changes in arterial wall tone occur almost instantaneously in response to energetic stimuli that affect the physical and psychological state of the body but do not enter into conscious awareness. Changes in VAS tone are believed to take place when postulated "neurohormones" resonate in response to subtle electromagnetic fields emitted by substances held in proximity to various parts of the human body. Particular substances induce specific resonance patterns and commensurate changes in the dynamic biophysical environment of the body. The brain responds to these changes at the level of the autonomic nervous system. Physical or psychological symptoms may result depending on the nature of resonant changes induced by different substances. Changes in arterial wall tone can be interpreted as VAS energetic signatures corresponding to the energetic patterns of different substances and their effects on the dynamic energy balance of the human body. In addition to assessing energetic causes of cognitive, emotional, and behavioral symptoms, analysis of the VAS reflex is used to assess potential adverse effects of treatments that are being considered. Analysis of the VAS is often performed to evaluate the nutritional status of a patient before acupuncture is administered to facilitate detoxification from alcohol or drugs. With continued research the VAS reflex may provide information about putative energetic imbalances associated with mental and emotional symptom patterns, suggesting treatments that address such identified imbalances.

Muscle Testing May Provide Clinically Useful Information in Some Cases

Muscle testing using an approach called applied kinesiology has been in widespread use in energy psychology and chiropractic since its invention in the United States several decades ago. Practitioners believe that subtle differences in muscle strength provide a precise indication of energetic imbalances in specific meridians corresponding to particular physical or emotional symptoms, including anxiety and depressed mood. On this basis, muscle testing is believed to provide useful information about energetic treatments that will most likely yield beneficial changes. Limited evidence suggests that applied kinesiology may provide useful clinical information about possible energetic imbalances related to some cases of mental or emotional symptoms. Pending further evidence from future observations and research, the skillful use of applied kinesiology may prove a useful adjunct to the assessment of certain mental or emotional symptoms. The diamond method of cantillation (Clifford, 1990) is an offshoot of applied kinesiology. Case reports suggest that information obtained through muscle testing is useful in determining beneficial energetic treatments; however, this technique has not been validated by double-blind, sham-controlled studies.

GDV is an Emerging Research Tool in Energy Medicine

In 2002 the National Institutes of Health (NIH) and the National Institute on Aging jointly sponsored a 2-day meeting dedicated to the scientific discussion of gas discharge visualization, a technology recently developed by Russian scientists that claims to measure human energy fields and to make medical diagnoses on the basis of those measurements (Francomano & Jonas, 2002). In this technique a high-intensity electric field is applied to the fingertips to stimulate emission of photons and electrons from living tissue. The emitted energy, in turn, results in a gaseous discharge that is photographed and analyzed with respect to an energetic model based on Chinese meridian theory. The postulated biophysical processes that GDV claims to detect have been described using quantum mechanics (Korotkov, Williams, & Wisneski, 2004). The GDV bioelectrography machine includes software that makes inferences about putative energetic factors associated with medical or psychiatric symptoms on the basis of the identified energetic pattern (Korotkov, 2002). At the NIH-sponsored meeting, research evidence for the existence of a human energy field was discussed, and GDV data for specific medical diagnoses were presented and reviewed. The meeting concluded with the development of a protocol for further research aimed at elucidating the physical mechanism underlying human energy field measurement and designing research protocols that will elucidate the accuracy and clinical usefulness of GDV and other apparatus that purport to measure human energy fields.

Table 5–2 lists representative established and emerging approaches that are used to assess the causes or meanings of mental or emotional symptoms.

A Future Integrative Mental Health Care Will Use Disparate Assessment Approaches

Nonconventional assessment methods will almost certainly influence the future evolution of Western psychiatry, eventually

Table 5–2 Nonconventional Assessment Approaches Used in Mental Health Care

Category	Assessment Modality	Comments
Biological assays of nutrients, blood, immunological markers, neurotransmitters, and metabolites	Serologic or RBC analysis of fatty acids, nutrients, trace metals, cytokines, etc.	Functional approaches will significantly improve specificity, leading to more accurate identification of causes of symptoms at level of molecular dysregulation.
		Case reports suggest possible correlations between neurotransmitter or functional approaches dysregulation and some mental or emotional symptoms
Monitoring forms of energy or information that are validated by current Western science	qEEG	Case reports and controlled studies suggest correlations between specific qEEG findings and depressed mood, mania, impaired attention, and other symptoms
	HRV monitoring	Case reports and studies suggest correspondences between HRV/qEEG monitoring and causes of mental or emotional symptoms
Monitoring forms of energy or information that are not validated by current Western science	Chinese, Ayurvedic, and Tibetan pulse diagnosis	Case reports and limited research findings suggest possible clinical use in clarifying causes of "energetic imbalances" associated with some mental and emotional symptom patterns
	Analysis of the VAS	
	GDV	
	Applied kinesiology	

RBC, red blood cell (count); GDV, gas discharge visualization; HRV, heart rate variability; qEEG, quantitative electroencephalography; VAS, vascular autonomic signal leading to integrative approaches incorporating advances in neuropharmacology, functional medicine, mind–body medicine, functional brain imaging, and possibly also energy medicine. Biological and electromagnetic assessment approaches are derived from conventional scientific theories and are thus susceptible to conventional research designs. Preliminary findings suggest that emerging approaches used to assess putative biological or electromagnetic factors associated with mental illness provide useful clinical information and may contribute to more accurate and specific understandings of the causes of symptoms and, by extension, more effective integrative treatment planning. In contrast, claimed mechanisms of action for subtle energy assessment methods are not susceptible to scientific study, and barring a radical paradigm shift in Western biomedicine, it is unlikely that these approaches will be empirically verified in the near future. As evidence for novel assessment methods accumulates, Western medical institutional barriers to novel ways of seeing and interpreting the causes or meanings of symptoms will soften in response to accumulating research findings and observational evidence. A future integrative medicine will incorporate novel assessment methods in ways that clarify the biological, energetic, or informational concomitants of mental or emotional symptoms.

◆ The Diagnostic Interview, Patient Contract, and Responsibilities of the Health Care Provider: Toward an Integrative Model

Goals of the initial interview or intake include obtaining a complete history, identifying the symptom pattern associated with distress or dysfunction, making a provisional assessment of causes or meanings of the patient's symptoms, determining the need for specialized assessment tests, and defining initial treatment goals. During the initial appointment, the clinician gathers pertinent information about the patient's medical, psychiatric, social, family, religious, and spiritual history. An integrative history is inherently difficult to take because practitioners trained in disparate systems of medicine generally have different opinions about historical information that is pertinent and how to conduct an intake interview. The absence of standardized integrative history-taking instruments interferes with cross-disciplinary communication between conventionally and nonconventionally trained medical practitioners. The findings of a recent survey suggest that the majority of nonconventional practitioners agree on questions that are important to include during an intake interview. This core group of questions may become the basis for future standardized interview tools in integrative medicine (Lindahl, Barrett, Peterson, Zheng, & Nedrow, 2005). The Mini-Mental State Exam is a useful screening tool when there are concerns over possibly severe impairment. Findings of the MMSE may point to the need for more extensive neuropsychological testing or a neurology consultation.

In the interest of economy of time, many clinicians ask new patients to bring medical or psychiatric records and to complete a self-assessment questionnaire before the first appointment. Asking new patients to bring medications and supplements to the interview will help ensure that doses and brands are accurately documented.

At the conclusion of the initial appointment, the clinician usually has enough information to make a formulation of possible causes or meanings of mental or emotional symptoms and to suggest useful approaches (if any) for further assessment. The practitioner should inform the patient of clinical findings and impressions within his or her conventional or nonconventional area of expertise only, recommend further assessment approaches (if any are indicated), and comment on reasonable treatment choices. A return appointment should be scheduled at an appropriate interval, depending on the severity of symptoms.

The chief responsibility of a Western physician is to establish the presence or absence of medical illness on the basis of the patient's self-reported history, collateral information, and assessment findings. As a conventionally trained Western physician, it is my strong view that treatment goals should be clarified and the evidence supporting reasonable conventional, nonconventional, and integrative treatments should be carefully reviewed before treatment is initiated or referrals are made to conventional or nonconventional practitioners. If a patient reports a history or symptoms that warrant urgent concern over a possibly emergent medical problem, including, for example, severe headaches, a history of untreated head injury, changes in the level of consciousness or other severe new-onset changes in mental functioning, nausea, vomiting, or other serious rapidly evolving complaints, he or she should be referred to an urgent care facility or emergency room immediately. When history and symptoms do not suggest the presence of a rapidly worsening medical problem, or in cases where a primary medical illness was previously suspected but has been ruled out by a Western-trained physician, it is reasonable for the patient to work primarily with his or her acupuncturist, herbalist, or other nonconventionally trained health care professional and to focus on one or more nonconventional treatments for which there is evidence. However, if a patient becomes medically ill while under the care of a nonconventional practitioner, he or she should be referred urgently to a Western-trained physician to avoid delays in the assessment and treatment of a possibly serious illness.

◆ The Logic of Integrative Assessment and Formulation: Overview

Certain assessment methods are more useful than others in clarifying the causes or meanings of a particular symptom. The evidence in favor of nonconventional assessment approaches with respect to many common mental or emotional symptoms is presented in the chapters of Part II. Determination of the optimum assessment approach for a specified symptom starts with a review of the evidence supporting the use of particular methods for clarifying the causes or meanings of specified symptom. The same logic is used to select appropriate conventional and nonconventional assessment approaches. The practitioner must first address the questions What is being looked for? What phenomena are believed to be pertinent to an accurate and complete understanding of the causes, course, conditions, or meanings of a particular symptom pattern? This inquiry goes to considerations of the phenomenal basis of illness, in other words, the kinds of social, psychological, biological, energetic, and possibly spiritual processes or events associated with mental or emotional symptoms. When considering the causes or meanings of a symptom pattern, it is useful to think in terms of their relative levels in a hierarchy of dynamic social, cultural, biological, neurobiological, and energetic factors. In many cases, multiple interrelated causes or meanings of a symptom exist at different hierarchic levels. Effective assessment strategies accurately identify core causes or meanings of the symptom pattern in question but may overlook more obscure causes or meanings.

Causes or Meanings of Symptoms Are Located at Interdependent Hierarchic Levels

There are multiple possible connections between the levels at which biological, informational, or energetic causes or meanings of symptoms exist and characteristics of treatments that will alleviate those causes. For example, a finding on qEEG analysis of abnormal left frontotemporal lobe activity in the mid-alpha frequency range (10–12 Hz) in a patient who complains of new-onset impairment in attention following a closed head injury suggests that treatments directed at "renormalizing" frontotemporal brain electrical activity in the mid-alpha range will probably result in improved attention. Reasonable treatment choices would then include certain EEG-biofeedback protocols, binaural sound, mind–body practices, certain natural products or synthetic drugs, and possibly also virtual reality exposure therapy. The logic of integrative treatment planning is explored in detail in Chapter 6.

The practitioner must ask what orthodox or nonconventional assessment approaches provide clinically useful, accurate, and reliable information about the causes or meanings of a specified symptom pattern in relation to the levels of possible causes in a hierarchy of dynamic factors. The practitioner must also consider what combination of conventional and nonconventional assessment methods yields the most accurate or most complete interpretation of causes or meanings. When the initial assessment is completed, the practitioner prepares a formulation illustrating both quantitative and qualitative evidence of social, cultural, psychological, biological, or energetic causes or meanings of the patient's complaint.

The optimum assessment strategy is that combination of approaches that will most reliably yield accurate and complete information about the causes or meanings of a symptom pattern. In most cases practical constraints of cost, availability, and patient preferences determine a realistic strategy. The most practical or realistic assessment plan sometimes combines several approaches in parallel. In other cases, a more practical solution is to use disparate assessment methods sequentially, depending on the nature or severity of a mental or emotional symptom, a review of medical or psychiatric history, and findings of the initial assessment. Criteria for determining whether to use two or more assessment methods at the same time (**parallel assessment**) or in succession (**sequential assessment**) are reviewed in the sections below. In most cases the integrative practitioner will select assessment methods after reviewing the evidence for different approaches with respect to the patient's history and principal symptom(s) in the context of practical constraints and patient preferences. The formulation includes history, findings, and observations that point to the causes or meanings of the principal symptom(s). Assessment continues on an as-needed basis for the duration of treatment. Response to treatment is assessed on successive return appointments. Changes in the principal symptom pattern, including worsening or newly emerging symptoms, may indicate a need for other assessment approaches to better characterize the causes or meanings of changes in the patient's mental or emotional state. Previously untried assessment methods sometimes result in significant new information and may suggest changes in the treatment plan that more adequately address the patient's symptoms.

When evaluating outcomes, it is sometimes useful to create a quality of life index, taking into account both personal and subjective factors, including attitude, self-esteem, level of autonomy (covering working capacity and activities of daily living), the quality of social relationships, sexual activity, considerations of financial security and home environment, and spiritual values and activities (Liverani, Minelli, & Ricciuti, 2000). Personal information adds an important qualitative dimension to the objective findings of randomized controlled trials.

The process of defining and redefining assessment and treatment is iterative and continues until the causes or meanings of the principal symptom pattern are accurately characterized and a practical and effective treatment plan is successfully implemented. Chapter 6 discusses the logical steps involved in translating the multimodal formulation into a suitable integrative treatment plan. Part II chapters contain symptom-focused algorithms for deriving realistic integrative assessment and treatment strategies addressing common cognitive, emotional, and behavioral symptoms.

Focusing on One Symptom or Many Symptoms

Assessment priority is often clear when a single symptom pattern has been identified as the primary cause of distress or impairment. However, at the time of the initial interview or during the course of treatment, a patient may report many symptoms at the same time or a progression of symptoms. In such cases, the clinician must decide whether to focus on one primary symptom or many core symptoms. In the clinician's judgment, causes or meanings of symptoms may be directly or indirectly related or independent of each other. The problem is reduced to determining how to prioritize assessment or treatment choices on the basis of measures of symptom severity or evidence that disparate symptoms are related. I have observed that most patients complain of many vague or specific symptoms but generally report one principal symptom pattern associated with severe distress or progressive impairment in social, intellectual, or occupational functioning. In such cases, the initial priorities of assessment and treatment planning are relatively clear. Evidence for the integrative management of common cognitive, emotional, and behavioral symptoms is discussed in Part II. A thorough intake will frequently reveal two or more principal symptoms associated with significant distress or impairment. The symptoms may be related in direct or indirect ways, or their causes or meanings may be independent of one another. In my own clinical experience as a psychiatrist treating or consulting on thousands of patients in private practice, outpatient managed care environments, inpatient psychiatric units, emergency rooms, hospital intensive care units, and inpatient medical-surgical services, I have encountered relatively few patients who complain of more than two primary unrelated mental or emotional symptoms. Chapter 6 discusses practical methods for treating patients who complain of two or more co-occurring mental or emotional symptoms.

*Choosing the Most Appropriate Integrative
Assessment Approach*

Because assessment generally involves passive monitoring of biological, biomagnetic, somatic, or "energetic" functioning, toxicities and adverse effects seldom occur. By the same token, there are no compelling reasons to avoid using a particular approach alone or in combination with other approaches. Determining the most appropriate assessment approaches to use when evaluating a patient depends on history, principal symptoms, the strength of evidence for different approaches, the availability of competent practitioners, cost, and patient preferences. In many cases there will be no apparent need for assessment beyond the initial interview and a brief mental state exam. When the practitioner decides to treat a patient without first using specialized assessment approaches, a poor or incomplete response to the initial treatment plan or a lack of clarity about the causes or meanings of symptoms may point to the need for specific assessment approaches in subsequent sessions.

◆ Deciding on the Type, Order, and Number of Assessment Approaches to Use

Depending on the complexity and severity of the patient's symptoms, an adequate formulation and treatment plan may be obtained on the basis of information obtained from the history and the clinical interview alone, a single assessment approach, or multiple sequential or parallel assessment approaches. It is reasonable to begin with an approach that will probably yield useful clinical information about the principal symptom pattern. In deciding how to assess a patient, there are always two basic choices: the use of one approach or the use of two or more approaches in parallel. These choices are discussed in the following sections.

Using One Assessment Approach or a Series of Single Approaches

Most clinicians use one assessment approach at a time because of practical constraints on cost and availability. The practitioner should start with the approach that will most likely yield reliable clinical information about causes or meanings of the principal symptom pattern(s). Evidence for the various methods used to assess common mental or emotional symptoms is summarized in Part II of this book. In cases where reliable information is obtained and a

multidimensional formulation has led to an effective treatment strategy, there is no need for further assessment. In cases where accurate information is not obtained from the initial assessment, the practitioner should carefully review the patient's symptoms and history to obtain salient information that may have been overlooked during the intake interview. Consulting the evidence tables in Part II for assessment methods pertaining to the principal symptom pattern will guide the practitioner to progressively more useful approaches. Practitioner and patient can then discuss choices in the context of practical cost and availability constraints and select an appropriate and realistic approach. This process continues until assessment findings clarify the causes or meanings of the patient's complaints, and an effective treatment plan is implemented.

The advantages of using single assessment approaches in sequence include reduced costs, simplicity, and the absence of potential safety issues when two or more approaches are combined. Using only one assessment approach avoids the risk of confounding the diagnostic picture with conflicting explanations of possible causes or meanings of a symptom in cases where disparate assessment approaches yield contradictory or inconsistent findings. Delay in the implementation of effective treatment is a potential disadvantage of using single assessment approaches one after another.

Using Two or More Assessment Approaches at the Same Time

The use of two or more assessment approaches in parallel is reasonable when a principal symptom has not improved or has worsened during the course of treatment or the clinical picture is complicated by newly emerging symptoms. These circumstances suggest that important information was overlooked in the initial history, or the initial assessment and treatment plan were not adequate. In such cases there is some urgency in accurately identifying the causes or meanings of the patient's complaint. The practitioner should first review the patient's history and current symptoms in detail to ensure that pertinent medical, psychological, or other problems have not been overlooked. In complicated cases, combining two or more assessment approaches may provide new information that will clarify the nature of persisting symptoms, permitting a more complete formulation, a more effective treatment plan, and improved outcomes. The practitioner should always take into account potential safety issues when combining two or more assessment approaches and document the patient's informed consent. When selecting assessment approaches, it is important to take the patient's cultural values and spiritual beliefs (if any) into account.

References

Ackerman, J. (2001). The biophysics of the vascular autonomic signal and healing. *Frontier Perspectives, 10*(2), 9–15.

Anthony, J. C. (2001). The promise of psychiatric enviromics. *British Journal of Psychiatry, 178*(Suppl. 40), 8–11.

Berrios, G., & Markova, I. (2002). Assessment and measurement in neuropsychiatry: A conceptual history. *Semin Clin Neuropsychiatry,7*(1), 3–10.

Beutler, L., & Malik, M. (Eds.). (2002). *Rethinking the DSM: A psychological perspective*. Washington, DC: American Psychological Association.

Bodeker, G. (2001). Evaluating Ayurveda. *Journal of Alternative and Complementary Medicine, 7*(5), 389–392.

Boerner, P. (2001). Functional intracellular analysis of nutritional and antioxidant status. *Journal of the American Nutraceutical Association, 4*(1), 27–41.

Clifford, T. (1990). *Tibetan Buddhist medicine and psychiatry: The diamond healing*. York Beach, ME: Samuel Weiser, Inc.

Cutrona, C. E., Cadoret, R. E., Suhr, J. A., et al. (1994). Interpersonal variables in the prediction of alcoholism among adoptees: Evidence for gene-environment interaction. *Comprehensive Psychiatry, 35,* 171–179.

Dantzer, R., Wollman, E., Vitkovic, L., & Yirmiya R. (1999). Cytokines and depression: Fortuitous or causative association? *Molecular Psychiatry, 4,* 328–332.

Delgado, P. L., & Moreno, F. A. (2000). Role of norepinephrine in depression. *Journal of Clinical Psychiatry, 61*(Suppl. 1), 5–12.

Eisenberg, D. (1997). Advising patients who seek alternative medical therapies. *Annals of Internal Medicine, 127,* 61–69.

Ernst, E., & Hentschel, C. (1995). Diagnostic methods in complementary medicine: Which craft is witchcraft? *International Journal of Risk and Safety in Medicine, 7,* 55–63.

First, M. (2002, Summer). A research agenda for DSM-V: Summary of the white papers. *Psychiatric Research Report,* pp. 10–13.

Francomano, C., & Jonas, W. (2002, April 17–18). *Measuring the human energy field: State of the science.* Paper presented at The Gerontology Research Center, National Institute on Aging, and National Institute of Health, Baltimore, MD.

Freud, S. (1909) Analysis of a phobia in a five-year-old boy. In J. Strachey (Ed. and Trans.), *Standard Edition of the Complete Psychological Works of Sigmund Freud* (vol. 10, pp. 5–147). London: Hogarth Press. (Original work published 1955)

Galton, F. (1876). The history of twins as a criterion of the relative powers of nature and nurture. *Journal of the Royal Anthropological Institute of Great Britain and Ireland, 6,* 391–406.

Gordon, E. (2002). Neuroimaging in neuropsychiatry. *Seminars in Clinical Neuropsychiatry, 7*(1), 42–53.

Gould, A., & MacPherson, H. (2001). Patient perspectives on outcomes after treatment with acupuncture. *Journal of Alternative and Complementary Medicine, 7*(3), 261–268.

Hammer, L. (2001). Qualities as signs of psychological disharmony. In: Hammer, L, ed. *Chinese pulse diagnosis: A contemporary approach* (pp. 539–594). Seattle, WA: Eastland Press.

Horrobin, D. (1996). Schizophrenia as a membrane lipid disorder which is expressed throughout the body. *Prostaglandins, Leukotrienes and Essential Fatty Acids, 55*(2), 3–7.

Horrobin, D. (1998). The membrane phospholipid hypothesis as a biochemical basis for the neurodevelopmental concept of schizophrenia. *Schizophrenia Research, 30,* 193–208.

Kendler, K. S. (1995). Genetic epidemiology in psychiatry: Taking both genes and environment seriously. *Archives of General Psychiatry, 52,* 895–899.

Kendler, K. S., Heath, A. C., Martin, N. G., et al. (1987). Symptoms of anxiety and depression: Same genes, different environments? *Archives of General Psychiatry, 44,* 451–457.

Korotkov, K. (2002). *Human energy field: Study with GDV bioelectrography.* Fairlawn, NJ: Backbone Publishing Co.

Korotkov, K., Williams, B., & Wisneski, L. (2004). Assessing biophysical energy transfer mechanisms in living systems: The basis of life processes. *Journal of Alternative and Complementary Medicine, 10*(1), 49–57.

Langevin, H., Badger, G., Povolny, B., et al. (2004). Yin and yang scores: A new method for quantitative diagnostic evaluation in traditional Chinese medicine research. *Journal of Alternative and Complementary Medicine, 10*(2), 389–395.

Lindahl, M., Barrett, R., Peterson, D., Zheng, L., & Nedrow, A. (2005). Development of an integrative patient history intake tool: A Delphi study. *Alternative Therapies in Health and Medicine, 11*(1), 52–56,

Lippman, A. (1992). Led (astray) by genetic maps: The cartography of the human genome and health care. *Social Science and Medicine, 35,* 1469–1476.

Liverani, A., Minelli, E., & Ricciuti, A. (2000). Subjective scales for the evaluation of therapeutic effects and their use in complementary medicine. *Journal of Alternative and Complementary Medicine, 6*(3), 257–264.

McDowall, M. E. (1987). *The identification of man-made environmental hazards to health: A manual of epidemiology.* London: Macmillan.

Merikangas, K. R., & Swendsen, J. D. (1997). Genetic epidemiology of psychiatric disorders. *Epidemiologic Reviews, 19,* 144–155.

Meyer-Lindenberg, J. (1991). The Holocaust and German psychiatry. *British Journal of Psychiatry, 159,* 7–12.

Owen, M., Cardno, A., & O'Donovan, M. (2000). Psychiatric genetics: Back to the future. *Molecular Psychiatry, 5,* 22–31.

Owen, M., Holmans, P., & McGuffin, P. (1997). Guest editorial: Association studies in psychiatric genetics. *Molecular Psychiatry, 2,* 270–273.

Plomin, R. (1994). *Genetics and experience: The interplay between nature and nurture* (pp. 1–40). Thousand Oaks, CA: Sage.

Regier, D., Kaelber, C., Rae, D., et al. (1998). Limitations of diagnostic criteria and assessment instruments for mental disorders: Implications for research and policy. *Archives of General Psychiatry, 55,* 109–115.

Reiss, D., Hetherington, M., Plomin, R., et al. (1995). Genetic questions for environmental studies: Differential parenting and psychopathology in adolescence. *Archives of General Psychiatry, 52,* 925–936.

Risch, N. (1997). Evolving methods in genetic epidemiology: Genetic linkage from an epidemiologic perspective. *Epidemiologic Reviews, 19,* 24–32.

Rosanoff, A. J., Handy, L. M., Plesset, I. R., et al. (1934). The etiology of the so-called schizophrenic psychoses with special reference to their occurrence in twins. *American Journal of Psychiatry, 91,* 247–286.

Sirovatka, P. (2004). APA launches DSM-V "Prelude" website. *Psychiatric News, 39,* 23–48.

Syldona, M., & Rein, G. (1999). The use of DC electrodermal potential measurements and healer's felt sense to assess the energetic nature of Qi. *Journal of Alternative and Complementary Medicine, 5*(4), 329–347.

Thomas, P., Romme, M., & Hamelijnck, J. (1996). Psychiatry and the politics of the underclass. *British Journal of Psychiatry, 169,* 401–404.

Vaddadi, K., Gilleard, C., Soosai, E., et al. (1996). Schizophrenia, tardive dyskinesia and essential fatty acids. *Schizophrenia Research, 20*(3), 287–294.

Wahlberg, K. E., Wynne, L. C., Oja, H., et al. (1997). Gene–environment interaction in vulnerability to schizophrenia: Findings from the Finnish Adoptive Family Study of Schizophrenia. *American Journal of Psychiatry, 154,* 355–362.

Wittchen, H., Hofler, M., & Merikangas, K. (1999). Toward the identification of core psychopathological processes: Commentary. *Archives of General Psychiatry, 5,* 929–931.

Zhang, & Chang-Lin. (2002). Skin resistance vs body conductivity: On the background of electronic measurement on skin. *Frontier Perspectives, 11*(2), 15–25.

Zhang, W., Zhen, J., Luo, F., et al. (2004). Evidence from brain imaging with fMRI supporting functional specificity of acupoints in humans. *Neuroscience Letters, 354*(1), 50–53.

6

Starting and Maintaining Integrative Treatment in Mental Health Care

◆ **Putting It All Together: Using Algorithms to Plan the Integrative Management of Cognitive, Emotional, and Behavioral Symptoms**

Algorithms incorporate three kinds of information

Integrative planning algorithms are based on an open design

The effectiveness and cost-effectiveness of conventional and nonconventional treatments, potential safety problems, patient preferences, and local availability of qualified practitioners are the most important issues to address when developing an integrative treatment plan. When mental health problems are viewed from the point of view of symptom patterns instead of disorders, emphasis is placed on treating core symptoms rather than diagnosing the patient according to criteria given in the *Diagnostic and Statistical Manual of Mental Disorders* (4th ed., *DSM-IV*), then treating a presumed disorder. Conventional treatments are briefly reviewed at the beginning of all Part II chapters; however, this book does not include a detailed discussion of the uses of conventional drugs and psychotherapy in mental health care. I am assuming that psychiatrists and other mental health professionals who use this book are already familiar with conventional treatment approaches. Excellent references summarizing the evidence for drug treatments and psychotherapy are available in American Psychiatric Association practice guidelines. The logic and clinical applications of treatment-planning algorithms are introduced in this chapter. All symptom-focused chapters of Part II include algorithms to help the practitioner plan integrative treatment strategies that incorporate appropriate conventional and nonconventional approaches, including considerations of psychotherapy and conventional drugs depending on the type and severity of symptoms. *Only Western-trained psychiatrists or primary care physicians should provide specific advice about the use of drugs to treat mental or emotional symptoms. It is sometimes appropriate for non–medically trained practitioners to suggest that conventional treatment may be beneficial and refer the patient to a Western physician for consultation.*

◆ **Overview**

The effectiveness and safety of many nonconventional therapies have been verified by consistently positive research findings of controlled, double-blind studies, systematic reviews and meta-analyses. Many so-called alternative therapies meet Western scientific criteria for efficacy and effectiveness but are not regarded as legitimate or mainstream for social or political reasons. Considerably more empirical evidence is available for nonconventional biological therapies because treatments based on a putative biological mechanism action have been more thoroughly investigated in controlled studies compared with therapies. Examples of nonconventional biological treatments of depressed mood that have been carefully evaluated include St. John's wort (*Hypericum perforatum*), *S*-adenosylmethionine (SAMe), 5-hydroxytryptophan (5-HTP), and folic acid. The majority of nonconventional therapies that do not postulate an explicit biological mechanism of action have not been evaluated as thoroughly as biological treatments, and there is comparatively less empirical evidence

supporting their use. Nonbiological approaches include mind–body therapies and treatments based on established or putative forms of energy or information. Electroencephalography (EEG) biofeedback is a kind of energy-information therapy based on current Western medical understandings of neurophysiology. In contrast, Reiki, qigong, and homeopathy are based on putative forms of energy or information that are not verified by current Western science. In spite of the absence of compelling evidence from Western-style research studies, these nonconventional treatments are nevertheless gaining acceptance because of increasing intellectual openness among conventionally trained medical practitioners and widespread popular interest. It is important to keep in mind that understandings of the clinical benefits of energy therapies are limited by small numbers of trials and the absence of compelling anecdotal evidence.

Many conventionally trained physicians believe that the beneficial effects of nonconventional treatments can be explained by the so-called ***placebo effect*** (a measurable improvement in health that is not attributable to effects of treatment). Although some nonconventional therapies are probably no more effective than placebos, the same argument can be applied to conventional biomedical treatments. In fact, the placebo effect is widely accepted in conventional biomedicine as playing a significant role in treatment for both medical and mental health problems (Dixon & Sweeney, 2000). Meta-analyses of controlled trials suggest that many conventional drugs used to treat depressed mood and other symptom patterns are no more effective than placebos (Kirsch, Moore, Scoboria, & Nicholls, 2002; Sussman, 2004; Thase, 2002). These observations are consistent with recent findings showing similar, presumably beneficial changes in regional brain activation after taking a conventional antidepressant or a placebo (Mayberg et al., 2002). Unresolved issues surrounding the role of placebo effects are shared concerns for both conventional and nonconventional practitioners. How placebos work to bring about the alleviation of symptoms is the subject of considerable research and debate. Until now there has been no agreed upon theory that adequately explains the so-called placebo effect. The general validity of the concept in fact continues to be questioned. A reanalysis of findings from hundreds of studies used to argue for the idea of placebo effects concluded that there is no compelling evidence for them (with the possible exception of some treatments of asthma) because of the absence of untreated control groups in the majority of studies (Kienle & Keane 1996, 1997). The controversy over placebo effects is complicated by the more recently described ***"nocebo" effects***—adverse effects associated with placebos—which may affect as many as 40% of individuals who take placebos (Tangrea, Adrianza, & Helsel, 1994). These findings suggest that many treatments probably have nonspecific effects that are beneficial or detrimental to health, including general effects on the body's immune, endocrinological, and central nervous system, but are not susceptible to rigorous empirical investigation. Intangible personal and interpersonal factors probably facilitate "self-healing" when patients undergo medical treatment. It is also important to consider the intriguing possibility that the effectiveness of many conventional and nonconventional treatments may be partly attributable to complex biological or energy-information mechanisms that cannot be adequately described using conventional biomedical concepts.

Conventional Western Psychiatry Will Continue to Benefit from Advances in Basic Neuroscience Research, but Market Issues and Safety Problems Are Slowing Growth

Advances in computing, electronic medical records, user-friendly database architectures and literature research methods, wireless networks, and human–computer interfaces will greatly enhance the capabilities of future mental health professionals and other practitioners to document patient progress and obtain reliable information when assessing and treating patients (Hsiung & Stangler, 2004). Broadband Internet links will soon lead to "virtual" consultations that will overcome current constraints of distance and time that delay or prevent medical care ("Virtual Second Opinions," 2004). These innovations will make it easier for practitioners to obtain current, accurate information about a wide range of treatment choices in a user-friendly format. Evolution in the technological infrastructure of medicine and medical informatics will lead to the acceleration of integrative medicine, resulting in general improvements in the quality of patient care. Basic neuroscience research will continue to yield important clinical advances, including new drugs, as well as treatments based on electricity and magnetic fields. Over 100 neurotransmitters have already been characterized, and many of these probably have significant roles in normal emotional or cognitive functioning. Future conventional drugs will target neurotransmitters, receptors, and intracellular signaling molecules (second messenger systems) that are presently understood in rudimentary ways. Examples include inositol triphosphate receptors, the immunophilins, and the so-called atypical neurotransmitters nitric oxide, carbon monoxide, and D-serine (Snyder, 2002).

In spite of progress in brain science, there is a widening gap between advances in basic neuroscience and pharmacology research and the introduction of promising new drugs. In recent years relatively few new psychopharmacologic medications have been developed and successfully brought to market, and costs of new drug development are soaring. In 2002, research and development spending on new drugs in the United States was $32 billion. In the same year the U.S. Food and Drug Administration (FDA) approved only 17 drugs based on novel active ingredients, equal to the lowest rate of new drug releases since 1983, when total research costs were only $3 billion. Pharmaceutical companies continue to invest heavily in new drug development. However, recent changes in FDA requirements have added complexity and cost to the process of getting a new drug to market. High development costs are passed on to patients and insurance companies, and many patients cannot afford medications that might alleviate their symptoms. This issue has become especially problematic for the poor, the elderly, and the chronically mentally ill. Problems associated with the growing cost of conventional health care represent opportunities for physicians and nonconventional practitioners to explore integrative treatment strategies that offer equal or greater effectiveness and, in many cases, greater cost-effectiveness compared with expensive conventional drugs ("Can Pfizer Deliver?," 2004).

The problems of limited new drug ideas and increasing drug prices are made worse by growing concerns over drug safety. In the United States alone, it is estimated that over 100,000 people die each year from properly prescribed medications (Lazarou, Pomeranz, & Corey, 1998). The likelihood of dying of a drug–drug interaction is directly proportional to the number of medications being taken. **Polypharmacy**—taking two or more drugs at the same time—increases the incidence and severity of adverse effects, medication prescribing errors, drug–drug interactions, hospitalizations, morbidity, mortality, and direct and indirect costs. Most patients who report mental or emotional symptoms use more than two treatments concurrently and seldom disclose this fact to their physicians or nonconventional practitioners (Eisenberg et al., 1998; Unutzer, 2002; Unutzer et al., 2000). Approximately one half of all elderly individuals admitted to a hospital take seven or more prescribed drugs, significantly increasing the risk of drug–drug interactions and potentially resulting in serious morbidity or death (Flaherty, Perry, Lynchard, & Morley, 2000). Elderly patients who take a psychotropic medication are 5 times more likely to have a motor vehicle accident compared with the general population, and this risk increases as doses go up (Ray, Fought, & Decker, 1992).

It is estimated that only 15 to 38% of patients undergoing psychotherapy are treated using evidence-based protocols (Sanderson, 2002). Specific psychological and social interventions are frequently beneficial treatments of cognitive, emotional, and behavioral symptoms. However, most mental health professionals do not use evidence-based psychological treatments in patient care. Reasons for this include lack of training in evidence-based therapies, the absence of a requirement for evidence-based treatments in continuing education, and negative practitioner biases against the use of evidence-based medicine. As many as one half of psychiatric patients fail to respond or respond partially to conventional treatments (Dubin, 2004). These patients are labeled "treatment-resistant" or "nonresponders." Treatment algorithms and consensus guidelines have been developed to address this widespread problem in conventional psychiatry. However, established algorithms do not take into account nonconventional assessment or treatment approaches, and do not significantly improve response rates for the following reasons:

◆ Brief 15-minute medication visits do not provide clinicians enough time to accurately identify target symptoms and develop adequate treatment plans.

◆ Conventional single-drug treatments are frequently changed to multiple-drug treatments without waiting for the patient to respond (and before trying nonconventional or integrative treatments).

◆ Polypharmacy addressing treatment resistance frequently leads to medication noncompliance and treatment failure.

◆ Co-occurring psychiatric symptoms are often missed during brief medicine-management sessions, and are therefore not adequately addressed.

♦ The role of psychotherapy is often devalued, especially in the management of severe symptom, including mania, severe depressed mood, and psychosis.

♦ Inpatient treatment generally emphasizes crisis intervention rather than treatment of core symptoms.

♦ Categories of Treatment and Levels of Evidence

By definition, mental or emotional symptoms are subjective and highly variable individual experiences of distress or dysfunction that are not susceptible to rigorous empirical analysis. Because of this, current research methods are sometimes inappropriate or inadequate tools for evaluating claims of a putative mechanism of action or verifying the effectiveness of both conventional and nonconventional treatments in mental health care. In spite of the limited amount of strong quantitative evidence, many conventional and nonconventional treatments remain in widespread use on the basis of qualitative evidence, professional consensus, or cultural traditions. Criteria used to select appropriate treatments in integrative medicine reflect both the rigor and relevance of available evidence. Quantitative findings from conventional biomedical research provide a useful index of rigor. Qualitative information obtained from patient interviews and some conventional and nonconventional assessment methods is an index of relevance. Integrative medicine strives to find a balance between the rigor of quantitative methods and the relevance of qualitative methods by combining objective and subjective information from history and assessment.

There are many ways to categorize interventions that are regarded as treatments in different systems of medicine. Philosophical issues related to establishing a typology of treatment categories are discussed in Chapter 2, Philosophical Problems. Chapter 4, Foundations of Clinical Methodology in Integrative Medicine, develops arguments for assessing levels and kinds of evidence in support of a putative mechanism of action or a claimed effect of a particular treatment. For purposes of this book, five categories of treatments are operationally defined: biological treatments, somatic treatments, mind–body practices, treatments based on scientifically validated forms of energy or information, and treatments based on putative forms of energy or information that are not validated by current Western science (i.e., energy medicine). Some treatments in each of the five general categories can be safely and effectively self-administered, whereas others require ongoing consultation and supervision by a conventionally or nonconventionally trained practitioner. With the exception of energy medicine, mechanisms of action or consistent beneficial outcomes have been empirically verified for treatments in each category. Some conventional and nonconventional treatments are maintained through consensus in the absence of compelling empirical data, whereas certain treatments remain in use on the basis of shared intuitions in spite of the absence of empirical evidence for a putative mechanism of action or a claimed therapeutic effect.

Depending on the available quantitative and qualitative evidence, a treatment can be regarded as substantiated, provisional, possibly effective, or refuted. It is important to note that claims of effectiveness can be made only with respect to a specified symptom pattern. In other words, it does not make sense to state that a particular treatment is "effective" or "ineffective" in general, but only to claim that that there is strong or weak evidence for a claimed effect with respect to a specified symptom pattern. A treatment is substantiated with respect to a principal symptom pattern when compelling quantitative or qualitative evidence supports the claim that the symptom pattern is alleviated when the treatment is skillfully applied. Provisional treatments are supported by significant but not compelling evidence, and there is limited or inconsistent evidence for treatments that are possibly effective for a specified symptom pattern. It is reasonable to regard a treatment as refuted with respect to efficacy claims for a specified symptom pattern when both quantitative and qualitative findings are consistently negative. Refuted treatments have no clinical value and are not discussed in this book. The chapters of Part II classify disparate treatments according to the relative strength of quantitative and qualitative evidence supporting their use for common mental or emotional symptom.

♦ Ethical and Liability Considerations in the Practice of Integrative Medicine

The ethical and legal relationship between any health care provider and any patient depends on the kinds of services provided and the implied or explicit purpose of the contract between them. The purpose of a relationship between a patient and a health care provider is contained in a contract or agreement to treat and to accept treatment. The relationship between a patient and a health care provider may consist of a limited one-time consultation, ongoing integrative treatment employing conventional or nonconventional treatment modalities, or an agreement to focus on spiritual issues, lifestyle changes, a medical disorder, or mental or emotional problems. In all cases the choice of treatment modalities defines the purpose of a contract between a patient and a health care provider. The health care provider is obligated to offer competent professional care, and the patient assumes responsibility for complying with the prescribed treatment plan or notifying the provider of adverse effects or other concerns that emerge during the course of treatment. The patient is also responsible for informing his or her health care provider in a timely manner of a decision to discontinue a recommended treatment.

Physicians and non–medically trained health care providers assume different risks and liabilities in working with patients or referring them to other providers (Cohen & Eisenberg, 2002; Studdert, Eisenberg, Miller, Curto, Kaptchuk, & Brennan, 1998). It is important for patients and health care providers to be familiar with legal and ethical requirements and norms within their professional group when treating patients or making referrals. The body of law pertaining to medical decision making in nonconventional or integrative treatments is in a state of flux. At present there is no clear ethical or legal framework that defines the scope of practice for physicians or nonconventionally trained health care providers who treat patients using alternative or integrative approaches (Adams, Cohen, Eisenberg, & Jonsen, 2002). In general, any health care provider has a legal and ethical duty to his or her patients. This duty includes the demonstration of professional competence when treating patients and the exercise of sound judgment when referring a patient for consultation with another health care provider. In general, medical practitioners who use interventions that are not recognized as falling within the scope of their professional competence may invite disciplinary action by the state medical board or other regulatory agencies if patients or professional peers make formal complaints to those bodies (Green, 1996). Disciplinary action may result in probation, suspension, or revocation of a professional license to practice. Western physicians who use alternative or integrative treatments should learn of any applicable restrictions imposed by the state medical board on the scope of medical practices within their medical subspecialty. The determination of acceptable scope of practice standards for a medical subspecialty requires a consideration of many complex legal issues. Medical practices regarded as legitimate in one state jurisdiction may be cause for probation or other disciplinary action in other states.

Making referrals poses important ethical and legal issues (Thorne, Best, Balon, Kelner, & Rickhi, 2002). When a patient's medical or mental health problem is outside the scope of a clinician's expertise and experience, the clinician is ethically obligated to refer the patient to an appropriate and competent provider. When a nonconventionally trained practitioner is the primary health care provider, it is appropriate to refer a patient to his or her primary care physician when there is a question of an unaddressed medical problem that cannot be adequately addressed by methods available to the practitioner. It is my strong opinion as a conventionally trained physician that giving medical advice to patients is always outside the reasonable scope of practice of nonconventionally trained practitioners who are not trained in Western medicine. This practice can result in inappropriate treatment, possibly harmful consequences, and delay appropriate, effective treatment. Any patient who has a potentially serious or rapidly progressing medical problem should be referred immediately to the closest urgent care facility. When a Western-trained physician is the managing health care provider, and there is no serious or rapidly progressing medical problem, and there is evidence that a nonconventional treatment will be beneficial, the physician is ethically obligated to refer the patient to an appropriate, qualified health care provider. Physicians should understand that when referring patients to nonconventional practitioners they assume liability for negative outcomes resulting from the referral, including harmful effects of treatment. For this reason, physicians should refer patients to nonconventionally trained practitioners only after confirming that the practitioner is reputable and qualified to practice in his or her specialty. Cohen's excellent book provides a concise review of ethical and legal issues that pertain to all health care professionals who practice alternative and integrative medicine (Cohen, 1998).

◆ Safety Issues in Integrative Mental Health Care

When considering any treatment for possible inclusion in an integrative treatment plan, it is important for the practitioner to be informed about safety concerns and appropriate monitoring requirements when managing self-treating patients and patients who are receiving conventional or nonconventional treatments under the supervision of a professionally trained provider. The evidence tables included in chapters in Part II comment on known safety issues associated with the modalities discussed. *Where particular combinations of conventional or nonconventional treatments are associated with known safety problems, those treatments or combinations should be avoided, or implemented in a way that minimizes risk after written informed consent has been obtained.*

It is important for the practitioner to provide all patients using conventional psychopharmacologic drugs or natural products with current, accurate information about possible safety issues even when the level of risk is relatively low. It is useful to provide the patient with a prepared handout or a clearly written note listing possible adverse effects or safety issues that may occur when a conventional drug or natural product is taken alone or in combination with other biologically active substances, including herbals, natural supplements, and certain foods. Conventional psychopharmacologic drugs frequently cause side effects and are potentially toxic when taken in combination with certain natural products or other conventional drugs. *All patients taking psychopharmacologic medications should be supervised by a psychiatrist or primary care physician. Only Western-trained physicians are qualified to advise patients on the management of adverse effects related to psychopharmacologic medications.*

In many cases, there is limited information about potential interactions between natural products and synthetic drugs. Chinese herbal medicines pose a special problem in this respect, as very little is known about safety issues when using Chinese herbal formulas concurrently with Western drugs (Lake, 2004). In contrast, many widely used Western herbal medicines have been extensively analyzed using biological assays, with the result that there is a substantial body of useful information about side effects and potential interactions when Western herbs are taken in conjunction with synthetic drugs (Bratman & Girman, 2003; Brinker, 1998; Harkness & Bratman, 2003; McGuffin, Hobbs, Upton, & Goldberg, 1997). Somatic and mind–body approaches as well as energy-information treatments are sometimes associated with unpleasant experiences but rarely cause serious safety problems. Safety issues resulting from the use of conventional or nonconventional treatments that are not based on a biological mechanism of action are generally minor, and can usually be resolved by adjusting the treatment protocol or changing the duration or frequency of sessions. For example, it is reasonable to advise a patient who complains of residual headache or dizziness following weekly EEG-biofeedback therapy to reduce the frequency of sessions. To ensure adequate care, it is important to notify patients undergoing any kind of treatment of potential risks associated with the approaches that are being used.

In general, different safety considerations apply to self-administered and professionally administered treatments. Self-administered treatments warrant an initial review of any associated risks, including advice about reputable brands of natural products, as well as activities or foods to avoid when practicing a particular mind–body technique or using a particular natural product. In contrast, professionally administered treatments often require ongoing supervision or monitoring to ensure the absence of unpleasant or unsafe side effects. This is particularly true of biologically active treatments, but it also applies in some circumstances to mind–body practices and energy-information treatments. All patients who are using unregulated natural products to treat mental or emotional symptoms should be provided with the names of specific reputable brands or encouraged to use Web-based resources that provide reliable information about brand quality and safety (two excellent resources are ConsumerLab.com at www.consumerlab.com and United States Pharmacopeia at http://usp-dsvp.org). Nonbiological treatments have few associated safety problems, and there is seldom a basis for potential interactions with conventional or nonconventional biological treatments. Important safety highlights are summarized in this section. Potential safety issues associated with the use of specific biological, somatic, mind–body, or energy-information treatments are discussed where applicable in Part II and are summarized in the relevant evidence tables.

A Western-trained physician should become familiar with the qualifications and skill of local nonconventionally trained practitioners before making specific patient referrals. Directories of professional societies for many nonconventional therapies are available through the National Center for Complementary and Alternative Medicine (NCCAM) and the Rosenthal Center for Integrative Medicine. Similarly, nonconventional practitioners should become familiar with the qualifications and skill levels of local Western medical specialists before referring a patient to a specific physician or other conventionally trained practitioner. Useful resources include the appropriate state medical board and the relevant professional medical association.

Uses of particular combinations of conventional and nonconventional treatments have not been well characterized by surveys or epidemiological studies; thus the magnitude and kinds of safety problems caused by combining conventional and nonconventional treatments has not been clearly defined. To date, few controlled studies have evaluated specific combinations of nonconventional and conventional approaches to determine levels of compatibility. In the absence of specific research findings, it is possible to make inferences about the compatibility of disparate treatments on the basis of what is known about the respective mechanisms of action of two or more treatments. Estimating relative degrees of compatibility can minimize the risk of potentially unsafe interactions by avoiding combinations of biological treatments based on mechanisms of action that are incompatible at one or more pharmacokinetic or pharmacodynamic levels of interaction in the body. By the same token, reasonable inferences can be made about combinations of biological treatments that are probably safe and beneficial based on knowledge of compatible or synergistic mechanisms of action.

There is always a possibility of unsafe interactions when herbs or other natural products are combined with conventional drugs. The findings of a systematic review of studies on herbal safety suggest that patients should be advised about possible toxicities or interactions when considering using a natural product concurrently with any conventional drug (Izzo & Ernst, 2001). All patients should be advised against using combinations for which potentially serious interactions have been documented, including concurrent use of St. John's wort (Hypericum perforatum) and an immunosuppressive agent, or Ginkgo biloba and warfarin. Because of methodological flaws and the absence of complete information about the bioactive constituents of many natural products, it is frequently difficult to distinguish between direct toxic effects of and adverse effects due to interactions between drugs and natural products.

Among herbs commonly used to treat mental health problems, few case reports of serious toxicities or interactions have been reported. These include two confirmed cases of spontaneous bleeding when Ginkgo biloba was combined with warfarin, and numerous case reports of potentially serious interactions between St. John's wort and immunosuppressive agents (including cyclosporin and indinavir), warfarin, theophylline, and selective serotonin reuptake inhibitors (SSRIs). Common side effects associated with St. John's wort include mild restlessness and gastrointestinal distress. A phototoxic rash has been rarely observed at doses higher than 900 mg/day. St. John's wort induces P450 liver enzymes, resulting in decreased serum levels of drugs metabolized by those enzymes, including anti-HIV drugs (protease inhibitors), warfarin (Coumadin), digoxin, oral contraceptives, and immunosuppressive drugs (Piscitelli et al., 2000; Ruschitzka et al., 2000). The use of St. John's wort is therefore contraindicated in patients taking any of these drugs. When in doubt about the safety of St. John's wort or any other biological treatment, the clinician should consult a reliable current textbook or refer the patient to a Western-trained physician or pharmacist. Although there are no confirmed cases of interactions with a class of antidepressants called monoamine oxidase inhibitors (MAOIs), patients should be advised to avoid concurrent use of St. John's wort and MAOIs. There is a slight risk of inducing mania or hypomania in bipolar patients, but this is not greater than with conventional antidepressant medications. A few cases of mild serotonin syndrome have been reported when typical doses of St. John's wort are taken with SSRIs (Gelenberg, 2000). One case report suggests that kava kava (Piper methysticum) preparations may interfere with the metabolism of the antiparkinsonian drug levodopa, and one case report suggests that kava may potentiate conventional benzodiazepines, causing excessive drowsiness. Valerian (Valeriana officinalis) can potentiate the sedating effect of benzodiazepines and other conventional drugs, and combined use of these biological treatments should be avoided.

Reports of mild serotonin syndrome have also been reported with therapeutic doses of L-tryptophan, but not 5-HTP. The judicious practitioner should consider combining L-tryptophan or 5-HTP with a conventional antidepressant only after the use of either agent alone has failed to improve mood. Patients taking L-typtophan or 5-HTP together with an SSRI or other conventional antidepressant should be monitored closely for signs of serotonin syndrome, including agitation, anxiety, perspiration, confusion, and autonomic arousal. All patients taking L-tryptophan or 5-HTP concurrently with a conventional antidepressant should be under medical supervision. It is important to note that L-tryptophan was banned in the United States in the early 1990s after several lethal cases of eosinophilia-myalgia syndrome (EMS) occurred in patients taking doses that were traced to one contaminated batch. This problem was soon corrected, and there have been no subsequent cases of EMS. There are some case reports of hypomania in bipolar patients taking either L-tryptophan or 5-HTP. Essential oils can potentially exacerbate preexisting medical conditions, including asthma and hypertension. Some essential oils, including those of parsley and nutmeg, have some MAOI activity, and should be avoided in patients who take MAOI antidepressants. There have been no reports of unpleasant or potentially dangerous interactions between SSRIs and essential oils. Medical history and current medications should be carefully reviewed before any treatment plan is started that includes aromatherapy.

◆ Safety Issues in Ayurvedic Medicine and Tibetan Medicine

In both Ayurvedic medicine and Tibetan medicine, there is a belief that poisons can be used as potent medicines if prepared correctly. The use of mercury and other potentially toxic metals, including arsenic and lead, as well as herbs that contain toxic compounds (e.g. *Aconitum ferox*, which contains a potentially lethal alkaloid), in both Ayurvedic and Tibetan medicine raises serious potential safety issues. Traditional approaches used to manufacture herbal products effectively minimize the risk of toxicities or adverse effects of commonly used medicinal preparations (Gogtay, Bhatt, Dalvi, & Kshirsagar, 2002). Recently introduced large-scale manufacturing processes have in turn introduced risks associated with incorrect selection or preparation of herbs, as well as contamination with heavy metals, pesticides, or pollutants (Saper et al., 2004). In India and China, good manufacturing practices are being embraced to reduce these risks to ensure that herbal products are regarded as safe and competitive on the world market. As for all traditions of herbal medicine, adverse effects or toxicities can occur when a patient uses inappropriate doses or combines herbals with a conventional drug.

All somatic therapies are potentially injurious if practiced in an unskilled way. To minimize liability and potential harm to patients, referring practitioners should refer patients to qualified body therapists. It is important for patients with medical problems, including chronic pain conditions and heart or lung disease, to consult with their family physicians before starting a rigorous exercise program or a mind–body practice that might place them at increased risk. To date, few significant safety concerns have been reported when scientifically validated energy-information treatments are used. However, some patients treated with virtual reality exposure therapy have reported transient discomfort. Fewer than 4% of individuals experience transient symptoms of disorientation, nausea, dizziness, headache, and blurred vision when in a virtual environment. "Simulator sleepiness" is a feeling of generalized fatigue that occurs infrequently. Intense sensory stimulation during virtual reality graded exposure therapy (VRGET) can trigger migraine headaches, seizures, or gait abnormalities in individuals who have these medical problems. VRGET is therefore contraindicated in these populations. Patients who have disorders of the vestibular system should be advised to not use VRGET. Anxious patients who are actively abusing alcohol or narcotics should not use VRGET. VRGET should be avoided in schizophrenics or others who have psychotic symptoms because immersion in a virtual environment can exacerbate delusions and potentially worsen reality testing (Wiederhold & Wiederhold, 2005). There are no known contraindications to the combined use of psychopharmacologic treatments and therapies based on forms of energy or information

described in current Western science (i.e., light, electricity, sound, and magnetic fields). There are no known contraindications to combining "subtle" energy therapies with other kinds of nonconventional or Western medical treatments. Intense or unskillful qigong practice and prolonged meditation are sometimes associated with transient psychosis in predisposed individuals, including patients diagnosed with schizophrenia, a dissociative disorder, or borderline personality disorder.

Conventionally trained physicians frequently use conservative strategies when combining drugs that may reasonably be inferred to be compatible on the basis of known mechanisms of action. Findings of compatibility or incompatibility are reported in the peer-reviewed medical literature, and eventually incorporated into the culture of accepted medical practice. Treatment planning in integrative medicine uses an analogous approach to determine degrees of compatibility when considering combinations of conventional and nonconventional treatments. Some treatments in biomedicine and nonconventional systems of medicine have general effects. Other treatments have specific effects. In many cases so-called general treatments can be safely combined with specific treatments with neutral or possibly synergistic outcomes. For example, a ***biological treatment*** (which operates at the level of a biochemical mechanism of action) can probably be safely combined with a ***somatic treatment*** (which operates through putative effects on the body at the level of the gross structure of the musculoskeletal system). In the same way, a treatment that employs a conventionally described form of energy or information (e.g., light or sound) can probably be safely combined with a somatic or subtle energy treatment, as the absence of a common mechanism ensures the absence of potential incompatibility when the treatments are used together.

◆ Unresolved Research Issues Influencing Integrative Approaches in Mental Health Care

Many conventional and nonconventional treatments remain in widespread use in spite of significant unresolved research issues. These include research design problems that limit the quality of controlled studies on many treatments, the undefined role of placebo effects in expectations and outcomes, and ambiguous criteria for verifying a putative mechanism of action or a claimed treatment effect. For example, most studies on St. John's wort in depressed mood pose design problems that have resulted in controversy over the significance of findings. At the time of writing, more than 10 controlled, double-blind studies have been conducted to assess the efficacy of St. John's wort as a treatment of depressed mood. Most studies have measured discrete biological markers in St. John's wort preparations on the assumption that a particular biologically active constituent is responsible for reported antidepressant effects. The situation is much more complex, and many bioactive constituents in St. John's wort probably have clinical effects on mood or general well-being. Research studies have compared nonstandardized preparations of St. John's wort to different kinds and doses of synthetic antidepressants. The findings of comparison studies are mixed,

Table 6–1   Research Issues Influencing Perceptions and Endorsement of Conventional and Nonconventional Treatments of Cognitive, Emotional, and Behavioral Symptoms

Treatment Category	Unresolved Research Issues
Biological treatments	Inconsistent results of well-designed studies due to absence of standardized preparations (e.g., St. John's wort)
	Unclear role of placebo effect on outcomes
	Difficult to assess general versus specific effects
	Problems measuring or correlating specific treatments (including conventional antidepressants, antipsychotics, and many natural products) with targeted biological change or functional brain states that are "therapeutic"
Somatic therapies	*Very* difficult to design controlled, blinded studies
	Difficult to recruit unbiased subjects
	Difficult to assess general versus specific effects
	Debate among nonconventional practitioners over best treatment protocols (e.g., craniosacral therapy)
Mind–body practices	Difficult to design controlled, blinded studies
	Difficult to assess general versus specific effects
	Constraints on outcomes measurements using existing technologies probably bias results
Treatments based on forms of energy or information that are verified by current Western science	Debate among nonconventional practitioners over best treatment protocols (e.g., EEG biofeedback, ECT, TMS, VNS)
	Problems measuring/correlating specific protocols with targeted changes in brain and desired clinical outcomes
	Difficult to assess general versus specific effects
Treatments based on forms of energy or information not verified by current Western science	Very difficult to design controlled, blinded studies (variables affecting outcomes unknown)
	Postulated mechanism of action outside of Western scientific paradigm constrains study design and outcomes measurement (qigong, Reiki, Healing Touch, etc.)
	Difficult to recruit unbiased researchers or subjects

ECT, electroconvulsive therapy; EEG, electroencephalography; TMS, transcranial magnetic stimulation; VNS, vagal nerve stimulation

reflecting nonstandard research designs and the absence of agreement over standardized preparations of St. John's wort. Research findings of studies on qigong, Therapeutic Touch, and other energy treatments are difficult to interpret because of ambiguous experimental controls and the absence of empirically testable hypotheses about putative mechanisms of action. Difficulties describing a putative mechanism of action and designing experiments that correlate clinical outcomes with energy treatments confound efforts to separate general effects from specific effects of a particular energy treatment.

Table 6–1 lists representative research problems that have affected perceptions and endorsement of both conventional and nonconventional biological, somatic, mind–body, and energy-information treatments.

Other Unresolved Issues Influencing Integrative Mental Health Care

Significant nonresearch issues are also influencing the acceptance and spread of both conventional and nonconventional treatments in mental health care. These include the absence of reimbursement for many treatments by health insurance providers, entrenched physician and institutional attitudes, the uneven availability of qualified conventional and nonconventional medical practitioners, and consumer ignorance about the evidence in support of specific conventional and nonconventional therapies. **Table 6–2** summarizes important factors that are slowing acceptance of both conventional and nonconventional treatments of mental health problems.

Table 6–2   Nonresearch Issues Influencing Perceptions and Endorsement of Conventional and Nonconventional Treatments of Mental or Emotional Symptoms

Treatment Category	Unresolved Nonresearch Issues
Biological treatments	Physician attitudes and ignorance
	Absence of standard products
	Most treatments are not covered by insurance
	Absence of accurate patient information on appropriate and safe indications
Somatic therapies	Qualified practitioners often unavailable
	Physician ignorance or attitudes in making referrals
	Liability issues if negative outcome
	Patient ignorance of treatment indications
Mind–body practices	Patients seek "rapid" solutions
	Patient ignorance of treatment indications
	Physician attitudes and ignorance
	Skilled instructors often unavailable
Treatments based on forms of energy or information that are verified by current Western science	Skilled therapists often unavailable
	Generally not covered by insurance
	Patient ignorance of treatment indications
	Physician attitudes and ignorance
Treatments based on forms of energy or information that are not verified by current Western science	Difficulty identifying skilled practitioners
	Physician attitudes and ignorance
	Patient attitudes and ignorance

◆ Methods and Evidence Ranking in Integrative Treatment Planning

Evidence rankings of treatments in medicine take into account empirical and subjective, quantitative and qualitative information. Detailed methods for evidence ranking are discussed in Chapter 4. Treatments are categorized as empirically verified, consensus-based, or intuitive approaches. As discussed above, four basic levels of evidence are then possible for any particular treatment in any category with respect to claims of efficacy for a specified mental or emotional symptom. By definition, intuitive treatments are not verifiable using contemporary biomedical methods, and shared beliefs or intuitions are the basis of efficacy claims. Putative mechanisms or claimed outcomes of some intuitive approaches are eventually verified by empirical means, and they emerge as consensus-based or empirically derived treatments. A recent example is the transition of some EEG-biofeedback protocols from intuitive to empirically derived treatments of anxiety and impaired attention. *I feel strongly that there are never legitimate reasons to recommend a treatment that is known to be ineffective or unsafe. Doing so may place the patient at risk and bring significant liability to the clinician. When there is reasonable doubt about the safety of a particular treatment modality, the practitioner should recommend against its use.* This approach to evidence ranking is useful for identifying reasonable treatment choices in the context of the patient's unique history, preferences, and constraints. The practitioner's judgment and clinical experience always play an important role in determining the most appropriate treatment plan.

◆ The Logic of Integrative Treatment Planning in Mental Health Care

The essential logic of integrative treatment planning can be conceptualized as taking place in several steps. The first step involves identifying particular treatments for which a mechanism of action or effectiveness has been verified with respect to a specified symptom on the basis of reasonable criteria. A clear formulation of plausible causes or meanings of a symptom is often necessary before this step can be taken in order that the putative mechanism of a treatment approach matches the putative cause of a target symptom. Professionally trained practitioners of Western medicine and nonconventional systems of medicine use both objective and subjective criteria to make decisions about treatment. Objective criteria include both quantitative and qualitative measures of putative mechanisms of action or claimed effects. It is important to note that quantitative and qualitative approaches used to assess treatment outcomes in both conventional Western medicine and many nonconventional systems of medicine incorporate disparate epistemological methods and assumptions, resulting in the selective inclusion or exclusion of certain kinds of information describing subjective or objective outcomes. (The implications of this issue for the evolution of medicine are addressed in Chapter 2.) In Western biomedicine objective criteria rest on quantitative measures of empirical observations, including replicable positive outcomes of controlled studies, consistent and statistically significant effects or effect sizes, and confirmatory

systematic reviews or meta-analyses of a claimed outcome or effect size. Qualitative measures include objective anecdotal reports by clinicians showing consistently positive outcomes, and subjective patient-centered reports of beneficial changes in individual, social, or occupational functioning in response to treatment. Western medicine relies largely on objective quantitative criteria to support claims that a particular treatment is efficacious with respect to a specified symptom pattern. Reliance on quantitative evidence in medical treatment planning rests on an implicit assumption that valid inferences about the causes of a symptom can be based on findings from an unrelated study population. In other words, positive findings from one or many studies are accepted as a legitimate and sufficient basis for using an empirically "verified" treatment in an individual with similar complaints, in spite of the absence of information about possible unique causes or meanings of a symptom in a particular case. In contrast to quantitative approaches, qualitative methods do not assume the validity of applying broad statistical conclusions from many studies to individual patients with similar complaints. Claims of efficacy of many conventional and nonconventional treatments of mental or emotional symptoms rely largely or exclusively on qualitative or subjective criteria.

Determining what criteria to use when selecting a treatment poses many complex issues. For example, some conventional or nonconventional treatments can be evaluated empirically, and a putative mechanism of action or claimed outcome can be verified in quantitative terms using contemporary biomedical methods. Western biomedicine regards empirically derived treatments as substantiated by the highest level of evidence, yet relatively few biomedical treatments fulfill criteria for this level of evidence, and therefore relatively few can be rigorously regarded as empirically derived according to the "gold standards" of Western science (see Chapter 4). Other treatments have become widely accepted because of consistently positive outcomes even when a putative mechanism of action cannot be empirically verified. Such treatments are maintained through professional consensus and are sometimes verified in terms of effectiveness even when a presumed mechanism of action is unsubstantiated. The majority of conventional and nonconventional treatments fall into this category. Still other treatments in Western medicine and nonconventional systems of medicine remain in use out of shared beliefs among patients or practitioners that a treatment "works," even in cases where consistently positive outcomes have not been reported and a putative mechanism or effect has not been confirmed. Treatments in this category continue to be used on the basis of shared intuitions among health care practitioners, patient values and social or cultural preferences, and economic factors. In contrast to Western biomedicine, integrative medicine considers evidence of effectiveness from the dual perspectives of both Western medicine and nonconventional systems of medicine. **Table 6–3** lists representative conventional and nonconventional treatments of cognitive, emotional, and behavioral symptoms in relation to three basic kinds of evidence used to substantiate claims of effectiveness. This list does not include specific claims of effectiveness with respect to a particular symptom pattern. The reader is referred to Part II for evidence tables showing the relative rankings of nonconventional treatments for the common mental and emotional symptom patterns covered in this book.

Table 6-3   Representative Conventional and Nonconventional Treatments of Cognitive, Emotional, and Behavioral Symptoms

Treatment Category	Mechanism or Effectiveness Verified by Both Biomedicine and Nonconventional Systems of Medicine	Mechanism or Effectiveness Verified by Nonconventional Systems of Medicine Only	Treatment in Use but Not Verified by Biomedicine or Nonconventional Systems of Medicine
Biological	Changes in nutrition Some Western herbals (e.g., St. John's wort, valerian) Some natural supplements (e.g., SAMe, omega-3 fatty acids)	Aromatherapy Homeopathy Caffeine/sugar elimination diets Macrobiotic diet	Most non-Western herbals (e.g., Chinese, Ayurveda, Tibetan, Kampo)
Somatic and mind–body approaches	Exercise Massage Yoga Animal-assisted therapy (includes use of horses, dolphins, and domestic pets)	Craniosacral therapy Ayurveda Applied kinesiology Alexander technique Trager approach to psychophysical integration	Rolfing Rubenfield synergy method
Modalities based on forms of energy or information validated by current Western science	Biofeedback (including EMG and EEG) Light therapy ECT, TMS, VNS, virtual reality exposure therapy	Music or sound therapy Cranioelectrotherapy stimulation (alpha stimulation)	Thermography
Modalities based on putative forms of energy or information not validated by current Western science	Acupuncture Meditation	Qigong Therapeutic Touch Healing Touch Reiki Prayer and directed intention	Bach flower essence therapies Polarity therapy

ECT, electroconvulsive therapy; EEG, electroencephalography; EMG, electromyography; SAMe, S-adenosylmethionine; TMS, transcranial magnetic stimulation; VNS, vagal nerve stimulation

◆ Nonconventional Treatments of Cognitive, Emotional, and Behavioral Symptoms

Important advances are taking place in nonconventional biological, somatic, mind–body, and energy-information approaches used to treat cognitive, emotional, and behavioral symptoms. This section introduces representative nonconventional treatments in current use in the four major categories.

Biological Treatments

Numerous herbs and nonherbal natural products including vitamins, minerals, and amino acids are in widespread use to treat cognitive, emotional, and behavioral symptoms. Putative mechanisms of action and evidence for their use in mental health care are reviewed in detail in the chapters of Part II.

Targeted amino acid therapy (TAAT) is an emerging treatment approach that postulates that specific deficiencies or imbalances in neurotransmitters are associated with mental and emotional symptom patterns and uses specific combinations of amino acids to therapeutically replace or "rebalance" neurotransmitters. Preliminary research findings suggest that targeted amino acid therapy results in sustained improvements in symptoms of insomnia, depressed mood, anxiety, fatigue, and inattention. Cumulative data from open trials of various amino acids (N = 322) suggest that over 90% of individuals who use amino acids for common symptom patterns report significant clinical improvement following 3 months of treatment using a

recommended TAAT protocol (personal communication, Neurosciences, Inc., January 2005). The researchers noted that 30 to 40% of individuals were taking at least one conventional drug concurrently. Comparisons with matched individuals taking only conventional medications were not performed. At present there are no findings supporting the use of specific doses or combinations of amino acids for specific symptom patterns.

Somatic and Mind–Body Approaches

Exercise and massage are beneficial for anxiety, depressed mood, and other symptoms. The evidence for these and other somatic approaches is reviewed in Part II. Yoga has been extensively researched for the treatment of specific mental and emotional problems, including obsessions and compulsions, depression, grief, phobias, dyslexia, insomnia, and substance abuse (Shannahoff-Khalsa, 2003). Research findings from open trials and case reports suggest that specific protocols combining different yogic postures, breathing practices, and meditation are beneficial for different symptom patterns. Symptom-focused applications of yoga in mental health care are reviewed in Part II.

Approaches Based on Forms of Energy or Information Validated by Current Western Science

Virtual Reality Graded Exposure Therapy

VRGET is a rapidly evolving computer-enhanced exposure therapy that combines advanced computer graphics, three-dimensional visual displays, and body-tracking technologies to create realistic virtual environments that simulate feared situations or objects. Virtual environments have been designed to provide visual, auditory, tactile, vibratory, vestibular, and olfactory stimuli to patients in highly controlled settings. Patients who undergo VRGET consistently report achieving "presence," a feeling of actual immersion in the reality being simulated (Wiederhold & Wiederhold, 2000). An important advantage of VRGET over conventional in vivo exposure therapy is that virtual environments that can be designed to provide graded levels of exposure, avoiding intense fear responses during therapy. During a virtual exposure session, the therapist monitors physiological indicators of stress, including heart rate and respirations, to closely track the patient's state of arousal. Biofeedback using this information is often combined with the therapist's comments to provide the patient with cues for using deep breathing or other stress-reducing behaviors with the goal of becoming desensitized to the anxiety-provoking stimulus in the virtual environment. Once the patient is desensitized to the virtual environment, he or she is ready to practice in vivo exposure to the feared object or situation.

Cranioelectrotherapy Stimulation and Paraspinal Square Wave Stimulation

Cranioelectrotherapy stimulation (CES) and paraspinal square wave stimulation (PSWS) are widely used to treat a range of pain and psychiatric symptoms. Both approaches are based on the external application of microcurrents to the brain or spinal cord. It has been postulated that beneficial effects are related to release of β endorphins during electrical stimulation. CES involves the application of weak electrical currents at various points on the head and neck. The mechanism of action probably involves induction of beneficial changes in EEG frequencies that correspond to clinical improvement in anxiety. Frequencies between 0.5 and 100 Hz are typically used. Research findings suggest that higher frequencies are associated with relatively greater EEG changes and more noticeable clinical improvements (Schroeder & Barr, 2001). In contrast to electroconvulsive therapy (ECT), the use of microcurrents takes place on an outpatient basis, avoids the requirement of general anesthesia, is not associated with significant adverse medical or psychiatric effects, and can be self-administered following initial training.

Approaches Based on Forms of Energy or Information That Are Not Validated by Current Western Science

Chinese Medicine, Ayurveda, and Tibetan Medicine

Chinese medicine, Ayurveda, and Tibetan medicine posit the existence of a subtle energy body and a manifest physical body, and address the complex energetic imbalances that are the causes or conditions of medical or mental illness using a combination of physical, psychological, and spiritual approaches (Clifford, 1990). The shared goal of all three systems of medicine is to restore balance in both the energetic and physical body, thus enhancing the body's capacity for self-healing. Afflictive emotions, including anxiety, anger, depressed mood, and psychosis, arise out of unskillful spiritual practice or humoral imbalances, and can be influenced by many internal and external factors (Bodeker, 2001). Chinese and Ayurvedic compound herbal medicines have been extensively studied and include

remedies for a range of mental and emotional symptom patterns. The compound herbal treatments used in Tibetan medicine are only beginning to be examined by Western-style research studies. Acupuncture is used in both Chinese medicine and Tibetan medicine, but not in Ayurveda. Increasing numbers of Western-style studies are verifying the therapeutic claims of acupuncture for a range of physical and psychiatric symptom patterns (Birch, 2004). Findings of sham-controlled studies show the benefits of acupuncture for depressed mood, anxiety, psychosis, and other mental and emotional symptom patterns. Self-healing through the skillful practice of visualization, meditation, listening to music, yoga, and the study of spiritual practices, including the exercise of compassion for oneself and others, are fundamental approaches in Ayurveda and Tibetan medicine systems (Goleman, 2004).

Spirituality, Prayer, Intention, Homeopathy, and Energy Medicine

In recent decades, many energy medicine techniques have come into increasing use for the treatment of medical and mental illnesses. These include acupuncture, qigong, homeopathy, Therapeutic Touch, Healing Touch, Reiki, prayer, and distant healing intention. Case reports, open trials, and increasing numbers of controlled studies suggest that acupuncture, qigong, and Therapeutic Touch are probably beneficial for anxiety and general emotional well-being. There is emerging evidence that Reiki is an effective treatment of depressed mood. Studies on the role of intention or putative subtle energies in health and illness are difficult to design because of problems clearly defining control conditions and measuring outcomes (see Chapter 3, Paradigms in Medicine, Psychiatry, and Integrative Medicine). Energetic techniques used in Chinese medicine have been investigated extensively, though controlled studies on acupuncture for specific mental and emotional symptom patterns have been inconsistent. Although some studies on acupuncture in depressed mood show efficacy similar to conventional antidepressants, others report no benefits or nonspecific effects that are equivalent to outcomes obtained using sham acupuncture protocols. Studies on the efficacy of distant healing or directed intention on depressed mood or other mental or emotional symptom patterns are still at an early stage, and debate continues in academic research communities over how best to design studies or measure outcomes. Findings from pilot studies, case reports, and recent controlled, double-blind trials suggest that measurable positive outcomes take place when healing intention (including prayer) is directed at healthy adults or individuals who complain of physical or emotional symptoms. These early findings have so far failed to substantiate a putative mechanism of action or specific effect of intention or subtle energies in health and illness. Available research findings do not support the use of a particular energy approach in the treatment of depressed mood or other mental or emotional symptoms. However, recent findings of apparent beneficial effects of Reiki on patients reporting depressed mood and stress have renewed discussion about possible mechanisms of directed intention in alleviating emotional symptoms. Controlled studies on energy therapies for cognitive, emotional, and behavioral symptoms are only beginning to take place. Intriguing case reports of beneficial effects in the context of widespread interest in the roles of energy and spirituality in health will eventually clarify the putative role of consciousness and spirituality in physical and mental health.

◆ **Homeopathy** Homeopathic preparations are widely used to self-treat a range of physical and psychiatric symptoms, but there is little information about outcomes from case reports or controlled studies. The determination of an effective homeopathic remedy is highly individualized and rests on a comprehensive biological, social, and psychological history and both a conventional and energetic assessment of symptom patterns. Because homeopathic remedies reflect the unique constitutional type of each patient, homeopathic treatments should be administered by a trained homeopathic physician. Controlled studies of standardized homeopathic preparations do not reflect complex variables that enter into the clinical practice of homeopathy because of individual constitutional differences that translate into unique remedies for each patient. This fact has led to considerable debate in the biomedical research community over the possible role of placebo effects. The peer-reviewed literature has reported on the controversy over the significance of homeopathic research findings for several decades. Some writers interpret meta-analysis findings as confirmation that homeopathy is based entirely on the placebo effect (Ernst & Resch, 1996), whereas others contend that meta-analyses point to beneficial treatment effects (Kleijnen, Knipschild, & Riet, 1991; Linde et al., 1997). Like Chinese medicine, Ayurveda, and other nonconventional systems of medicine, homeopathy assumes the existence of a vital force or energy. Energetic imbalances manifest as different symptom patterns. Conventional biomedicine cannot explain a putative mechanism of action or measure claimed clinical effects of homeopathic remedies, which are typically diluted beyond the point of possible biological action according to classical understandings of cause and effect. This problem has been addressed by recent assessment approaches that take into account perceived changes in mental, emotional, and spiritual functioning following treatment (Bell, Lewis, Lewis, Brooks, Schwartz, & Baldwin, 2004).

Similarities exist between basic principles in homeopathy and modern psychiatry, including the postulated role of self-healing and a possible "microdose effect" of treatments that permit the subsequent use of low doses to elicit therapeutic responses (Davidson, 1994). In recent decades this conceptual overlap has led to increasing uses of homeopathic remedies in mental health care. Emerging models based on complex systems theory, nonlinear dynamics, or quantum information may help to elucidate the mechanism of action associated with beneficial effects in homeopathic treatment (Schwartz & Russek, 1997; Schwartz & Russek, 1997; Smith, 2004). Homeopathy may eventually prove to rest on the induction of subtle changes in energy or information that influence the energetic or biological systems of the body in beneficial ways.

◆ **Religious and spiritual values and beliefs** Relationships between religious, spiritual, or existential values or beliefs and physical or mental health have been examined in hundreds of studies over more than a century. Religious or spiritual beliefs are of central importance to many patients, and often improve coping and resilience during stressful periods (Larson & Milano, 1996). A meta-analysis of recent studies suggests that regular involvement in a religious or spiritual practice is often associated with improved mental health in general (Gartner, Larson, & Allen, 1991). Sociological, psychological, behavioral, and biological models have been advanced to explain the beneficial effects of religious or existential attitudes on mental health (Levin, 1996). Existential well-being is highly correlated with good mental health in general (Tsuang, Williams, Simpson, &

Lyons, 2002). A meta-analysis of 12 clinical and epidemiological studies on the health benefits of religious or spiritual involvement showed that risk of depressed mood was inversely related to religiosity (Koenig & Futterman, 1995). Highly evolved neural circuits may underlie the capacity for transformative spiritual experiences (d'Aquili & Newberg, 1993). Although social or biological models can explain some aspects of improved mental health related to religious or spiritual involvement, they cannot potentially explain reported effects of intercessory prayer and other spiritual or energy healing methods.

◆ **Prayer, intention, and energy healing** Approximately one in three U.S. adults prays in an effort to improve health, and more than two thirds of those who pray believe that prayer is beneficial to their health (McCaffrey, Eisenberg, Legedza, Davis, & Phillips, 2004). Significantly, only 10% of those who pray for improved health mention this fact to their physicians. It is estimated that almost 80% of patients believe that their religious or spiritual beliefs influence their physical or mental health. In contrast, fewer than 20% of physicians ask patients about their religious beliefs (King & Bushwick, 1994). Almost 40% of family physicians pray with patients, and most who do so believe that praying has beneficial effects on common medical problems (Anderson, Anderson, & Felsenthal, 1993). Positive findings were reported in 60% of studies included in a systematic review of controlled trials on prayer and other forms of healing intention used as treatments of a medical or psychiatric disorder (Astin, Harkness, & Ernst, 2000). The biological effects of intercessory prayer at a distance have been studied extensively in cell cultures, animals, and humans (Dossey, 1997).

Evaluating research findings on intercessory prayer, healing intention, and energy healing methods is a difficult task. The scientific evaluation of putative effects of intercessory prayer in healing presents complex methodological challenges because of subjective differences between patients' and healers' beliefs and inherent problems identifying and controlling for variables that potentially interfere with study designs or influence outcomes. A systematic review of randomized controlled trials on prayer, healing intention, and other approaches that purport to ameliorate symptoms by directing subtle energy into patients was inconclusive because of research design problems, small study sizes, and poor reporting of studies in the medical literature (Abbot, 2000). However, extensive case reports, findings from open studies, and some controlled trials provide strong evidence for consistent beneficial effects of intention, prayer, and other spiritual healing techniques that cannot be adequately explained by current science (Benor, 2002). Interpersonal belief in the efficacy of prayer probably plays a significant role (Palmer, Katerndahl, & Morgan-Kidd, 2004). However, there is emerging evidence that prayer and other forms of healing intention result in health benefits. Studies on the effects of prayer on medical illnesses often include measures of depressed mood before and after the period of active intercessory prayer. A landmark study on prayer in healing showed that patients with advanced AIDS exhibited improved immunologic status and improved mood following several weeks of intercessory prayer (Sicher, Targ, Moore, & Smith, 1998).

The evidence for specific beneficial effects of various energy medicine approaches in mental health is reviewed in Part II. Healing intention probably has beneficial psychological effects and may also have subtle influences on complex living systems at the levels of physiology, energetics, or information (Zahourek, 2004). Evidence from case reports and small controlled trials suggests that above-chance correlations exist between EEG activity and brain metabolic activity based on functional magnetic resonance imaging (fMRI) findings in sensory-isolated human beings (Radin, 2004; Standish, Johnson, Kozak, & Richards, 2003). The size of this effect may be stronger when there is empathic union between two or more subjects (Grinberg-Zylberbaum, Delaflor, & Goswami, 1994). Continued research in this area will help clarify a putative mechanism of action for some reports of nonlocal healing associated with directed intention, including Reiki, Healing Touch, and prayer.

◆ **Reiki, healing touch, and therapeutic touch** Reiki is an energy healing practice that was introduced to the West from Japan in the 19th century; however, its ancient origins may have been in Tibet. Practitioners of Reiki assert that a fundamental energetic principle, ki, promotes physical or psychological healing when guided by a skilled practitioner. Like many forms of energy healing, physical contact between practitioner and patient is not believed to be necessary for beneficial effects to take place. In contrast to Healing Touch or Therapeutic Touch, the Reiki practitioner does not consciously direct healing intention to specific regions of the body, but serves as a "conduit" for ki to "flow into" the patient to restore healthy energetic functioning. Reiki treatments can be administered directly to the patient or across considerable distances. Claims of a distant healing effect rest on a postulated role of consciousness that cannot be explained by contemporary scientific models. Findings of a controlled study suggest that regular Reiki treatments reduce symptoms of depressed mood and stress (Shore, 2004). Emerging research findings suggest that conventionally understood mechanisms involved in hands-on Reiki include beneficial changes in autonomic regulation and EEG activity associated with sustained deep relaxation, reduced heart rate, and blood pressure (Mackay, Hansen, & McFarlane, 2004; Wirth & Cram, 1994).

Healing Touch is described as a form of energy medicine administered by trained practitioners in North America and Europe to treat a range of physical and emotional symptoms. Several specific techniques are used, including "charka spreading," "magnetic unruffling," "mind clearing," and "stopping." The mechanism of action is not yet clearly established, but Healing Touch practitioners and many patients who seek this treatment believe that direct spiritual or energetic contact between the practitioner and patient results in relief from physical and emotional symptoms. The Healing Touch practitioner positions the hands over certain parts of the body but does not actually touch the patient's body. In contrast, in Therapeutic Touch, there is gentle physical contact. Healing Touch is available on request to pain or cancer patients in many hospitals, and increasing numbers of nurses are becoming certified as Healing Touch or Therapeutic Touch practitioners. A critical review of research on Healing Touch and Therapeutic Touch can be found in Benor (2002).

Energy Psychology: Thought Field Therapy, Emotional Freedom Techniques, and Somatoemotional Release

Other spiritual or energy healing methods used to treat cognitive, emotional, and behavioral symptoms include energy psychology, shamanic healing rituals, spiritual methods in Ayurvedic and Tibetan medicine, and the use of crystals to amplify or focus healing energy. There is ongoing speculation and debate about meanings of energy, including concepts from quantum mechanics and quantum field theory that may help to explain postulated subtle effects of human intention on health and illness (Feinstein, 2003; Hankey, 2004). It is likely that expectation plays a role in disparate forms of energy medicine. Chronically ill individuals who wish to be treated by a spiritual or distant healing technique and believe they are being treated report improvements in the quality of life (Wiesendanger, Werthmuller, Reuter, & Walach, 2001).

Energy psychology is an emerging field in clinical psychology based on the assumption that imbalances in subtle energy fields cause cognitive, emotional and behavioral symptoms (Gallo, 1999). It is an eclectic combination of Western psychological theory and Chinese meridian theory which posits that energetic imbalances in the meridians are associated with different emotional or mental symptom patterns. Thought field therapy (TFT) and Emotional Freedom Techniques (EFT) are energy psychology approaches used to treat a range of mental and emotional symptom patterns, including anxiety and depressed mood. Both approaches are based on Chinese meridian theory and posit that physical or emotional symptoms reflect underlying energetic imbalances. In TFT the patient is first assessed using applied kinesiology or another form of muscle testing. In contrast, EFT treatments are administered on the basis of presumed energetic imbalances without first assessing the patient through muscle testing. In TFT the patient is asked to invoke a "thought field" associated with depressed mood, a traumatic memory, or other principal symptom patterns. The TFT practitioner then reattunes energetic imbalances associated with that symptom by tapping on specific acupuncture points in a specified manner, resulting in relief from distressing symptoms. TFT is based on shared beliefs among its practitioners and limited findings from case reports. The few controlled studies that have been conducted to date have resulted in negative or inconsistent findings. EFT is a simplified version of TFT that involves only one routine for stimulating acupuncture points. There is even less evidence for EFT from case reports or controlled studies.

Somatoemotional release is an energy therapy method developed by two researchers in the 1970s that purports to "release" pathological energetic states that accumulate in the body in the form of "energy cysts" following physical injury. The technique involves "facilitation by touching" the patient's body in various places while gently guiding the patient to assume positions that stimulate body memories of an alleged past trauma. The approach is believed to result in the release of a pathological energy cyst caused by trauma, alleviating associated physical and emotional symptoms. No sham-controlled studies have been done on this modality. However, data are available from case reports and intensive treatment programs.

◆ Integrative Mental Health Care: Overview of Basic Principles

In managing any emotional or mental complaint, the primary goal in integrative mental health care is to identify the most substantiated treatment that is acceptable to the patient, affordable, and locally available from a qualified practitioner, and to develop an effective and realistic integrative strategy around this core treatment. Cognitive, emotional, and behavioral symptoms are unique subjective experiences of distress or impairment that are difficult to describe in empirical terms. The integrative management of mental health problems begins with a thorough history, including documentation of the severity and course of symptoms, identification of other psychiatric or medical problems, and a review of biological, psychological, cultural, and possibly spiritual causes or meanings associated with the symptom pattern. Based on the patient's unique history, the assessment of probable psychological, biological, or energetic factors leads to a multilevel formulation and an initial integrative treatment plan. The most appropriate integrative plan is subsequently determined on the basis of the evidence tables, taking into account the patient's history of response to previous conventional or nonconventional treatments, pertinent assessment findings, financial or insurance constraints, availability of local competent providers of a recommended modality, and the patient's preferences.

Different strategies are appropriate when managing moderate versus severe cognitive, emotional, and behavioral symptoms. When a severely symptomatic patient is initially seen by a conventionally trained physician, it is appropriate to refer him or her to a nonconventional medical practitioner when it is established that the patient is not actively suicidal, homicidal, or grossly psychotic, and has provided informed consent for referral to a qualified local practitioner of the recommended modality.

Establishing a suitable integrative treatment plan involves linking the patient's history and assessment findings with treatments that address the causes or meanings of symptoms. Integrative treatment planning takes into account hierarchical relationships between causes or meanings of the principal symptom pattern. In the absence of a complete or accurate picture of relationships between factors associated with mental or emotional symptoms, the formulation will remain obscure and of limited value. Consequently, the practitioner will not have sufficient information on which to base a treatment plan that effectively addresses the causes or meanings of a specific symptom pattern in a particular patient. The result will be an inadequate or inappropriate treatment plan and a poor outcome.

Criteria used to select appropriate treatments in integrative medicine reflect both rigor and relevance of available evidence. Quantitative information from conventional biomedical research is a useful index of rigor. Qualitative information obtained from patient interviews and some conventional and nonconventional assessment methods is an index of relevance. Integrative medicine strives to find a balance between the rigor of empirical research and the relevance of personal information through the use of both quantitative and qualitative information during assessment and treatment planning. Integrative treatment planning matches pertinent information from the patient's history and assessment findings with treatments that address probable psychological, biological, somatic, or energetic causes or meanings of symptom patterns. Treatment planning takes into account conventional and nonconventional approaches that have been tried previously, and the strength of evidence for treatments that have not been tried in the context of patient preferences and realistic constraints on cost and availability. The optimum treatment plan is the ideal combination of treatments addressing the causes or meanings of a symptom pattern. There will often be a discrepancy between the optimum integrative treatment plan and a realistic plan that takes into account patient preferences, financial constraints, availability of competent conventional or nonconventional practitioners, and so on. The practitioner should encourage the patient to initially use treatments for which there is compelling evidence for the

principal symptom pattern(s) being addressed. For example, aerobic exercise and improved sleep hygiene should be recommended if a moderately depressed patient is reluctant to take supplements or is not interested in trying a mind–body practice. It is important at the outset that the practitioner and patient agree on criteria for assessing beneficial changes and a time frame in which improvement can be reasonably expected.

Conventional drugs and the nonconventional treatments discussed in this book should not be viewed as substitutes for psychotherapy. Even in cases where conventional drugs or nonconventional treatments are very successful, important psychodynamic issues are frequently present. Patients who are motivated to do psychological work and have the capacity for insight should be encouraged to consider ongoing psychotherapy. Journal writing should be encouraged so that progress can be tracked and the patient can accurately monitor symptoms and provide feedback to the practitioner about the effectiveness of treatment and safety issues. At regular follow-up appointments, the practitioner and patient should review progress and modify the treatment plan if symptoms have not improved significantly within a mutually agreed-upon time frame, or when the patient is not motivated to use a recommended treatment because of adverse effects or other reasons. If a symptom pattern of moderate severity worsens or remains unimproved after an agreed-upon time has passed, it is reasonable to discuss biological treatment choices, including conventional medications and natural products. When treating severe mental or emotional symptoms, follow-up appointments should be scheduled weekly if possible, *and the patient should be instructed to contact the nearest emergency room or go to an urgent care center in the event of suicidal thoughts or psychotic symptoms.* Assuming that serious medical problems have been ruled out as possible causes of symptoms, the treatment plan should be reviewed and modified as needed at successive follow-up appointments until an effective and realistic integrative plan is identified.

When a symptom or symptom pattern has worsened, evolved, or has not responded to treatment following a period of time in which it is reasonable to expect improvement, it is appropriate to review and clarify both the medical and psychiatric differential diagnoses. Referrals to Western or nonconventional medical specialists may be helpful to rule out confounding but undiagnosed problems that are interfering with treatment response, including, for example, hypothyroidism, other endocrinological disorders, other medical disorders, or a putative energetic imbalance. It is important to invite the severely symptomatic patient to actively participate in all treatment decisions to provide encouragement and to monitor compliance.

The practitioner's recommendations should be based on evidence of the comparative effectiveness or cost-effectiveness (where data are available) of conventional medications, natural products or mind–body approaches that are reasonable candidate treatments of the principal symptom pattern. Treatment recommendations should always take into account the patient's history of responses to previous conventional or nonconventional treatments, including adverse effects, allergies, and interactions with drugs or natural products. For example, many patients experience gastrointestinal distress or reduced libido when taking SSRI antidepressants and soon discontinue these in spite of beneficial effects. Others may report a history of "nervousness" or insomnia when taking SAMe, or hypersomnolence when starting a trial on 5-HTP. It is important to take this information into account to ensure compliance when formulating a realistic treatment plan. After formulating the optimum treatment plan, the clinician and patient should agree on a realistic plan that is acceptable to the patient, affordable, and does not pose potential safety issues when combined with therapies that are currently being used.

Assuming that a complete history has been taken and an adequate assessment has been performed, putting together an effective integrative treatment plan involves several basic steps:

◆ Identifying or prioritizing the principal symptom pattern that is being addressed

◆ Selecting the optimum treatment or combination of treatments from the relevant evidence table

◆ Deciding whether to use a single treatment or two or more treatments in parallel

◆ Verifying compatibility between the selected treatments (i.e., when a parallel treatment strategy is being used)

◆ Determining a realistic integrative treatment plan in view of patient preferences, local availability of competent practitioners, and any financial constraints

◆ Implementing the treatment plan (including referrals to conventional or nonconventional practitioners) with the patient's informed consent

◆ Following the patient at regular intervals to assess response to treatment and modify the plan if indicated in view of significant new information from history or assessment

Table 6–4 illustrates the flow of information from history to assessment and formulation to treatment planning and ongoing assessment in an individual who complains of depressed mood. Hierarchical levels at which possible causes or meanings

Table 6–4　Integrative Management, Including History Taking, Assessment, Formulation, Treatment Planning, and Ongoing Assessment

	History	Assessment	Formulation	Optimum Integrative Plan	Assessment (Ongoing)
Social	Relationship problems; history of alcohol abuse	Complete social history focusing on relationship and alcohol abuse	Primary relationship problem related to low self-esteem worse when drinking	Encourage brief couples therapy; encourage positive social activities around spiritual beliefs	Review social issues and alcohol use in ongoing therapy
Lifestyle	Doesn't exercise; watches TV late; craves sweets	Previously runner; poor sleep habits cause fatigue; eats refined carbohydrates to self-treat mood(?)	Diminished motivation to exercise when depressed and relationship problems	Encourage improved nutrition, addressing carbohydrate craving; instruct in sleep hygiene; review realistic exercise plan	Review progress in lifestyle changes in ongoing therapy
Biological	History of slightly low thyroid (free T4); chronic poor nutrition; progressive weight problem	Repeat TFTs; add CBC, liver panel (alcohol abuse), fasting glucose; and consider glucose tolerance test	Borderline low FT-4; other laboratory tests within normal limits	Replace thyroid hormone; endocrinology consult; trial on biological agent for depressed mood (see evidence table for depressed, mood, Chapter 8)	Review emerging medical data; determine clinical correlations with thyroid replacement and/or antidepressant treatment
Psychological	Recurrent major depressive episodes beginning age 18; no history of mood swings; no history of psychosis; social anxiety improved with alcohol	Conventional mental status examination; conventional biopsychosocial history	Father was alcoholic; significant "adult child of alcoholic" issues, including low self-esteem; avoidant social pattern	Individual supportive psychotherapy focusing on relationship issues; CBT directed at alcohol relapse triggers and social anxiety; instruct in guided imagery	Ongoing review of progress in CBT for anxiety reduction, avoidance of relapse triggers and improved relationship dynamics
Cultural, spiritual, and energetic	Strong values around Buddhist beliefs; meditates daily, though less often when depressed; "not centered" recently, and decreased "sense of meaning"	Complete history of spiritual beliefs, values, and practices	Regular Buddhist meditation previously helped patient to reframe stressful life experiences in positive ways and use healthy lifestyle habits to manage stresses; patient has avoided meditation and other spiritual practices since becoming depressed	Encourage patient to resume meditation practice with meditation group; encourage patient to read spiritual texts for insight and encouragement; consider energy treatment	Ongoing review of benefits of spiritual practice

CBC, complete blood count; CBT, cognitive-behavioral therapy; FT-4, free thyroxine; TFT, thyroid function tests of symptoms are "located" include social and lifestyle issues and biological, psychological, and energetic factors.

◆ **Starting and Maintaining an Effective Integrative Treatment Plan**

Following the initial consultation, integrative mental health care continues in a stepwise manner and includes new assessment approaches, changes in the original formulation, and modifications of the initial treatment plan. If history or current symptoms suggest the need for formal assessment beyond a comprehensive interview and a Mini-Mental State Examination, the evidence tables are used to identify substantiated assessment approaches that may provide accurate information about the causes of a symptom pattern. The patient should be referred to an appropriate laboratory for biological assessments that are indicated, including urine or serum studies. Referrals are made to qualified nonconventionally trained practitioners when other assessment approaches are indicated by history. Potentially beneficial treatments should be reviewed with the patient together with ongoing assessment.

When evaluating treatment choices, it is always prudent to consider substantiated treatments first. In cases where a highly substantiated treatment was previously tried but ineffective or poorly tolerated, and the patient's history suggests that it was not tried at an adequate dose or duration, or under appropriate supervision to achieve beneficial effects, it is reasonable to recommend trying the same modality again. In cases where a particular substantiated conventional or nonconventional treatment has previously been effective, it is reasonable to recommend resuming the same treatment. However, many patients who have benefited from a particular conventional or nonconventional treatment express ambivalence about resuming the treatment because of concerns over adverse effects. In such cases the evidence tables in this book are used to identify the highest ranked treatments that have not been previously tried, and alternative approaches are identified on the basis of the evidence.

Chronic or severe symptoms, significant new assessment findings, or incomplete responses to previous treatments frequently lead to new treatment choices. As treatment continues, emerging assessment findings or newly reported history suggests changes in the treatment plan until symptoms are alleviated or realistic treatment choices are exhausted. Considerations that enter into recommendations for one treatment versus two or more treatments in parallel are discussed below. Follow-up appointments are scheduled at intervals that reflect the severity of symptoms and requirements (if any) for symptom monitoring. I have found that patients generally improve more rapidly when engaged in supportive psychotherapy or cognitive-behavioral therapy together with the conventional and nonconventional approaches discussed in this book. When symptoms are moderate, it is generally reasonable and appropriate to schedule regular follow-ups roughly every 2 to 4 weeks, until the patient reports significant sustained reduction in severity of the principal symptom pattern(s). More severe symptoms generally warrant more frequent appointments. In all cases it is important for the practitioner and patient to agree on how often it is necessary to meet for ongoing assessment and treatment, including psychotherapy if that is a part of the treatment plan. **Table 6–5**

summarizes important steps in starting and maintaining an effective integrative program for mental health problems.

The integrative treatment of cognitive, emotional, and behavioral symptoms may initially involve a single approach, or a combination of disparate psychological, biological, somatic, mind–body, or energetic treatments. The most suitable plan for a particular symptom pattern will probably vary from patient to patient. The most realistic, effective, or preferred treatment plan for one patient complaining of moderate anxiety may involve taking supplements and following a self-directed mind–body program, for example, the daily practice of yoga. The most effective or appropriate treatment plan for another patient with similar symptoms may involve different supplements, drug therapy, and a referral to an expert alternative medical practitioner. There are pros and cons associated with recommending a single approach versus multiple treatments in parallel, and self-treatment versus expert referral. Issues of compatibility between two or more treatments must be taken into account. Issues pertaining to safety and compatibility are addressed in the evidence tables. Potentially unsafe treatment combinations should always be avoided and actively discouraged, and safe combinations that are known to produce synergistic benefits for the principal symptom pattern should be strongly encouraged. Examples of synergistic treatment combinations for the management of depressed mood include exercising while exposed to bright light and taking omega-3 fatty acids or folate with a conventional antidepressant or SAMe. Moderately symptomatic anxious or depressed patients should be encouraged to initially try combining self-directed approaches including exercise, improved nutrition, appropriate supplements, and mind–body practices in parallel before taking conventional or natural product–derived treatments. Combining these approaches can reasonably be expected to improve moderately depressed mood, anxiety, or insomnia as effectively as conventional drugs, while avoiding the potential adverse effects of drugs. Self-directed changes in lifestyle and nutrition empower the patient to pursue a range of healthy nutritional or mind–body practices with demonstrated efficacy against mild to moderate symptoms. Furthermore, there are no contraindications to combining lifestyle changes with antidepressants or nonconventional biological treatments. If a patient who complains of mild to moderate symptoms elects to start a conventional biological treatment after considering the range of effective and available treatment options, safety issues, including adverse effects and potential incompatibilities between the conventional drug and any natural products that are being used, should be reviewed by a conventionally trained physician or other qualified Western medical practitioner. *The integrative practitioner should always obtain and document informed consent regarding risks associated with the selected treatment.*

Severely symptomatic patients should be encouraged to initially try a substantiated conventional or nonconventional core biological treatment in combination with supplements known to provide synergistic benefits, lifestyle changes, and beneficial nonconventional treatments that are congruent with their values, locally available, and affordable. Severely symptomatic patients who do not respond to substantiated biological treatments and who do not complain of significant adverse effects should be encouraged to continue the biological treatment regimen while starting a trial on a natural product known to work synergistically with the core treatment, and also trying at least one other nonbiological approach that may be beneficial for the

Table 6–5   Starting and Maintaining Effective Integrative Mental Health Care

Goals of the Initial Consultation

Comprehensive social, family, medical, psychiatric, cultural, and religious or spiritual history; review of pertinent medical and psychiatric symptoms; and identification of mental or emotional symptoms

IMPORTANT: *Always assess suicide risk and urgently refer suicidal patients to the nearest emergency room with friend or relative.*

Order laboratory studies if indicated by history (see algorithm for principal symptom).

Refer patient to Western medical specialist if symptoms and history suggest underlying undiagnosed or rapidly progressing medical illness.

Identify the highest ranked treatment that has not been tried for the principal symptom pattern being addressed. In cases where most or all substantiated treatments have already been tried without benefit, confirm that they were done correctly, for an adequate period of time, and administered by qualified practitioner (where applicable).

In cases where all realistic substantiated treatments have already been tried for the principal symptom pattern, it is reasonable to consider provisional and possibly effective treatments in combination with more substantiated treatments.

Identify the highest ranked integrative treatment strategy centered around a core treatment that has not yet been tried or has been previously effective for the specified symptom pattern in the same patient. This is the optimum integrative treatment plan.

Check evidence tables in companion Web site (www.thieme.com/mentalhealth) to ensure current accurate information for assessment and treatment approaches.

Work with patient to identify a realistic treatment plan that reflects the patient's values and preferences, financial constraints, and local availability of qualified practitioners. For mild to moderate symptoms, the initial treatment plan should emphasize lifestyle changes, improved nutrition, mind–body practices, exercise, and supplements. For severe symptoms, the initial treatment plan should emphasize biological agents, including conventional drugs and natural product–derived treatments. Discuss psychotherapy if appropriate and patient is motivated.

Review potential safety issues and document informed consent, including informed consent to any referrals to conventional or nonconventional practitioners. Implement the plan and schedule appropriate follow-up.

Summarize treatment plan for the patient verbally and in writing; obtain and document informed consent if treatment is initiated or referral is made.

Clarify expectations of time course and reasonable expectations of improvement.

Goals of the Initial Follow-up Visit

Review interval changes in symptom pattern(s) and assess compliance with treatment plan and changes in principal symptom pattern(s).

Assess and treat emerging mental or emotional symptoms.

Review significant positive or negative laboratory findings or new medical or psychiatric history or symptoms with patient.

Consult symptom-specific algorithm to identify appropriate integrative treatment options in view of new information.

Review treatment plan in detail with patient to gauge progress, problems, etc.

IMPORTANT: *Be sure the patient clearly understands the treatment plan. (if the patient does not understand, the onset of treatment will be delayed and symptoms may worsen).*

Encourage patient commitment to selected treatment, including positive lifestyle changes.

Work with patient to modify plan as needed with respect to new history, emerging symptoms, new assessment findings, and partial or failed treatment response.

Establish phone contact with other health care providers involved in patient care (if indicated). Schedule next two follow-up appointments.

Goals of Subsequent Follow-up Visits

Review interval changes in mental, emotional, or medical symptoms and assess compliance and progress.

Consult symptom-focused algorithm to identify appropriate options, including possible modification of current treatment plan.

If psychopharmacologic treatment is indicated, (Western physicians should) consult established psychopharmacology treatment algorithms. **Only conventionally trained practitioners should give advice about conventional drugs.**

Collaborate with patient to develop optimum integrative plan, always taking into account effectiveness, safety, financial constraints (if any), and patient preferences.

Review treatment plan in detail, answering any questions or concerns about treatment goals, side effects, etc.

Obtain patient release as indicated to exchange information with other Western or nonconventional practitioners to coordinate treatment plan and reduce risk of inappropriate or unsafe treatment combinations.

Treatment and assessment continue until symptoms resolve or reasonable and realistic treatment strategies have been exhausted.

principal symptom pattern, including exercise, a mind–body practice, biofeedback, or bright light exposure. Examples of natural products that enhance the efficacy of conventional drugs include folate, thiamine and vitamin B_{12}, 5-HTP, and omega-3 fatty acids. In many cases elements in an integrative treatment plan will be influenced by the severity of the patient's functional impairment and his or her level of motivation to pursue treatments that may be beneficial. Recommending a substantiated nonconventional treatment when a qualified practitioner of that modality is not available locally, or the treatment is unaffordable or unacceptable for other reasons, may delay or compromise patient care. Provisional approaches should be considered as reasonable core treatments only after substantiated approaches have been exhausted, the patient refuses treatments that are more likely to succeed for legitimate reasons (e.g., cultural issues or concerns about adverse effects), or the treatment is unavailable or unaffordable. In some cases, combining a provisional treatment that is supported by limited evidence with a substantiated treatment is more effective than using a single substantiated approach. The potential efficacy of possibly effective treatments can be evaluated using an "*N* of 1" approach when most substantiated or provisional treatments have been tried with limited success (see section Emerging Research Methodologies in Chapter 4). Response to treatment (or lack thereof), newly emerging symptoms, new assessment findings, or significant new history is taken into account during follow-up appointments. Assessment and treatment continue in reciprocal fashion until the most effective realistic integrative plan is achieved.

At some point during treatment, the practitioner and patient decide whether to continue maintenance therapy or discontinue treatment. It is reasonable to consider discontinuing treatment when symptoms have diminished significantly, social or occupational functioning has markedly improved, and the patient has adopted lifestyle changes that effectively address his or her original complaint. Discontinuing a particular treatment should also be considered in cases where the appropriate and skillful use of a particular approach has failed to alleviate symptoms following a mutually agreed-upon period in which it is reasonable to expect improvement. This will probably vary significantly depending on the treatment, symptom severity, and the preferences and overall resilience of the patient.

The practitioner implicitly assumes liability when referring a patient to any other medical practitioner. Thus the prudent integrative practitioner should carefully review basic material about the efficacy and safety of any recommended treatment before making a referral. For example, a moderately depressed patient who is interested in receiving acupuncture treatment should be informed that the evidence supports the use of acupuncture assuming that a qualified Chinese medical practitioner is available to administer the treatment. However, a severely depressed individual should not be advised to seek acupuncture treatment, because research evidence at this time does not support the use of acupuncture for symptoms of severe depressed mood.

The evidence tables for the common symptom patterns in Part II include integrative treatment strategies that are sometimes more effective than individual conventional or nonconventional treatments. When a complex symptom pattern involves two or more principal symptoms, the clinician should initially use treatments that address both symptom patterns (i.e., when such treatments exist). Integrative strategies that address complex symptom patterns are included in the algorithms given in Part II. The evidence tables are updated quarterly in the companion Web site to this book (www.thieme.com/mentalhealth) starting from the date of publication. A realistic treatment plan that is acceptable to the patient is determined on the basis of the patient's openness to trying the recommended treatment, cost or insurance considerations, and local availability of a qualified practitioner (i.e., when a practitioner is required for the recommended treatment). In cases where all substantiated treatments have apparently been tried and failed or are unavailable, unaffordable, or unacceptable to the patient, the patient should be encouraged to consider combinations of substantiated and provisional or possibly effective approaches, including lifestyle changes and a regular mind–body practice. The reader is encouraged to go to the companion Web site before finalizing any treatment plan to check the updated evidence tables for significant new research information on assessment or treatment approaches. Important new findings are published on an almost continuous basis. In some cases the strength of evidence supporting

the use of an established assessment or treatment approach will have changed significantly in a positive or negative direction. It is the practitioner's responsibility to the patient to ensure that assessment and treatment recommendations are based on the most current information available.

There is always a risk of confusion or miscommunication surrounding the recommended treatment plan when the patient is being seen concurrently by two or more practitioners. This problem can be avoided when one practitioner takes responsibility for coordinating patient care, and the patient provides his or her written permission for all practitioners to exchange information. The managing practitioner should accurately document all conventional and nonconventional treatments being used in the patient's chart. Good record keeping safeguards against potentially incompatible treatment combinations. Patients generally benefit from contact between their various health care providers, and coordinated care often avoids inappropriate or delayed treatment.

◆ Integrative Management of Mild to Moderate Cognitive, Emotional, and Behavioral Symptoms

A patient complaining of mild to moderate depressed mood, anxiety, cyclic mood changes, disturbed sleep, diminished wakefulness, or cognitive problems should be regarded as a candidate for nonconventional treatments only after possible medical causes have been excluded by a conventionally trained psychiatrist or primary care physician. Evidence for appropriate conventional and conventional approaches should be presented to the patient during the initial consultation. The patient should be referred to a qualified practitioner of a nonconventional treatment unless his or her physician has training in that approach. For example, a moderately depressed patient who is interested in receiving acupuncture treatment should be informed that controlled studies and extensive case reports suggest that acupuncture will probably be beneficial. However, a patient who requests acupuncture treatment for severe depressed mood should be advised against acupuncture on the basis of insufficient research findings to support the use of acupuncture for this indication.

The question of combining two or more approaches in an initial integrative treatment plan versus successive single treatments should be discussed. If the patient elects to try only one approach initially, he or she should be encouraged to explore therapies that are substantiated by the highest level of evidence for the principal symptom pattern. For example, specific nutritional, somatic, or mind–body approaches should be encouraged if the patient is reluctant to take supplements or conventional medications. Conventional and nonconventional biological therapies can be tried later if mild to moderate symptoms do not improve following a reasonable investment of time and effort. Constraints on availability and affordability of both conventional and nonconventional treatments, and patient preferences should always be taken into account. The practitioner and patient should agree on benchmarks for monitoring changes in symptom severity, as well as a time frame in which it is reasonable to expect improvement. Expectations are always present, and talking about them gives patient and practitioner a framework in which to develop a collaborative dialogue with the patient about perceived progress or delays in treatment.

Patients who request conventional or natural product–derived treatments for mild to moderate symptoms should be encouraged to initially use self-directed approaches that are substantiated by strong evidence. Depending on the principal symptom being addressed, these may include improved nutrition, lifestyle changes, supplements, and mind–body practices in parallel before using either conventional or nonconventional biological treatments. Combining self-directed approaches can reasonably be expected to improve symptoms of mild to moderate severity as effectively as conventional medications or natural products, while avoiding potential problems of adverse effects and noncompliance associated with conventional drugs. Self-directed changes in lifestyle and nutrition frequently motivate patients to pursue a range of healthy nutritional, exercise, or mind–body practices with demonstrated efficacy for the management of mild to moderate cognitive, emotional, and behavioral symptoms. Furthermore, incompatibility issues resulting in safety problems and noncompliance do not arise when combining self-directed lifestyle changes or mind–body practices with biologically active agents because there are no potential contraindications. If the patient elects to start a (conventional or natural product–derived) biological treatment after considering available treatment options for symptoms of mild to moderate severity, he or she should be referred to a psychiatrist, primary care physician, or qualified nonconventional practitioner to discuss the risks and benefits of substantiated treatment choices, as well as potential adverse effects and incompatibilities between conventional drugs, natural products, and other biological treatments being used. *Informed consent should always be obtained (and documented) regarding potential risks associated with the selected biological treatment and its concurrent use with other medications, if any.*

In some cases it is appropriate to encourage the patient to engage in regular supportive psychotherapy or cognitive-behavioral therapy directed at reducing the severity of the principal symptom pattern. Cognitive-behavioral therapy is frequently beneficial for anxiety and depression. Supportive psychotherapy is especially helpful when the patient is motivated to explore dynamic or interpersonal issues. Journal writing often helps patients monitor the effectiveness of different treatments. The practitioner and patient should review progress and problems with the current treatment plan at regular follow-up appointments, and modify the plan if reasonable expectations for improvement are not met. Some patients are not motivated to pursue certain treatments because of adverse effects, lack of motivation, or personal reasons. In cases where mild or moderate symptoms worsen or remain unimproved following 1 month of consistent self-directed efforts including lifestyle changes, improved nutrition, and a regular somatic or mind–body practice, it is appropriate to encourage the patient to consider biological treatment options that are substantiated for the principal symptom pattern, including conventional drugs and natural products. Conversations about conventional medications should always be deferred to a psychiatrist or primary care physician. Considerations of herbals, other natural products, or homeopathic preparations should be referred to qualified naturopathic physicians, herbalists, or homeopathic physicians. In all cases where biological treatments are being considered, the practitioner's recommendations should be based on a thorough review of the evidence in the context of patient preferences and realistic constraints on availability and cost.

When considering biological treatments, the clinician's recommendations should take into account the patient's history of response to previous conventional and nonconventional biological agents, including reports of sensitivity to side effects when using specific conventional drugs or natural product–derived treatments. For example, some patients experience significant gastrointestinal distress when taking certain conventional drugs and soon discontinue their use. Others may report agitation after taking even small doses of SAMe, or feelings of sedation or lethargy when starting on a trial of 5-HTP. To minimize the risk of an unfavorable outcome or noncompliance, it is important to obtain a thorough history of treatment responses and adverse effects associated with previous biological treatments. This information will assist the clinician in formulating an integrative plan that will be well tolerated and beneficial. After presenting recommendations to the patient based on the above considerations, the clinician and patient should agree on a treatment plan that does not pose safety or incompatibility issues with respect to other therapies that are currently being used. Many natural products that are beneficial for the treatment of mild to moderate mental or emotional symptoms augment the effectiveness of conventional medications, including, for example, folate, thiamine, vitamin B_{12}, 5-HTP, and certain omega-3 fatty acids. Use of many natural substances in conjunction with a conventional drug frequently improves treatment response. In many cases this strategy will permit the patient to eventually reduce the dose of a conventional drug with a commensurate reduction in adverse effects but without loss of effectiveness.

◆ Integrative Management of Severe Cognitive, Emotional, and Behavioral Symptoms

In contrast to mild or moderate symptoms, the preferred initial approach to severe mental or emotional symptoms is built around a core conventional or nonconventional biological treatment that is substantiated for the principal symptom pattern. Depending on the patient's circumstances, motivation, and preferences, it may be appropriate to recommend self-directed changes in nutrition, exercise, stress reduction, specific supplements, psychotherapy, or a mind–body practice. However, severely impaired individuals are frequently unmotivated or lack the capacity to engage in regular exercise or pursue a mind–body practice. During the initial consultation, the practitioner should determine whether there is an urgent or undiagnosed medical problem, and refer the patient appropriately. Finding out whether a patient is suicidal, potentially dangerous, or unable to care for his or her basic needs is the single most important task when evaluating a patient who presents with severe mental or emotional symptoms. A patient who is homicidal, grossly psychotic, or actively contemplating suicide should be monitored closely to ensure safety, and accompanied to the nearest emergency room or urgent care center for urgent evaluation and possible hospitalization. Patients who complain of psychotic symptoms, severe or rapidly progressing anxiety, depressed mood, cognitive impairment, or disturbed sleep or wakefulness, but who do not require hospitalization, should be promptly referred to a psychiatrist or primary care physician for evaluation and consideration of conventional medication management.

As in the evaluation of mild to moderate mental or emotional symptoms, the initial consultation with a severely symptomatic patient ideally includes a thorough medical, social (including alcohol and substance abuse), cultural and psychiatric history, and appropriate laboratory tests (e.g., thyroid studies, electrolytes, and complete blood count [CBC]) to rule out possible contributing medical problems. A thorough history will clarify the medical-psychiatric differential diagnosis, and establish or exclude a history of mood swings, psychotic symptoms, progressive cognitive decline, the presence of alcohol or substance abuse, or evolving medical or neurologic illness. The proactive psychiatrist or primary care physician should make referrals to appropriate medical specialists when laboratory studies are abnormal. A commonly cited example is the association between abnormal levels of thyroid hormones (elevated thyroid-stimulating hormone or low free thyroxine) and persisting depressed mood. Anemias or other disorders of the blood, electrolyte or metabolic derangements, and other markers of medical illness are often associated with reports of depressed mood. Correcting primary medical problems frequently results in symptomatic improvement. Evolving neurological symptoms and a known history of cancer or heart disease warrant automatic referrals to specialists in these areas of Western medicine prior to the consideration of nonconventional treatments. Patients who are actively abusing alcohol or an illicit substance should be referred to an appropriate rehabilitation program.

Assuming that medical causes and substance abuse have been excluded, follow-up appointments should be scheduled in 1- to 2-week intervals. The patient should be given clear written instructions to contact the nearest emergency room or call 911 in the event of worsening psychotic symptoms or homicidal or suicidal thoughts. When two or more principal symptom patterns are present at the same time, the clinician and patient must consider whether to treat them in parallel or sequentially. In most cases a core symptom will probably constitute the focus of clinical attention at any time during treatment, and a treatment plan will be directed at that principal symptom pattern. When two principal symptoms are being addressed at the same time, it may be necessary to combine disparate treatment approaches, especially when no single approach is efficacious against both principal symptoms. The algorithms in Part II of this book identify assessment and treatment approaches that are useful when common cognitive, emotional, and behavioral symptoms occur together. The patient should be encouraged to initially try only conventional, nonconventional, or integrative approaches that have been substantiated as effective for the principal symptom(s). In cases where most substantiated approaches have been tried with little benefit, it is reasonable to consider combinations of two or more substantiated approaches, or combinations of substantiated and provisional or possibly effective treatments. This approach is analogous to "augmentation" strategies in conventional psychiatry, and continues until an effective integrative plan is achieved or all reasonable and realistic treatment combinations have been exhausted and the patient has not improved. Reasonable integrative strategies will vary depending on the principal symptom pattern being treated, as well as patient preferences and constraints. The practitioner who is managing the patient's care should obtain the patient's written consent to exchange information with other practitioners who are seeing the patient. The treatment plan should be carefully reviewed and modified at follow-up appointments until the most effective and realistic combination of conventional and nonconventional treatments is identified.

In cases where severe mental or emotional symptoms fail to respond following a period of time in which it is reasonable to expect improvement, or the patient is noncompliant with treatment because of adverse effects or lack of motivation, it is appropriate to carefully review and clarify both the medical and psychiatric history. In such cases it may be helpful to refer the patient to a Western medical specialist or nonconventional practitioner to rule out the possibility of undiagnosed psychological, medical, or energetic causes or meanings of symptoms that are not being adequately addressed. These may include, for example, self-defeating psychological defense patterns, hypothyroidism, other endocrinological disorders, degenerative neurological disorders, and cancer, as well as energetic imbalances or spiritual problems as described in Chinese medicine or Ayurveda. It is important to invite the severely symptomatic patient to take an active role in all treatment decisions to improve the clinician–patient alliance, improve patient autonomy and motivation, and enhance compliance.

◆ Determining the Optimum Realistic Integrative Treatment Plan

Determining the optimum combination of treatments when addressing a particular mental or emotional symptom pattern is the first step in developing a successful integrative treatment plan. In many cases the strength of evidence for disparate treatments will be comparable. In such cases the practitioner identifies treatments that reflect an appropriate integrative plan in view of the patient's history, preferences, values, and any financial constraints. Some highly rated treatment approaches may be unavailable, unaffordable, or unacceptable to the patient. If the history or assessment findings indicate that the patient would benefit from a particular treatment, but a qualified practitioner of the recommended treatment is not locally available, it makes little sense to suggest that treatment unless the patient has the financial resources to obtain the treatment from a qualified practitioner elsewhere. A skilled nonconventional practitioner may be available but unaffordable because of the absence of insurance coverage for his or her services. In other cases, a qualified local nonconventional practitioner may provide services that are covered by insurance (e.g., acupuncture), but the patient is hesitant to accept the recommended treatment for other reasons. Some patients are hesitant to receive acupuncture treatment because of fears or misconceptions about what is involved in the treatment "process." By the same token, it is inappropriate to recommend a conventional antidepressant as a first-line treatment for a moderately depressed patient who has a long history of noncompliance with antidepressants because of poor tolerance of adverse effects, or who is opposed to taking antidepressants on the basis of strong personal values or beliefs. A patient who is clearly opposed to conventional treatment will probably refuse treatment or become noncompliant, and may discontinue his or her relationship with the prescribing psychiatrist or primary care physician. From the perspectives of integrative medicine, it is generally more appropriate to recommend to patients who are mildly or moderately depressed the use of nonconventional treatments that have equivalent efficacy to conventional antidepressants.

Many patients will have previously tried a potentially beneficial conventional or nonconventional treatment but discontinued prematurely because of adverse effects. In conventional mental health care, poor compliance with an otherwise appropriate and effective treatment is often the cause of treatment failure. Patients sometimes "forget" to follow advice about treatments, resulting in incomplete response. For example, a patient taking an SSRI for depressed mood may experience significantly greater improvement when taking folate at the same time, but may often forget to take folate. It is often useful in this context to explore possible psychodynamic meanings or purposes of forgetting. For example, the patient may be conflicted about getting well, and "forgetting" may reflect unconscious resistance. Forgetting can also imply a problem with memory or organization, suggesting the need for continued assessment. Clarifying the patient's experience of forgetting will often improve compliance or provide useful clues about other viable treatment choices.

Determining a realistic integrative treatment plan that will probably be effective for a specified symptom pattern and acceptable to a particular patient requires a thorough history, including a complete and accurate record of previous treatments and responses, ongoing efforts to obtain additional pertinent information, and a relationship of trust and cooperation between practitioner and patient. Practical and personal factors should always be taken into account before the practitioner makes specific recommendations. Working as a team, the practitioner and patient will probably identify appropriate treatment choices relatively quickly. In this way, the process of treatment selection progresses from an initial optimum integrative plan to a plan that is both realistic and acceptable to the patient. Integrative medical management sometimes requires more time and effort than is customary for conventional medical or mental health care. However, compared with the standard Western psychiatric treatment, the personal attention and efforts of the integrative practitioner often translate into a more complete history, more reliable assessment findings, a more comprehensive treatment plan, and improved or more rapid response to treatment.

After the practitioner and patient have consulted the most current version of the evidence tables and have selected treatments that are effective, realistic, and acceptable for consideration in the initial integrative treatment plan, the next step is to determine whether to recommend individual versus multiple treatments in parallel or sequentially. Sections below discuss factors involved in these clinical decisions, including measures of compatibility, efficacy, cost-effectiveness, and others.

General Considerations

Deciding whether to recommend a single treatment, separate treatments in sequence, or many treatments at one time is based on the same logical and empirical approaches used in integrative assessment planning (see Chapter 5, History Taking, Assessment, and Formulation in Integrative Mental Health Care). Decisions in favor of one approach over another ultimately rest on considerations of safety and effectiveness in the broader context of a patient's history, local availability of a qualified practitioner of the recommended treatment, patient values and preferences, and any financial constraints. The probability, type, and magnitude of risk associated with combining two or more modalities is related in a general way to the kinds of treatments being considered, and in an exact way to the specific treatments that are candidates for integration. Decisions about safe or appropriate combinations of different kinds of treatments and specific treatments are based on empirical methods and logical inference. Modalities that belong to a general treatment category are based on related, sometimes identical mechanisms of action. Disparate treatment categories rely on different kinds of empirically demonstrated or putative underlying mechanisms. When the mechanisms of action for two or more treatments are understood, reasonable inferences can sometimes be made about expected degrees of compatibility, even in the absence of supporting empirical evidence for compatibility. When the mechanisms of two or more modalities are not understood, or when only one mechanism is clearly defined, inferences about compatibility are more tenuous, and the practitioner must rely on outcomes data from studies or case reports. When a putative mechanism of action is not understood, and there are no associated gross biological effects of the treatment (as is true of all modalities that purport to use subtle energy or information, and most treatments based on scientifically validated forms of energy or information), it is likely that the modality in question can be safely combined with other treatments for which there is an established biological mechanism of action. In such cases, direct amplification of the effects of one treatment by the other cannot potentially occur because the respective mechanisms of action are unrelated. However, when biological mechanisms of action have been established for two or more treatments being considered for combined use, there is often a risk of harmful or unpleasant effects. In such cases, the magnitude of risk depends on functional relationships between mechanisms of action associated with the respective treatments that will determine the potential for harmful "amplifying" or antagonistic biological effects if the treatments are combined. The picture becomes more complex when one considers that the same treatment can have quite different effects at different hierarchic levels of structure or function, possibly mediated by disparate mechanisms of action, depending on how the treatment is used, the target symptom pattern, and the presence of synergistic or interfering influences of other treatments being used concurrently.

Disparate treatment approaches are regarded as compatible or incompatible when used in combination depending on the degree of similarity or synergy between their respective mechanisms of action, evidence for enhanced effectiveness, and the absence of significant safety issues when they are combined. Approaches to combining empirically derived, intuitive, and consensus-based treatments differ in important ways. In the case of empirically derived treatment approaches, degrees of compatibility are a matter of cumulative evidence from basic or clinical research, or anecdotal reports showing that combining two or more treatment approaches results in desirable synergistic effects in the absence of safety concerns. On the basis of literature reviews or expert consultation, conventionally trained physicians typically attempt to determine degrees of compatibility before combining empirically derived treatments. The same approach can be used when evaluating the compatibility of empirically derived nonconventional treatments and is helpful in determining the suitability of disparate treatments for inclusion in an integrative treatment plan. For example, if the evidence for a particular naturopathic herbal treatment for depressed mood reveals that the herb contains bioactive constituents that function as weak serotonin reuptake inhibitors, and the herb has an established safety record over decades when used alone or in combination with conventional SSRIs, there is substantial evidence for probable compatibility between that particular herb and conventional antidepressants that work as SSRIs. Conventionally designed studies have examined the effectiveness of intuitive approaches, including qigong, Reiki, and Healing Touch, in the treatment of medical and psychiatric symptom patterns. There is substantial anecdotal information but limited research evidence for the effectiveness of these approaches. In contrast to empirically based approaches, two or more intuitive treatment approaches cannot be compared using analytical methods because their foundational principles cannot be reduced to propositions about empirically verifiable claims of a putative mechanism of action. The mechanisms of action of intuitive approaches are not susceptible to empirical analysis, and there are no existing means for determining when it is beneficial or safe to combine them with other treatments. In other words, clinical judgments pertaining to combinations of two or more intuitive approaches, or combinations of an intuitive approach and an empirically derived approach, are necessarily ambiguous because of the absence of verifiable empirical evidence for their putative mechanisms of action.

Compatibility problems generally do not occur when two or more assessment approaches are combined because assessment involves the passive measurement of psychological, physiological, energetic, or informational processes to obtain pertinent information about putative causes or meanings of symptom patterns. However, when intuitive or empirically based assessment methods affect psychological, physiological, or energetic processes, the practitioner must consider whether changes induced by disparate assessment approaches are potentially incompatible or mutually interfering. In a practical vein, considerations of potential incompatibility have little bearing when the integration of intuitive assessment or treatment approaches with other intuitive or empirically based assessment or treatment approaches is being considered. Intuitive assessment and treatment approaches have been used together with other intuitive or empirically based approaches for centuries in the absence of serious safety concerns. As noted previously, mental or emotional symptoms of mild or moderate severity frequently respond to lifestyle changes, including stress management, exercise, improved sleep, and changes in nutrition. Severe mental or emotional symptoms may also benefit from healthy changes in lifestyle, assuming the patient is motivated to pursue them or is not impaired in his or her capacity to do so. However, severe symptoms seldom respond to lifestyle changes alone. After consulting the relevant evidence tables, the patient and practitioner agree on changes in exercise habits or nutrition to which the principal symptom pattern might reasonably be expected to respond. There are no potential contraindications to combining self-directed lifestyle changes with other treatments. Therefore, when the patient is motivated or is not profoundly impaired, it is almost always appropriate to recommend self-directed approaches in combination with other treatments for the management of severe symptoms.

Going beyond general advice on nutrition, sleep, and exercise, it is reasonable to begin with a particular approach when there is substantial evidence in favor of that treatment for a principal symptom pattern, and that modality has not previously been tried. The updated evidence tables provide the practitioner with a list of substantiated, provisional, and possibly effective approaches that have not previously been tried and constitute legitimate treatment choices. Exceptions to this general rule include cases where a patient has a history of noncompliance due to side effects caused by treatments that are similar to untried approaches but have already been tried, a qualified local practitioner of a recommended treatment is unavailable, or the patient has strong preferences or values that render the treatment unacceptable.

At the start of treatment, the practitioner and patient should agree on a time frame in which it is reasonable to expect beneficial changes in response to the selected treatment. Assuming good compliance, the appropriate evidence tables are used to select another modality with a high probability of alleviating the target symptom in cases where the patient does not respond adequately after a reasonable period of time. This process continues in conjunction with any indicated ongoing assessment until an effective treatment plan is achieved. Depending on symptom severity, the presence of two or more principal symptom patterns, and practical considerations of cost, patient preferences, convenience, and so on, the practitioner and patient may elect to try other treatment combinations when the patient has not responded to the initial integrative plan.

In addition to these general considerations, patient preferences should always be honored, and autonomy should be encouraged. The importance of lifestyle should be stressed, including a healthy diet, regular exercise, and possibly a mind–body practice. Patients who complain of chronic relationship or work stress should be encouraged to consider psychotherapy.

The patient who does not respond adequately to single treatments in sequence may benefit from two or more treatments in parallel depending on symptom severity, response, preferences, local availability of qualified practitioners, and financial considerations. Integrative treatment planning always proceeds from the initial formulation and is subject to modification depending on pertinent new information from history and ongoing assessment. The optimum integrative approach for one patient with moderately depressed mood may include daily aerobic exercise, a consistent yoga practice, improved nutrition, and folic acid supplementation. Another moderately depressed patient with a different treatment–response history, different financial resources, and different preferences might benefit most from weekly psychotherapy, meditation, and a conventional antidepressant. The central goal of integrative treatment planning is to identify the optimum realistic plan for every patient.

Sequential versus Parallel Treatments

Mild or moderate cognitive, emotional, and behavioral symptoms often respond to single treatments. A stepwise or sequential approach to treatment minimizes potential safety concerns by separating treatments in time, while providing the patient with a straightforward plan that is usually more cost-effective compared with more complicated integrative treatment approaches. Because few or no biological or other dynamic (e.g., biomagnetic, electromagnetic, or other energetic) interactions are possible when treatments are used at different times, safety issues of potential incompatibility seldom need to be addressed. Exceptions and caveats to this general principle are mentioned in the symptom-focused chapters in Part II (e.g., avoiding use of an MAOI antidepressant within 2 weeks following discontinuation of fluoxetine, tricyclic antidepressants, or other long half-life conventional drugs). When formulating an appropriate integrative treatment plan, the practitioner should refer to the relevant evidence table in Part II to identify the most substantiated treatments for a specified symptom. In cases where a symptom does not respond adequately following a reasonable trial period, other appropriate treatments can be identified using the relevant evidence table. Continued assessment is sometimes useful in identifying significant factors that may have been overlooked during the initial workup.

During the course of treatment, new assessment findings sometimes suggest treatments that more adequately address the causes or meanings of symptoms. In my experience, combining two synergistic treatments is often beneficial in cases where the principal symptom pattern has failed to respond to two or more sequential treatments. Many patients respond to combinations of treatments from two or more disparate categories, including, for example, a conventional or nonconventional biological treatment, exercise or a mind–body practice, and an appropriate energy-information treatment. Managing several treatments in parallel is always more complicated than monitoring the patient's response to single treatments administered sequentially. However, I have found that combining treatments frequently results in more rapid relief when symptoms are severe, and may therefore be more cost-effective compared with single treatments one after another. The practitioner should consider initially using two or more treatments together for severe mental or emotional symptoms if the patient is motivated and has the capacity to follow an involved treatment plan. Recommending two or more treatments in parallel is also appropriate for moderate or severe symptoms when there is a history of nonresponse to multiple trials of single treatment approaches.

◆ Determining Safety and Degrees of Compatibility When Combining Two or More Treatment Modalities

The general goals of developing an effective treatment plan must be balanced by measures taken to minimize potential risk to the patient Therefore, as in conventional Western medicine, the skillful integrative clinician should always follow the ancient dictum *Primum non nocere* ("Above all, do no harm"). Clinical decisions to combine conventional or nonconventional medicinal agents, especially when they are from disparate systems of medicine, must be made with caution, with reference to reliable medical literature, and always on a case-by-case basis. Combinations of treatments that are appropriate and carry low risk for one patient may, for reasons related to differences in genetic or bioenergetic constitution, different cultural backgrounds, or personal histories of allergies or drug sensitivities, carry considerable risk for another patient. Considering differences in personal history in estimating risk is an accepted "background" principle in the practice of conventional biomedicine, and it is also a responsible

and conservative principle that should guide the professional practice of integrative medicine.

Before recommending the combined use of two or more biologically active agents, the absence of potential contraindications should ideally be established from controlled studies (and preferably on the basis of systematic reviews or meta-analyses of well-done randomized controlled trials) verifying the absence of harmful interactions. In the absence of definitive clinical trials data, basic research findings confirming the mechanisms of action for two or more specified medicinal agents can provide a basis for inferring that the specified medicines do not potentially interact, or interact in nonharmful ways. In the absence of both clinical and basic research data, reasonable inferences can sometimes be made about probable risk when two or more specified conventional or nonconventional modalities are combined if consistent anecdotal evidence demonstrates their safe combined use by large numbers of patients—preferably in different parts of the world—over long periods of time. In view of the above considerations and caveats, any two or more medicinal agents or biologically active natural products should be used in combination only when there is an acceptably small risk that their combined use may result in toxicities or adverse effects, and only when there is evidence of additive or synergistic effects of the specified combination of modalities.

In some cases it is appropriate to try untested combinations of biologically active agents when the effectiveness and safety of their combined use can reasonably be inferred in cases of persisting symptoms following sequential treatments using single conventional or nonconventional medicinal agents. It is reasonable and defensible in such cases to risk possible safety concerns by combining two or more potentially interacting treatments, assuming the patient has provided informed consent and remains under close supervision. In fact, this approach has become accepted medical practice among conventionally trained psychiatrists when evaluating whether to combine two or more psychopharmacologic drugs in treatment-resistant patients. In such cases, the "*N* of 1" approach is helpful in establishing a treatment protocol that is both safe and effective.

In all the cases discussed here, decisions about integrative medical management must weigh probable benefits of improvement against probable risks of undesirable or unsafe outcomes in the context of reliable medical evidence or reasonable inferences of compatibility when a specified integrative treatment approach is used. Therefore, as in Western biomedicine, treatment choices in integrative medicine are ultimately based on practitioners' and patients' judgments of acceptable risk.

◆ Identifying Compatible Treatments

Enhancing Outcomes through Additive or Synergistic Effects Is a Basic Goal of Integrative Treatment

The last step in formulating a suitable integrative treatment strategy is to identify specific compatible treatments that potentially enhance outcomes when combined. Certain modalities that are compatible can be safely combined to enhance treatment outcomes, while many treatments that may be safely combined demonstrably do not improve outcomes. When planning integrative treatment, equal emphasis must be given to safety and effectiveness. After using the evidence-ranking tables in Part II to select the preferred treatment or treatments that adequately address the patient's principal symptom pattern, the next step in identifying potentially useful combinations of treatments is to determine combinations that are both safe and effective. To ensure that the optimum integrative formula is achieved for the principal symptom pattern, determining the degree of compatibility between treatments under consideration must take place before specific recommendations are made to the patient.

Compatibility between treatment methods can be conceptualized as existing along a continuum in which replicated controlled studies compose the most compelling evidence of compatibility, and accepted standards of practice in the absence of supporting studies correspond to the weakest evidence for compatibility. Using this approach, degrees of incompatibility or risk are graded on a continuum, starting from documented toxicities when specific approaches are combined, and progressing to combinations that are safe but neutral, to specific treatment combinations that provide additive or synergistic benefits. Methods for combining empirically based treatments and intuitive approaches are different because mechanisms of action and claims of effectiveness have not been established for intuitive approaches (see Chapter 4). Therefore, knowledge of mechanisms of action or outcomes cannot provide a basis for selecting intuitive methods when planning treatment. Criteria for determining when to combine intuitive treatment approaches with other kinds of treatments are discussed below.

The combined use of compatible treatments can result in neutral, additive, or synergistic effects. Compatible treatments that are neutral with respect to one another are safe when used together but result in little or no incremental improvement in outcomes. In contrast, combining treatments that are additive or synergistic with respect to one another typically results in improved outcomes. The distinction between additive and synergistic effects is at the level of underlying mechanisms of action. Two or more treatments are additive with respect to each other when there is a common or overlapping mechanism of action, and their combined use has biological, energetic, or other effects that enhance treatment outcomes. For example, 5-HTP and a conventional antidepressant that functions as a serotonin agonist have additive neurobiological effects at the level of brain serotonin receptors. Two or more treatments can be described as synergistic with respect to one another when they operate on the basis of mechanisms of action that are nonoverlapping but reinforce one another in a described biological, energetic, or informational way, resulting in improved outcomes.

In some cases, biological treatments may reinforce or be reinforced by treatments that result in changes at the level of dynamic biomagnetic activity of the brain. SAMe and folic acid, for example, are compatible treatments that are synergistic at a biological level on the basis of disparate mechanisms of action that work together to enhance outcomes. EEG-biofeedback and conventional antidepressants are probably synergistic through reciprocally reinforcing neurobiological and electromagnetic effects on certain brain circuits.

It is frequently difficult to ascertain whether treatments are compatible in ways that are additive or synergistic because mechanisms of action have not been clearly elucidated. Furthermore, two or more additive or synergistic biological or

nonbiological treatments may reinforce one another at many functional levels, including gross physiology, neurobiology, bioenergetics, and informational. Disparate treatments can be additive or synergistic with respect to each other to varying degrees. Claims of compatibility between treatments are supported by both quantitative and qualitative evidence, including controlled studies or reliable observations confirming that two (or more) treatments are unsafe in combination, safe but neutral when used together, synergistic when combined, or additive in their effects on the basis of improved outcomes in the absence of apparent synergy because of disparate established mechanisms of action.

The four basic levels of compatibility to consider when combining empirically based modalities are (1) two or more treatments are established to be incompatible, and their combined use is therefore contraindicated; (2) two or more specified treatments can be safely combined in a neutral way, but there are no apparent beneficial additive or synergistic effects; (3) two or more specified treatments have beneficial additive effects when combined with respect to a principal symptom pattern; and (4) two or more treatments are compatible, and are also synergistic with respect to beneficial effects on a principal symptom pattern. Identifying a proposed integrative treatment strategy as contraindicated or neutral does not require knowledge of the respective mechanisms of action of the treatments involved. However, confirming that a particular integrative strategy includes treatments that are additive or synergistic requires knowledge of their respective mechanisms of action. **Table 6–6** provides an overview of possible levels of compatibility between any two or more empirically derived treatment approaches following the above.

Table 6–6 Levels of Compatibility for Any Two or More Empirically Derived Treatments

Level of Compatibility	Example
Contraindicated: Two or more treatments are demonstrated to be incompatible or pose unacceptable safety risks	Concurrent use of MAOI and SSRI antidepressants risks serotonin syndrome, hypertension, stroke, etc.
Neutral: Two or more treatments are compatible but are not additive or synergistic with respect to a particular principal symptom pattern	Aerobic exercise and Tai Chi in a patient with generalized anxiety disorder
Additive: Two or more treatments complement each other and enhance outcomes through common or overlapping mechanisms of action	Combining 5-HTP with an SSRI or other conventional antidepressant that affects brain serotonin activity
Synergistic: Two or more treatments mutually interact to enhance outcome on the basis of nonoverlapping but reinforcing mechanisms of action	Using EEG-biofeedback together with SAMe or a conventional antidepressant

EEG, electroencephalography; 5-HTP, 5-hydroxytryptophan; MAOI, monoamine oxidase inhibitor; SAMe, S-adenosylmethionine; SSRI, selective serotonin reuptake inhibitor

Issues of Compatibility: When and When Not to Combine Two or More Treatments

It is good medical practice to recommend concurrent use of two or more treatments only when there is a reasonable basis for assuming minimum risk of potential incompatibility resulting in unpleasant or harmful effects. Both quantitative and qualitative criteria are used to determine the degree of compatibility between two or more treatments. When compatibility has been empirically demonstrated or inferred, it is reasonable to suggest two or more treatments concurrently when their combined use results in beneficial synergistic or additive effects with respect to a specified target symptom. It is appropriate to recommend safe but neutral treatment combinations when approaches likely to have additive or synergistic effects have been attempted and failed, do not exist for the principal symptom pattern in question, or are excluded from consideration for other reasons (e.g., known history of poor tolerance, treatment is unavailable or unaffordable, or viable combinations conflict with patient values or preferences). Depending on the starting dates and durations of two or more treatments, it is sometimes difficult to infer whether treatments are neutral or synergistic in combination. This is especially true in cases where empirical data from studies or clinical observations are limited or unavailable.

Three basic levels or ratings of compatibility are defined for any two or more treatments: compatible and advantageous in combination because of synergistic or additive effects, compatible and neutral in combination, and incompatible and contraindicated in combination. Determinations of additive and synergistic degrees of compatibility are discussed in detail below. Certain treatment combinations are inherently compatible because of fundamentally unrelated mechanisms of action that do not potentially interfere with one another, whereas other particular combinations can be regarded as incompatible because of documented or inferred contraindications, including toxic biological or other consequences of their combined use.

In some cases, compatibility between two or more treatments can be reasonably inferred from extensive anecdotal reports of their safe and effective combined use. For example, it is reasonable to infer that lifestyle changes, including improved nutrition and exercise or relaxation training, can be used safely in combination with all biological, somatic, or mind–body practices, and energy-information therapies can be safely combined with most other treatments.

Assessing compatibility between more than two treatments poses special problems. There is a greater chance of both positive and negative interactions with three or more treatments compared with two treatments. This becomes especially problematic when biological treatments are combined. In conventional Western medicine, the concurrent use of multiple medications has become a contentious issue in many medical specialties, including psychiatry, where combining two or more medications is frequently associated with significant risk of toxic interactions. Psychiatrists must often balance the potential benefits of combining particular medications against the risk adverse effects to the patient. When treating severe symptoms, psychiatrists often accept risks associated with combining two or more drugs. In my experience, the use of single psychopharmacologic medications is generally as effective as combining two or more medications. Furthermore, relatively few large controlled studies have demonstrated superior efficacy when two or more conventional drugs are combined in the treatment of mental health problems, while there is frequently increased risk of toxicity from interactions. For this reason, conventionally trained Western psychiatrists are trained to verify (e.g., using databases on drug interactions) acceptable levels of risk before combining two or more medications.

As discussed above, it is reasonable to consider combining two biological treatments when a patient has not responded to trials on two or more single conventional or nonconventional biological treatments, and reasonable combinations of biological treatments and appropriate lifestyle changes, somatic, mind–body, or energy-information therapies have failed to alleviate the principal symptom pattern(s). In Western psychiatry, assuming there is empirical evidence for the effectiveness of a specified combination of two drugs, the standard of practice is to begin the second medicine at a very low dose and gradually increasing the dose until a therapeutic response is achieved while monitoring the patient for signs of toxicity. This empirical approach assumes that psychiatrists are trained to make judicious choices on the basis of current information, that they keep current on emerging safety information, and that they are proactive and engaged when treating patients. When skillfully done, this is an effective and safe approach to patient care in general, and can be extended to considerations of nonconventional treatments in the integrative management of mental or emotional symptoms.

Only practitioners who are trained in a particular system of medicine should advise patients on the use of combinations of specialized treatments within that tradition. This is especially true when combinations of synthetic medicines or natural products are being considered because of inherently greater risks of toxicities when combining biologically active treatments compared with somatic, mind–body, or energy-information modalities. Questions about specific medications (including synthetic drugs and herbals used as medicines) should be deferred to a clinician who is professionally trained in the relevant system of medicine. Because of a lack of training, misunderstandings, or negative bias, practitioners of one professional system of medicine are seldom able to give competent advice about treatments in other professional systems of medicine. Therefore, Western physicians who are not dually trained in Chinese medicine should not comment or give advice on uses of Chinese herbs, acupuncture, or moxibustion. By the same token, it is not appropriate for licensed Chinese medical practitioners to comment on or give advice about uses of psychopharmacologic medicines. Special considerations when combining Chinese and Western medical treatments in the management of mental or emotional symptoms are especially relevant in Western countries, where Chinese medicine is the dominant nonconventional system of medicine. These are discussed in some detail elsewhere (Lake, 2004), and will not be repeated here.

When the evidence tables, history, and patient preferences suggest that combining two or more specific approaches will be beneficial and safe, it is reasonable to start with treatments that are additive or synergistic. The optimum integrative strategy uses the most compatible treatments that will most likely result in beneficial changes in the principal symptom pattern. The practitioner should carefully review potential safety issues when considering recommending two or more specific treatments in parallel. It is important for the practitioner and patient to agree on an acceptable level of risk when combining approaches that potentially result in unpleasant effects and to document informed consent in the patient's chart. It is especially important to obtain informed consent in cases where combinations of biological treatments are being considered for which there are known risks of potentially harmful interactions. For example, concurrent use of some conventional drugs and some natural product–derived medicines is inadvisable or frankly contraindicated because of safety issues that are well documented or predictable on the basis of identified mechanisms of action. Examples include the potential risk of a serotonin syndrome when combining an SSRI and a natural product that promotes the synthesis of serotonin in the brain, including L-tryptophan and 5-HTP. Combining St. John's wort with a protease inhibitor or warfarin (or other medicines that interfere with platelet aggregation) can significantly lower serum levels of both drugs, placing the patient at considerable medical risk. Combinations of many biologically active substances potentially result in unpleasant effects. However, when used judiciously by an experienced practitioner, most biological treatments do not interact in ways that potentially result in contraindications for safety reasons. Serious medical contraindications to combining natural products with conventional drugs (or other natural products) occur infrequently when reasonable practice guidelines are followed.

In sum, the judicious integrative practitioner bases treatment recommendations on guidelines that take into account possible contraindications when combining two or more conventional drugs or natural products. When combining two or more biological treatments is demonstrably safe, and reliable evidence supports a specific combination of two or more substances in the treatment of a specified symptom pattern, it is often reasonable to do so when the patient has been informed about potential risks, a conservative dosing strategy is used, and the patient is closely monitored for complaints that may suggest treatment-emergent safety concerns. Examples of integrative strategies based on disparate categories of treatments that do not potentially interact include combinations of self-directed treatments (including lifestyle changes, mind–body practices, and energy healing methods) and an appropriate natural or synthetic biological agent.

Use Only One Medicinal Treatment Whenever Possible

To minimize risk while optimizing the probability of a beneficial response to any integrative plan, it is prudent to recommend initially the use of only one biological treatment for the management of a mental health problem. In this context, conventional drugs, some herbals, and compound herbal formulas are considered "biological treatments" depending on how they are used, dosing, and frequency of use. Many natural products that are generally not considered biological treatments can be safely taken in combination with potent conventional drugs or herbal medicines. For example, substantial evidence supports a synergistic effect when certain B vitamins are combined with conventional antidepressants. Natural products that ameliorate mental or emotional symptoms include some vitamins and minerals, amino acids and their precursors, some fatty acids, and some hormones. The distinction between a "biological treatment" and a "supplement" is frequently ambiguous, reflecting different use traditions in disparate systems of medicine. For our purposes, a ***biological treatment*** is a biologically

active substance that has a specified, sometimes potent, therapeutic effect on a particular symptom pattern and is an effective treatment in the context of a particular system of medicine. In contrast, a ***supplement*** is a natural substance that may have beneficial effects on physical or mental health in general but does not alleviate a specific symptom pattern. Natural substances used as supplements are frequently included in healthy diets, and have general beneficial effects on physical and mental health. A particular conventional or nonconventional biological treatment is frequently an important component of integrative treatment addressing severe symptoms. As noted earlier in this chapter, biological treatments are often unnecessary when treating symptoms of mild to moderate severity, or when there is a risk of toxicity when combining two or more biological treatments. However, when symptoms are severe, it is reasonable to initiate treatment using a biological approach. In all cases the most appropriate choice is determined by reviewing the evidence in the context of patient history, personal preferences, and any constraints on treatment cost or availability. The integrative practitioner determines appropriate combinations of treatments on a case-by-case basis after consulting the relevant evidence and discussing realistic options with the patient.

Even in cases where it is reasonable to expect that combining three or more biological treatments will yield outcomes that are significantly better than one or two treatments, practical considerations sometimes militate against this strategy. For example, patients who suffer from severe symptoms of depressed mood, anxiety, or psychosis are frequently too impaired to pursue more than one treatment approach, especially when a recommended treatment requires a capacity for organized thought, motivation, or insight. In such cases it is reasonable to consider appropriate combinations of biological treatments, including conventional drugs and some natural products, depending on the principal symptom pattern(s) being addressed. In contrast, recommending the pursuit of a mind–body practice, cognitive-behavioral therapy, or ongoing EEG-biofeedback therapy, although sometimes beneficial for some patients, would probably be of limited practical value for the management of severe symptoms, at least not in the initial phase of treatment.

Inferring Compatibility of Empirically Based Modalities When Mechanisms of Action Are Established but There Is Limited Safety Information

When the mechanisms of action for two or more conventional or nonconventional biological treatments have been verified, the problem of demonstrating compatibility goes back to the distinction between quantitative and qualitative evidence in medical research. This approach rests on an understanding of the respective mechanisms of action of medical practices that are candidates for possible integration. In cases where there is little or no information from randomized controlled trials or observational studies confirming compatibility, a knowledge of mechanisms of action can be used to infer degrees of compatibility between any two or more empirically derived treatment approaches being considered for combined use. In this context, mechanism of action refers to biochemical, physiological, energetic, or other processes that are known to be the means by which a desired outcome is achieved. Accurate understanding of the mechanism of action underlying a specified treatment leads to reasonable (but not always correct) inferences about potentially compatible combinations of the specified approach with another treatment for which the mechanism of action is also clearly established. A specified approach that is based on a well-described mechanism of action will probably be compatible with another treatment based on a different mechanism of action if the respective mechanisms of action do not potentially interfere with each other in ways that reduce the effectiveness of one or both treatments or result in harmful biochemical, physiological, energetic, or other consequences. Incompatibilities that are possible when disparate treatments are combined can be described as a "canceling out" of beneficial effects or the induction of "pathological changes" in structure or function.

Determining Compatibility When the Mechanism of Action Is Unknown

In cases where a purported mechanism of action has not been clearly delineated for one or more treatment approaches being considered for combined use, a review of available research data, or anecdotal reports of adverse effects can help to determine whether there is a significant risk of incompatibility. Reports of similar adverse effects or toxicities of disparate treatments imply that similarities in underlying mechanisms of action exist with respect to treatment effects on structure or function. On the basis of similar adverse effects or toxicities that pose significant safety concerns, disparate modalities should not be combined in the absence of convincing information from controlled trials or reliable observational studies. In such cases a high probability of clinically significant incompatibility can reasonably be inferred from an understanding of mechanisms of action.

The "N of 1" randomized trial has gained recent attention as a method for determining the effectiveness and safety of a specified nonconventional treatment (or combination of nonconventional and conventional approaches), and is useful when formal research studies are impractical or unaffordable. This approach avoids many limitations inherent in randomized controlled trials and bypasses the requirement for inferring the likelihood of specific beneficial effects or specific safety concerns in a particular patient from statistically averaged therapeutic effects or risks observed in a group of patients exposed to the treatment in question. Questions of potential incompatibility can generally be resolved in a straightforward way in cases where established nonconventional treatments are being considered. The conservative practitioner can use an "N of 1" controlled trial on a particular patient to estimate the potential benefits and risks of a particular integrative strategy.

Combining Intuitive Treatments with Empirically Based Treatments

The method for determining when to combine an intuitive treatment with an empirically based treatment cannot rely on knowledge of mechanisms of action. When determining whether to combine an intuitive approach with an empirically derived treatment, or whether to combine two or more intuitive approaches, the practitioner must rely on reports of effectiveness and adverse effects when the specified treatments have previously been used together. Possible levels of compatibility between any specified intuitive treatment and any other specified treatment are similar to those for empirically based

treatments. Some nonconventional treatments are presently regarded as intuitive because contemporary technologies cannot verify or refute a purported mechanism of action. These include treatments that probably have a general biological effect on the organism but have not been shown to have specific beneficial effects on mental or emotional symptoms. Examples of such intuitive approaches include aerobic exercise and music therapy for moderately anxious or depressed patients. Other intuitive treatments have no identified or apparent biological basis of action and can probably be safely combined with other intuitive or empirically derived methods. Examples include combining regular qigong exercises with massage therapy or light exposure therapy when treating a moderately depressed patient. It is likely that both kinds (i.e., those for which there is probably a general biological mechanism of action and those for which there is no apparent biological basis) of intuitive treatments can be safely combined with other conventional or nonconventional modalities. When combining an intuitive approach with any other treatment, it is frequently possible to make reasonable inferences about contraindications and neutral or additive effects on the basis of research findings or clinical observations, but it is never possible to infer the existence of synergy—the highest level of compatibility—because the mechanism of action is undefined for any intuitive treatment. There can be no empirical basis for predicting complementary effects when an empirically derived treatment based on a known mechanism of action is combined with an intuitive treatment based on an unknown mechanism of action. Therefore, levels of compatibility for combinations of intuitive and empirically based treatments can be determined only on the basis of inference from outcomes studies or clinical observations.

◆ Putting It All Together: Using Algorithms to Plan the Integrative Management of Cognitive, Emotional, and Behavioral Symptoms

An algorithm is a problem-solving method that takes into account many factors and different kinds of information. Algorithms show the flow of information from initial conditions to a series of outcomes through progressively branching steps or decisions. The steps are guided by different criteria, including logical considerations, empirical information, analytical judgments, and subjective considerations. Clinically useful algorithms guide the practitioner in the skillful management of a specified symptom pattern by clarifying the most effective, appropriate, and realistic assessment or treatment approaches while also taking into account each patient's unique history, preferences, and financial constraints. Practical algorithms for clinical problem solving focus on the management of a core symptom pattern while identifying factors that may interfere with the patient's response to treatment.

The kinds of information and choices that enter into integrative assessment and treatment planning are described in this section. The quality of information that enters into an algorithm will determine the quality and effectiveness of unique clinical solutions. Inaccurate or incomplete patient information will result in a suboptimal plan. Conversely, accurate and complete information about history, symptoms, and patient preferences or circumstances will lead to a practical integrative strategy that reflects optimum realistic assessment and treatment approaches for a principal symptom pattern of a specific patient. A realistic integrative strategy is derived on the basis of evidence of effectiveness and compatibility in the context of medical and psychiatric history, current symptoms, patient preferences and values, and the availability and affordability of medical resources. Considerations of qualitative and quantitative evidence and constraints related to patient preferences or the cost or availability of treatment choices are built into the algorithms.

I have argued above that there is no standard or best integrative approach incorporating specific assessment or treatment modalities for all patients who report similar mental or emotional symptom patterns. Each patient is defined by unique history, symptoms, preferences, values, geographical location, and financial circumstances. The optimum integrative formula thus depends on the individual circumstances, preferences, and values in the context of locally available medical resources, and the judgment and experience of the managing practitioner. This point leads to a fundamental distinction between conventional Western biomedicine and the philosophy of integrative medicine. In contrast to Western biomedicine, integrative medicine has no standard or universal guidelines for addressing a particular symptom in different patients. As discussed in Chapter 4, the basic methods and specific approaches that compose integrative medicine evolve continuously. Future optimum integrative strategies addressing a specified symptom pattern will be determined relative to the available empirical evidence in the context of the preferences, cultural and financial circumstances of particular patients, and the professional judgment and experience of the practitioner. Integrative medicine rests on the assumption of unique psychological, biological, and energetic constitutions of every patient, and the corollary assumption that unique causes or meanings of symptoms are present in different patients. This model naturally leads to a highly individualized approach to assessment and treatment planning.

The algorithms in Part II are intended to be used from the perspective of presumed psychological, biological, and energetic individuality, with the goal of guiding the practitioner in developing integrative strategies that take into account the complex and unique characteristics and circumstances of every patient. The algorithms are not intended as a device for deriving simple shortcuts in patient care.

Algorithms used in Western medicine are limited in many ways. They are generally global in scope and thus fail to address individual patient circumstances, needs, and preferences. Conventional treatment-planning algorithms are seldom closely coupled with assessment findings and frequently based on consensus opinions that reflect biases about particular treatment approaches rather than objective medical evidence. Unlike algorithms used in conventional Western medicine, integrative planning algorithms do not provide a means for identifying standardized health care approaches. Indeed, that idea would clearly be at odds with the basic principles of sound integrative medical care.

Algorithms Incorporate Three Kinds of Information

The algorithms are constructed to take into account three kinds of information or inputs: assessment or treatment choices supported by the best available evidence following a review of the pertinent conventional and nonconventional medical literature;

my professional judgment based on my own clinical experience and my discussions with expert practitioners; and patient preferences, values, or practical financial or other constraints dictated by individual circumstances. As described above, the detailed contents of the evidence tables in Part II was determined by a comprehensive literature research supplemented by secondary sources, including personal communications with researchers or expert practitioners, conferences, symposia, and Web-based discussion groups pertaining to clinical uses of particular modalities. Assessing the compatibility of disparate approaches is a critical step when making informed clinical judgments about both safety and effectiveness in integrative treatment planning. The evidence tables guide the clinician through reasonable choices of compatible treatments with respect to many common mental and emotional symptom patterns. Assessment or treatment choices are selected on the basis of the empirical evidence for particular approaches in the context of current symptoms and history of previous treatments and treatment responses. This method takes into account previously unrecognized or evolving symptom patterns as the patient progresses from intake to assessment to formulation and treatment. The patient goes through multiple "phases" of history taking, assessment, formulation, and treatment until an optimum realistic integrative strategy is identified. Several sessions are sometimes required to gather all pertinent historical and current information pertaining to possible causes or meanings of the patient's complaints, to incorporate assessment findings into the treatment plan, and to evaluate the safety and effectiveness of treatment. The algorithms provide a practical method for planning assessment and treatment in the context of new assessment findings, emerging history, and changes in symptoms or responses to treatment.

Integrative Planning Algorithms Are Based on an Open Design

The algorithms incorporate an open design, permitting inputs at many points during assessment, formulation, and treatment planning. The point at which an algorithm is modified when planning integrative mental health care for a particular patient depends on the principal symptom pattern(s), symptom severity, the presence of co-occurring medical or psychiatric symptoms, patient preferences or values, and financial or other constraints that affect practical implementation of a treatment plan. Unique assessment and treatment choices are generated when an algorithm addressing a specified symptom pattern is applied to a particular patient. Case presentations at the end of the chapters in Part II illustrate representative assessment and treatment approaches that are derived when the algorithms are used to generate integrative strategies on the basis of the unique clinical information, preferences, and constraints of an individual complaining of a mental health problem.

When considering what approaches to recommend, the practitioner should keep in mind that the detailed contents of the evidence tables will change on a continuous basis as new evidence accumulates for both conventional and nonconventional approaches. In some cases, emerging evidence will support the use of a particular assessment or treatment approach, whereas other findings will cast doubt on conventional, nonconventional, or integrative approaches used to assess or treat a particular symptom pattern. As new findings emerge, the evidence tables will be modified (see www.thieme.com/mentalhealth),

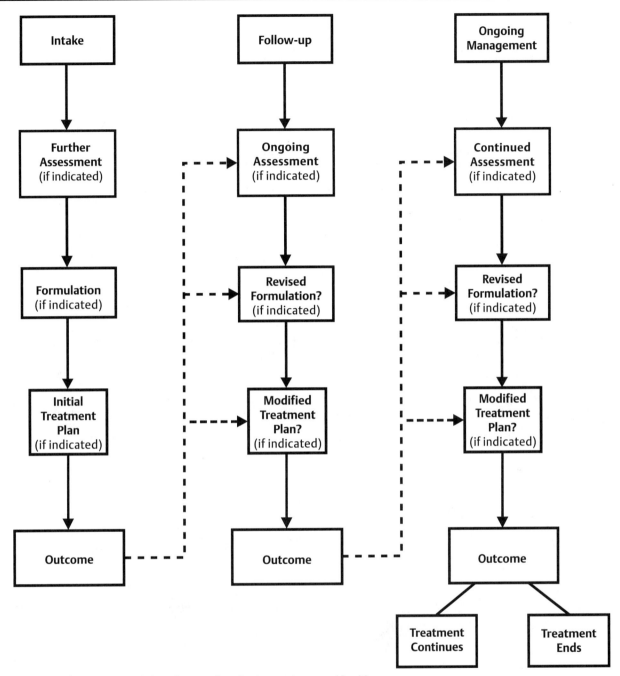

Figure 6–1 The logical structure of algorithms used to plan integrative mental health care.

thus permitting the practitioner to identify the most effective assessment and treatment approaches addressing a specified symptom pattern. It is likely that future content changes in the evidence tables will sometimes result in significant changes in integrative strategies generated by the algorithms.

Algorithms for integrative treatment planning include different pathways based on the above considerations for matching symptoms, treatment response history, newly acquired assessment findings, patient preferences, and other factors to the most appropriate combined or sequential treatment strategies addressing a principal symptom pattern. The translation of emerging research findings or newly disclosed history into appropriate modifications of the treatment plan is a central part of skillful integrative care. The failure of a specified treatment to ameliorate a particular symptom pattern in a particular

patient will translate into new inputs in the algorithm that will generate new recommendations. This process will result in ongoing modifications in integrative treatment guidelines addressing the same symptom pattern and the same patient at different times in treatment. The use of algorithms in this way facilitates an evolving, flexible approach to treatment planning. Novel parallel or sequential treatments are generated until symptoms improve, resolve, or remain unchanged in cases where available realistic treatment choices are exhausted.

With the above general considerations in mind, **Fig. 6–1** illustrates the logical structure of algorithms for planning the integrative management of cognitive, emotional, and behavioral symptoms. Algorithms addressing the common symptom patterns discussed in this book are included in the chapters of Part II.

References

Abbot, N. (2000). Healing as a therapy for human disease: A systematic review. *Journal of Alternative and Complementary Medicine, 6*(2), 159–169.

Adams, K., Cohen, M., Eisenberg, D., & Jonsen, A. (2002). Ethical considerations of complementary and alternative medical therapies in conventional medical settings. *Annals of Internal Medicine, 137,* 660–664.

Anderson, J., Anderson, L., & Felsenthal, G. (1993). Pastoral needs for support within an inpatient rehabilitation unit. *Archives of Physical Medicine and Rehabilitation, 74,* 574–578.

Astin, J. A., Harkness, E., & Ernst, E. (2000). The efficacy of "Distant Healing": A systematic review of randomized trials. *Annals of Internal Medicine, 132*(11), 903–910.

Bell, I., Lewis, D., Lewis, S., Brooks, A., Schwartz, G., & Baldwin, C. (2004). Strength of vital force in classical homeopathy: bio-psycho-social-spiritual correlates within a complex systems context. *Journal of Alternative and Complementary Medicine, 10*(1), 123–131.

Benor, D. (2002). Spiritual Healing: Scientific validation of a healing revolution, professional supplement. In *Healing Research* (Vol. 1). Southfield, MI: Vision Publications.

Birch, S. (2004). Clinical research on acupuncture: 2. Controlled clinical trials, an overview of their methods. *Journal of Alternative and Complementary Medicine, 10*(3), 481–498.

Bodeker, G. (2001). Evaluating Ayurveda. *Journal of Alternative and Complementary Medicine, 7*(5), 389–392.

Bratman, S., & Girman, A. M. (2003). *Mosby's handbook of herbs and supplements and their therapeutic uses.* St. Louis, MO: Mosby.

Brinker, F. (1998). *Herb contraindications and drug interactions* (2nd ed.) Portland, OR: Eclectic Medical Publications.

Clifford, T. (1990). *Tibetan Buddhist medicine and psychiatry: The diamond healing.* York Beach, ME: Samuel Weiser, Inc.

Cohen, M. (1998). *Complementary and alternative medicine: Legal boundaries and regulatory perspectives.* Baltimore, MD: Johns Hopkins University Press.

Cohen, M., & Eisenberg, D. (2002). Potential malpractice liability associated with complementary and integrative medical therapies. *Annals of Internal Medicine, 136,* 596–603.

d'Aquili, E., & Newberg, A. (1993). Religious and mystical states: A neuropsychological substrate. *Zygon, 28,* 200–277.

Davidson, J. (1994). Psychiatry and homeopathy: basis for a dialogue. *British Homeopathic Journal, 83,* 78–83.

Dixon, M., & Sweeney, K. (2000). *The human effect in medicine: Theory, research and practice.* Oxford: Radcliffe Medical Press.

Dossey, L. (1997). *Healing words: The power of prayer and the practice of medicine.* New York: HarperCollins.

Dubin, W. (2004). *Clinical practices that lead treatment resistance* (Abstract 81D, Symposium 81). Paper presented at the annual meeting of the American Psychiatric Association, New York.

Eisenberg, D., Davis, R., Ettner, S., et al. (1998). Trends in alternative medicine use in the United States, 1990–1997: Results of a follow-up national survey. *Journal of the American Medical Association, 280*(18), 1569–1575.

Ernst, E., & Resch, K. (1996). Clinical trials of homeopathy: A re-analysis of a published review. *Forschende Komplementarmedizin, 3,* 85–90.

Feinstein, D. (2003). Subtle energy: Psychology's missing link. *IONS Noetic Sciences Review,* 1716–35.

Flaherty, J., Perry, H., Lynchard, G., & Morley, J. (2000). Polypharmacy and hospitalization among older home care patients. *Journals of Gerontology, Series A: Biological Sciences and Medical Sciences, 55*(10), M554–M559.

Gallo, F. (1999). *Energy psychology: Explorations at the interface of energy, cognition, behavior and health.* Boca Raton, FL: CRC Press.

Gartner, J., Larson, D., & Allen, G. (1991). Religious commitment and mental health: A review of the empirical literature. *Journal of Psychology and Theology, 19,* 6–25.

Gelenberg, A. J. (2000). St. John's wort update. *Biological Therapies in Psychiatry, 23,* 22–24.

Gogtay, N. J., Bhatt, H. A., Dalvi, S. S., & Kshirsagar, N. A. (2002). The use and safety of non-allopathic Indian medicines. *Drug Safety, 25*(14), 1005–1019.

Goleman, D. (2004). *Destructive emotions: How can we overcome them? A scientific dialogue with the Dalai Lama.* New York: Bantam Books.

Green, J. (1996). Integrating conventional medicine and alternative therapies. *Alternative Therapies in Health and Medicine, 2*(4), 77–81.

Grinberg-Zylberbaum, J., Delaflor, M., & Goswami, A. (1994). The Einstein/Podolsky/Rosen paradox in the brain: The transferred potential. *Physics Essays, 7*(4), 422–428.

Hankey, A. (2004). Are we close to a theory of energy medicine? *Journal of Alternative and Complementary Medicine, 10*(1), 83–86.

Harkness, R., & Bratman, S. (2003). *Mosby's handbook of drug-herb and drug-supplement interactions.* St. Louis: Mosby.

Hsiung, R. & Stangler, R. (2004). *The office of the future: Technology in psychiatry* (American Association for Technology in Psychiatry Issue Workshop 2). Presented at the annual meeting of the American Psychiatric Association, New York.

Izzo, A., & Ernst, E. (2001). Interactions between herbal medicines and prescribed drugs: A systematic review. *Drugs, 61*(15), 2163–2175.

Kienle, G. S., & Kiene, H. (1996). Placebo effect and placebo concept: A critical methodological and conceptual analysis of reports on the magnitude of the placebo effect. *Alternative Therapies in Health Medicine, 2,* 39–54.

Kienle, G. S., & Kiene, H. (1997). The powerful placebo effect: Fact or fiction? *Journal of Clinical Epidemiology, 50,* 1311–1318.

King, D., & Bushwick, B. (1994). Beliefs and attitudes of hospital inpatients about faith-healing and prayer. *Journal of Family Practice, 39,* 349–352.

Kirsch, I., Moore, T., Scoboria, A., & Nicholls, S. (2002). The emperor's new drugs: An analysis of antidepressant medication data submitted to the U.S. Food and Drug Administration. *Prevention and Treatment, 5*(23). Available at journals.apa.org/prevention/volume5/toc-jul15–02.html

Kleijnen, J., Knipschild, P., & Riet, G. (1991). Clinical trials of homeopathy. *British Medical Journal, 302,* 316–323.

Koenig, H., & Futterman, A. (1995, March 16–17). *Religion and health outcomes: A review and synthesis of the literature.* Paper presented at the Conference on Methodological Advances in the Study of Religion, Health and Aging, Kalamazoo, MI.

Lake, J. (2004). The integration of Chinese Medicine and Western medicine: Focus on mental illness. *Integrative Medicine: Integrating Conventional and Alternative Medicine, 3*(4), 20–28.

Larson, D., & Milano, M. (1996, March/April). Religion and mental health: Should they work together? *Alternative and Complementary Therapies,* pp. 91–98.

Lazarou, J., Pomeranz, B., & Corey, P. (1998). Incidence of adverse drug reactions in hospitalized patients: A meta-analysis of prospective studies. *Journal of the American Medical Association, 279*(15), 1200–1205.

Levin, J. (1996). How religion influences morbidity and health: Reflections on natural history, salutogenesis and host resistance. *Social Science and Medicine, 43,* 849–864.

Linde, K., Clausius, N., Ramirez, G., Melchart, D., Eitel, F., Hedges, L., & Jonas, W. (1997). Are the clinical effects of homeopathy placebo effects? A meta-analysis of placebo-controlled trials. *Lancet, 350,* 834–843.

Mackay, N., Hansen, S., & McFarlane, O. (2004). Autonomic nervous system changes during Reiki treatment: A preliminary study. *Journal of Alternative and Complementary Medicine, 10*(6), 1077–1081.

Mayberg, H., Silva, J., Brannan, S., Takell, J., Mahurin, R., et al. (2002). The functional neuroanatomy of the placebo effect. *American Journal of Psychiatry, 159,* 728–737.

McCaffrey, A., Eisenberg, D., Legedza, A., Davis, R., & Phillips, R. (2004). Prayer for health concerns: Results of a national survey on prevalence and patterns of use. *Archives of Internal Medicine, 164,* 858–862.

McGuffin, M., Hobbs, C., Upton, R., & Goldberg, A. (1997). *Botanical safety handbook.* Boca Raton, FL: CRC Press.

Palmer, R., Katerndahl, D., & Morgan-Kidd, J. (2004). A randomized trial of the effects of remote intercessory prayer: Interactions with personal beliefs on problem-specific outcomes and functional status. *Journal of Alternative and Complementary Medicine, 10*(3), 438–448.

Piscitelli, S. C., Burstein, A. H., Chaitt, D., et al. (2000). Indinavir concentrations and St John's wort. *Lancet, 355,* 547–548.

Radin, R. (2004). Event-related electroencephalographic correlations between isolated human subjects. *Journal of Alternative and Complementary Medicine, 10*(2), 315–323.

Ray, W., Fought, R., & Decker, M. (1992). Psychoactive drugs and the risk of injurious motor vehicle crashes in elderly drivers. *American Journal of Epidemiology, 136*(17), 873–883.

Rotman, D. Can Pfizer deliver? (2004 February). *Technology Review, 58*–65.

Ruschitzka, F., Meier, P. J., Turina, M., et al. (2000). Acute heart transplant rejection due to Saint John's wort. *Lancet, 355,* 548–549.

Sanderson, W. (2002). Are evidence-based psychological interventions practiced by clinicians in the field? *Medscape Mental Health, 7*(1). Available at www.medscape.com/Medscape/psychiatry/journal/2002/v07.n01/mh011 1.01.sand/mh0111.01.san-01.html

Saper, R. B., Kales, S. N., Paquin, J., Burns, M. J., Eisenberg, D. M., Davis, R. B., & Phillips, R. S. (2004). Heavy metal content of ayurvedic herbal medicine products. *Journal of the American Medical Association, 292*(23), 2868–2873.

Schroeder, M. J., & Barr, R. E. (2001). Quantitative analysis of the electroencephalogram during cranial electrotherapy stimulation. *Clinical Neurophysiology, 112*(11), 2075–2083.

Schwartz, G., & Russek, L. (1998, Winter). The plausibility of homeopathy: The systemic memory mechanism. *Journal of Alternative and Complementary Medicine, 4*(4), 336–337.

Schwartz, G., & Russek, L. (1997). The challenge of one medicine; Theories of health and eight world hypotheses. Advances: *The Journal of Mind–Body Health, 13*(3), 7–23.

Shannahoff-Khalsa, D. (2003). Kundalini Yoga meditation techniques in the treatment of obsessive compulsive and OC spectrum disorders. *Brief Treatment Crisis Intervention, 3,* 369–382.

Shore, A. G. (2004). Long-term effects of energetic healing on symptoms of psychological depression and self-perceived stress. *Alternative Therapies in Health Medicine, 10*(3), 42–48.

Sicher, F., Targ, E., Moore, D., & Smith, H. (1998). A randomized double-blind study of the effect of distant healing in a population with advanced AIDS. *Western Journal of Medicine, 169*(6), 356–363.

Smith, C. (2004). Quanta and coherence effects in water and living systems. *Journal of Alternative and Complementary Medicine, 10*(1), 69–78.

Snyder, S. (2002). Forty years of neurotransmitters: A personal statement. *Archives of General Psychiatry, 59,* 983–994.

Standish, L. J., Johnson, L. C., Kozak, L., & Richards, T. (2003). Evidence of correlated functional magnetic resonance imaging signals between distant human brains. *Alternative Therapies in Health Medicine, 9*(1), 122–125.

Studdert, D., Eisenberg, D., Miller, F., Curto, D., Kaptchuk, T., & Brennan, T. (1998). Medical malpractice implications of alternative medicine. *Journal of the American Medical Association, 280,* 1610–1615.

Sussman, N. (2004, July). The "file-drawer" effect: Assessing efficacy and safety of antidepressants. *Primary Psychiatry,* p. 12.

Tangrea, J., Adrianza, E., & Helsel, W. (1994). Risk factors for the development of placebo adverse reactions in a multicenter clinical trial. *Annals of Epidemiology, 4,* 327–331.

Thase, M. (2002). Antidepressant effects: The suit may be small, but the fabric is real. *Prevention and Treatment, 5*(32). Available at journals.apa.org/prevention/volume5/toc-jul15–02.html

Thorne, S., Best, A., Balon, J., Kelner, M., & Rickhi, B. (2002). Ethical dimensions in the borderland between conventional and complementary/alternative medicine. *Journal of Alternative and Complementary Medicine, 8*(6), 907–915.

Tsuang, M., Williams, W., Simpson, J., & Lyons, M. (2002). Pilot study of spirituality and mental health in twins. *American Journal of Psychiatry, 159*(3), 486–488.

Unutzer, J., et al. (2002). Surveys of CAM: Part V—Use of alternative and complementary therapies . . . psychiatric and neurologic diseases. *Journal of Alternative and Complementary Medicine, 8*(1), 93–96.

Unutzer, J., Klap, R., Sturm, R., Young, A., Marmon, T., et al. (2000). Mental disorders and the use of alternative medicine: Results from a national survey. *American Journal of Psychiatry, 157,* 1851–1857.

Virtual second opinions: Breaking barriers of time and place. (2004, February). Available at www.mdng.com

Wiederhold, B., & Wiederhold, M. (2000). Lessons learned from 600 virtual reality sessions. *Cyberpsychology and Behavior, 3*(3), 393–400.

Wiederhold, B., & Wiederhold, M. (2005). Side effects and contraindications. In *Virtual reality therapy for anxiety disorders: Advances in evaluation and treatment* (chapter 5). Washington, DC: American Psychological Association.

Wiesendanger, H., Werthmuller, L., Reuter, K., & Walach, H. (2001). Chronically ill patients treated by spiritual healing improve in quality of life: Results of a randomized waiting-list controlled study. *Journal of Alternative and Complementary Medicine, 7*(1), 45–51.

Wirth, D. P., & Cram, J. R. (1994). The psychophysiology of nontraditional prayer. *International Journal of Psychosomatics, 41*(1–4), 68–75.

Zahourek, R. P. (2004). Intentionality forms the matrix of healing: A theory. *Alternative Therapies in Health Medicine, 10*(6), 40–49.

Part II

Integrative Management of Common Mental and Emotional Symptoms

7

Symptom-Focused Integrative Mental Health Care

This brief chapter introduces the clinical part of the book. The other chapters of Part II provide critical reviews of nonconventional and integrative assessment and treatment approaches used in mental health care. The following core symptom patterns are covered:

◆ Depressed mood
◆ Mania and cyclic mood changes
◆ Anxiety
◆ Psychosis
◆ Cognitive impairment
◆ Substance abuse and dependence
◆ Disturbances of sleep and wakefulness

Each chapter begins with an overview of the social and financial costs associated with the core symptom pattern that is being addressed. The sections on assessment and treatment begin with concise reviews of the effectiveness and safety of established conventional approaches. Nonconventional biological, somatic, and energy-information approaches used to assess the core symptom pattern are addressed. This is followed by a review of the evidence pertaining to nonconventional treatment approaches and includes comments on safety problems and contraindications where relevant. Evidence for integrative treatments combining conventional and nonconventional approaches is discussed in this section. The clinical material is organized by level of evidence and category of modality. All assessment and treatment approaches are assigned to one of three basic levels of evidence: substantiated, provisional, and possibly accurate (for assessment approaches) or possibly effective (for treatment approaches). Substantiated approaches are in current use and are supported by compelling evidence. Provisional approaches are in current use and are supported by strong evidence. Possibly effective approaches may be in current use and are supported by inconsistent or limited evidence.

For each level of evidence, nonconventional assessment approaches are organized into four general categories: biological approaches, somatic approaches, methods based on forms of energy or information validated by current Western science, and methods based on putative forms of energy or information not validated by Western science. Nonconventional treatments are organized according to these four categories in addition to a fifth category, mind–body approaches.

Exhibits summarize significant research findings, specific clinical protocols, and safety issues. These evidence tables contain the essential clinical information on which integrative management should be based. The evidence tables are updated on a regular basis with significant new research findings in the companion Web site (www.thieme.com/mentalhealth). Based on emerging evidence, some nonconventional or integrative approaches that are now provisional will be designated as "substantiated," while others will be moved to the category of "possibly effective" treatments. Likewise, certain assessment or treatment approaches that are "possibly effective" based on current evidence will emerge as "provisional" or "substantiated." Whenever possible, the reader should consult the companion Web site to obtain the most current research findings for a particular modality with respect to the mental health problem that is being treated.

All chapters contain algorithms intended to guide the practitioner in planning the integrative assessment and treatment of the core symptom patterns discussed. Case vignettes illustrate the integrative management of the symptom pattern being addressed, taking into account the evidence for both conventional and nonconventional approaches.

◆ Integrative Mental Health Care: An Overview

This section contains a concise overview of clinical methods in integrative mental health care. (Methods in integrative assessment and treatment planning are discussed in detail in Chapters 5, History Taking, Assessment, and Formulation in Integrative Mental Health Care, and 6, Starting and Maintaining Integrative Treatment in Mental Health Care.) Integrative management begins with a consideration of the most substantiated assessment and treatment approaches for a target symptom pattern and systematically progresses to provisional and possibly effective modalities in the context of the patient's previous treatment history, practical constraints of location or cost, and patient preferences. Possibly effective approaches are sometimes reasonable choices when substantiated and provisional approaches have failed, are unavailable or unaffordable, or when there is anecdotal evidence that a particular integrative strategy incorporating a possibly effective treatment may improve outcomes. Patients who express a preference for a possibly effective modality should be encouraged to first try more substantiated conventional or nonconventional approaches or to begin a trial on a possibly effective treatment while also continuing to use a substantiated treatment that is synergistic. When starting a patient on a possibly effective treatment, the practitioner should ideally follow an "N of 1" protocol to obtain pertinent clinical information about the patient's response at the early stages of treatment.

Before finalizing any integrative treatment plan, the reader is encouraged to go to the companion Web site (www.thieme.com/ mentalhealth) to check the updated evidence tables for pertinent new information on relevant assessment or treatment approaches. The Web site is organized like the book by core symptoms. Updates to the evidence tables are based on published research findings, as well as systematic reviews, case reports, and reviews of research in progress. In some cases the quality of evidence supporting the use of an established assessment or treatment approach for a particular core symptom will have changed significantly in either a positive or negative direction. *It is the practitioner's responsibility to the patient to ensure that specific assessment and treatment recommendations are based on the most current and most reliable information available.*

◆ Starting and Maintaining an Integrative Treatment Plan

The integrative management of cognitive, affective, and behavioral symptoms begins with a thorough history, including documentation of the severity and course of the symptom pattern, accurate identification of co-occurring mental health or medical problems, and a review of biological, psychological, cultural, and possibly energetic or spiritual causes or meanings of symptoms. Based on the patient's unique history, assessment leads to a multilevel formulation (see Chapter 5) and an initial integrative treatment plan (see Chapter 6). The most appropriate and realistic integrative strategy for each patient is subsequently determined on the basis of the evidence tables for a specified core symptom pattern, taking into account the patient's history of response to previous conventional, nonconventional, or combined treatments, pertinent assessment findings, the patient's preferences (which may reflect individual cultural or socioeconomic differences) or financial constraints, and local availability of a qualified provider of a recommended conventional or nonconventional modality. When a patient is initially seen by a conventionally trained physician, it is appropriate to refer him or her to a nonconventional medical practitioner only after the risk of suicide or a life-threatening medical problem has been ruled out, informed consent has been obtained and documented in the patient's chart, and a qualified local practitioner of the recommended modality has been identified.

When history or current symptoms suggest the need for assessment beyond a comprehensive interview and a Mini-Mental State Examination (MMSE), the practitioner uses the evidence tables to identify the highest ranked assessment approaches that provide specific diagnostic information. Check the companion Web site (www.thieme.com/mentalhealth) for regular updates of the evidence tables showing different assessment approaches. The patient should be referred to an appropriate laboratory for biological assessments, including urine or serum studies. Appendix B provides Web sites and other resources that will help you locate reliable resources for the various assessment approaches discussed in this book. Assessment and treatment planning are usually discussed in parallel during the initial consultation.

When deriving an integrative treatment plan, it is always prudent to first consider using substantiated treatments. In cases where a previously tried substantiated treatment was ineffective, the patient's history suggests that an adequate dose or duration were not used, significant adverse effects led to noncompliance, or the patient was not treated by a skilled practitioner, it is reasonable to encourage the patient to try the same modality again, while following a more effective protocol or working with a more qualified practitioner. In cases where a previously used substantiated conventional or nonconventional treatment has been effective, it is reasonable to recommend resuming the same treatment. Important exceptions to this general rule include cases in which a patient responded to a particular conventional or nonconventional treatment but is ambivalent about resuming the treatment because of concerns over adverse effects or cannot afford the treatment. In such cases the relevant evidence tables are used to identify the highest ranked treatments that have not been previously tried. Check the companion Web site to ensure that the information on which you are basing the treatment plan is current and accurate. The evidence tables in the Web site are updated on a regular basis. The highest ranked modalities are presented to the patient as the most viable treatment alternatives. In most cases more than one substantiated modality can serve as the core treatment of the optimum integrative treatment plan for a particular patient. A realistic treatment plan is subsequently determined on the basis of the patient's openness to trying one or more recommended treatments, cost or insurance considerations, and local availability of a qualified practitioner (i.e., when a practitioner is required for the recommended treatment).

Appendix B lists resources that will help you locate reliable sources of the various nonconventional treatments discussed in this book, and includes Web-based directories of practitioners trained in diverse nonconventional modalities. In cases where all substantiated treatments have already been tried and proven ineffective, are unacceptable to the patient, unavailable locally, or unaffordable, the practitioner should encourage the patient to consider specific synergistic treatment combinations (i.e., when there is evidence for combinations), including at least one substantiated conventional or nonconventional modality together with at least one provisional or possibly effective approach. The evidence tables include comments on synergistic treatment combinations reviewed in detail in the text that are sometimes more effective than individual conventional or nonconventional treatments.

In most cases provisional treatments are considered after appropriate substantiated conventional and nonconventional approaches have been exhausted. The patient may refuse to consider certain substantiated treatments because of concerns over adverse effects, or a recommended treatment may be unaffordable or unavailable where the patient lives. Recommending a specific nonconventional treatment when a qualified practitioner of that modality is not available locally, or the treatment is unaffordable or is unacceptable for other reasons, may delay or compromise patient care. In some cases, combining a provisional treatment with a substantiated treatment is more effective than using a single substantiated conventional or nonconventional approach alone. Evidence supporting specific combinations of substantiated and provisional approaches is summarized in the evidence tables. It is generally appropriate to consider treatments that are regarded as possibly effective in cases where substantiated and provisional treatment choices have been exhausted or excluded for reasons discussed above. The practitioner is encouraged to check the companion Web site for updates, as some treatments listed as possibly effective may have become substantiated by new research findings. The same logic is employed when selecting possibly effective treatments to use in combination with other provisional or substantiated modalities, as when considering whether to combine different substantiated or provisional treatments. Changes in symptoms, emerging assessment findings, or significant new history are taken into account during follow-up appointments. Assessment and treatment continue until an effective individualized integrative strategy is achieved.

As in conventional psychiatric treatment planning, in some cases treatment fails when all appropriate modalities and reasonable treatment combinations have been tried without success. In such difficult cases it is often helpful to work collaboratively with other practitioners to ensure that the patient's symptoms are thoroughly evaluated, and to consider creating new assessment or treatment strategies.

I have argued in the first part of this book that the methodology and clinical methods of integrative mental health care cannot potentially provide the deep insights achieved through long-term psychotherapy, a supportive relationship with a loved one, or ongoing spiritual work. It is thus important to encourage patients who do not respond to the approaches discussed in this book to consider undergoing long-term psychotherapy if they are not already doing so.

The integrative practitioner should always keep in mind that he or she implicitly assumes liability when referring a patient to any other medical practitioner. This is especially true for conventionally trained physicians making referrals to nonconventional medical practitioners. Thus any integrative practitioner should carefully review with the patient what is known about the effectiveness and safety of any recommended treatment before making a referral. A brief note in the patient's chart should be made to document that informed consent has taken place. A moderately depressed patient who wishes to receive acupuncture treatment, for example, should be informed that several studies and extensive anecdotal reports suggest that acupuncture will probably be beneficial assuming that a qualified Chinese medical practitioner is available to administer the treatment. However, a severely depressed individual should not be advised to seek acupuncture treatment, because current research evidence does not strongly support the use of acupuncture for the management of severe depressed mood.

The integrative treatment of a cognitive or emotional symptom may initially involve a single approach, or a combination of two or more particular biological, somatic, mind-body, and energetic treatments. The most suitable treatment plan will probably vary from patient to patient. The preferred treatment plan for one patient may involve taking supplements and following a self-directed mind–body program, for example, the daily practice of yoga. The optimum realistic treatment plan for another patient with similar symptoms may involve a referral to an expert nonconventional medical practitioner. The pros and cons of choosing a single approach versus multiple approaches in parallel, as well as self-treatment versus expert referral, are discussed in Chapter 6.

Potentially unsafe treatment combinations should always be avoided and actively discouraged, whereas safe combinations that produce synergistic benefits should be strongly encouraged. Examples of synergistic combinations in the treatment of depressed mood include exercising while exposed to bright light, and taking essential fatty acids or folate with a conventional antidepressant or S-adenosylmethionine.

Moderately symptomatic patients should be encouraged to initially try combining self-directed approaches, including exercise, improved nutrition, appropriate supplements, and mind–body practices, in parallel before taking conventional or natural product–derived treatments. Combining these approaches can reasonably be expected to improve moderate symptoms as effectively as conventional medications, while avoiding adverse effects of drugs. Self-directed changes in lifestyle and nutrition empower the patient to pursue a range of healthy nutritional or mind–body practices with demonstrated efficacy against mild to moderate symptoms. Furthermore, there are no contraindications to combining lifestyle changes with conventional medications or nonconventional biological treatments. If a moderately symptomatic patient elects to start a conventional medication after considering the range of effective and available treatment options, safety issues, including adverse effects and potential incompatibilities between the drug and any natural products that are being used concurrently, should be reviewed by a conventionally trained physician or other qualified Western medical practitioner. In all cases the practitioner should obtain and document informed consent regarding risks associated with the selected treatment. Severely symptomatic patients should be encouraged initially to try a substantiated biological treatment alone or in combination with supplements known to provide synergistic benefits for the core symptom pattern. Exercise, relaxation, and substantiated nonconventional treatments that are congruent with the patient's cultural values or beliefs should also be recommended when the patient is motivated to pursue these approaches and the treatments are affordable. Severely symptomatic patients who do not respond to a substantiated biological treatment or a conventional medication and do not complain of adverse effects should be encouraged to continue their conventional treatment while starting a trial on a natural product that works synergistically with their current biological treatment.

In some cases it is beneficial to try at least one other approach that addresses the target symptom, including modifying nutrition, regular exercise, a mind–body practice, and bright light exposure. In many cases treatment recommendations will depend largely on the degree of the patient's functional impairment, as well as his or her level of interest in a novel approach. Natural products that enhance the efficacy of conventional psychiatric drugs include folate, thiamine, vitamin B_{12}, 5-hydroxytryptophan, and essential fatty acids.

Severely symptomatic patients frequently experience other cognitive, emotional, or behavioral symptoms concurrently, including anxiety, psychosis, cognitive impairment, depressed mood, or disturbances of sleep or wakefulness. When treating a severely symptomatic patient who presents with a complex symptom pattern, it is important to consider appropriate assessment and treatment strategies that address the symptoms of greatest concern. Treatment-planning algorithms in each chapter are linked to exhibits showing assessment and treatment approaches that can be used when two or more core symptom patterns are being addressed at the same time.

◆ Algorithms: An Introduction to Their Use

All symptom-focused chapters include algorithms based on assessment and treatment methods pertinent to the core symptom pattern being discussed. **Figure 7–1** illustrates the

Intake
- Chief complaint [major presenting symptom(s)]
- Complete medical, ψ, social, family, cultural Hx
- Review of medical and ψ Sx
- Document previous Rx and Rx response for recurring Sx
- Structured clinical interview (similar to DSM-4)

Urgent medical or ψ referral ① if suicidal/homicidal/gradely disabled or potentially urgent medical problem

Further Assessment (if indicated by history) ②
- Indicated in cases where primary Sx pattern is vague or causes unclear from intake + Hx
- See evidence tables in Part II chapters
- Assessment targets are one or more psychological, biological, somatic, or validated or non-validated energy-information causes of Sx "X"

Note: There is often a provisional formulation while additional studies are pending.

If >1 primary ψ Sx is present, use table for integrative planning ③

Formulation ④
- Core Sx pattern(s) identified
- Multifactorial, biological, somatic/mind-body, energy-information causes or conditions underlying Sx pattern are postulated from Hx and assessment

Integrative Treatment Plan (initial) ⑤
- (See below when >1 core Sx)
- Ideal integrative Rx plan follows formulation and best evidence (See Part II evidence tables). Review detailed evidence tables and updates on website (www.thieme.com/mentalhealth) before making final plan
- "Realistic" integrative Rx plan based on any constraints and patient preferences
- Clinician and patient agree on desired outcomes and reasonable timeframe for Rx response
- Review safety issues. Obtain signed consent.
- Make referrals, if indicated
- Issues addressed include: self-Rx vs. professional Rx, single "core" Rx vs. multiple Rx, CAM vs. conventional vs. integrative Rx plan

(*Note*: when conventional drugs indicated, patient should follow directions given by physician)

If >1 primary ψ ③ Sx is present, use table for integrative Rx planning

Outcome (initial) ⑥
- Change in Sx (better or worse)
- Quantifiable outcomes achieved (e.g., significant improvement in Sx severity on standardized scale)
- Qualitative outcomes achieved (improved life quality, etc.)

① Urgent referral to the closest emergency room or urgent care facility is always indicated when a patient is suicidal, homicidal, unable to care for basic needs of food, clothing, or shelter, or has a serious medical problem that is not being treated by a Western M.D.

② Formal assessment is not always indicated (e.g., in cases where Hx or previous Rx-response have already been clearly established).

③ All Sx-focused algorithms in Part II chapters include evidence tables showing assessment and treatment approaches addressing complex Sx patterns (i.e., when 2 or more core Sx occur together).

④ Significant new findings, emerging Sx, or newly disclosed Hx lead to changes in formulation. However the initial formulation may remain unchanged in the absence of new information.

⑤ Moderate Sx often respond to lifestyle changes, mind-body practices, and energy-information therapies, in addition to biological treatments.

When treating severe Sx, emphasis should be on biological therapies including conventional drugs, natural products, and evidence–based combinations that target the core Sx pattern. Other treatments including somatic, mind-body, and energy-information modalities, are sometimes beneficial alone or in combination with conventional drugs (see evidence tables for core symptom).

Cycles of assessment, formulation, and treatment continue until the target Sx resolves or Sx persists after all reasonable Rx have been tried. The practitioner and patient then consider goals of continued maintainence therapy versus treatment termination.

⑥ Useful outcome measures in mental health care can be quantitative or qualitative.

Figure 7–1 Algorithm for integrative assessment and treatment planning (general). See the companion Web site (www.thieme.com/mentalhealth) for updates before finalizing plans. See evidence tables and text for complete reviews of evidence-based options. Note that integrative management can proceed to further assessment and changes in formulation if indicated, but may also go directly to a modified treatment plan. Dx, diagnosis; Hx, history; Rx, treatment; Sx, symptoms; TK, psychological.

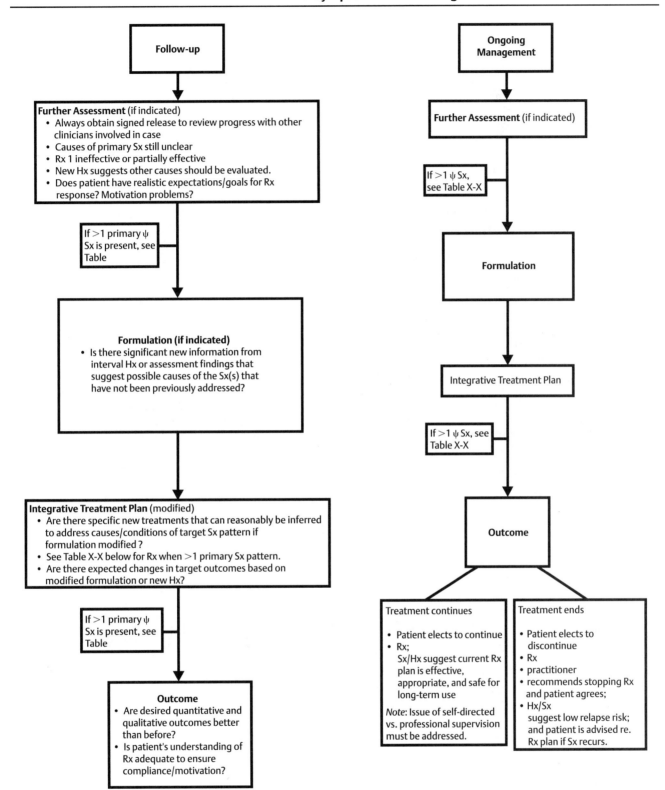

Figure 7–1 *(Continued)*

features of algorithms and how they are used. The algorithms are intended to provide practitioners with the necessary conceptual tools to develop individualized integrative assessment and treatment strategies for a particular patient on the basis of the evidence discussed in the symptom-focused chapters (and updated in the companion Web site).

Integrative management guidelines are derived from the medical, social, family, psychiatric, and spiritual history in the context of what is known about the patient's response to previous conventional or nonconventional treatments, and the highest ranked assessment or treatment approaches that have not yet been tried for a specified core symptom pattern. Both conventional and nonconventional assessment and treatment approaches are identified where relevant. Conventional assessment approaches include the MMSE, structured clinical interviews, and biological assays of the urine and blood. Conventional treatments include psychotherapy, synthetic drugs, and electroconvulsive therapy. Representative nonconventional assessment approaches include functional assessment of the serum or urine, quantitative electroencephalography (qEEG) mapping of electrical brain activity, analysis of the vascular autonomic signal, and Chinese pulse diagnosis. Representative nonconventional treatment approaches include Western herbals; Chinese, Ayurvedic, and other herbal formulas; acupuncture; homeopathic remedies; somatic therapies and mind–body practices; and emerging technology-based approaches, for example, virtual reality graded exposure therapy and EEG biofeedback. In addition to these formalized treatment approaches, exercise, dietary modifications, relaxation, and guided imagery are included where relevant. The algorithms can be used to formulate parallel and sequential treatment strategies for the core symptom patterns discussed. During the course of treatment, integrative management progresses from the most substantiated approaches to provisional or possibly effective combinations of disparate biological, somatic, mind–body, or energy-information treatments.

The algorithms in this book expand on the basic empirical methodology and criteria used in conventional psychiatric treatment guidelines, and are used to determine the most effective and appropriate integrative strategies with respect to a particular symptom pattern in the context of the patient's unique history, circumstances, and preferences. They are based on quantitative and qualitative, empirical and nonempirical criteria. The general methodology for evaluating the quality and relevance of clinical information and ranking evidence" is developed in Chapter 4, Foundations of Clinical Methodology in Integrative Medicine.

An optimum integrative treatment plan is developed for every patient, taking into account the evidence for a range of conventional and nonconventional assessment and treatment choices. A practical or realistic treatment plan is subsequently identified on the basis of patient preferences, financial or insurance constraints, and local availability of qualified conventional or nonconventional practitioners.

The clinical content and logical structure of the algorithms will evolve over time in response to conceptual advances in medicine, emerging clinical methods, and new research findings pertaining to existing assessment and treatment techniques. Significant changes in the structure or content of the algorithms will be included in updates to the companion Web site.

8

Integrative Management of Depressed Mood

Energy-information approaches validated by Western science

Energy-information approaches not validated by Western science

◆ **Integrative Management Algorithm for Depressed Mood**, 166

◆ **Integrated Approaches to Consider When Two or More Core Symptoms Are Present**, 168

Case vignette

This chapter covers the integrative management of depressed mood only. Mania and cyclic mood changes are addressed in Chapter 9.

◆ Economic and Social Costs of Depression

Depression is one of the most serious and costly health problems facing the world today. Because of the high incidence of suicide and other medical or mental illness in depressed individuals, depression is regarded as the leading cause of death and disability from adolescence through middle age. The total economic burden of depression in the United States alone in terms of direct costs, mortality costs from depression-related suicides, and lost workplace productivity grew from $52.9 billion in 1990 to $83.1 billion in 2000. During the same 10-year period, direct treatment costs for depression increased from $19.9 billion to $26.1 billion (Greenberg et al., 2003). Approximately 15% of adults will experience severe depressed mood during their lifetimes, and ~15% of these will eventually commit suicide.

Available conventional treatment approaches do not adequately address depressed mood. In the medical community and the public at large there is growing debate over the efficacy and safety of conventional antidepressants. Controversy over the efficacy of conventional antidepressants deepened in 2004 because of allegations of a "file drawer" effect that may positively bias outcomes data on antidepressants and other conventional pharmacological treatments in psychiatry. When published research data are analyzed together with findings that were previously classified by the U.S. Food and Drug Administration (FDA), the effect sizes of many conventional antidepressants are substantially reduced (Sussman, 2004). On this basis it has been argued that many antidepressants are probably no more effective than placebo. This becomes even more concerning when high placebo response rates of most large controlled studies on antidepressants are taken into account. The U.S. House Oversight and Investigations Subcommittee of the Energy and Commerce Committee recently criticized the pharmaceutical industry for selectively publishing only studies with positive outcomes. Legislation is now pending that will require drug companies to post clinical trials data in a timely manner (The Fair Access to Clinical Trials Act HR 5252). During the same hearings the FDA was criticized for its failure to disclose negative findings of many industry-sponsored drug studies on antidepressants and other psychiatric medications (Bender, 2004; Sussman, 2004). In October 2004, the FDA issued a black box warning on the use of all antidepressants in children and adolescents on the basis of a meta-analysis of 24 placebo-controlled trials on antidepressants involving more than 4000 children, claiming that children and adolescents who use these drugs have an 80% greater risk of attempting suicide compared with children taking a placebo ("FDA Black Box Warning," 2004). Two retrospective analyses of large cohorts taking conventional antidepressants failed to confirm an above-chance correlation between increased risk of suicide and any age group, including children and adolescents (Isacsson, Holmgren, & Ahlner, 2005; Martinez et al., 2005). Both studies cite confounding factors not addressed in the original meta-analysis that resulted in the FDA black box warning that probably affect the risk of suicide. Another retrospective review of U.S. suicides between 1996 and 1998 found a positive relationship between tricyclic antidepressants and suicide risk but no correlation between selective serotonin reuptake inhibitors (SSRIs) or other nontricyclics and suicide (Gibbons, Bhaumik, & Mann, 2005).

At the time of this writing debate is ongoing over the relationship between conventional antidepressant use and increased suicide risk in the general population, particularly children and adolescents. In response to concerns over the safety of antidepressants and other conventional drugs, in early 2005 the FDA directed the Institute of Medicine to undertake a formal review of procedures used by pharmaceutical manufacturers to monitor drug safety, especially after a new drug has gone to market (Mechcatie, 2004). The *Journal of the American Medical Association* and other leading peer-reviewed medical journals have responded to these safety concerns by requiring that all studies considered for publication after July 1, 2005, must first be posted in a clinical trials registry that is open to the public.

◆ The Western Medical Model of Depressed Mood

In Western medicine there is still no dominant theory explaining the pathogenesis of depressed mood. Research findings suggest that chronic depressed mood is probably associated with many psychological, biological, and environmental factors, including dysregulation at the level of neurotransmitters and their receptors, problems in endocrinological and immune functioning and other medical illnesses, environmental toxins, adverse effects of prescribed drugs, substance abuse, and chronic stress. Because of the multiplicity of factors associated with depressed mood, it is often difficult to distinguish between causes and effects. For example, brain-imaging studies have confirmed atrophy in a part of the brain (the hippocampus) that may predispose individuals to depressed mood—and associated neuropsychological impairments—or result from prolonged cortisol elevation related to chronic stress (Schatzberg, 2002). Western psychiatry describes many distinct affective disorders in which persisting core symptoms of depressed mood occur in the context of a broader symptom pattern that may include psychosis, or lesser or greater degrees of mania (e.g., euphoric, agitated, or irritable mood; racing thoughts; and diminished need for sleep). For purposes of formulating an appropriate and effective integrative treatment plan addressing mood symptoms, it is important to distinguish individuals who report depressed mood only from those who are depressed in the context of an underlying medical illness or ongoing substance abuse, or who also experience symptoms of mania, hypomania, or psychosis. The fourth edition of *Diagnostic and Statistical Manual of Mental Disorders–Text Revision* (*DSM-IV-TR*) describes two principle patterns, or "disorders," of depressed mood depending on the course and severity of symptoms: major depressive disorder and dysthymic disorder. Western psychiatry defines **dysthymic disorder** as a symptom pattern in which chronic depressed mood of moderate intensity persists at least 2 years, together with two or more of the following symptoms: change in sleep, change in appetite, fatigue, agitation or slowing, diminished concentration, and feelings of worthlessness (but *not* thoughts of death or suicide). In contrast, **major depressive disorder** is a symptom pattern in which recurring episodes of severe depressed mood, including thoughts of suicide or death, last at least 2 weeks, together with at least five of the above symptoms. The diagnosis is confirmed through history, clinical presentation, and the elimination of possible confounding medical problems or substance abuse. In spite of differences in naming and classifying mood symptoms, most Western systems of medicine address symptoms that resemble the subjective experience of chronic depressed mood as it is generally reported by patients.

According to *DSM-IV* criteria, when sustained euphoric or irritable mood (i.e., a manic or hypomanic episode) is present, the principle diagnosis cannot be dysthymia or major depressive disorder. When recurring depressive episodes of variable severity and duration are interspersed with brief periods of moderate or severe euphoria or irritability and longer periods of sustained normal or "euthymic" mood, the Western diagnosis is cyclothymic or bipolar disorder, Unipolar depressed mood, also called major depressive disorder, is characterized by depressive mood episodes of varying duration and severity. In contrast, a diagnosis of cyclothymic disorder is made when the patient complains of mild to moderate depressive mood changes interspersed with episodes of hypomania. According to the DSM criteria, Bipolar Disorder is a syndrome characterized by more severe depressive and manic cycles. Symptom patterns described as psychotic disorders or severe personality disorders in conventional psychiatric nosology may also include depressed mood as a prominent feature. However, in those cases depressed mood is typically not the focus of clinical attention. The *DSM-IV-TR* stipulates that specific criteria must be fulfilled to diagnose a particular mood disorder; however, the longitudinal course of chronic depressed mood is highly variable, and over the course of their illness patients generally experience minor or severe episodes of depression interspersed with quiescent periods or other concurrent psychiatric symptoms (Judd, 2004).

about medical, psychiatric, family, and social history that may be related to a patient's complaint of depressed mood. The Mini-Mental State Exam (MMSE), Beck Depression Inventory, and Hamilton Depression Inventory are structured interview tools commonly used to assess the relative severity of symptoms as well as the social and psychodynamic factors associated with depressed mood. In addition to the clinical interview, laboratory screening studies are sometimes used to assess possible endocrinological, infectious, or metabolic causes of depressed mood. Bioassays that identify underlying medical causes of depressed mood include thyroid studies (free thyroxine, or T4 [FT4], and thyroid-stimulating hormone [TSH]), fasting blood glucose, liver enzymes, complete blood count (CBC), serum iron levels, serum electrolytes, blood urea nitrogen (BUN), and urinary creatinine. When an underlying medical problem, substance abuse, or medication side effects contribute to mood changes, these are treated directly. When depressed mood does not resolve after a suspected medical cause has been treated, assessment continues until underlying psychological or medical causes are adequately addressed.

Conventional Assessment Is Limited by Flawed Standardized Symptom Rating Instruments and Poorly Defined Criteria

A meta-analysis of 70 studies on the Hamilton Depression Scale suggests that this standardized instrument is conceptually flawed and does not reliably measure treatment outcomes (Babgy, Gyder, Schuller, & Marshall, 2004) In 2003 a panel of experts submitted recommendations to the American College of Neuropsychopharmacology (ACNP) in hopes of quantifying the definitions of these terms (Boschert, 2003). The panel agreed that an improvement of less than 25% constitutes a **nonresponse,** that an improvement in symptoms between 26 and 49% is a **partial response,** and that clinically significant responses can be reliably assessed only if they last at least 3 weeks (in contrast to a previously used criterion that defined a **response** as a significant reduction in symptoms lasting at least 1 week). The same expert panel defined **remission** as significant clinical improvement lasting at least 3 consecutive weeks in which no more than 2 of the 9 symptoms designated in the *DSM-IV* for a major depressive episode are present. A **partial remission** in a major depressive episode takes place when there is at least a 50% reduction in baseline symptoms, but the full criteria for remission are not met. When a patient in remission does not experience recurring symptoms for at least 8 consecutive weeks, he or she fulfills criteria for **recovery.** The response rates of most patients to conventional antidepressants are not well defined because most studies do not quantify treatment outcomes using these formal criteria. Furthermore, relatively few psychiatrists are aware of, or regularly employ, stringent research criteria to assess clinical outcomes when treating depressed patients.

◆ The Integrative Assessment of Depressed Mood

Conventional assessment approaches in current use provide largely ambiguous information about the putative biological or other causes of depressed mood. Western-trained psychiatrists rely on structured interviews to obtain salient information

◆ Overview of Nonconventional Approaches Used to Assess Depressed Mood

Serum folate levels are consistently low in depressed patients and predict nonresponse to conventional antidepressants and increased relapse risk. Research findings suggest that red blood cell (RBC) fatty acid composition is a useful predictor of differential response rates of depressed mood to different biological treatments, including dietary changes, omega-3 fatty acid supplementation, and conventional antidepressants. Assays of RBC membrane composition of certain fatty acids will probably come into common use in the assessment of depressed mood. A total serum cholesterol level below 150 mg/dL is strongly correlated with severe depression and increased risk of violent suicide attempts and will probably become a standard assessment approach in this population. Serum homocysteine levels are potential indicators of metabolic imbalances associated with depressed mood, and this bioassay will probably come into increasing use in the assessment of underlying metabolic causes of depressed mood. This assessment approach is attracting research interest because of the close relationship between elevated serum homocysteine levels, depressed mood, and heart disease. Quantitative urinary and serum analysis of neurotransmitter metabolites (including serotonin and γ-aminobutyric acid [GABA]) may provide useful information about neurochemical or metabolic factors associated with depression that will establish an empirical basis for future conventional and integrative treatment strategies. Quantitative electroencephalography (qEEG) brain mapping holds significant promise as a clinically useful predictor of differential response rates to conventional antidepressants based on disparate mechanisms of action. Advances in qEEG brain mapping will probably become a standard approach in the neuropsychiatric assessment of treatment-resistant depression. Preliminary findings suggest that low serum levels of phenylethylamine (PEA) and phenylacetic acid (PAA) occur in some cases of depressed mood, indicating the need for specific amino acid supplementation strategies. At present, limited research evidence supports the use of Chinese pulse diagnosis, analysis of the vascular autonomic signal (VAS), applied kinesiology, and homeopathic constitutional analysis, but these approaches may help to clarify energetic imbalances associated with some cases of depressed mood. **Table 8–1** summarizes substantiated and provisional nonconventional approaches in current use to assess depressed mood.

Table 8–1 Substantiated and Provisional Nonconventional Approaches Used to Assess Depressed Mood

	Assessment Approach	Evidence for Specific Diagnostic Information	Positive Finding Suggests Efficacy of This Treatment
Substantiated			
Biological	Serum levels of certain vitamins Serum triglyceride and cholesterol levels	Low serum folate predicts nonresponse to conventional and nonconventional treatments Low B$_{12}$ and vitamin E levels often found in depressed patients Low total serum triglycerides and cholesterol levels correlate with more severe depressed mood and higher risk of suicide *A total serum cholesterol level lower than 150 mg/dL is a specific indicator of significant risk of violent suicide attempt*	Deficiency states indicate need to supplement with folate, vitamins B$_{12}$ or E *Always check serum lipid levels in severely depressed, treatment refractory, or suicidal patients* Reasonable modifications in diet, and possibly also changes in cholesterol-lowering medications, should be explored when addressing total cholesterol levels lower than 160 mg/dL
Energy-information assessment methods validated by Western science	qEEG and AER	Increased α or θ, decreased interhemispheric coherence in unipolar depression Reduced α and increased β in bipolar depression High AER predicts improved response to SSRIs Negative prefrontal cordance predicts improved response to SSRIs and homeopathic treatments	Abnormal qEEG findings suggest specific treatment strategies and differentiate unipolar from bipolar depressed mood
Provisional			
Biological	RBC fatty acids	Low RBC omega-3 fatty acids are correlated with more severe depressed mood	Augmentation of conventional Rx with omega-3 fatty acids may improve response
Energy-information assessment approaches validated by Western science	qEEG	qEEG changes in responders correspond to therapeutic concentrations of hyperforin in St. John's wort	Specific qEEG findings may predict differential response to certain kinds of antidepressants
Energy-information assessment approaches in use but not validated by Western science	None at time of writing		

AER, auditory evoked response; qEEG, quantitative electroencephalography; RBC, red blood cell (count); Rx, treatment; SSRI, selective serotonin reuptake inhibitor

◆ Substantiated Approaches Used to Assess Depressed Mood

Low Serum Folate Levels Are Common in Depressed Patients

Low serum folate levels predict more severe depressed mood and nonresponse to fluoxetine (Prozac), other conventional antidepressants, lithium augmentation, and thyroid hormone (Fava et al., 1997; Papakostas et al., 2004a,b). A significant percentage of severely depressed patients have low serum folate levels (Bottiglieri, 1996). Many treatment refractory depressed patients respond to conventional or nonconventional treatments when folate in the form of folinic acid is added to their existing regimen (Papakostas, 2004b). Furthermore, low serum folate levels are associated with an increased risk of relapse in patients who have successfully responded to fluoxetine and other conventional antidepressants (Papakostas, 2004a). On this basis it is prudent to check the serum folate level in any patient who does not respond to a conventional or nonconventional treatment of depressed mood.

qEEG Is Helpful in Differentiating Unipolar and Bipolar Depressed Mood

Abnormal EEG findings occur in up to 40% of depressed patients (Small, 1993). EEG changes described as "small, sharp spikes" are often present in severely depressed suicidal patients (Small, 1993). Basic research is ongoing to develop normative databases to enhance diagnostic accuracy when psychiatric symptoms are evaluated using EEG or qEEG (Thatcher, 1998). Quantitative electroencephalography analysis of unipolar depressed patients typically reveals increased alpha (α) or theta (θ) power, and decreased interhemispheric coherence (Nieber & Schlegel, 1992; Princhep et al., 1990). In contrast, bipolar depressed patients often have reduced α activity and increased beta (β) power (John, 1988). Many bipolar patients come to treatment after experiencing a single major depressive episode but have not yet had a manic episode. In such cases a qEEG map provides valuable diagnostic information that can inform the most appropriate treatment. Although there are no definitive correlations between specific qEEG findings and different categories of depressed mood, reduced α activity and increased β power point to the likelihood of an evolving bipolar picture. The clinician and patient can then plan appropriate treatment strategies. In contrast, findings of increased α or θ power suggest that the correct diagnosis is probably unipolar depression, and appropriate conventional or integrative treatments can be aggressively instituted.

Abnormal High AER or Decreased Prefrontal Cordance Predicts Enhanced Antidepressant Response Rates

Response rates to conventional antidepressants can be predicted on the basis of differences in brain electrical activity evoked by sounds of various intensities. The brain's response to an auditory signal is called an auditory evoked response (AER). Relatively greater AERs correspond to lower activity of brain serotonin and predict improved response of unipolar depressed patients (Gallinat et al., 2000) to SSRIs. This finding has been corroborated by prospective studies examining the relationship between *cordance* and response to antidepressants that increase brain serotonin levels (Suffin et al., 1997). Cordance is a measure of localized electrical brain activity relative to averaged brain EEG patterns. Numerous studies have established a correlation between cordance and measures of brain perfusion or regional metabolic activity as shown by functional magnetic resonance imaging (MRI) and positron emission tomography (PET). Significant reductions in brain serotonin levels and associated slowing in EEG activity take place when healthy volunteers drink a tryptophan-depleting mixture of amino acids (Knott, Howson, Perugini, Ravindran, & Young, 1999). This finding has been substantiated by clinical data. Over half of patients with severe depressed mood who subsequently had the highest response rates to SSRIs showed significant decreases in prefrontal cordance during the first 48 hours of therapy, suggesting that improvement was due to normalization of low brain serotonin levels (Cook et al., 2002; Demott, 2002). In contrast, nonresponders to SSRIs or placebo did not show negative prefrontal cordance following treatment, suggesting that low serotonin was not the primary cause of depressed mood in these cases. Differences in prefrontal EEG cordance also predict response differences of depressed patients to homeopathic remedies (Bell et al., 2004).

◆ Provisional Approaches Used to Assess Depressed Mood

Low RBC Membrane Fatty Acids May Be Correlated with Increased Severity of Depressed Mood

Red blood cell membrane levels and serum levels of docosahexaenoic acid (DHA), an omega-3 fatty acid, are consistently lower in depressed individuals (Peet, Murphy, Shay, & Horrobin, 1998; Tiemeier, van Tuijl, Hofman, Kiliaan, & Breteler, 2003). Preliminary findings suggest that the average dietary ratio of omega-6 to omega-3 essential fatty acids is correlated with incidence of depression. Lower dietary intake of foods rich in omega-3 fatty acids resulted in relatively higher ratios of arachidonic acid (AA) (an omega-6) to ecosapentanoic acid (EPA) (an omega-3) in red blood cells, which in turn were positively correlated with greater severity of depressed mood (Edwards, Peet, Shay, & Horrobin, 1998). The relationship between RBC levels of omega-3s and depressed mood remains unclear because of the high rate of smoking among depressed patients (Quattrocki, Baird, & Yurgelun-Todd, 2000). Smoking has been correlated with both diminished consumption of foods rich in omega-3s and abnormally low omega-3 tissue levels (Leng et al., 1994).

Low Serum Cholesterol Levels Are Correlated with Severity of Depressed Mood and Suicide Risk

Depressed patients who attempt suicide have abnormal low serum total cholesterol and triglyceride levels, which may provide future clinical markers for suicide risk (Bocchetta, 2001). Low serum lipid levels are associated with persistently low platelet serotonin levels in depressed suicidal patients (Steegmans et al., 1996). Low cholesterol levels indirectly lead to reduced brain serotonin because of the requirement of adequate cholesterol in nerve cell membranes to maintain the functional integrity of serotonin receptors (Sarchiapone 2001;

Steegmans et al., 1996). Total serum cholesterol and triglyceride levels are significantly decreased in patients who are considering suicide or who have recently attempted suicide (Yong-Ku, 2003). This observation is consistent with a high rate of severe depression and suicide attempts in individuals afflicted with a rare genetic syndrome that causes an enzyme deficiency resulting in abnormal low serum cholesterol (Lalovic et al., 2004). The findings of a large case-control study suggest that an inverse relationship exists between the severity of depressed mood and serum total cholesterol (Kim & Myint, 2004). Nonsuicidal depressives tend to have cholesterol levels in the range of 180 mg/dL, and severely depressed suicidal patients tend to have serum total cholesterol levels in the range of 150 mg/dL. On the basis of these findings, it is prudent to check cholesterol levels of severely depressed patients, to make appropriate dietary recommendations, and to address issues related to the use of cholesterol-lowering medications. In addition, suicide precautions should be undertaken when managing a severely depressed patient with a serum total cholesterol level of 150 mg/dL or lower.

◆ Determining Causes of Depressed Mood

Table 8–2 outlines the following assessment approaches that may provide specific diagnostic information about the causes of depressed mood.

Positive Dexamethasone Suppression Test is Found in Women but not Men

Serum cortisol levels are suppressed following dexamethasone in women but not men. A placebo-controlled study of 74 depressed inpatients showed that low levels of cortisol following dexamethasone correlated with severity of depressed mood in pre- or postmenopausal women but not in men (Osuch et al., 2001). This finding suggests important hormonal differences in the etiology of depression in men and women, and has implications for differential treatment effects of both conventional and nonconventional treatments. The dexamethasone suppression test (DST) is probably not a useful indicator of the pathophysiological basis of depressed mood in men.

Urinary Metabolites of Neurotransmitters may be Correlated with Severity of Depressed Mood

Both norepinephrine and serotonin probably have important roles in depressed mood. To date, consistent correlations have not been found between depressed mood and specific neurotransmitter metabolites in the urine or serum (Delgado, 2000). Neurotransmitter dysregulations associated with depressed mood are probably highly idiosyncratic and related to multiple genetic, dietary, and other environmental factors (personal communication, Kellerman, Neuroscience Inc., February 2005).

Table 8–2 Assessment Approaches That May Provide Specific Diagnostic Information about Causes of Depressed Mood

Category	Assessment Approach	Evidence for Specific Diagnostic Information	Comments
Biological	DST Urinary PEA and PAA	Serum cortisol levels are suppressed following dexamethasone in severely depressed women but not in men PEA and PAA acid levels may be consistently low in bipolar depressed mood	Suggests differential efficacy of same treatments in men and women Low PEA (or PAA) suggests dietary amino acid deficiency or metabolic problem
Somatic	None at time of writing		
Energy-information assessment approaches validated by Western science	None at time of writing		
Energy-information assessment approaches not validated by Western science	Chinese medical pulse diagnosis and VAS reflex Homeopathic constitutional assessment Applied kinesiology	Recent grief, anguish, agitated depression, and hysterical depression are associated with distinctive pulse characteristics according to TCM theory VAS reflex may provide useful information for identifying effective conventional treatments in nonresponsive patients Specific constitutional types may correspond to different symptom patterns of depressed mood Muscle testing using applied kinesiology may provide useful information about energetic causes of depressed mood	A specific energetic pattern obtained using pulse diagnosis or VAS may suggest the most effective energetic or conventional treatment for depressed mood Constitutional analysis may permit identification of most effective homeopathic remedies Findings on applied kinesiology testing suggest certain kinds of energetic treatments

DST, dexamethasone suppression test; PAA, phenylacetic acid; PEA, phenylethylamine; TCM, traditional chinese medicine; VAS, vascular autonomic signal

Abnormal Low Urinary PEA Levels Are Seen in Bipolar Depression

Mean plasma and urine concentrations of PEA and its metabolite PAA may be consistently low in depressed individuals diagnosed with bipolar disorder (Sabelli et al., 1986), suggesting that a dietary deficiency or metabolic dysregulation affecting brain availability of phenylalanine (the amino acid precursor of PEA) may be an important etiologic factor in some cases of depressed mood.

Abnormal Electrolyte Levels Are Associated with Depressed Mood

Depressed mood is sometimes associated with abnormal high or low serum levels of calcium and magnesium, and abnormal low levels of potassium (Alarcon & Franceschini,1984; Kirov, Birch, Steadman, & Ramsey, 1994; Reiser & Reiser, 1985; Webb & Gehi, 1981).

Energy-Information Assessment Approaches That Are Not Validated by Western Science

Chinese Pulse Diagnosis and VAS

According to Chinese medical theory, depressed mood is frequently associated with kidney qi and yang essence deficiency (Flaws & Lake, 2001). Hammer (2001) has observed that recent grief or anguish is distinguishable from long-term or repressed grief on the basis of subtle pulse differences. Agitated depressed mood and hysterical depression are also associated with distinctive features of the pulse at many positions in the body. The accurate discrimination of subtle differences in the pulse provides information that is useful in planning acupuncture or herbal treatments that effectively address disparate energetic types of depressed mood.

Recent research on a phenomenon associated with the pulse called the vascular autonomic signal (VAS) reflex may ultimately validate claims of traditional pulse assessment methods in Chinese medicine, Ayurveda, and Tibetan medicine. Case report findings suggest that the VAS reflex provides clinically useful information about conventional treatments of depressed mood that are poorly responsive to conventional approaches. In one case VAS analysis determined that a 36-year-old woman who complained of irritable, depressed mood had an estrogen deficiency and identified specific doses of estrogen and L-tryptophan that reportedly resulted in a consistent improvement in her mood (Ackerman, 1989).

Homeopathic Constitutional Assessment

Homeopathy classifies individuals into different constitutional types based on a multifactorial assessment that takes into account physical, cognitive, and emotional traits. There is some evidence that certain constitutional types are more likely to experience depressed mood (Gaylord & Davidson, 1998). Furthermore, individuals who are predisposed to depressed mood may respond more to homeopathic remedies addressing specific energetic imbalances that are characteristic of those constitutional types. The constitutional analysis of individuals who are depressed because of grief may provide useful information for selecting specific homeopathic remedies addressing their specific constellation of emotional, physical and energetic symptoms (Gaylord & Davidson, 1998).

◆ The Integrative Treatment of Depressed Mood

Conventional Treatments of Depressed Mood Have Limited Efficacy and Unresolved Safety Problems

Emerging evidence suggests that the use of most conventional antidepressants for moderate or severe depressed mood is supported by provisional or ambiguous research findings. A meta-analysis of 15 randomized double-blind controlled trials concluded that conventional antidepressants are probably effective in the short-term management of dysthymic disorder (Silva de Lima, 2003). Several independent analyses have concluded that most trials of antidepressants sponsored by pharmaceutical companies fail to show significant response differences between conventional antidepressants and placebos (Hollon, DeRubeis, Shelton, & Weiss, 2002; Jacobson Roberts, Berns, & McGlinchey, 1999; Kirsch, Moore, Scoboria, & Nicholls, 2002; Thase, 2002). There is ongoing debate over the validity of antidepressant trial designs, and it has been suggested that standardized research methods bias outcomes in favor of antidepressants (Fisher & Greenberg, 1997; Quitkin, Rabkin, Gerald, Davis, & Klein, 2000). In the United States and Western European countries, more than two thirds of depressed patients never receive adequate treatment with conventional antidepressants (Girolamo et al., 2004; Remick, 2002). This is due to both inadequate screening by physicians and underreporting by patients (Simon, Fleck, Lucas, & Bushnell, 2004). Over half of all patients who use conventional antidepressants are not treated by psychiatrists and have never been formally diagnosed with depression (Frei, 2004). Of those who are diagnosed and receive recommended doses of conventional antidepressants, between 40 and 70% fail to respond (Keitner, 2004). The issue of nonresponse to conventional antidepressants is complicated by reports of overall worsening of depressed mood with long-term treatment (Fava, 2003). An analysis of 27 studies showed that there was no advantage to prolonged treatment with conventional antidepressants in terms of reduced risk of relapse, and that individuals taking conventional antidepressants for longer periods are more likely to relapse (Viguera, Baldessarini, & Friedberg, 1998). Approximately one half of individuals who fully recover from an episode of severe depressed mood relapse within 2 years regardless of whether they are taking a conventional antidepressant (Schrader 1994; Hasin et al., 1996). The findings of a placebo-controlled multicenter study showed that approximately one third of patients who stop taking conventional antidepressants after responding to them subsequently failed to respond to the same antidepressant when it was given (Schmidt et al., 2002). These findings have raised concerns about *treatment-refractory depression,* defined as the absence of a 50% or greater reduction in symptoms using a standardized rating scale during a 4-week trial on an antidepressant at a recommended dose. Systematic reviews of studies on treatment-refractory depression found little evidence to support conventional pharmacological treatments (including combined drug regimens) or psychological treatments of treatment-refractory depression (Lam, Wan, Cohen, & Kennedy, 2002; Stimpson, Agrawal, & Lewis, 2002). "Treatment-resistant" patients are twice as likely to be hospitalized, have more outpatient visits, and use more psychotropic drugs compared with patients who respond to conventional antidepressants (Crown et al., 2002). Research findings suggest that conventional antidepressants may have limited beneficial effects because they do not address impairments in neuroplasticity or neurogenesis that may underlie chronic depression (Jacobs, van Praag, & Gage, 2000; Manji, Moore, Rajkowska, & Chen, 2000). These findings suggest that future antidepressant agents with neurotrophic or neuroprotective effects (similar to lithium carbonate) may be more effective than contemporary drugs that target specific neurotransmitters but do not stimulate synaptic growth or reduce nerve cell loss or atrophy believed to be associated with chronic depressed mood (Elkis, Friedman, Wise, & Meltzer, 1995).

Recent allegations of a "file drawer" effect (see discussion above) cast further doubt on the overall efficacy of conventional antidepressants (Sussman, 2004). Most individuals who relapse following remission do so within the first 6 months. A Cochrane systematic review found that differences between patients taking antidepressants and placebos were small, and concluded that the risks associated with conventional antidepressant therapy "are less likely to be outweighed by their benefits than is currently believed to be the case" (Moncrieff, 2004). A meta-analysis of 32 randomized placebo-controlled trials concluded that recommended doses of SSRIs achieve full remission in about one third of patients, compared with a 28% remission rate in patients receiving a placebo. The same meta-analysis found a 45% remission rate in patients treated with venlafaxine, an antidepressant that targets both serotonin and norepinephrine. The response difference between SSRIs and placebo lacks statistical significance; however, this analysis showed a significant difference between placebo and venlafaxine. A Cochrane meta-analysis of 33 double-blind controlled studies of conventional antidepressants in moderate and severe depressed mood concluded that patients improved on average by 53% on the basis of standardized symptom rating scales when taking recommended doses of all classes of conventional antidepressants (Bollini, 1999). This finding is significant in view of the fact that standardized research paradigms define remission as a 50% or greater improvement in symptom severity. Furthermore, high antidepressant doses are associated with significantly increased risk of adverse effects but do not correlate with improved efficacy, whereas lower doses are associated with a slightly reduced response rate but significantly reduced adverse effects. The reviewers commented that "more research is needed on cheaper and, perhaps, more effective interventions aimed at retaining depressed patients on treatment, by managing adverse reactions and improving the therapeutic relationship between patient and physician."

The high cost of prescription drugs has become an important issue for many patients who take conventional antidepressants. In this context it is significant that the cost-effectiveness of more expensive SSRIs is equivalent to that of the older inexpensive tricyclic antidepressants (Peveler, Kendrick, Thompson, & Buxton, 2004).

The controversy surrounding conventional antidepressants was recently increased by alarming reports that the chronic use of most antidepressants in children and adolescents may be associated with increased risk of suicide. The FDA and the American Psychiatric Association are advising psychiatrists to closely monitor pediatric patients when prescribing conventional antidepressants (Hinton & Melonas, 2004; Weller, Kang, & Weller, 2004). It is significant that many nonconventional treatments of depressed mood, including St. John's wort (*Hypericum perforatum*), *S*-adenosylmethionine (SAMe), continue to be viewed with skepticism in the Western medical community because of disputed claims of antidepressant efficacy. This debate is taking place in the context of an ideological divide between orthodox biomedical psychiatry and established nonconventional approaches, and will eventually be resolved by well designed studies, rigorous analysis, and complete, unbiased disclosure of research findings for both conventional and nonconventional treatments of depressed mood.

◆ Overview of Contemporary Biomedical Treatments of Depressed Mood

Contemporary Western psychiatric treatments of depressed mood employ algorithms that guide the clinician in the logical selection of different classes of pharmaceutical agents or psychotherapy on a case-by-case basis (American Psychiatric Association, 1993, Trivedi & Kleiber, 2001). Although a mood disorder is formally diagnosed on the basis of a persisting pattern of symptoms, the selected treatment targets the core symptom or symptoms that cause the greatest impairment in social or intellectual functioning. Symptoms that constellate around depressed mood define the particular symptom-focused treatment plan that is used. For example, certain conventional antidepressants with a sedating side-effect profile are typically used for "agitated" depression, whereas drugs with stimulating adverse effects are generally used to treat "vegetative" depressed mood. Previous treatments and outcomes, symptom severity, and complicating medical problems (if any) are also taken into account. Research trials on many promising synthetic antidepressant medications are ongoing and will probably result in a new generation of safe and effective conventional treatments. Electroconvulsive therapy (ECT) is often effective when severe depressed mood has not responded to medications. Emerging conventional treatments that hold promise include transcranial magnetic stimulation (TMS) and vagal nerve stimulation (VNS). Repetitive transcranial magnetic stimulation (rTMS) may be an effective treatment of depressed mood; however, findings to date are inconsistent (Speer et al., 2000). A Cochrane review of 16 small sham-controlled studies concluded that responses of depressed patients to rTMS versus sham TMS did not differ significantly (Martin et al., 2004). More recent studies incorporating more specific treatment protocols show beneficial effects of rTMS. In contrast, exposure to low-frequency rTMS (1 Hz) causes diminished regional cerebral blood flow and does not improve mood. In a 4-week randomized prospective trial, 25 severely depressed patients randomized to repetitive TMS or ECT experienced comparable improvements in mood (Janicak, Dowd, & Martis, 2002). Repetitive pulsed TMS was administered to the left prefrontal cortex, while ECT was administered bitemporally. The mean improvement in Hamilton Depression Inventory ratings in patients who received 10 to 20 rTMS treatments was 55%, compared with an average improvement of 64% in patients who received 4 to 12 ECT treatments during the same 4-week period. In contrast to favorable findings in unipolar depressed mood, a sham-controlled study of rTMS in bipolar depressed patients did not show a benefit (Nahas, Kozel, Li, Anderson, & George, 2003).

Current "integrative" approaches in Western psychiatry include combined uses of medications and psychotherapy but exclude most nonconventional therapies. Although cognitive therapy or supportive psychotherapy is often recommended for major depression, contemporary biomedical psychiatry strongly endorses medication management as the central goal of psychiatric treatment. However, large prospective studies comparing psychotherapy to conventional antidepressants have demonstrated roughly equivalent efficacy, and patients who remain in psychotherapy may have significantly lower relapse rates compared with matched patients taking antidepressants (Elkin et al., 1989; Blackburn, Eunson, & Bishop, 1986; Casacalenda, Perry, & Looper, 2002). Conventional drugs are more effective when taken in conjunction with psychotherapy. A systematic review of 16 randomized trials concluded that patients who take antidepressants while engaged in regular psychotherapy respond more rapidly and have more sustained improvement in depressed mood compared with patients who use either approach alone (Pampallona, Bollini, Tibaldi, Kupelnick, & Minizza, 2004).

◆ Substantiated and Provisional Nonconventional Treatments of Depressed Mood

Many nonconventional treatment modalities of depressed mood have been validated by consistent positive results from controlled, double-blind studies, and in some cases, systematic reviews or meta-analyses. Combining conventional antidepressants with certain nonconventional treatments accelerates the rate of treatment response or improves outcomes overall. Nonconventional treatments that have been studied in combination with antidepressants include exercise, changes in nutrition, bright light exposure, somatic, and mind–body techniques, as well as certain nonconventional biological treatments. Many nonconventional treatments have been empirically validated and fulfill biomedical criteria for efficacy and safety but are not in widespread use in Western countries because of economic, social, or ideological factors, including limited postgraduate training in the use of nonconventional treatments in mental health care, the dominant role of the pharmaceutical industry, and widespread acceptance of conventional antidepressants. Examples of empirically validated nonconventional biological treatments of depressed mood include St. John's wort, SAMe, 5-hydroxytryptophan (5-HTP), folic acid, ecosapentanoic acid (EPA, an omega-3 essential fatty acid), and, to a lesser extent, acetyl-L-carnitine, and dehydroepiandrosterone (DHEA). Placebo-controlled double-blind studies and meta-analyses of controlled studies consistently show that SAMe has equivalent or superior antidepressant efficacy compared with tricyclic antidepressants. In contrast, most nonconventional treatments that are not based on an explicit pharmacological mechanism of action have not been rigorously examined by Western science, and therefore have relatively weaker scientific evidence supporting claims of efficacy.

St. John's wort, SAMe, 5-HTP, EPA, and acetyl-L-carnitine have been evaluated for their antidepressant efficacy alone or in combination with synthetic antidepressants. Advantages of augmenting a synthetic antidepressant with one of these natural products include equivalent response rates at reduced antidepressant doses, improved tolerance and compliance, and faster response rates. Many studies have validated the safety and efficacy of combining SAMe with a synthetic antidepressant. Folate and vitamin B_{12} are cofactors in the synthesis of SAMe and should be taken together with SAMe. Severely depressed patients found to have low serum folate levels are significantly less likely to respond to antidepressants; therefore, all depressed patients should be encouraged to take folate. Folate alone, in doses from 200 μg to 15 mg, has been shown to result in sustained improvement in depressed mood. EPA has been shown to be effective against moderate depressed mood in doses of 1, 2, or 4 g/day when used alone or in combination with an antidepressant. However, emerging evidence suggests that another omega-3 fatty acid, DHA, does not significantly improve depressed mood. Depressed patients taking SAMe or EPA should be monitored for signs of hypomania, which has been reported in a few cases. Depressed mood also responds to 5-HTP alone or in combination with a synthetic antidepressant. 5-HTP crosses the blood–brain barrier, where it is converted to serotonin. Similar to SAMe and antidepressants, 5-HTP and a synthetic antidepressant potentiate each other, sometimes resulting in a more complete or rapid response. However, when combining 5-HTP with an SSRI, the clinician should monitor for signs of a serotonin syndrome, although no reports of this potentially serious side effect have been reported in the peer-reviewed literature at the time of writing. Acetyl-L-carnitine has been studied in placebo-controlled double-blind trials in severely depressed patients, elderly depressed patients, and depressed demented patients. Although fewer studies have been done on acetyl-L-carnitine than other natural products used to treat depressed mood, and no studies have compared it with synthetic antidepressants, results to date are promising. Nonbiological treatments of depressed mood include exercise and somatic and mind–body therapies, from general relaxation training to yoga, Tai Chi, and qigong, as well as treatments based on empirically validated forms of energy or information (e.g., EEG biofeedback and bright light exposure).

Research on many nonconventional treatments is at an earlier stage. Provisional nonconventional treatments of depressed mood include EEG biofeedback, certain acupuncture protocols, and mind–body techniques. Chinese medical treatments of depressed mood, including acupuncture and electroacupuncture, show promising results, although the mechanism of action remains unclear. One large prospective controlled study showed equivalent antidepressant efficacy of a particular electroacupuncture protocol and amitriptyline. **Table 8–3** summarizes the available evidence for substantiated and provisional nonconventional approaches used to treat depressed mood.

Table 8–3   Substantiated and Provisional Nonconventional Treatments of Depressed Mood

	Treatment Approach	Evidence for Modality or Integrative Approach	Comments (Including Safety Issues or Contraindications)
Substantiated treatments			
Biological	St. John's wort (*Hypericum perforatum*)	A standardized preparation (300 mg tid) of St. John's wort is comparable to conventional antidepressants for moderate depressed mood. Case reports of severe depression responding to higher doses (up to 1800 mg/day)	***Caution:*** St. John's wort is contraindicated in patients taking protease inhibitors, immunosuppressive agents, theophylline, and oral contraceptives. It should be avoided in pregnancy and in patients taking MAOI antidepressants
	S-adenosylmethionine (SAMe)	SAMe 400 to 1600 mg/day has comparable efficacy to conventional antidepressants. SAMe has synergistic beneficial effects when combined with folate (1 mg), vitamin B_{12} (800 μg), or conventional antidepressants. SAMe accelerates response, improves outcomes, and may lower effective doses of conventional antidepressants. Case reports of response in treatment-refractory patients	***Note:*** SAMe may be safely combined with conventional antidepressants ***Caution:*** SAMe may cause transient arousal or agitation during titration to therapeutic dose. Rare cases of hypomania have been reported in bipolar patients
	Vitamins (including folate, B_6, B_{12}, C, D, and E)	Folate 0.5 to 1.0 mg/day augments the effects of conventional antidepressants, and SAMe patients with normal B_{12} serum levels respond better to conventional antidepressants than patients who are B_{12} deficient. Large doses of vitamin D (100,000 IU) may be more effective than bright light therapy in seasonal depressed mood.	Thiamine and vitamins B_6, C, and E may augment conventional antidepressants. Vitamins do not cause adverse effects at doses recommended for depressed mood
	Omega-3 fatty acids	Combining omega-3 fatty acids (especially EPA) 1–2 g/day with conventional antidepressants improves response and may accelerate response rate. Case reports of EPA effective in severe depressed mood. A common mechanism of action may underlie antidepressant effects and beneficial effects in coronary artery disease	***Note:*** Reports of gastrointestinal adverse effects with omega-3s; may alter glucose metabolism in diabetics, and one case report of prolonged bleeding time when taken with warfarin (Coumadin)
Somatic and mind–body approaches	Exercise	Regular exercise at least 30 minutes 3 times a week is as effective as conventional antidepressants, St. John's wort, and cognitive therapy for moderate depressed mood. Exercising under bright light is more effective than exercise or bright light alone	***Note:*** Medically ill or physically impaired patients should consult with their physician before starting a strenuous exercise program
Approaches based on forms of energy information validated by Western science	Bright light exposure	Regular bright light exposure (10,000 lux for 30–40 minutes/day) improves depressed mood and may have more rapid onset than conventional antidepressants. Bright artificial and natural light are equally effective. Benefits are greater when there is a seasonal pattern. Safe as part of conventional treatment of depression in pregnant women. Exposure to bright light when exercising is more effective than either approach alone	***Note:*** Evening bright light exposure may cause insomnia. Rare cases of hypomania have been reported in bipolar patients. Transient mild adverse effects include jitteriness, headaches, and nausea
Energy-information approaches not validated by Western science	None at time of writing		

Table 8–3 Substantiated and Provisional Nonconventional Treatments of Depressed Mood *(Continued)*

	Treatment Approach	Evidence for Modality or Integrative Approach	Comments (Including Safety Issues or Contraindications)
Provisional treatments			
Biological	Dietary modifications	Restricting caffeine and refined sugar and increasing consumption of fatty fish and whole foods rich in B vitamins may improve depressed mood or reduce the risk of becoming depressed	Vitamin or omega-3 supplements should be encouraged in patients who are unable to modify their diets
	Ayurvedic herbs	Several Ayurvedic herbs and compound herbal formulas are probably beneficial	Patients taking Ayurvedic herbs should be supervised by an Ayurvedic physician
	5-hydroxytryptophan (5-HTP)	5-HTP 300 mg/day is probably as effective as conventional antidepressants for moderate depressed mood. Some cases of treatment-refractory depression improve when 5-HTP 300 to 600 mg/day is combined with carbidopa or conventional antidepressants	***Note:*** 5-HTP causes moderate sedation, and doses larger than 100 mg should be taken at bedtime
	L-tryptophan	L-tryptophan 1–2 g may be equivalent to imipramine 150 mg and other conventional antidepressants. L-tryptophan 2 g augments fluoxetine 20 mg and improves sleep quality. L-tryptophan 1–2 g combined with bright light therapy is more effective than either approach alone in seasonal depressed mood	***Note:*** Patients who benefit from L-tryptophan should be tried on 5-HTP, which more readily crosses the blood–brain barrier, is more efficiently converted to serotonin, and has fewer side effects than L-tryptophan. L-tryptophan can cause sedation and should be dosed at bedtime. Uncommon side effects of L-tryptophan include dry mouth and blurred vision ***Warning:*** Serious adverse effects have been reported when L-tryptophan is combined with MAOI antidepressants
	Acetyl-L-carnitine (ALC)	ALC 1–3 g/day in divided doses may be beneficial in elderly depressed or depressed demented patients. ALC should be considered when depression is related to post-traumatic brain injury or age-related cognitive decline	ALC does not have adverse effects at therapeutic doses for depression. Gastrointestinal side effects often occur at doses of inositol that are therapeutic in depressed mood
	Inositol	Inositol 12–20 g/day may be beneficial in both unipolar and bipolar depressed mood. Inositol may have synergistic effects when combined with conventional mood stabilizers	
	Dihydroepiandrosterone (DHEA)	DHEA 90 to 450 mg/day in mild to moderate depressed mood. DHEA has synergistic effects when combined with conventional antidepressants and may be an effective monotherapy for moderate depressed mood. DHEA may be beneficial when depressed mood occurs together with anxiety, psychosis, or cognitive impairment	***Warning:*** DHEA should be avoided in women with a history of estrogen receptor–positive breast cancer. DHEA supplementation may increase the risk of prostate cancer in men who are at risk
	Cortisol-lowering agents	Cortisol-lowering agents including ketoconazole, aminoglutethimide, and metyrapone may be beneficial	***Note:*** Drugs that lower cortisol are probably ineffective when depression occurs together with psychosis. Systemic antifungal drugs inhibit cytochrome P_{450} enzymes, interfering with the synthesis of cortisone and the sex hormones, resulting in gynecomastia, menstrual irregularities, infertility, and adrenal insufficiency

(Continued)

Table 8–3   Substantiated and Provisional Nonconventional Treatments of Depressed Mood *(Continued)*

	Treatment Approach	Evidence for Modality or Integrative Approach	Comments (Including Safety Issues or Contraindications)
Somatic and mind–body treatments	Total or partial sleep deprivation	One night of total sleep deprivation followed by sleep phase advance is effective in severe depressed mood. Partial sleep deprivation improves moderate depressed mood. Partial sleep deprivation combined with maintenance lithium therapy and morning bright light exposure may be more effective than either approach alone in bipolar depression	Combining periodic partial sleep deprivation with a conventional antidepressant in severely depressed patients is probably more effective than either approach alone
	Mindfulness training and yoga	Mindfulness training is probably as effective as cognitive therapy in moderate depressed mood. Regular yoga (breathing or postures) practice may be as effective as conventional antidepressants in severe depressed mood	Combining mindfulness training or guided imagery with conventional antidepressants is more effective than conventional treatments alone
Energy-information approaches validated by Western science	High-density negative ions	Regular daily exposure to high-density negative ions is probably an effective treatment of seasonal depressed mood	Antidepressant effects of exposure to high-density negative ions and bright light may be equivalent. *Note:* Low-density negative ions are probably ineffective
	Dim green, blue, or red light	Regular exposure to dim red or blue light may be as effective as bright light exposure in seasonal depression. Dim green light 2 hours before exposure to natural light may accelerate response to conventional antidepressants	Predawn exposure to dim red light may improve depressed mood in abstinent alcoholics
	Music or binaural sound	Attentive listening to music probably improves moderately depressed mood. Combining music with guided imagery is more beneficial than either approach alone. Listening to binaural sounds in the beta frequency range (16–24 Hz) may improve depressed mood	*Note:* Music and patterned sounds may produce positive or negative emotional effects depending on culture and individual preferences
	EEG biofeedback and heart rhythm variability (HRV) biofeedback	Combined EEG–HRV biofeedback ("energy cardiology") training may improve depressed mood	Effective EEG-biofeedback training is generally highly individualized
Energy-information approaches not validated by Western science	Acupuncture, electroacupuncture (EA), and computer-controlled EA (CCEA)	Conventional acupuncture may be effective against severe depressed mood. EA alone may be as effective as EA combined with amitriptyline or other conventional antidepressants. CCEA using high-frequency currents may be more effective than conventional or standard EA	Rare cases of HIV, hepatitis B and C, pneumothorax, and cardiac tamponade have been reported in patients treated with acupuncture
	Homeopathic preparations	Homeopathic remedies may be beneficial in some cases depending on constitutional findings	Homeopathic preparations are generally too dilute to cause adverse effects, but rare cases of toxicity have been reported
	Spirituality and religious beliefs	Spirituality and religious beliefs are associated with reduced risk of depressed mood	Regular support groups with spiritual-religious themes reduce the severity of depressed mood and increase emotional well-being
	Healing Touch (HT) and Therapeutic Touch (TT)	Regular HT or TT treatments may reduce the severity of depressed mood and bereavement	HT and TT probably have equivalent efficacy
	Qigong	Regular qigong practice results in generally improved emotional well-being	*Caution:* Brief psychotic episodes have been reported during qigong in histrionic or psychotic patients and individuals diagnosed with personality disorders

EEG, electroencephalogram; EPA, ecosapentanoic acid; HIV, human immunodeficiency virus; MAOI, monoamine oxidase inhibitor

Substantiated Treatments of Depressed Mood

Biological Treatments

◆ Medicinal herbs

St. John's wort (Hypericum perforatum) is an effective treatment of mild to moderate depressed mood   In Western Europe and the United States, St. John's wort is the most widely used natural product to treat depressed mood. Debate continues over the antidepressant mechanism of action of St. John's wort, but individual constituents have different effects that are probably synergistic and benefit depressed mood in many ways. Animal studies suggest that constituents of St. John's wort function as serotonin reuptake inhibitors, decrease binding to benzodiazepine receptors, weakly inhibit monoamine oxidase (MAO), and possibly also bind to N-methyl-D-asparate (NMDA) receptors (Cott, 1997). Hyperforin probably contributes more to the antidepressant effect of St. John's Wort than hypericin (Muller et al., 1998), but many commercial preparations continue to be standardized to 0.3% hypericin. A large 6-week randomized placebo-controlled study confirmed a dose–response relationship between hyperforin content and antidepressant efficacy of St. John's wort preparations in moderately depressed individuals (Laakman, Dienel, & Kieser, 1998). Speculation about the primary antidepressant role of hyperforin has led to problems when comparing recent studies with early studies that did not control for that constituent. In response to these concerns, many St. John's wort preparations are now standardized to both hypericin and hyperforin. However, commercially available preparations continue to have uneven quality and inconsistent standardization because of the absence of federal requirements for manufacturing herbal products in the United States under the Dietary Supplement Health and Education Act of 1994 (DSHEA; De Smet & Nolen, 1996).

Claims of an antidepressant effect of St. John's wort have been more rigorously investigated than the efficacy claims of any other herbal medicine (Upton, 1997). At the time of writing, more than 30 double-blind controlled trials on St. John's wort in depressed mood have been conducted. A Cochrane systematic review of 27 trials involving over 2200 patients, 17 of which were placebo-controlled, concluded that St. John's wort is significantly more effective than placebo for the treatment of mild to moderate depressed mood (Linde & Mulrow, 2004). Other meta-analyses have concluded that the antidepressant effect of standardized St. John's wort preparations is comparable to conventional antidepressants in moderately depressed patients (Ernst, 1995; Kim, Streltzer, & Goebert, 1999; Linde, Ramirez, Mulrow, Pauls, Weidenhammer, & Melchart, 1996). However, a recent meta-analysis using more stringent inclusion criteria that controlled for publication bias and small study effects found a significantly smaller antidepressant effect than reported in previous meta-analyses (Werneke, Horn, & Taylor, 2004). Ten placebo-controlled studies demonstrated equivalent efficacy to tricyclic antidepressants, and three recent studies have confirmed equivalent efficacy to SSRIs: fluoxetine (Schrader, 2000), sertraline (Davidson & the Hypericum Depression Trial Study Group, 2002), and paroxetine (Szegedi, Kohnen, Dienel, & Kieser, 2005). A few double-blind studies have demonstrated the efficacy of St. John's wort in severe depressed mood (Vorbach, Arnoldt, & Hubner, 1997). A large multicenter study sponsored

by the National Institutes of Health (NIH) showed that St. John's wort and sertraline were equally ineffective in the treatment of severe depressed mood, and that neither treatment was more effective than placebo (Davidson & the Hypericum Depression Trial Study Group, 2002). The validity of the NIH study findings has been questioned because of concerns over serious design flaws, including the use of subtherapeutic doses of both St. John's wort and sertraline for the target population, and selective recruitment of severely depressed patients who had previously been refractory to most conventional treatments, short duration, and lack of statistical power. In a follow-up study, the majority of nonresponders ($N = 95$) to a standardized St. John's wort preparation responded to conventional antidepressants with significant improvements in depressed mood (Gelenberg et al., 2004). This finding suggests that conventional antidepressants are more effective than St. John's wort in refractory depressed mood and reopens the question of a possibly significant placebo effect.

Adverse effects with St. John's wort   In most studies comparing St. John's wort with conventional antidepressants, patients receiving St. John's wort reported fewer and less serious side effects and were more likely to complete the study than patients treated with conventional antidepressants. In one large study 23% of patients taking high-dose St. John's wort (1800 mg/day) reported mild side effects in contrast to 41% of patients taking imipramine, many of whom discontinued the trial because of severe side effects (Vorbach et al., 1997). Uncommon side effects include upset stomach, feelings of restlessness, and mild sedation. There are no published cases of serotonin syndrome or other serious side effects when St. John's wort is used at recommended doses, but there are several case reports of possible serotonin syndrome when St. John's wort and a conventional antidepressant were used together (Lantz, Buchalter, & Giambanco, 1999). Pregnant women should be advised against the use of St. John's wort. Although no case reports have definitively linked the herb to serious interactions with MAOI antidepressants, their combined use should be avoided. Significant safety concerns exist when St. John's wort is used concurrently with certain anti–human immunodeficiency virus (HIV) drugs (protease inhibitors) (Piscitelli et al., 2000), immunosuppressive agents, Coumadin (warfarin), digoxin, and oral contraceptives. However, millions of individuals who self-treat depressed mood with St. John's wort preparations report infrequent serious side effects or herb–drug interactions. In the mainstream biomedical literature, published commentaries describing safety concerns should therefore be examined in the context of misrepresentation or distortion of the actual magnitude of adverse effects associated with St. John's wort by large pharmaceutical companies (McIntyre, 2000). Compelling evidence from high-quality studies, meta-analyses, and systematic reviews consistently show the efficacy of standardized St. John's wort preparations in moderate depressed mood. Pending the results of ongoing studies, the available data continue to support the use of standardized St. John's wort preparations in the treatment of mild or moderate depressed mood.

◆ Amino acids and their precursors

S-adenosylmethionine (SAMe) is an effective treatment of moderate and possibly severe depressed mood   The antidepressant effects of S-adenosylmethionine (SAMe) are probably achieved by increased brain levels of serotonin, dopamine, and norepinephrine. The synthesis of these neurotransmitters by SAMe requires both B$_{12}$ (1 mg) and folate (800 μg) (Crellin, Bottiglieri, & Reynolds, 1993). Many depressed patients are deficient in B vitamins (Bottiglieri et al., 1990), and all patients taking SAMe should be encouraged to take B$_{12}$ and folate concurrently. This integrative approach has been shown to result in improved outcomes when SAMe is used. The cerebrospinal fluid of depressed patients has been found to be deficient in SAMe (Bottiglieri et al.,1990). Controlled studies (Criconia et al., 1994; Fetrow & Avila, 2001) and one meta-analysis of the efficacy of SAMe in depression (Bressa, 1994) have demonstrated efficacy and safety that are equal or superior to conventional antidepressants (Agency for Healthcare Research and Quality, 2002). SAMe can be used orally and intravenously. The effective dose is significantly smaller when administered by injection, and few adverse effects have been reported. Some studies suggest comparable efficacy to conventional antidepressants in the treatment of refractory severe depressed mood (De Vanna & Rigamonti, 1992; Rosenbaum et al., 1990). In spite of its long-established use as an antidepressant, most controlled studies on SAMe in depressed mood have been conducted since 1994. The most significant findings from a large 7-week multicenter double-blind randomized controlled trial which showed that SAMe (1600 mg/day), given orally, and imipramine (150 mg/day) had equivalent efficacy, and SAMe was associated with significantly fewer adverse effects (Delle Chiale, Panc- cheri, & Scapicchio, 2000). Another multicenter study demonstrated equivalent efficacy between SAMe (400 mg IV) and oral imipramine (150 mg; Delle Chiale et al., 2000).

Advantages of SAMe include relatively rapid onset of action, usually within 1 week of starting treatment, the absence of clinically significant interactions with synthetic drugs, and relatively few side effects compared with conventional antidepressants. Moderate feelings of arousal or agitation are common when SAMe is being titrated to a therapeutic dose, but side effects typically resolve within a few weeks. A common dosing strategy is to begin treatment at 200 mg twice daily, and to gradually increase to 400 mg twice daily, monitoring for side effects and therapeutic response. The standard maintenance regimen for depressed mood is between 800 and 1600 mg in two to four divided doses. Absorption is improved when SAMe is taken before meals. Controlled studies and case reports have demonstrated that SAMe augments the effects of conventional antidepressants in the absence of safety issues (Alvarez, Udina, & Guillamat, 1987; Berlanga, Ortega-Soto, Ontiveros, & Senties, 1992; Friedel, Goa, & Benfield, 1989; Torta et al., 1988). Findings of a small open trial suggest that combining SAMe (800 to 1600 mg/day) with a conventional antidepressant results in improved overall response, is effective in patients who had been refractory to conventional antidepressants, and may accelerate the rate of response (Alpert, 2004). This integrative approach has been shown to result in improved outcomes while also permitting a reduction in the dose of the conventional antidepressant by as much as 30% in some cases. Advantages of reducing the dose of the conventional antidepressant include fewer side effects and improved compliance.

The putative mechanism of action by which SAMe augments the effects of conventional antidepressants to which a patient has become nonresponsive may involve reexternalizing neurotransmitter receptors that have been internalized by the nerve cell membrane during prolonged exposure to a conventional antidepressant (Brown, Gerbarg, & Bottiglieri, 2002). The butane–disulfonate product has significantly greater bioavailability than the tosylate form, and is available an an enteric-coated tablet for longer shelf life. Although SAMe is well tolerated, transient anxiety, insomnia, gastrointestinal side effects, dry mouth, and dizziness have been reported. Cases of hypomania have been reported in patients diagnosed with bipolar disorder (Carney, Chari, Bottiglieri, Reynolds, & Toone, 1987).

Other Natural Products

◆ **Vitamins**

Folate and B$_{12}$ improve response to conventional antidepressants and SAMe Findings from controlled trials and case reports support the use of certain vitamin and mineral supplements as adjunctive treatments of depressed mood. Among these are folate, thiamine, and vitamins B$_{12}$, B$_6$, E, and C (Benton, Haller, & Fordy, 1995). Refractory depressed mood is often associated with low serum levels of folate and B$_{12}$ (Bottiglieri, 1996; Bottligliери, Hyland, et al., 1990), and depressed mood is one of the most common symptoms associated with folate deficiency (Alpert & Fava, 1997). Folate is an essential cofactor in the synthesis of S-adenosylmethionine, which has well-established antidepressant effects. The response of depressed patients treated with an SSRI together with 0.5 to 1.0 mg of folinic acid, a form of folate that more readily crosses the blood–brain barrier, was as much as 30% greater than patients treated only with an SSRI (Papakostas et al., 2004b). A Cochrane review of three controlled studies involving a total of 247 individuals concluded that "folate may have a potential role as a supplement to other (conventional) treatments" of depressed mood (Taylor, Wilder, Bhagwagar, & Geddes, 2004). Patients who took 1 mg of folate with a conventional antidepressant experienced incrementally greater reductions in depressed mood compared with conventional drugs alone. However, one study failed to show a differential effect when folate was combined with trazodone, a widely used antidepressant.

In spite of the neutral comments of the Cochrane reviewers, many studies continue to support the use of folate in conjunction with conventional antidepressants. For example, the efficacy of fluoxetine (Prozac) and other conventional antidepressants is significantly enhanced by the addition of daily folate. Folate is a widely recommended adjunctive treatment of depressed mood, and it has been my clinical experience that depressed patients improve more rapidly and report increased feelings of vitality when taking folate (1 mg) and B$_{12}$ (1 mg), together with a conventional antidepressant or SAMe. Depressed patients who have higher serum levels of B$_{12}$ respond more completely to conventional antidepressants than patients with low B$_{12}$ levels (Hintikka, Tolmunen, Tanskanan, & Viinamäki, 2003), suggesting that B$_{12}$ supplementation is an important adjunctive therapy. Some depressed patients report improved mood and energy with a daily thiamine supplementation of 50 mg (Benton, Griffiths, & Halter, 1997). Vitamin D (400–800 IU/day) noticeably improved mood in patients diagnosed with seasonal affective disorder after 5 days of daily use (Lansdowne & Provost, 1998). Supplementation with large doses of vitamin D (100,000 IU/day) may be more effective than bright light therapy in the treatment of seasonal depressed mood (Gloth & Hollis, 1999).

Omega-3 Fatty Acids

Research findings suggest that several mechanisms of action may underlie the putative antidepressant effects of omega-3 fatty acids, including increased central nervous system (CNS) serotonin activity (Hibbeln et al., 1998), anti-inflammatory effects (Calder, 1997), suppression of phosphatidylinositol second messenger activity (Kinsella, 1990), and possibly increased heart rate variability (Villa et al., 2002). The mechanism of action may be similar to that of conventional antidepressants including tricyclics and SSRIs, which are known to suppress release of many pro-inflammatory cytokines by immune cells, possibly causing beneficial changes in the brain that manifest as improved mood (Maes, Smith, Christophe, Cosyns, Desnyder, & Meltzer, 1998). Increased production of pro-inflammatory cytokines takes place in the initial or acute phase of severe depressed mood (Maes et al., 1996). Direct administration of the same cytokines into the brain causes dysregulation in serotonin metabolism that mirrors changes observed in depressed individuals. Reports that omega-3 fatty acids may reduce the incidence of coronary artery disease (Hibbeln, 1995) by influencing the production of pro-inflammatory cytokines in the heart may help to explain the observed correlation between heart disease and major depressive disorder. Adding EPA, an omega-3 fatty acid, to conventional antidepressants improves overall response, and may accelerate the response rate (Nemets, Stahl, & Belmaker, 2002). Findings to date suggest that an effective antidepressant dose of EPA is probably at least 2 g/day. Case reports and a few small clinical trials suggest that EPA is beneficial in depressed mood when combined with conventional antidepressants in whole foods (see discussion below) or when taken as a supplement.

To date, only one small double-blind study has evaluated the efficacy of DHA alone as a treatment of severe depressed mood (Marangell et al., 2003). Patients treated with DHA (2 g/day) or placebo improved at the same rate. A case report claimed rapid dramatic improvement in a severely depressed, suicidal patient who had been refractory to multiple antidepressant trials, including lithium augmentation (Puri, 2002). The patient reported sustained improvement in mood over a 9-month period while maintained on EPA (4 g/day) alone. No adverse effects were reported.

At the time of writing, three small double-blind controlled studies had evaluated omega-3s in combination with conventional antidepressant medications (Nemets et al., 2002; Peet & Horrobin, 2002; Su, Huang, Chiu, & Shen, 2003). In two studies EPA (1 or 2 g/day) was added to the ongoing conventional treatment. In the third study patients were treated with a mixture of EPA and DHA (9.6 g/day) in addition to their conventional medication. In all three studies treatment response was significantly greater in the combined omega-3/antidepressant groups compared with groups treated with antidepressants only. Some patients who had previously been refractory to conventional antidepressants improved significantly when omega-3s were added to their conventional treatments. Patients in the combined omega-3/antidepressant groups reported significant improvements in insomnia,

and reduced feelings of guilt and worthlessness. Severe side effects were not reported in the combined treatment groups or the conventional treatment groups. The above findings support the use of EPA in combination with conventional antidepressants, including patients who are refractory to conventional antidepressants. However, it remains unclear whether EPA (or specific ratios of EPA to DHA) has an independent antidepressant effect or possibly enhances the efficacy of conventional antidepressants via second messenger systems in a manner that is similar to the postulated mechanism for lithium augmentation (Nemets et al., 2002). On the basis of available data, depressed patients should be encouraged to take EPA (1–2 g/day) as an augmentation strategy in conjunction with their current antidepressant regimen.

Although results of the only study to date on omega-3s as a stand-alone treatment of depressed mood were negative, many questions about fatty acid composition, dosing, treatment duration, and severity of symptoms have not been answered. Confirmation of the significance of an augmentation or stand-alone effect in the treatment of depressed mood and clarification of the antidepressant mechanism of action of fatty acids will require long-term prospective trials designed to answer these questions. Gastrointestinal side effects have been reported (Stoll et al., 1999), and omega-3s may interfere with glucose metabolism in diabetic patients (Glauber, Wallace, Griver, & Brechtel 1988). There is one case report of increased bleeding risk when omega-3 fatty acids are used together with Coumadin (Buckley, Goff, & Knapp, 2004).

Somatic and Mind–Body Approaches

Regular Exercise Is as Effective as Most Conventional and Nonconventional Biological Treatments of Depressed Mood

Case reports, randomized controlled trials, and two meta-analyses confirm that regular exercise has beneficial effects on depressed mood (Lawlor & Hopker, 2001; Tkachuk & Martin, 1999). Increased brain levels of mood-elevating endorphins, dopamine, norepinephrine, and serotonin following sustained exercise have been proposed as possible antidepressant mechanisms. Regular exercise also enhances self-sufficiency and ensures positive social interactions with other people. It is difficult to separate beneficial effects of exercise from other lifestyle factors, and it is possible that exercise contributes to overall feelings of wellness while not having specific mood-elevating effects. The optimum duration or frequency of exercise in depressed mood has not yet been determined but probably varies with age and conditioning. Both aerobic exercise and nonaerobic strengthening exercises are equally efficacious. Exercise is probably comparable to individual cognitive therapy and group therapy for depressed mood (Tkachuk & Martin, 1999). The antidepressant effects of running or fast walking are equivalent to cognitive-behavioral therapy and conventional antidepressants in moderately depressed individuals (Fremont & Craighead, 1987). Conventional antidepressants and exercise probably have equivalent effects on moderate depressed mood (Blumenthal et al., 1999). The therapeutic benefits of regular exercise are also comparable to validated nonconventional biological treatments of depressed mood, including St. John's wort (Ernst, Rand & Stevinson, 1998). Running 45 minutes twice each week, regular relaxation, meditation, or group psychotherapy probably have equivalent antidepressant effects (Lutz, 1986).

Depressed patients who exercise in a brightly lit (2500–4000 lux) indoor environment experience more significant improvements in mood and greater feelings of vitality compared with depressed individuals who exercise indoors in ordinary room light (400–600 lux) (Partonen, Leppamaki, Hurme, & Lonnqvist, 1998). Depressed women patients who combined exercise with bright light exposure while taking a daily vitamin regimen reported significant improvements in mood (Brown, Goldstein-Shirley, Robinson, & Casey, 2001). A study is ongoing to determine the amount, type, and frequency of exercise that is needed for sustained improvement in depressed mood in the absence of other treatments (Dunn et al., 2002).

In a 16-week study 156 depressed patients over the age of 50 were randomized to aerobic exercise 3 times a week, medications (sertraline/Zoloft, up to 200 mg), or exercise and medications (Blumenthal et al., 1999). All groups had improved significantly by the end of the study, and there were no significant differences in response rates using standardized symptom rating scales to assess mood, self-esteem, negative thoughts, and so on. Patients taking an antidepressant only improved faster initially than the other two groups, but patients who exercised only had a lower 6-month relapse rate. Sixty percent of patients who exercised only experienced complete remission, versus 65% of patients taking sertraline and 69% of patients who exercised and took a conventional antidepressant. Differences in these outcomes are not significant.

Energy-Information Approaches That Are Validated by Western Science

Regular Morning Exposure to Bright Light Improves Seasonal Depressed Mood

Light of different intensities and colors is widely used in conventional biomedicine and many nonconventional systems of medicine to treat a range of medical and psychological symptoms. There is no agreed-on theory supporting the use of light as a therapy, and many mechanisms of action are probably involved, including regulation of melatonin and neurotransmitters, especially the monamines (Neumeister, 2004). Recent theoretical work suggests that the beneficial effects of light may be consistent with meridian theory in Chinese medicine (Cocilovo, 1999). Most studies show that exposure to bright light (10,000 lux) for 1 to 2 hours daily over several weeks has therapeutic effects in moderately or severely depressed patients. This effect is especially robust in patients who report recurring seasonal depressed mood changes. A systematic review of controlled studies confirmed an antidepressant effect of bright light exposure therapy in seasonal depressed mood, but provided only limited evidence supporting bright light as a treatment of nonseasonal unipolar depressed mood (Jorm, Christensen, Griffiths, & Rodgers, 2002). A more recent meta-analysis of controlled studies concluded that bright light exposure or dawn simulation for seasonal depressed mood, and bright light exposure (but not dawn simulation) for nonseasonal depression have comparable efficacy to conventional antidepressants (Golden, et al., 2005). Morning exposure and evening exposure to bright light are probably equally effective

in seasonal depressed mood; however, there are reports of insomnia with evening exposure (Meesters, Jansen, Lambers, Bouhuys, Beersma, and Van de Hoffdakker, 1993). The antidepressant effects of bright light exposure may have more rapid onset than conventional antidepressants (Levitt, Joffe, & Kennedy, 1991). Findings of a small randomized trial suggest that bright light therapy may be an effective alternative to conventional antidepressants in pregnant depressed women (Epperson et al., 2004). Depressed patients who exercised regularly improved more when exposed to bright light than ordinary room light (Partonen et al., 1998). Exposure to natural sunlight, especially in the early morning, also has a significant antidepressant effect, and may reduce the length of hospital stays in severely depressed inpatients (Benedetti, Colombo, Barbini, Campori, & Smeraldi, 2001). Some patients exposed to bright morning light (10,000 lux) on a regular basis report transient side effects, including mild jitteriness or headaches (10%) and mild nausea (16%; Terman & Terman, 1999). Sporadic cases of hypomania have been reported, especially in winter depressives or bipolar patients exposed to early morning bright light (Bauer, Kurtz, Rubin, & Marcus, 1994). Almost two thirds of patients who use bright light exposure therapy in the evening report insomnia (Labbate, Lafer, Thibault, & Sachs, 1994). Because of the risk of insomnia with evening bright light exposure, all patients who choose bright light exposure to treat depressed mood should be encouraged to use this approach in the morning only. Bright light exposure therapy using an artificial light is relatively inexpensive and easy to use following an initial consultation to educate the patient about the most effective daily protocol, and the importance of obtaining a full-spectrum light of the required brightness.

Provisional Treatments of Depressed Mood

Biological Treatments

◆ Diet

Foods rich in B vitamins are beneficial in depressed mood   Observational trials show consistent relationships between good nutrition and improved mood. Reducing or eliminating consumption of refined sugar and caffeine significantly improves mood in some depressed patients, but research findings are inconsistent (Christensen, 1991). Foods rich in B vitamins, especially folate, pyridoxine (B_6), and methylcobalamin (B_{12}) are especially beneficial. These vitamins work as enzyme cofactors and facilitate the production of endogenous neurotransmitters, including serotonin, dopamine, and norepinephrine, whose deficiencies are hypothesized to be associated with depressed mood. Foods rich in B vitamins include whole grains and dark green leafy vegetables. Depressed patients should be encouraged to optimize their diets to ensure adequate consumption of foods rich in vitamins and other nutrients (see discussion above) known to influence brain functioning in depression. In some cases, taking vitamin or mineral supplements will provide additional benefits. Patients who prefer not to modify their diets should be encouraged to take appropriate doses of vitamins, minerals, or other supplements that are known to be beneficial in depressed mood.

Diets high in omega-3 fatty acids are associated with lower prevalence rates of depression   Food preferences influencing fatty acid consumption may be directly related to different rates of depressed mood when industrialized countries are compared with more traditional cultures. Epidemiological surveys have demonstrated an inverse correlation between the risk of depressed mood and fish consumption. Countries where fish is an important part of the average diet are characterized by significantly lower rates of depressed mood and suicidality (Hibbeln et al., 1998; Silvers & Scott, 2002; Tanskanen, Hibbeln, Hintikka, Haatainen, Honkalampi, & Viinamäki, 2001). For example, in Japan, where fish consumption is very high, only 0.12% of the population experiences depressed mood in a given year. In contrast, New Zealanders, who consume relatively little fish, report a 6% annual rate of depression.

Although epidemiological studies show correlations, definitive evidence for a causal relationship between essential fatty acids found in fish oil or other foods and depressed mood can only be achieved through prospective controlled trials. A large Dutch study showed that the incidence of depressed mood declined as dietary intake of omega-3 fatty acids increased relative to omega-6 fatty acids (Tiemeier et al., 2003). Significantly, relatively greater intake of omega-3 fatty acids was correlated with lower C-reactive protein levels, suggesting an overall reduction in inflammation.

Negative findings from recent studies continue to obscure the relationship between a high-fish diet and the risk of depressed mood. In one study, 452 men with histories of cardiovascular disease and angina were randomized to a diet high in fatty fish (or fish oil supplements) or "no fish advice" over a 6-month period (Ness et al., 2003). At the end of the study period, there were no significant group differences in new cases of anxious or depressed mood, and in fact more patients in the high-fish group reported depressed mood or anxiety. Principal sources of omega-3s include salmon, halibut, other deep-sea fish, and flaxseed oil.

◆ Medicinal herbs

Certain Ayurvedic herbs are probably effective for moderate depressed mood   As in Chinese herbal medicine, most Ayurvedic herbal treatments are compounded from several herbs. Research findings suggest that several herbs used in Ayurvedic compound herbal formulas, including *Withania somnifera, Mucuna pruriens, Acorus calamus, Convolvulus pluricaulis,* and *Celestrus panniculatus,* probably have antidepressant effects (Gupta & Singh, 2002; Koirala, 1992; Kushwaha & Sharma, 1992). A widely used compound herbal formula called Mentat probably has beneficial effects in moderate depressed mood (Sharma, Kushwaha, & Sharma, 1993). Recent concerns have been raised about heavy metal contaminants in some Ayurvedic herbal preparations, but serious adverse effects have not been reported in trials of Ayurvedic herbals for depressed mood. A patient who wishes to try an Ayurvedic herbal treatment should be referred to a qualified Ayurvedic physician.

◆ Amino acids and their precursors

5-HTP in combination with conventional antidepressants is probably an effective treatment in some cases of refractory depressed mood   5-hydroxytryptophan and L-tryoptophan are amino acid precursors of serotonin. Both have been evaluated for their antidepressant efficacy. 5-HTP is generally preferred over L-tryptophan because it crosses the blood–brain barrier at a

higher rate, is converted into serotonin more efficiently than L-tryptophan, and has a more marked antidepressant effect. 5-HTP begins to have an antidepressant effect at doses between 100 and 300 mg/day. More than 15 controlled studies have demonstrated consistent positive effects of 5-HTP in moderate depressed mood (Birdsall, 1998). However, most studies on 5-HTP in depressed mood are small, and study design problems preclude definitive conclusions at present. A Cochrane review of 5-HTP and L-tryptophan in depressed mood identified 108 studies, but analysis of findings was limited to only two studies involving 64 patients that met strict inclusion criteria (Shaw, Turner, & Del Mar, 2004). On the basis of those limited findings, the Cochrane reviewers concluded that 5-HTP is probably more effective than placebo for depressed mood. Although the conclusions of the Cochrane review must be taken into account, 5-HTP should be regarded as a provisional treatment of depressed mood on the basis of consistent positive results from many controlled studies in the context of continued strong anecdotal evidence of its safety and clinical efficacy.

Some research protocols combine 5-HTP with MAOI antidepressants or carbidopa in efforts to increase the amount of 5-HTP that crosses the blood–brain barrier. Carbidopa is a peripheral decarboxylase inhibitor that increases CNS availability of 5-HTP by interfering with the enzyme that breaks down 5-HTP in the blood (van Praag, 1984). 5-HTP is used alone or in combination with conventional antidepressants. In an open trial, two thirds of depressed patients treated with 5-HTP at 50 to 300 mg/day improved before the third week of treatment (Sano, 1972). In an early small double-blind trial, 5-HTP at 375 mg/day and imipramine at 150 mg/day had equivalent antidepressant efficacy (Angst, Woggon, & Schoepf, 1977). Sixty-three depressed patients randomized to fluvoxamine (150 mg) or 5-HTP (300 mg) experienced similar improvements in mood (Poldinger Calanchini, & Schwarz, 1991). Case reports show that treatment-refractory patients sometimes improve when 5-HTP (300 mg) is combined with carbidopa, tricyclic antidepressants, MAOIs, or SSRIs (Kline & Sacks, 1980; Mendlewicz & Youdim, 1980; Nardini et al., 1983; Sargent, Williamson, & Cowen, 1998; van Hiele, 1980; van Praag, 1984). In an open study, almost half of 100 patients who had been refractory to conventional antidepressants responded to 5-HTP (up to 600 mg/day) in combination with carbidopa (150 mg/day) over a period of weeks to months (van Hiele, 1980). Findings from another open trial suggest that 5-HTP at 300 mg/day is more effective against bipolar depression than unipolar depressed mood (Fujiwara & Otsuki, 1974). Rapid clinical improvement in depressed mood has been reported in patients treated by intravenous 5-HTP at 25 to 50 mg who are already taking oral MAOIs (Kline & Sacks, 1980). 5-HTP is moderately sedating, and doses greater than 100 mg are typically taken at bedtime.

L-tryptophan combined with a conventional antidepressant, vitamins B6 and C, or bright light is probably beneficial in moderate depressed mood   L-tryptophan has been used to treat depressed mood in many European countries for decades. It can be safely combined with most conventional antidepressants with appropriate supervision, but serious adverse effects can result when combined with MAOIs (see discussion below). L-tryptophan is present in many foods and is naturally synthesized into 5-HTP in the body. 5-HTP (see discussion above), in turn, is the immediate precursor of serotonin, one of the principle neurotransmitters implicated in depressed mood. The use of L-tryptophan to treat depressed mood originated in response to findings that serum L-tryptophan levels are often low in depressed patients and tend to normalize following successful response to treatment (Luchins, 1976). However, the therapeutic benefits of L-tryptophan as a stand-alone treatment of depressed mood remain unverified because of inconsistent findings, small trial sizes, and flawed study designs.

At the time of this writing at least 30 studies on L-tryptophan have demonstrated efficacy in moderate but not severe depression. Several double-blind placebo controlled studies have yielded negative findings for L-tryptophan as a stand-alone treatment of depressed mood (Cooper & Datta, 1980; Mendels et al., 1975). However, most of these studies were small, of short duration, did not use standardized L-tryptophan preparations or fixed doses, or included patients with complicated diagnostic pictures, including mania. Several early studies showed that L-tryptophan does not potentiate the antidepressant effects of tricyclics (Lopez-Ibor Alino et al., 1973; Shaw, Johnson, & MacSweeney, 1972); however, patients taking MAOI antidepressants and L-tryptophan had higher response rates than patients using either approach alone (Coppen, Coppen, Shaw, & Farrell, 1963; Glassman & Platman, 1969). Serious side effects (serotonin syndrome) have been reported when MAOIs are combined with L-tryptophan, including orthostatic hypotension, hyperreflexia, diaphoresis, and delirium (Lopez-Ibor Alino et al., 1973; Pope et al., 1985). Therefore, this combined approach should be considered only after other integrative approaches with fewer associated risks have failed, and only with the patient's (documented) informed consent, and only under close medical supervision.

Several studies suggest that L-tryptophan is beneficial in patients with seasonal depressed mood. Findings suggest that L-tryptophan and bright light exposure have similar antidepressant effects, and that combining L-tryptophan (1–3 g/day) and bright light exposure is more efficacious than either treatment alone (Lam et al., 1997). Two early double-blind, placebo-controlled studies concluded that L-tryoptophan at 6 to 9 g/day and imipramine at 150 mg/day have an equivalent antidepressant effect (Coppen et al., 1972; Jensen et al., 1975). L-tryptophan in combination with vitamins B_6 and C may be as effective as imipramine for moderate depressed mood (Rao & Broadhurst, 1976). Sixteen medication-free patients with seasonal depressed mood were treated alternately with bright light exposure and L-tryptophan. One half were treated with L-tryptophan first, and one half were initially treated with bright light exposure. Fifty-four percent of patients in each group experienced significant improvements in depressed mood. When treatment was discontinued at the end of the 7-week study, patients in both groups relapsed, but relapse was less rapid in the group receiving L-tryptophan following light exposure (Ghadirian, Murphy, & Gendron, 1998).

L-tryptophan is typically used at night because of its sedating properties, and is dosed between 1500 and 5000 mg, depending on therapeutic response. Combining L-tryptophan (2 g) with fluoxetine (Prozac, 20 mg) resulted in a more rapid antidepressant response and improved sleep quality in depressed patients complaining of chronic insomnia (Levitan, Shen, Jindal, Driver, Kennedy, & Shapiro, 2000). No cases of serotonin syndrome or other serious adverse effects were reported with this combined approach.

Rare side effects of L-tryptophan include drowsiness, dry mouth, and blurred vision. Some 1500 cases of eosinophilia-myalgia syndrome (EMS) and 37 deaths in patients taking L-tryptophan were reported in the late 1980s and early 1990s. All cases were traced to contaminants in a single batch of one over-the-counter L-tryptophan preparation (Kilbourne et al., 1996). The manufacturing problem that resulted in the contaminated batch was identified and rapidly corrected. There have been no subsequent reports of EMS associated with L-tryptophan.

Acetyl-L-carnitine is probably beneficial when depression occurs with cognitive impairment Acetyl-L-carnitine has been studied in double-blind, placebo-controlled trials in severely depressed patients, elderly depressed patients, and depressed demented patients (Bella, Biondi, Raffaele, & Pennisi, 1990; Garzya, Corallo, Fiiore, Lecciso, Petrelli, & Zotti, 1990. It has general neuroprotective effects, and mediates improved mood and possibly reduction in the severity of cognitive impairments in normal aging, dementia, or traumatic brain injury by enhancing mitochondrial energy production and partially compensating for deficits in CNS cholinergic activity. Most studies conducted to date have evaluated acetyl-L-carnitine in elderly depressed patients and have demonstrated a consistent antidepressant effect after about 1 month of treatment (Pettegrew, Levine, & McClure, 2000). In a 2-month placebo-controlled study, demented depressed patients treated with acetyl-L-carnitine at 3 g/day in divided doses experienced significantly greater improvements in mood and global functioning compared with patients taking a placebo (Bella et al., 1990). In a double-blind, placebo-controlled study, almost half of elderly severely depressed patients ($N = 28$) treated with acetyl-L-carnitine at 500 mg qid experienced full remission, and previously elevated serum cortisol levels normalized (Garzya, et al., 1990). In a small double-blind crossover study of hospitalized elderly depressed patients, acetyl-L-carnitine had superior antidepressant efficacy compared with placebo, but comorbid anxiety symptoms did not improve (Tempesta, Casella, Pirrongelli, Janiri, Calvani, & Ancona, 1987). Fewer studies have been done on acetyl-L-carnitine than other natural products used to treat depressed mood, and no studies have compared it with synthetic antidepressants. Most studies on depressed mood report few or no adverse effects. Acetyl-L-carnitine may be safely used in combination with conventional antidepressants, but studies have not been done to demonstrate possible synergistic effects. It is reasonable to consider a trial on acetyl-L-carnitine starting at 500 mg/day and gradually advancing to 2 g/day in divided doses in demented depressed patients or in cases where conventional antidepressants are not effective or have been discontinued because of adverse effects.

◆ Other biological treatments

Inositol is probably beneficial in bipolar depressed mood Inositol is a B vitamin that has been reported to improve depressed mood in large doses up to 20 g/day and probably works by normalizing desensitized serotonin receptors (Benjamin, et al., 1995; Levine, Barak, & Ganzalves et al., 1995; Levine, Barak, Kofman, & Belmaker, 1995). In contrast to 5-HTP and other natural precursors of neurotransmitters, inositol is synthesized into phosphatidyl inositol (PI), an important second messenger that is required for normal nerve cell function. Desirable effects of lithium in depressed mood, mania, and possibly other symptoms are probably mediated through inhibition of the enzyme required for synthesis of PI in certain brain regions, including the hippocampus (Belmaker, 1996). A stereoisomer of inositol called epi-inositol may be the most effective form of this natural compound (Einat, Shaldubina, & Belmaker, 2000). A Cochrane review concluded that inositol when used as a primary or adjunctive treatment of depressed mood cannot be recommended on the basis of completed double-blind studies (Taylor, Carney, Geddes, & Goodwin, 2004). However, it is important to note that the reviewed studies were of short duration and involved few patients. Larger studies of longer duration are required to determine the antidepressant efficacy of inositol. In a small 4-week double-blind, placebo-controlled study, 28 depressed patients were randomized to inositol 12 g/day versus placebo (Levine, Barak, & Gonzalves et al., 1995). The inositol group reported significantly greater improvement in mood compared with the placebo group. Responders in the inositol group relapsed rapidly when they stopped taking inositol, whereas patients who improved with placebo did not relapse when they stopped taking a placebo (Levine, Barak, Kofman et al., 1995). This finding supports the view that the beneficial effects of inositol in depressed patients are based on an active mechanism of action, and not a placeo effect. In a small 6-week double-blind, randomized trial, 24 bipolar depressed patients were randomized to receive conventional mood stabilizers plus inositol 12 g/day or placebo (Chengappa et al., 2000). By the end of the study, half (6) of the patients in the combined inositol–mood stabilizer group reported at least a 50% reduction in depressed mood symptoms, compared with only 3 patients (25%) in the placebo group. No significant side effects of inositol were reported at the doses used in this study. Larger studies are needed to confirm the apparent synergistic effect of inositol when used with conventional antidepressants or mood stabilizers. Gastrointestinal side effects at doses that are effective in depressed mood have resulted in limited use of inositol in spite of its therapeutic potential.

DHEA may be an effective monotherapy of moderate depressed mood and should be considered when depression occurs together with psychosis, anxiety, or cognitive impairment The putative antidepressant mechanism of DHEA remains unclear but may involve androgen receptors, estrogen receptors, or well-defined neurotransmitter systems, including serotonin, GABA, NMDA, and norepinephrine. Physiological replacement doses of DHEA (i.e., 30 to 90 mg/day, a dose range corresponding to DHEA serum levels that are normal in people younger than age 40) probably improve mood in middle-aged or elderly depressed patients (Wolkowitz et al., 1997). In a small 6-week study ($N = 22$), DHEA administered in an escalating dose (30 mg/day for 2 weeks, followed by 30 mg twice a day for 2 weeks and 30 mg three times daily for 2 weeks) resulted in significant improvements in mood compared with placebo (Wolkowitz et al., 1999). Two thirds of patients in both groups continued on their conventional antidepressants; however, 3 patients in the DHEA group and 4 patients in the placebo group did not take medications during the study. Depressed mood scores in half of patients in the DHEA group improved by 50% or more using standardized rating scales. A larger follow-up study suggests that higher doses are probably more

effective when DHEA is used as a monotherapy. In a 6-week double-blind, randomized, placebo-controlled crossover study ($N = 46$), moderately depressed adults were randomized to DHEA at 90 mg/day for 3 weeks, followed by DHEA at 450 mg/day (150 mg tid) for 3 weeks versus placebo (Schmidt et al., 2005). None of the patients used conventional antidepressants concurrently with DHEA. A 50% or greater reduction in depressive symptoms was observed in the majority of patients in the DHEA group, which also reported improvements in baseline sexual functioning. Significantly, most patients who responded to DHEA remained asymptomatic at 12-months follow-up. Further research is needed to replicate these findings, evaluate DHEA for severe depressed mood, and clarify the mechanism of a synergistic or independent antidepressant effect of DHEA.

Depressed HIV-positive patients experienced significant improvements in mood and fatigue when taking DHEA at 200 to 500 mg/day (Rabkin, Ferrando, Wagner, & Rabkin, 2000). Serum testosterone levels and CD4 T-cell counts were not affected.

Psychotic or demented patients often experience significant comorbid depressed mood. DHEA should be considered when depressed mood occurs together with anxiety, psychosis, and cognitive impairment. Research findings suggest that DHEA supplementation reduces the rate of cognitive deterioration in Alzheimer's disease, and may improve anxiety and negative psychotic symptoms in schizophrenics (see Chapter 11, Integrative Management of Psychosis, and Chapter 12, Dementia and Mild Cognitive Impairment). In a double-blind, placebo-controlled study, 30 schizophrenic inpatients treated with DHEA at 100 mg/day in addition to their conventional antipsychotic medications experienced significant improvements in depressed mood, anxiety, and negative psychotic symptoms (Strous et al., 2003). Women improved more than men, and serum cortisol levels did not change during treatment. DHEA may promote cancer in women who have a history of estrogen receptor–positive breast cancer (Calhoun et al., 2003) and should be avoided in this population. However, a metabolite of DHEA called 7-keto-DHEA is not converted into androgens or estrogens and can probably be safely used in this population. Preliminary findings suggest that DHEA supplementation may increase the risk of prostate cancer in men with early or undetected prostate cancer (Arnold, Le, McFann, & Blackman, 2005). Combining DHEA with conventional psychiatric medications is a reasonable integrative approach to co-occurring depressed mood, anxiety, and psychosis.

Drugs that lower cortisol may have antidepressant effects A Cochrane review of two randomized controlled trials and seven case studies found evidence of improved mood in depressed patients treated with cortisol-lowering agents, including the antifungal drug ketoconazole (200 to 1200 mg/day) and the anti-adrenal drugs aminoglutethimide (750 mg–1 g/day) and metyrapone (200 mg–2 g/day; Brown, Bobadilla, & Rush, 2001). Reduction in the severity of depressed mood was not dose related. Findings to date suggest that depressed patients who are psychotic do not respond to cotisol-lowering agents. Systemic antifungal drugs frequently cause gastrointestinal upset. These drugs—especially ketoconazole—inhibit cytochrome P_{450} enzymes, interfering with the synthesis of cortisone and the sex hormones, resulting in gynecomastia, menstrual irregularities, infertility, and adrenal insufficiency. Rare cases of fatal arrhythmias have been reported. The antiadrenals sometimes cause dizziness, drowsiness, headache, lightheadedness, and nausea.

Somatic and Mind–Body Approaches

Total and Partial Sleep Deprivation Improves Unipolar and Bipolar Depressed Mood

Total sleep deprivation often results in immediate and dramatic improvement of severely depressed mood, but improvements are difficult to sustain after the patient returns to a normal sleep pattern. A putative mechanism of action is related to increased brain levels of dopamine and possibly also serotonin following total sleep deprivation. One night of total sleep deprivation followed by a gradual phase advance of sleep onset results in sustained improvements in mood in up to 75% of responders (Riemann et al., 1999). In this technique, the patient is instructed to go to sleep at 5:00 P.M. on the day following total sleep deprivation, and to advance the time of sleep onset by 1 hour every night until he or she has returned to a normal sleep pattern. Bipolar depressed patients who combine total sleep deprivation with morning bright light exposure and maintenance lithium therapy report significantly improved mood compared with patients taking lithium only or lithium in combination with total sleep deprivation (Colombo, Lucca, Benedetti, Barbini, Campori, & Smeraldi, 2000). Total sleep deprivation is sometimes used in cases of severe depression. Ten hospitalized bipolar depressed patients were randomized to fluoxetine (Prozac) alone or fluoxetine and total sleep deprivation (Benedetti, Barbini, Lucca, Campori, Colombo, & Smeraldi, 1997). Patients who underwent sleep deprivation while taking Prozac improved more rapidly than patients taking Prozac alone. Bipolar depressed patients who were subjected to total sleep deprivation in conjunction with morning bright light exposure experienced significant and sustained improvement in mood independently of whether they were continued on conventional lithium therapy (Colombo et al., 2000). On the basis of these findings, combining bright light exposure with periodic total sleep deprivation may be an effective alternative strategy for the management of bipolar depressed mood.

Partial sleep deprivation by restricting sleep by several hours every 4 to 5 days may improve moderately depressed mood (Leibenluft, Moul, Schwartz, Madden, & Wehr, 1993). Combining partial sleep deprivation with conventional antidepressants may have a greater antidepressant effect than either approach alone. In a double-blind, randomized trial, depressed patients who engaged in partial sleep deprivation while taking amitriptyline at 150 mg reported more sustained improvements in mood compared with matched patients taking antidepressants but not restricting sleep (Kuhs, Farber, Borgstadt, Mrosek, & Tolle, 1996).

Mindfulness Training and Somatic Therapies Improve General Emotional Well-being

Controlled studies and case reports suggest that certain somatic or mind–body practices improve general emotional well-being and enhance mood. Improved capacity for focused attention and reflection has been proposed as an important nonspecific psychological benefit of mind–body practices.

Animal-facilitated psychotherapy probably improves general emotional well-being in depressed individuals (Odendaal, 2002). Mindfulness training includes many styles of meditation and guided imagery. Mind–body practices include Tai Chi, qigong, Yoga, and the Hakomi body-centered method. Guided imagery is widely used as a treatment of depressed mood in Western countries. The regular practice of a mind–body skill may be as beneficial as cognitive-behavioral therapy and conventional antidepressants in the management of moderately depressed mood (Murphy, Carney, Knesevich, Wetzel, & Whitworth, 1995). Mindfulness training combined with cognitive therapy may enhance outcomes compared with cognitive therapy alone (Mason & Hargreaves, 2001). In an open trial 60 women with postpartum depressed mood and anxiety experienced significant relief during the first 4 weeks following childbirth using a combined relaxation-guided imagery protocol (Rees, 1995). Depressed patients who had previously been diagnosed with somatoform disorders experienced greater improvements in mood when guided imagery was combined with antidepressants than with conventional medications alone (Bernal, Cercos, Fuste, Vallverdu, Urbieta Solana, & Montesinos Molina, 1995).

Yoga Is Probably Beneficial in both Moderate and Severe Depressed Mood

Of the various mind–body disciplines used to obtain relief from psychiatric symptoms, more studies have been done on yoga than any other discipline (Shannahoff-Khalsa, 2004). The mechanism of action of Yogic breathing might be similar to the effects of vagal nerve stimulation, in that both approaches involve modulation of the balance of parasympathetic and sympathetic autonomic tone. Yogic breathing achieves desirable changes through a variety of specific exercises that differentially affect the brainstem and limbic system, whereas VNS relies on a weak electrical current to achieve desirable changes in brain autonomic activity that mediate improved mood or reduced anxiety. Like Yogic breathing techniques, the regular practice of various yoga postures (asanas) probably results in beneficial changes in the autonomic nervous system, leading to improved cardiorespiratory performance and increased feelings of psychological well-being (Harinath et al., 2004).

Many styles of yoga are probably beneficial in depressed mood. A particular style of Yogic breathing called Sudarshan Kriya (SK) yoga has been extensively evaluated as a potential treatment of depressed mood and other cognitive and affective symptoms (Shannahoff-Khalsa et al., 1999). Moderately depressed patients improved significantly by the end of a 5-week yoga class (Woolery, Myers, Sternlieb, & Zeltzer, 2004). In a group of severely depressed hospitalized patients, improvements associated with SK breathing practice were comparable to responses from conventional antidepressants and only slightly less robust than patients receiving electroconvulsive therapy (Janakiramaiah et al., 2000). Emerging evidence suggests that the regular practice of forms of yoga that do not include specialized breathing exercises also improve depressed mood, including Hatha yoga, Omkar meditation, and Iyengar yoga. Regular practitioners of Hatha yoga and Omkar meditation also had significant increases in melatonin secretion, possibly related to increased serotonin, an established benefit of meditation (Walton, Pugh, Gelderloos, & Macrae, 1995). In a small randomized case-control study, mildly depressed practitioners of Iyengar yoga reported significant improvements in mood following semiweekly yoga practice for 5 weeks (Woolery et al., 2004).

A significant limitation of studies on yoga or any mind–body practice is the absence of double-blinding, as enrolled patients are necessarily aware of engaging in specific movements or breathing exercises of a particular mind–body practice. Many depressed patients have difficulty becoming motivated to start a mind–body practice; they should be gently encouraged to take classes at the start of their practice, and slowly transition to a daily self-directed program if they find it beneficial to their mood and general state of well-being.

Treatments Based on Scientifically Validated Forms of Energy or Information

Provisional treatments of depressed mood incorporating forms of energy or information that are validated by contemporary Western science include high-output negative ions, exposure to dim light, music and binaural sound, and different forms of biofeedback.

Regular Exposure to High-Density Negative Ions Is Beneficial in Seasonal Depressed Mood

Research findings from double-blind, controlled trials show that regular daily exposure to high-density negative ions is an effective treatment of depressed mood when there is a seasonal pattern of occurrence. This approach may have comparable efficacy to bright light exposure for this condition. In one study 25 depressed patients with seasonal depressed mood were randomized to high-density negative ions (2.7×10^6 ions/cm^3) versus low-density negative ions (1×10^4 ions/cm^3) using in-home ion generators 30 minutes daily for 3 weeks (Terman & Terman, 1995). Fifty-eight percent of patients exposed to high-density negative ions experienced significant improvements in mood on standardized rating scales compared with 15% of patients exposed to low-density negative ions. In a randomized, controlled trial, 158 patients with seasonal depressed mood were randomly assigned to bright light exposure (10,000 lux) at different times of day versus high-density or low-density negative ions for 2 weeks (Terman, Terman, & Ross, 1998). Patients exposed to high-density negative ions or bright light experienced significant and equivalent improvements in mood. There was a differential beneficial effect of morning versus evening bright light exposure. In a 5-week open study, 32 patients diagnosed with seasonal major depressive disorder were randomized to daily bright light therapy, high-density negative ions, or low-density negative ions. Significant improvements in mood were observed in patients receiving bright light or high-density negative ions, but not low-density ions (Goel, 2004).

Adverse effects were not associated with regular daily exposure to negative ions following the protocols used in these studies.

Regular Morning Exposure to Dim Light Is Beneficial for Nonseasonal Depressed Mood

Recent studies suggest that regular exposure to dim red or blue light might be as efficacious as bright light, especially in the management of seasonal depressed mood. In a single-blind study, 57 patients diagnosed with seasonal affective disorder were randomized to daily bright light or dim red light exposure over 4 weeks. Both groups experienced a 40% reduction in symptoms using standardized rating scales (Wileman et al., 2001). Exposure to dim light simulating sunrise in the early morning (250 lux) might improve depressed mood in abstinent alcoholics who experience seasonal mood swings (Avery, Bolte, & Ries, 1998). Recent findings suggest that low-intensity (7 lux) blue light (446–477nm) has beneficial effects in seasonal depressed mood that are comparable to those obtained from standard therapies using full-spectrum bright light (10,000 lux). Blue light is particularly effective in suppressing melatonin and phase shifting the circadian pacemaker (Warman, Djik, Warman, ARendt, & Skene, 2003). In a small study researchers compared the melatonin suppression effect of dim red versus dim blue light in 24 subjects who had been diagnosed with major depression with a seasonal pattern according to *DSM-IV* and were at least moderately depressed and reported normal sleeping patterns. Subjects were exposed to early morning dim blue or red light for 45 minutes every morning between 6:00 and 8:00 for 3 weeks (Glickman, Byrne, Pineda, & Brainard, 2004). Fifty-four percent of subjects exposed to dim blue light had achieved full remission by the end of the study. Exposing depressed patients to low-intensity artificial light ~2 hours before they would naturally be exposed to daylight may increase the speed of response to conventional antidepressants. Thirty depressed inpatients, 9 of whom were diagnosed as bipolar, who were being treated with 40 mg of citalopram (Celexa) were randomized to dim green light (400 lux) in the early morning or a sham non-light-emitting device during the first 2 weeks of drug treatment (Benedetti, Colombo, Pontiggia, Bernasconi, Florita, & Smeraldi, 2003). Patients in the combined citalopram–light exposure group improved more and faster on standardized symptom rating scales compared with patients taking citalopram alone or placebo. Adverse effects have not been reported with regular exposure to dim light.

Music and Binaural Sound Probably Have Beneficial Effects on Depressed Mood

Many studies have examined the mood-enhancing effects of music; however' most protocols combine music with relaxation techniques or body-centered therapies. Subsequently, a specific antidepressant effect of music has not been established. The available evidence suggests that certain musical tones alone or in combination with somatic or mind–body therapies have a nonspecific beneficial effect on mood.

Listening to music or soothing sounds may reduce the severity of depressed mood. Many depressed patients intuitively listen to music or patterned sounds in efforts to alleviate mood symptoms. Frequent listening to music probably has beneficial effects on endorphins and other neurotransmitters that mediate improvements in depressed mood (Drohan, 1999). Different categories of music affect the neurochemical basis of depressed mood in different ways; some styles and rhythmic patterns of music or sound produce beneficial changes, whereas some apparently result in negative mood changes (Smith & Noon, 1998). Case reports suggest that binaural sounds (i.e., different sound frequencies presented separately to each ear) in the beta frequency range (16–24 Hz) improve mood (Lane, Kasian, Owens, & Marsh, 1998; Milligan &

Waldkoetter, 2000). Music therapists take these differences into account when making specific recommendations to depressed patients in view of psychiatric history, cultural background, and individual musical preferences.

The findings of controlled trials suggest that music alone or in combination with guided imagery has beneficial effects on standardized mood scales in depressed cancer patients. Soon after listening to tranquil music, depressed outpatients experienced significant improvements in mood, as well as beneficial changes in heart rate and blood pressure (Lai, 1999). Cancer patients who participated in weekly sessions of combined music and guided imagery reported greater improvements in depressed mood and overall quality of life compared with patients in a "wait-list" group (Burns, 2001). Cancer patients who received music therapy while undergoing autologous stem cell transplantation reported significantly greater improvements in both anxiety and depressed mood compared with patients who did not receive music therapy (Cassileth, Vickers, & Magill, 2003). I frequently encourage depressed patients to incorporate listening to music in their daily routines and to regard this as an important part of their therapy. For depressed or anxious patients, regular attentive listening to soothing music can strengthen emotional resilience in the face of the day's anticipated problems and stresses.

EEG Biofeedback Using Photic Stimulation Probably Reduces the Severity of Depressed Mood

Many kinds of biofeedback, including electromyogram (EMG), galvanic skin response (GSR), and electroencephalogram (EEG), have been examined in open and double-blind studies of depressed mood. The mechanism of action underlying these treatment modalities has yet to be confirmed; however, indirect evidence suggests that changes in the levels of serotonin and perhaps other neurotransmitters are associated with improved mood. Sustained "shifts" in the dynamic equilibrium of electrical brain activity have been proposed as the therapeutic mechanism underlying EEG biofeedback. Case reports and studies show reductions in the severity of depressed mood using photic stimulation (Kumano, Horie, Shidara, Kuboki, Suematsu, & Yashushi, 1996) or α asymmetry EEG biofeedback protocols (Baehr & Rosenfeld, 2003; Baehr, Rosenfeld, & Baehr, 2001; Rosenfeld, 2000). EEG biofeedback has been successfully used to treat depressed mood in chronic alcoholics and to reduce relapse rates (Peniston & Kulkosky, 1989; Saxby & Peniston, 1995; Waldkoetter, & Sanders, 1997). Larger double-blind studies are needed to confirm a consistent and robust effect of EEG biofeedback in depressed mood.

Energy Cardiology—Combining Feedback from EKG and EEG

Measures of heart rate variability (HRV) provide the basis for biofeedback directed at changing the brain's autonomic activity. This approach is called HeartMath and is based on the theory that positive emotional states result in increased coherence of several physiological aspects of heart rhythm, and that feedforward and feedback loops between the heart, brainstem, and neocortex have beneficial modifying effects on complex relationships between specific emotional or cog-

nitive states and specific patterns of heart rate variability (McCraty & Atkinson, 1999). Case reports suggest that this approach improves depressed mood and other symptoms that result from chronic stress (McCraty, Atkinson, & Tomasino, 2001). Findings suggest that correlations between electrocardiogram (EKG) and EEG activity provide evidence for complex feedback loops between the heart and brain that regulate emotion (McCraty et al., 2001; Schwartz & Russek, 1996). This integrative approach is called energy cardiology. Future mood-enhancing therapies will probably combine biofeedback from the electrical activity of the heart and brain.

Nonconventional Treatments Based on Postulated Forms of Energy or Information That Are Not Validated by Western Science

Acupuncture is Probably Beneficial in Moderate and Severe Depressed Mood

Controlled studies and case reports suggest that acupuncture has beneficial effects on depressed mood, including conventional needle acupuncture, electroacupuncture (Hechun et al., 1990), and computer-controlled electroacupuncture (CCEA) (Hechun et al., 1993). Evaluating the clinical efficacy of acupuncture in depressed mood poses many methodological problems because of heterogeneity in the severity and comorbidity of cognitive, affective and physical symptom patterns, concurrent uses of other conventional or nonconventional treatments in patients receiving acupuncture, the fact that Western diagnostic categories do not correspond to Chinese medical diagnoses, and the use of different acupuncture treatment protocols depending on the patient's unique energetic formulation (MacPherson, Thorpe, Thomas, & Geddes, 2004). This section provides a brief overview of significant recent research. The evidence base for acupuncture treatments of depressed mood is extensively reviewed elsewhere (Flaws & Lake, 2001; Schnyer & Allen, 2001). Findings of a double-blind, sham-controlled study suggest that traditional acupuncture (i.e., in the absence of electrical current) is an effective treatment of severely depressed outpatients (Allen, Schnyer, & Hitt, 1998). By the end of this 8-week study, 68% of 33 female outpatients treated with an acupuncture protocol directed at depressed mood had achieved full remission. Interestingly, depressed women patients in the wait-list group who received no treatment showed equivalent improvement in mood. In a large six-week multicenter study, 241 depressed inpatients were randomized to receive electroacupuncture plus placebo or electroacupuncture plus amitriptyline (Luo, Meng, Jia, & Zhao, 1998). Both groups experienced equivalent improvement in depressed mood. Factor analysis using the Hamilton Rating Scale for Depression (HRSD) showed that electroacupuncture was superior to amitriptyline when there was comorbid anxiety. Patients treated with electroacupuncture had significantly elevated plasma norepinephrine concentrations following a 6-week course of treatment, suggesting that electro-acupuncture may stimulate release of norepinephrine in the brain (Riederer, Tenk, Werner, Bischko, Rett, & Krisper, 1975). Depressed patients who failed to respond to electroacupuncture did not show significant changes in serum norepinephrine levels (Fanqiang et al., 1994). A recent innovation in acupuncture uses computer-guided modulation of the frequency and waveform of the current delivered through acupuncture needles. Findings from open trials of CCEA suggest that high frequencies (1000 Hz) yield responses in depressed patients that are superior to both conventional acupuncture and electroacupuncture (Hechun et al., 1993, 1995).

Although acupuncture is associated with few adverse effects, a meta-analysis of studies of complications related to acupuncture identified infrequent cases of infection with HIV and hepatitis B and C due to the use nonsterilized needles. Rare cases of pneumothorax and cardiac tamponade have been reported as a result of the accidental puncturing of lungs or the pericardium (Ernst & White, 1997).

Homeopathic Remedies Are Probably Effective in Some Cases

Many case reports (Hein, 1991, 1992; Sevar, 1995; Zaren, 1995), a few open studies (Davidson, Morrison, Shore, Davidson, & Beday, 1997), but no controlled trials suggest that homeopathic treatments are beneficial in some cases of depressed mood. Both short- and long-term constitutional remedies are used, depending on symptom severity and the energetic pattern that is being treated. The specific constitutional treatment for depressed mood depends on findings of a careful medical, family, and social history and an assessment of the patient's personality, food preferences, and any problems with heat or cold intolerance and other subjective indicators of "energetic imbalances." Different remedies are used to address specific differences in personality factors associated with depressed mood. For example, the angry depressed patient is energetically different from the resentful, weepy, or indifferent depressed patient, and there are commensurate differences in the most appropriate treatment for these disparate symptom patterns (Spence, 1990). Davidson and colleagues (1997) suggested that acute or severe symptoms of depressed mood should be initially managed using conventional antidepressants. When severe symptoms have subsided, it is reasonable to consider a homeopathic preparation if constitutional assessment by a homeopathic physician suggests that ongoing energetic imbalances can be effectively addressed in this way.

Homeopathic remedies are generally too dilute to potentially cause adverse effects; however, rare cases of toxicity have been reported when low dilutions of arsenic, cadmium, or other heavy metals are used (Ernst, 1995). Concerns about possible carcinogenic effects of remedies containing *Aristolochia* have been raised, and there are rare reports of allergic reactions.

Spirituality, Prayer, and Energy Healing Methods

◆ **Religiosity and spiritually focused group therapy** It has been established that religiosity and spiritual values predict good mental health in general, including reduced risk of depressed mood and lower rates of anxiety (Kendler, Liu, Gardner, McCullough, Larson, & Prescott, 2003). Individuals who have strong religious practices report fewer and less severe symptoms of depressed mood (Smith, McCullough, & Poll 2003; Smith, McCullough, & Poll, 2004). Possible

explanations include an improved sense of social identity through religious affiliation, and the regular expression of feelings of thankfulness and forgiveness. Depressed severely mentally ill patients who attended regular weekly support groups emphasizing these themes reported improved mood, reduced anxiety, increased insight, and improved capacity for forgiveness (Sageman, 2004). Group members became progressively more articulate when expressing feelings of loneliness or isolation, and disclosed increased confidence in the future and hopefulness at "moving beyond old traumas." The researchers, who were also group facilitators, felt that regular opportunities to reflect on general religious and spiritual themes led to an increased capacity for forgiveness and compassion, including forgiving others who had caused suffering in the past, and cultivating a general sense of forgiveness and compassion through identification with a forgiving God.

◆ **Healing Touch and Therapeutic Touch** Practitioners of these energy healing methods claim the capacity to intuit energetic imbalances in the body and direct healing energy to specific bodily regions or functions to correct those imbalances. Preliminary findings from case reports and two small nonblinded studies suggest that Healing Touch has beneficial effects on depressed mood. In an open study 30 moderately to severely depressed patients were randomized to receive Healing Touch or assigned to a wait list (Bradway, 2003). The treatment group received two Healing Touch sessions weekly for 3 weeks. Control patients received no treatment, including no exposure to a sham Healing Touch treatment. By the end of the study, patients in the treatment group experienced significantly improved mood that was reportedly sustained at 1-month follow-up. The significance of these findings is limited by the small study size and the absence of a sham treatment group. Regular HealingTouch may be beneficial in bereaved patients (Robinson, 1996). Healthy female volunteers who were randomly assigned to receive Therapeutic Touch reported significantly greater reductions in their overall level of emotional distress compared with wait-listed women. Serum levels of nitric oxide were significantly lower in the Therapeutic Touch group compared with controls, suggesting a possible mechanism of the reported mood enhancing and antinausea effects of Therapeutic Touch (Lafreniere et al., 1999). Regular Healing Touch treatments resulted in significant reductions in despair, depersonalization, and somatization in grieving mothers who had recently lost a child (Kempson, 2000–2001).

◆ **Qigong** Qigong is an ancient method of treatment or self-treatment in Chinese medicine that has its origins before written language. Qigong and other energy practices may represent the earliest historical attempts of humans to heal. Like prayer, Healing Touch, and Reiki, qigong is used to treat both physical and psychological symptoms. Depressed patients can engage in a regular qigong practice or receive "emission qigong" treatments from a qigong master. Most studies on qigong have examined the effectiveness of regular qigong practice on general indicators of physical or psychological health (Wang, 1993). Findings of open trials on the efficacy of qigong or Tai Chi as treatments of "neuroticism" showed that indicators of anxiety, depressed mood, and quality of sleep were significantly better in patients who had consistently practiced qigong or Tai Chi for at least 5 years compared with individuals who had not practiced either mind–body technique (Tang et al., 1990). Another open study (Schwartzman, 1998) demonstrated improved mood in depressed patients who practiced qigong consistently for at least 2 years. Patients who followed a regular daily practice of qigong reported general improvement in their baseline emotional state, including improved indicators of mood. In a 2-month open pilot study, 39 patients with a *DSM-IV* diagnosis of major depressive disorder, dysthymic disorder, or bipolar disorder received qi "emission" treatments administered by qigong masters (Gaik, 2003). Half of the subjects engaged in the regular daily practice of qigong. Standardized ratings of depressed mood for all subjects had improved by the end of the study, and there was not a significant differential response rate in patients who received qi "emission" treatments while practicing qigong. Findings of this study cannot be generalized because a control group and a sham-treatment protocol were not part of the design.

The unskillful or excessive practice of qigong, or qigong practice in the absence of adequate guidance, can result in significant psychological or psychosomatic symptoms (Lake, 2001). The *DSM-IV* describes psychotic symptoms that can occur as a consequence of erroneous qigong as a kind of culture-bound syndrome, "qigong psychotic reaction." To minimize these risks, patients who tend to be histrionic or patients who have a history of psychosis or who have been diagnosed with personality disorders should be advised to practice qigong moderately and only under the guidance of a skilled instructor.

◆ Possibly Effective Nonconventional Treatments of Depressed Mood

Possibly effective nonconventional biological treatments of depressed mood include a Siberian herb called *Rhodiola rosea* when used alone, *Ginkgo biloba* (when used adjunctively with a conventional antidepressant), and the amino acids L-tyrosine and L-phenylalanine. *R. rosea* (golden root) is now widely used in Russia and Western Europe, and has mood-enhancing properties similar to *Panax ginseng* and the other adaptogens. Preliminary evidence suggests that targeted amino acid therapy using L-tyrosine or L-phenylalanine may be beneficial in cases where there are specific neurotransmitter deficiencies. Prayer, Reiki, and other "energy" treatments of depressed mood are gaining acceptance because of growing popular interest in Western countries and gradually accumulating evidence supporting their efficacy and safety. Although spiritual healing, directed intention, and "energy medicine" are being increasingly used to treat depressed mood in North America and Europe, evidence supporting their use is limited by inherent study design problems resulting in largely ambiguous findings. **Table 8–4** reviews the evidence for nonconventional treatments that are possibly effective in the management of depressed mood.

Medicinal Herbs

Rhodiola Rosea (Golden Root)

The findings of an extensive research program in the former Soviet Union point to many potential uses of *Rhodiola rosea* in

psychiatry (Brown & Gerbarg, 2004). *R. rosea* (golden root) is a traditionally used Siberian herb that has been demonstrated to increase brain levels of 5-hydroxytryptophan and reportedly has antidepressant and cognitive enhancing effects (Saratikov & Krasnov, 1987). It can be safely taken with conventional antidepressants, and there is preliminary evidence of an augmentation effect. Typical doses range from 200 to 400 mg/day. *R. rosea* may be safely combined with conventional antidepressants, and serious adverse effects have not been reported.

Ginkgo Biloba

Preliminary evidence suggests that *Ginkgo biloba* may augment conventional antidepressants in treatment-resistant depressed mood (Schubert & Halama, 1993).

Nonherbal Natural Products

L-tyrosine

Although L-tyrosine is not an essential amino acid, it plays many fundamental roles in human physiology. L-tyrosine is obtained directly through diet or synthesized from phenylalanine. It is also a necessary precursor to the synthesis of three neurotransmitters implicated in depressed mood: epinephrine, norepinephrine, and dopamine. Tyrosine is required for synthesis of nerve growth factor (NGF) and thyroxin, the most important thyroid hormone. Tyrosine deficiency is frequently associated with depressed mood (Grevet et al., 2002). Effective doses in depressed mood range from 500 to 1500 mg/day. Large doses of tyrosine may promote growth of malignant melanoma or other cancers (Harvie, Campbell, Howell, & Thatcher, 2002).

L-Phenylalanine

Depressed patients found to be deficient in phenylethylamine (PEA), a neurotransmitter synthesized from L-phenylalanine, improved significantly when treated with supplements of this amino acid (Sabelli et al., 1986). This finding is consistent with the hypothesis that low brain levels of PEA manifest as depressed mood.

Selenium and Rubidium

Supplementation with rubidium and selenium may be beneficial in some cases of depressed mood. In an open study 50 depressed patients who were deficient in selenium experienced significant improvements in mood and anxiety following daily selenium supplementation at 100 μg (Benton & Cook, 1991). Small open trials suggest that daily supplementation with rubidium in the form of rubidium chloride at doses between 180 and 720 mg has beneficial effects in depression that may be equivalent to conventional antidepressants (Calandra & Nicolosi, 1980; Williams, Maturen, & Sky-Peck, 1987). Adverse effects of rubidium have not been reported at doses that are therapeutic in depressed mood. Recommended doses of mineral supplements may be safely taken in combination with conventional antidepressants or natural products used to treat depressed mood, including SAMe.

Table 8–4 Possibly Effective Nonconventional Treatments of Depressed Mood

Category	Treatment Approach	Evidence for Claimed Treatment Effect	Comments
Biological	*Rhodiola rosea* (golden root)	*R. rosea* 200 to 400 mg/day increases brain serotonin levels and may have antidepressant effects	*R. rosea* may augment conventional antidepressants
	Ginkgo biloba	*G. biloba* may augment conventional antidepressants in treatment-refractory patients	*G. biloba* may provide a safe alternative to conventional augmentation strategies. **Caution:** *G. biloba* should not be taken with warfarin or other drugs that affect bleeding time
	L-tyrosine	L-tyrosine 500 to 1500 mg may have antidepressant effects	**Caution:** Large doses of l-tyrosine may promote growth of malignancies
	L-phenylalanine	L-phenylalanine may be beneficial in depressed patients with low serum PEA levels	Targeted amino acid therapy uses specific combinations of amino acids to treat identified neurotransmitter deficiencies
	Mineral supplements	Supplementation with selenium 100 μg or rubidium chloride 180 to 720 mg may be beneficial in some cases	**Note:** Supplementation with selenium or rubidium may be effective when these elements are deficient in the diet
Somatic and mind–body	Massage	Regular massage therapy probably improves general emotional well-being and is beneficial in premenstrual and postpartum depression	Chiropractic and the Alexander technique may be beneficial in some cases
Energy-information approaches validated by Western science	Cranioelectrotherapy stimulation (CES)	Daily 40-minute CES treatments may be beneficial in some cases	CES may reduce alcohol or substance abuse in depressed alcoholics or addicts
Energy-information approaches not validated by Western science	Reiki	Regular Reiki treatments may be beneficial for depressed patients	Distant Reiki and hands-on Reiki treatments may be equally effective
	Prayer and distant healing intention	Individuals who pray and those prayed for may benefit from shared beliefs	**Note:** Intercessory prayer had no effect on depressed mood
	Energy psychology	Energy psychology methods, including Emotional Freedom Technique and body-centered psychotherapy, may be beneficial in some cases of depressed mood	Recent studies suggest a significant placebo effect
	Combining crystals with conventional energy-information approaches	Crystals worn in conjunction with conventional energy-information treatments and healing intention were associated with significant improvements in depressed mood	**Note:** Patients who wore glass or quartz crystals reported equivalent improvements. Impossible to determine a specific effect related to intention and wearing a crystal

PEA, phenylethylamine

Somatic and Mind–body Approaches

Case reports suggest that many body-centered approaches are beneficial for mental health in general. Massage, chiropractic, the Alexander technique, and other somatic therapies are based on assumptions that gentle manipulations of certain parts of the body result in beneficial "shifts" in emotional or spiritual equilibrium that improve mood. Controlled studies on somatic techniques are difficult to perform, and placebo effects may play a significant role. Limited research findings suggest that massage therapy improves moderately depressed mood associated with chronic fatigue, and may ameliorate premenstrual or postpartum depression (Field et al., 1997; Hernandez-Reif et al., 2000; Mantle, 2002).

Energy-Information Approaches Validated by Western Science

Cranial Electrotherapy Stimulation

Findings from many small studies of cranial electrotherapy stimulation (CES) in depressed alcoholics or drug abusers

suggest that regular daily 40-minute to 1-hour treatments are associated with significant improvements in mood, as well as diminished alcohol or drug use (Smith, Tiberi, & Marshall, 1994).

Energy-Information Approaches Not Validated by Western Science

Hands-On and Distant Reiki Treatments

Studies of Reiki as a treatment of emotional distress in chronic pain patients suggest beneficial effects (Dressen & Singg, 1998). Findings of a double-blind, sham-controlled trial support the hypothesis that regular hands-on or distant Reiki treatments are associated with significant improvements in mood and stress based on standardized symptom rating scales (Shore, 2004). Following standardized pretest assessment of mood and stress, 73 volunteers were recruited using newspaper and radio ads. All volunteers complained of depressed mood or stress; however, few met *DSM-IV* criteria for major depressive disorder. Fifty volunteers completed the study, including 1-year post-treatment follow-up. Volunteers were randomized to receive weekly $1^1/_2$-hour hands-on Reiki, distant Reiki, or distant sham Reiki treatments over a 6-week period. The same Reiki master served as both the Reiki healer and sham healer, depending on randomized instructions, to "send healing energy" or to remain passive. Patients who received hands-on or distant Reiki treatments improved significantly and to the same degree on standardized ratings of depressed mood and stress, exhibiting improvements in feelings of hopelessness and reductions in overall stress. Improvements were sustained at 1-year follow-up in the absence of continuing Reiki treatments. Patients who received sham Reiki treatments did not improve. Compared with conventional psychopharmacological treatments, the findings of this preliminary study suggest that Reiki may be an effective and cost-effective energy treatment of patients complaining of depressed mood.

Prayer and Distant Healing Intention

In a 3-month controlled study on the effects of intercessory prayer on depressed mood, subjects where not told whether they were assigned to a wait list or the group that was prayed for several times each week. Interestingly, individuals who prayed and patients who were prayed for reported similar beneficial changes in mood. The findings of this study are limited by the fact that standardized mood-rating scales were not used. Positive findings in both subjects and individuals who prayed were attributed to shared beliefs in the healing efficacy of prayer (O'Laoire, 1997). A study on distant healing in patients diagnosed with major depression who remained on conventional antidepressants did not find a differential effect of prayer compared with conventional antidepressants alone (Greyson, 1996).

Energy Psychology, Body Psychotherapy, and Other Subtle Energy Healing Methods

Emotional freedom technique (EFT) is a simplified version of thought field therapy (TFT) that is used to treat psychological symptoms resulting from traumatic experiences. Few controlled studies have been conducted on EFT. Findings of one sham-controlled study suggest that there is no difference between established EFT approaches and sham treatments of depressed mood (Waite & Holder, 2003). Body psychotherapy is a form of energy psychology that is popular in Germany, Switzerland, the Netherlands, and other European countries. More research has been done on this technique than TFT or EFT. Case studies and retrospective case reviews suggest that some depressed patients experience generally improved feelings of well-being following body psychotherapy. In some cases of depressed mood, energy psychology approaches may

be effective because of positive expectations; however, negative findings of the only sham-controlled trial to date do not provide a basis for recommending TFT or EFT as a specific treatment of depression.

Combining Crystals with Conventional Energy-Information Methods

In one study 141 chronically depressed patients who had failed to respond to conventional antidepressants were randomly assigned to carry glass or quartz crystals for 3 months while undergoing different kinds of conventional energy-information treatments, including cranial electrotherapy stimulation (CES), autogenic training, photostimulation, music, and brain wave synchronization using EEG biofeedback training (Shealy et al., 1993). All patients were instructed to "program" their crystals by "breathing healing thoughts" into the crystals, which were kept in satin pouches placed about their necks. All subjects remained off conventional antidepressants during the study. Significant and equivalent improvements in mood (using standardized mood-rating scales) were reported 2 weeks into the study in patients wearing both the glass and the quartz crystals. Several nonconventional healing methods were employed in parallel in this study; therefore, it is not possible to attribute an antidepressant effect solely to crystals, other more conventional treatments, or shared positive healing intentions of patients or therapists.

Although a group placebo effect is clearly a possible explanation of positive outcomes, the impressive magnitude of improvement in depressed mood renders the findings of this study significant. Further research is warranted to identify possible synergistic influences of the various healing approaches employed.

◆ Integrative Management Algorithm for Depressed Mood

Figure 8–1 is the integrative management algorithm for depressed mood. Note that specific assessment and treatment approaches are representative examples of reasonable choices. Moderate symptoms often respond to exercise, dietary modification, mind–body practices, and energy-information therapies. When managing severe symptoms, emphasize biological therapies. Encourage exercise and other lifestyle changes in motivated patients. Consider conventional, nonconventional, and integrative approaches that have not been tried.

See evidence tables and text for complete reviews of evidence-based options.

Before implementing any treatment plan, always check evidence tables and Web site updates at www.thieme.com/mentalhealth for specific assessment and treatment protocols, and obtain patient informed consent.

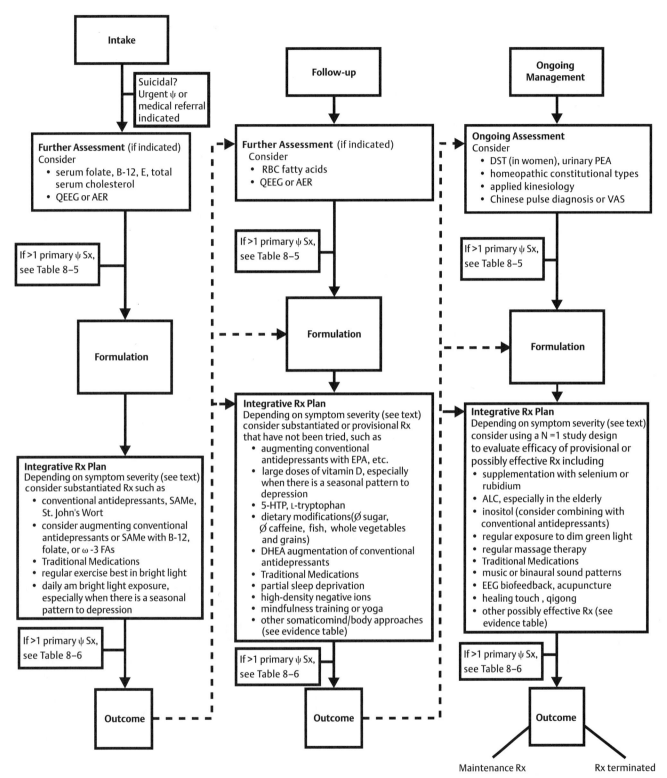

Figure 8–1 Integrative management algorithm for depressed mood. Note that specific assessment and treatment approaches are representative examples of reasonable choices. Rx, treatment; Sx, symptoms.

◆ Integrated Approaches to Consider When Two or More Core Symptoms Are Present

Table 8–5 shows the assessment approaches to consider using when depressed mood is the focus of clinical attention and one or more other symptoms are being assessed concurrently.

Table 8–6 outlines the treatment approaches to consider using when depressed mood is the focus of clinical attention and one or more other symptoms are being treated concurrently.

Table 8–5   Assessment Approaches to Depressed Mood When Other Symptoms Are Being Assessed Concurrently

Other Symptom(s) Being Assessed Concurrently	Assessment Approach	Comments
Mania or cyclic mood changes	Serologic studies	Low serum folate predicts nonresponse to both conventional and nonconventional treatments of depressed mood.
		Low serum B_{12} and vitamin E levels are often found in depressed patients.
		Low RBC omega-3 fatty acids are correlated with more severe depressed mood.
		Low total serum triglycerides and cholesterol levels correlate with more severe depressed mood and higher risk of suicide.
		Abnormal low RBC folate levels (but normal serum folate levels) are common in bipolar patients.
		Low trace lithium levels (i.e., from low nutritional intake) are common in acute mania.
		High pretreatment serum homovanillic acid (HVA) levels predict improved response to lower doses of conventional antipsychotics in acute mania.
		Limited evidence suggests that PEA and phenylacetic acid levels are consistently low in bipolar depressed mood.
	qEEG brain mapping	Abnormal qEEG findings suggest specific treatment strategies and differentiate unipolar from bipolar depressed mood.
		Specific qEEG findings may predict differential response to certain conventional antidepressants, including SSRIs, and some nonconventional antidepressants.
		Limited evidence suggests that pretreatment qEEG in manic or cycling patients facilitates selection of the most effective conventional drug treatment.
	Chinese medical pulse diagnosis and VAS reflex	Limited evidence suggests that Chinese pulse diagnosis and analysis of the VAS provide accurate information when evaluating mania, cyclic mood changes, and depressed mood. Both approaches may provide clinically useful information when planning the conventional and nonconventional treatment of depressed mood and mania.
Anxiety	Serologic studies	Limited evidence suggests that total serum cholesterol is elevated in chronically anxious patients.
		Limited evidence suggests that deficiencies of niacin and vitamins B_6, C, and E are associated with generalized anxiety.
		Limited evidence suggests that deficiencies of magnesium, selenium, and phosphorus are associated with chronic anxiety.
		Limited evidence suggests that high urinary glutamate levels are correlated with general anxiety.
	qEEG brain mapping	Limited evidence suggests that specific qEEG findings can be used to guide treatment selection in anxious patients, including conventional drugs and EEG biofeedback training.
Psychosis	Serologic studies	Low RBC omega-3 fatty acids are correlated with more severe depressed mood, and limited evidence suggests that consistently low RBC levels of two fatty acids (arachidonic acid and DHA) correspond to low brain levels of these fatty acids in chronic psychosis
	qEEG brain mapping	Limited evidence suggests that specific qEEG findings correlate with differential response rates of psychosis to both conventional and nonconventional treatments.
	Analysis of VAS reflex	Limited evidence suggests that the VAS reflex provides useful information when identifying conventional medications and specific doses that will be effective in previously nonresponsive psychotic patients.
Cognitive impairment	qEEG brain mapping, VEP, and AER	qEEG mapping provides useful information when planning EEG biofeedback protocols addressing cognitive impairment in general.
		qEEG mapping can be used to evaluate response to conventional and nonconventional cognitive enhancing treatments.
		Limited evidence suggests that qEEG mapping, VEP, and AER studies permit early diagnosis and more aggressive treatment of early Alzheimer's and mild cognitive impairment.

Table 8–5 Assessment Approaches to Depressed Mood When Other Symptoms Are Being Assessed Concurrently *(Continued)*

Other Symptom(s) Being Assessed Concurrently	Assessment Approach	Comments
Substance abuse or dependence	Serologic studies	In alcohol abuse the magnitude of serum deficiencies of vitamins A and C, some B vitamins, as well as zinc, magnesium, and essential fatty acids is an indicator of the severity of malnutrition.
	AER	Conventional treatments of heroin detoxification normalize AER findings.
	qEEG brain mapping	Limited evidence suggests that qEEG brain mapping provides useful information when planning specific EEG biofeedback protocols for relapsing alcoholics or narcotics abusers.
	Chinese medical pulse diagnosis and VAS reflex	Limited evidence suggests that VAS analysis provides useful information when planning detoxification protocols based on acupuncture and conventional medications.
Disturbance of sleep or wakefulness	Serologic studies	Deficiencies in vitamins C, E, B_{12}, and folic acid are correlated with increased daytime sleepiness and insomnia.
		Abnormal low serum levels of magnesium and zinc are often associated with increased daytime sleepiness.
	Chinese pulse diagnosis	Limited evidence suggests that Chinese pulse diagnosis provides clinically useful information about energetic imbalances that manifest as daytime sleepiness or nighttime wakefulness.

AER, auditory evoked response; DHA, docosahexaenoic acid; EEG, electroencephalography; PEA, phenylethylamine; qEEG, quantitative electroencephalography; RBC, red blood cell (count); SSRI, selective serotonin reuptake inhibitor; VAS, vascular autonomic signal; VEP, visual evoked potential

Table 8–6 Treatment Approaches to Depressed Mood When Other Symptoms Are Being Treated Concurrently

Other Symptom(s) Being Treated Concurrently	Treatment Approach	Comments
Mania or cyclic mood changes	St. John's wort	Standardized St. John's wort preparations 300 mg tid have comparable efficacy to conventional antidepressants for moderate depressed mood.
		Limited evidence suggests that St. John's wort at higher doses (up to 1800 mg/day) is effective against severe depressed mood.
		Caution: St. John's wort is contraindicated in in patients taking protease inhibitors, immunosuppressive agents, theophylline, and oral contraceptives. It should be avoided in pregnancy and in patients taking MAOI antidepressants.
		St. John's wort may be an effective treatment of SAD.
		Combining St. John's wort with bright light exposure may be more effective against SAD than either approach alone.
	Folate	Folate 0.5 to 1 mg/day augments the effects of conventional antidepressants and SAMe.
		Folic acid 200 μg/day may augment the effects of lithium in mania.
	Omega-3 essential fatty acids	Combining omega-3 fatty acids (especially EPA) 1 to 2 g/day with conventional antidepressants improves response and may accelerate response rate.
		Limited evidence suggests that EPA alone is an effective treatment of severe depressed mood.
		EPA 1 to 2 g/day in combination with conventional mood stabilizers may reduce severity and frequency of manic episodes.
	5-HTP and L-tryptophan	5-HTP 300 mg/day is probably as effective as conventional antidepressants for moderate depressed mood.
		Some cases of treatment-refractory depression improve when 5-HTP 300 to 600 mg/day is combined with carbidopa or conventional antidepressants.
		L-tryptophan 1 to 2 g may be equivalent to imipramine 150 mg and other conventional antidepressants.
		L-tryptophan 2 g augments fluoxetine 20 mg and improves sleep quality.
		L-tryptophan 1 to 2 g combined with bright light therapy is more effective than either approach alone in SAD.
		Limited evidence suggests that L-tryptophan reduces the frequency of depressive mood swings and also reduces the severity of mania in bipolar patients.
		Limited evidence suggests that L-tryptophan 3 g tid added to lithium improves symptoms of mania more than lithium alone.
	Mindfulness training	Mindfulness training is probably as effective as cognitive therapy in moderate depressed mood.
		Certain meditation practices promote calmness and may be beneficial in mania or hypomania.

Table 8–6   Treatment Approaches to Depressed Mood When Other Symptoms Are Being Treated Concurrently *(Continued)*

Other Symptom(s) Being Treated Concurrently	Treatment Approach	Comments
Anxiety	Dietary changes	Limited evidence suggests that restricting caffeine and refined sugar and increasing consumption of fatty fish and whole foods rich in B vitamins improves depressed mood and reduces the risk of becoming depressed.
		Limited evidence suggests that avoiding refined sugar and caffeine and increasing protein and foods containing tryptophan reduce symptoms of generalized anxiety and panic.
	L-tryptophan and 5-HTP	L-tryptophan 2 to 3 g/day or 5-HTP 25 to 100 mg up to 3 times a day is probably an effective treatment of generalized anxiety.
		Limited evidence suggests that 5-HTP prevents panic attacks.
	Exercise	Regular exerce at least 30 minutes 3 times a week is as effective as conventional antidepressants, St. John's wort, and cognitive therapy for moderate depressed mood.
		Exercising under bright light is more effective against depression than exercise or bright light alone.
		Regular aerobic or strengthening exercise reduces generalized anxiety symptoms, and there is limited evidence that it may reduce both the frequency and severity of panic attack.
	Acupuncture	Conventional acupuncture may be effective against severe depressed mood.
		Electroacupuncture alone may be as effective as electroacupuncture combined with amitriptyline or other conventional antidepressants, and there is limited evidence that computer-controlled electroacupuncture using high-frequency currents is more effective than conventional or standard electroacupuncture.
		Some acupuncture and electroacupuncture protocols probably reduce symptoms of generalized anxiety.
	Music and binaural sound	Attentive listening to music probably improves moderately depressed mood.
		Combining music with guided imagery is more beneficial than either approach alone.
		Limited evidence suggests that listening to binaural sounds in the beta frequency range (16–24 Hz) improves depressed mood.
		Regular listening to soothing music or certain binaural sounds can significantly reduce generalized anxiety
	Combining HRV and EEG biofeedback	There is limited evidence that combined EEG-HRV biofeedback ("energy cardiology") training improves depressed mood.
		EEG, EMG, GSR, and thermal biofeedback are effective treatments of generalized anxiety, and there is emerging evidence that regular biofeedback permits dose reductions of conventional drugs.
		Combining GSR biofeedback and relaxation is more effective against anxiety than either approach alone.
		Biofeedback training using HRV probably reduces symptoms of generalized anxiety
Psychosis	Omega-3 essential fatty acids	Limited evidence suggests that the omega-3 essential fatty acid EPA (1–4 g) alone or in combination with conventional antipsychotics (and especially clozapine) improves psychotic symptoms. Beneficial effects may be more robust in the early acute phase of psychotic illnesses.
Cognitive impairment	Dietary changes	Moderate wine consumption, reduced saturated fats, and reduced total caloric intake are correlated with reduced risk of developing Alzheimer's disease.
		Limited evidence suggests that diets high in fish or other sources of omega-3 fatty acids and low in omega-6 fatty acids are associated with a reduced risk of developing dementia.
	Folate and vitamin B_{12}	Limited evidence suggests that folate 50 mg/day improves mood and cognition in depressed demented individuals.
		Daily folate, vitamin B_{12}, or thiamine supplementation may be beneficial in some cases of age-related cognitive decline and Alzheimer's disease.
	Acetyl-L-carnitine (ALC)	Limited evidence suggests that ALC 1 to 3 g/day in divided doses is beneficial in elderly depressed demented patients.
		ALC should be considered when depression is related to post-traumatic brain injury or age-related cognitive decline.
		Limited evidence suggests that ALC 1500 to 3000 mg is beneficial for mild cognitive decline and Alzheimer's disease.
		ALC may improve cognitive performance in healthy adults, as well as in depressed individuals and abstinent alcoholics
	DHEA	DHEA 90 to 450 mg/day in mild to moderate depressed mood.
		DHEA has synergistic effects when combined with conventional antidepressants and may be an effective monotherapy for moderate depressed mood.
		DHEA may be beneficial when depressed mood occurs together with anxiety, psychosis, or cognitive impairment.

Table 8–6   Treatment Approaches to Depressed Mood When Other Symptoms Are Being Treated Concurrently *(Continued)*

Other Symptom(s) Being Treated Concurrently	Treatment Approach	Comments
	Music and binaural sound	Regular music therapy probably enhances global functioning in demented individuals, reduces agitation and wandering, enhances social interaction, improves depressed mood, increases cooperative behavior, and increases baseline cognitive functioning Binaural sounds in the beta frequency range may enhance cognitive functioning in healthy adults.
	Healing Touch (HT) and Therapeutic Touch (TT)	Limited evidence suggests that regular HT or TT treatments reduces agitation, improves global functioning, improves sleep schedule, and enhances compliance with nursing home routines.
		Patients who receive regular HT treatments may require lower doses of medications for agitated behavior
Substance abuse or dependence	Dietary changes	Alcoholics who improve their diets, including reduced intake of refined sugar and caffeine and increased intake of omega-3 fatty acids and protein, probably have an increased chance for maintaining sobriety.
	Exercise	Limited evidence suggests that regular aerobic exercise or strength training in abstinent alcoholics improves general emotional well-being.
	Mindfulness training	Abstinent alcoholics and addicts who engage in a regular mindfulness practice or meditation probably have a reduced risk of relapse.
		Spiritually focused support groups probably reduce relapse risk.
	Acupuncture	Some points and protocols are probably more effective than others in reducing symptoms of alcohol or cocaine withdrawal.
Disturbance of sleep or wakefulness	Dietary changes	Alcohol use at bedtime causes rebound insomnia.
		Caffeine in beverages or medications causes insomnia; caffeine withdrawal causes daytime sleepiness and fatigue.
		Refined sugar snacks at night cause rebound hypoglycemia and disturbed sleep.
	L-tryptophan and 5-HTP	Combining L tryptophan 2 g with a conventional antidepressant probably enhances. antidepressant response and improves sleep quality.
		5-HTP and L-tryptophan probably reduce symptoms of mild or situational insomnia.
		5-HTP increases sleep duration in obstructive sleep apnea and narcolepsy.
	Bright light exposure	Regular carefully timed bright light exposure resynchronizes phase advanced or phase delayed sleep to the patient's time zone.
	Acupuncture	Some acupuncture and auriculotherapy protocols probably reduce the severity of sleep disturbances, including insomnia related to depression or other emotional problems.

DHEA, dehydroepiandrosterone; EEG, electroencephalography; EMG, electromyography; EPA, ecosapentanoic acid; GSR, galvanic skin response; 5-HTP, 5-hydroxytryptophan; HRV, heart rate variability; MAOI, monoamine oxidase inhibitor; SAD, seasonal affective disorder; SAMe, *S*-adenosylmethionine

Case Vignette

History and Initial Presentation

Paul is a 57-year-old retired broker with a complicated medical history, including coronary artery disease, and adult onset non-insulin-dependent diabetes. He was recently started on a statin for elevated cholesterol. He is a recovering alcoholic and has been sober for 11 years. Recently, he has "been less interested" in life and seldom goes out. He has three grown children and two grandchildren. Paul first experienced severe depressed mood at the age of 18. At that time his symptoms included persistent feelings of hopelessness and worthlessness, severe daytime fatigue, loss of appetite, and frequent thoughts of suicide. He remained sober but began to have cravings for alcohol. Paul did not seek professional help at that time and recalls "gutting it out," and eventually feeling better after several months. Afterwards, his mood was "OK" for 3 years, when he again experienced severe depressed mood and suicidal thoughts. There have been no episodes of mania or hypomania. He was eventually diagnosed with major depressive disorder and started on fluoxetine (Prozac) at 20 mg. His mood improved dramatically after 6 weeks, but he experienced adverse effects including dizziness and diminished libido. Paul discontinued Prozac after 1 year because of these adverse effects. Two years later he became depressed again. A psychiatrist started him on sertraline (Zoloft) at 100 mg, but his mood continued to worsen, and he was eventually hospitalized for 3 days because of intrusive suicidal thoughts. While hospitalized, Paul was started on lithium carbonate and continued on Zoloft, which was increased to 200 mg. Following discharge, his mood remained stable, but he experienced a 30-pound weight gain during the first 3 months on lithium, and "the tremor and nausea were also annoying." After 3 years, against his psychiatrist's advice, Paul decided to stop taking lithium, but continued taking Zoloft. His psychiatrist eventually tried paroxetine (Paxil), nefazadone (Serzone), bupriprion (Wellbutrin), venlafaxine (Effexor), trazadone (Desaryl), and, most recently, citalopram (Celexa). Paul discontinued Effexor after a few days because of severe unremitting headaches. He was recently started on mirtazapine (Remeron), and has experienced carbohydrate cravings. Paul describes most conventional antidepressants as "working for a while . . . then they peter out. . . ." One year ago he chose to retire early and left "the fast lane. . . ." Paul recently heard about a local clinic where both conventional and nonconventional mental health care is available. He was intrigued, and after his frustrating experiences with conventional treatments, he was open to new approaches.

Assessment, Formulation, and Integrative Treatment Plan

Mary, a nurse practitioner trained in Western psychiatry and acupuncture, takes a thorough medical, psychiatric, and social history, including a detailed review of Paul's treatment-response history to conventional antidepressants and his history of adverse effects. Mary confirms that the most recent episode of severe depressed mood was about 2 years ago, and since then Paul has been moderately depressed most of the time. She examines Paul's tongue and eyes and performs a Chinese medical pulse diagnosis, which confirms stagnant liver qi as a probable underlying cause of depressed mood. Paul notes recent weight gain on mirtazapine 15 mg at bedtime. He is concerned that he has been eating too many sweet foods, which have been increasing his blood sugar readings. Paul discloses anxiety over "my existential issues" and discloses that he is considering trying "some kind of mind–body thing" to address these concerns. Mary assesses Paul's current mood as moderately depressed according to *DSM-IV* criteria, which is consistent with his Chinese medical diagnosis of stagnant liver qi. She confirms the absence of suicidal thoughts and decides to order conventional biological screening tests, including serum total cholesterol and triglycerides, RBC folate level, and thyroid studies. She briefly reviews the evidence showing relationships between Paul's medical problems and depressed mood, and notifies Paul of mood worsening side effects described in the *Physician's Desk Reference* (*PDR*) for an antihypertensive medication that he is taking. Paul expresses his disappointment and frustration over incomplete responses to conventional antidepressants and a long history of adverse effects. Mary reviews substantiated nonconventional approaches for moderate depressed mood, including lifestyle changes, acupuncture, and other therapies that improve mood when used alone or in combination with conventional antidepressants.

Paul is clearly skeptical about Chinese medicine, and Mary decides not to pursue this direction. He expresses strong interest in nonconventional biological treatments. The initial treatment plan includes continuation on the current dose of mirtazapine, a trial on adjunctive SAMe, vitamin supplements, daily aerobic exercise, improved diet, and regular stress management. Mary uses a standard reference to confirm that SAMe may be safely used in patients with heart disease and informs Paul of possible adverse effects, including mild agitation or sedation, and gastrointestinal distress during the initial weeks of treatment. Using the clinic's computer, Mary quickly goes online to search an expert database on natural products (Natural Medicine Comprehensive Database) and confirms the absence of documented interactions between SAMe, mirtazapine, and Paul's other medications. She documents her review of safety issues and Paul's informed consent in the intake note. She recommends a quality brand of SAMe and tells Paul where he can find it. They agree on a trial of SAMe starting at a dose of 200 mg daily, gradually

increasing the dose every week to the recommended therapeutic range (800–1600 mg/day) while monitoring for side effects. Mary recommends taking folate and vitamin B_{12} with SAMe, and explains that these vitamins are important cofactors when taking SAMe. Paul agrees with the recommended treatment plan and signs a release authorizing Mary to notify his psychiatrist of the new plan. Paul appears to have limited insight and is not psychologically minded, and Mary decides to not refer him to a psychotherapist. She advises Paul to obtain a medical release from his family practice physician before starting to exercise and suggests that he begin a program of gradually increasing exercise under medical supervision. Paul agrees to begin exercising and to start a daily routine of listening to relaxing music. Paul is given a hand-written note outlining the treatment plan. Initial follow-up is scheduled in 3 weeks, and Paul is invited to call for an earlier appointment if he has problems taking the SAMe or his symptoms worsen before then.

Follow-Up

After 3 weeks, Paul returns, frustrated that "nothing is working. . . . I'm going downhill fast." He complains of feeling sad most of the time, continues to crave sweets, and remarks that overeating and weight gain are still problems. He denies suicidal thoughts, but he feels demoralized and appears anxious. He has not kept up a regular exercise program, but he has been listening to music several times a day and has been working in his garden. Paul has started taking a multivitamin, but he has not purchased the other recommended vitamin supplements. His RBC folate level returned in the low-normal range, and serum total cholesterol level was 155 mg/dL. Thyroid studies are in the normal range. Mary tells Paul about recent studies showing the relationship between abnormal low total cholesterol and the severity of depressed mood, and suggests that he discuss adjusting the dose of his statin with his family practice doctor. On reviewing the events of the previous few weeks, Mary learns that Paul did not select the quality brand of SAMe she recommended and has not increased his dose according to the original plan. He continues to take only 200 mg of SAMe in the morning. Mary reminds Paul that when he reaches an adequate dose of SAMe, assuming there are no significant adverse effects and his mood improves, it will be reasonable to consider discontinuing the mirtazapine in consultation with his psychiatrist, which will probably eliminate his nighttime cravings, resulting in desired weight loss.

Two weeks later, Paul appears brighter and is noticeably more rested. He seems calmer and appears to have lost some weight. He smiles as he explains that his internist has given him "a clean bill of health" to exercise, and he has been riding a bicycle almost every day. His family practice doctor recommended lowering the dose of his statin, and his repeat total cholesterol level is now 180 mg/dL, "but the LDL [low-density lipoprotein] to HDL [high-density lipoprotein] ratio is still in the safe zone. . . ." Paul has found the recommended brand of SAMe and has continued to titrate his dose as agreed. At 400 mg he experienced mild restlessness, but this went away after a few days at that dose. He currently takes 400 mg before breakfast and lunch, and there are no adverse effects. Paul reports that he began to experience consistent improvement in depressed mood after taking this dose (800 mg/day) for about 1 week.

About a week ago Paul met with his psychiatrist, who agreed that it is reasonable to discontinue the mirtazapine if he continues at his present baseline for 1 month. Regular exercise has resulted in a 5-pound weight loss over the past 3 weeks. His most recent blood pressure reading was moderately lower than before, and his internist is considering taking him off the oral hypoglycemic agent if he continues to exercise

and lose weight. Paul enjoys music every day and has started to play golf again. He is comfortable with the idea of returning every 2 months for the next 6 months for routine follow-up appointments. He agrees to continue taking SAMe at his current dose, and Mary asks Paul to call her with an update about 1 month after he stops taking the mirtazapine under his psychiatrist's supervision.

References

Ackerman, J. (1989). A study of device technology based on acupuncture meridians and chi energy. *Conference Proceedings: Energy Fields in Medicine, 156.*

Agency for Healthcare Research and Quality, U.S. Department of Health and Human Services. (2002). *Evidence Report/Technology Assessment: S-adenosyl-l-methionine for Treatment of Depression, Osteoarthritis, and Liver Disease* (No. 64). Available at www.ahrq.gov

Alarcon, R. D., & Franceschini, J. A. (1984). Hyperparathyroidism and paranoid psychosis: Case report and review of the literature. *British Journal of Psychiatry, 145,* 477–486.

Allen, J., Schnyer, R., & Hitt, S. (1998). The efficacy of acupuncture in the treatment of major depression in women. *Psychological Science, 9*(5), 397–401.

Alpert, J., & Fava, M. (1997). Nutrition and depression: The role of folate. *Nutrition Reviews, 55*(5), 145–149.

Alpert, J. (2004). *Oral S-adenosyl methionine (SAMe) for antidepressant augmentation: An open-label trial* (Abstract no. 72). Paper presented at the annual meeting of the American Psychiatric Association, New York.

Alvarez, E., Udina, C., & Guillamat, R. (1987). Shortening of latency period in depressed patients treated with SAMe and other antidepressant drugs. *Cell Biology Reviews, 1,* 103–110.*

American Psychiatric Association. (1993). Practice guidelines for major depressive disorders in adults. *American Journal of Psychiatry, 150*(Suppl. 4), 1–26.

Angst, F., Woggon, B., Schoepf, J. (1977). The treatment of depression with L-5-hydroxytryptophan versus imipramine. Resutls of two open and one double-blind study. *Archives of Psychiatry and Neurology, 224*(2), 175–186.

Arnold, J. T., Le, H., McFann, K. K., & Blackman, M. R. (2005). Comparative effects of DHEA vs. testosterone, dihydrotestosterone, and estradiol on proliferation and gene expression in human LNCaP prostate cancer cells. *American Journal of Physiology Endocrinology and Metabolism, 288*(3), E573–E584.

Avery, D. H., Bolte, M. A., & Ries, R. (1998). Dawn simulation treatment of abstinent alcoholics with winter depression. *Journal of Clinical Psychiatry, 59,* 36–44.

Baehr, E., Rosenfeld, J. P., & Baehr, R. (2001). Clinical use of an Alpha asymmetry neurofeedback protocol in the treatment of mood disorders: Follow-up study one to five years post therapy. *Journal of Neurotherapy, 4,* 11–18.

Baehr, E., & Rosenfeld, J. P. (2003). Mood disorders. In D. Moss, A. McGrady, T. Davies, & I. Wickramasekera (Eds.), *Handbook of mind–body medicine for primary care* (pp. 377–392). Thousand Oaks, CA: Sage.

Bagby, R., Gyder, A., Schuller, D., & Marshall, M. (2004). The Hamilton depression rating scale: Has the gold standard become a lead weight? *American Journal of Psychiatry, 161,* 2163–2177.

Bauer, M. S., Kurtz, J. W., Rubin, L. B., & Marcus, J. G. (1994). Mood and behavioral effects of four-week light treatment in winter depressives and controls. *Journal of Psychiatric Research, 28,* 135–145.

Bell, I. R., Lewis, D. A. II., Schwartz, G. E., Lewis, S. E., Caspi, O., Scott, A., Brooks, A. J., & Baldwin, C. M. (2004). Electroencephalographic cordance patterns distinguish exceptional clinical responders with fibromyalgia to individualized homeopathic medicines. *Journal of Alternative and Complementary Medicine,10*(2), 285–299.

Bella, R., Biondi, R., Raffaele, R., & Pennisi, G. (1990). Effect of acetyl-L-carnitine on geriatric patients suffering from dysthymic disorders. *International Journal of Clinical Pharmacological Research, 10*(6), 355–360.

Belmaker, R. H. (1996, June). *The inositol depletion hypothesis: Promise and problems* [Conference abstract]. Paper presented at the Twentieth Collegium Internationale Neuro-psychopharmacologicum, Melbourne, Australia.

Bender, K. (2004, December). Study to reveal drug study reforms. *Psychiatric Times,* p. 1.

Benedetti, F., Barbini, B., Lucca Campori, E., Colombo, C., & Smeraldi, E. (1997). Sleep deprivation hastens the antidepressant action of fluoxetine. *European Archives of Psychiatry and Clinical Neuroscience, 247*(2), 100–103.

Benedetti, F., Colombo, C., Barbini, B., Campori, E., & Smeraldi, E. (2001). Morning sunlight reduces length of hospitalization in bipolar depression. *Journal of Affective Disorders, 62*(3), 221–223.

Benedetti, F., Colombo, C., Pontiggia, A., Bernasconi, A., Florita, M., & Smeraldi, E. (2003). Morning light treatment hastens the antidepressant effect of citalopram: A placebo-controlled trial. *Journal of Clinical Psychiatry, 64*(6), 648–653.

Benjamin, J., Agam, G., Levine, J., et al. (1995). Inositol treatment in psychiatry. *Psychopharmacology Bulletin, 31*(1),167–175.

Benton, D., & Cook, R. (1991). The impact of selenium supplementation on mood. *Biological Psychiatry, 29*(11), 1092–1098.

Benton, D., Griffiths, R., & Halter, J. (1997). Thiamine supplementation, mood and cognitive functioning. *Psychopharmacology (Berlin), 129*(1), 66–71.

Benton, D., Haller, J., & Fordy, J. (1995). Vitamin supplementation for 1 year improves mood. *Neuropsychobiology, 32,* 98–105.

Berlanga, C., Ortega-Soto, H. A., Ontiveros, M., & Senties, H. (1992). Efficacy of S-adenosyl-L-methionine in speeding the onset of action of imipramine. *Psychiatry Research, 44*(3), 257–262.

Bernal, I., Cercos, A., Fuste, I., Vallverdu, R., Urbieta Solana, R., & Montesinos Molina, I. (1995). Relaxation therapy in patients with anxiety and somatoform disorders in primary care [Spanish]. *Aten Primaria, 5,* 499–504.

Birdsall, T. C. (1998). 5-hydroxytryptophan: A clinically-effective serotonin precursor. *Alternative Medicine Review, 3*(4), 271–280.

Blackburn, I. M., Eunson, K. M., & Bishop, S. (1986). A two-year naturalistic follow-up of depressed patients treated with cognitive therapy, pharmacotherapy, and a combination of both. *Journal of Affective Disorders, 10,* 67–75.

Blumenthal, J. A., Babyak, M. A., Moore, K. A., Craighead, W. E., Herman, S., Khatri, P., et al. (1999). Effects of exercise training on older patients with major depression. *Archives of Internal Medicine, 159*(19), 2349–2356.

Bocchetta, A., Chillotti, C., Carboni, G., et al. (2001). Association of persona nd familial suicide risk with low serum cholesterol concentration in male lithium patients. *Acta psychiatrica Scandinavica, 104*(1), 37–41.

Bollini, P., Pampallona, S., Tibal G., et al. (1999). Effectiveness of antidepressants. Meta-anylose-effect relationships in randomized clinical trials. *British Journal of Psychiatry, 174,* 303.

Boschert, S. (2003). Preliminary report aimed at improving depression treatment. *Clinical Psychiatry News,* p. 40.

Bottiglieri, T. (1996). Folate, vitamin B_{12}, and neuropsychiatric disorders. *Nutrition Reviews, 54,* 382–390.

Bottiglieri, T., Godfrey, P., Flynn, T., et al. (1990). Cerebrospinal fluid S-adenosylmethionine in depression and dementia: Effects of treatment with parenteral and oral S-adenosylmethionine. *Journal of Neurology, Neurosurgery, and Psychiatry, 53,* 1096–1098.

Bottiglieri, T., Hyland, K., Laundy, M., Godfrey, P., Carney, M. W., Toone, B. K., & Reynolds, E. H. (1990). Enhancement of recovery from psychiatric illness by methylfolate. *Lancet, 336*(8730), 1579–1580.

Bradway. (2003). The effects of Healing Touch on depression. In: *Healing Touch Research Summary.*

Bressa, G. M. (1994). S-adenosyl-L-methionine (SAMe) as antidepressant: Meta-analysis of clinical studies. *Acta Neurologica Scandinavica Supplementum, 154,* 7–14.

Brown, R. P., & Gerbarg, P. L. (2004). *The rhodiola revolution: Transform your health with the herbal breakthrough of the 21st century.* Emmaus, PA: Rodale.

Brown, R. P., Gerbarg, P. L., & Bottiglieri, T. (2002). S-adenosylmethionine (SAMe) for depression. *Psychiatric Annals, 32*(1), 29–44.

Brown, E. S., Bobadilla, L., & Rush, A. J. (2001). Ketoconazole in bipolar patients with depressive symptoms: A case series and literature review. *Bipolar Disorders, 3*(1), 23–29.

Brown, M. A., Goldstein-Shirley, J., Robinson, J., & Casey, S. (2001). The effects of a multi-modal intervention trial of light, exercise, and vitamins on women's mood. *Journal of Women's Health, 34*(3), 93–112.

Buckley, M. S., Goff, A. D., & Knapp, W. E. (2004). Fish oil interaction with warfarin. *Annals of Pharmacotherapy, 38*(1), 50–52.

Burns, D. S. (2001). The effect of the Bonny method of guided imagery and music on the mood and life quality of cancer patients. *Journal of Music Therapy, 38*(1), 51–65.

Calandra, C., & Nicolosi, M. (1980). *Comparison of the pharmacological actions of the antidepressants: Rubidium chloride and chlorimipramine* [Italian]. Paper presented at the 34th Congress of the Italian Society of Psychiatry, Catania, Italy.

Calder, P. C. (1997). N-3 polyunsaturated fatty acids and cytokine production in health and disease. *Annals of Nutrition and Metabolism, 41*, 203–234.

Calhoun, K. E., Pommier, R. F., Muller, P., et al. (2003). Dehydroepiandrosterone sulfate causes proliferation of estrogen receptor–positive breast cancer cells despite treatment with fulvestrant. *Archives of Surgery, 138*, 879–883.

Carney, M., Chari, T., Bottiglieri, T., Reynolds, E., & Toone, B. (1987). Switch mechanism in affective illness and oral S-adenosylmethionine (SAMe). *British Journal of Psychiatry, 150*, 724–725.

Casacalenda, N., Perry, C., & Looper, K. (2002). Remission in major depressive disorder: A comparison of pharmacotherapy, psychotherapy and control conditions. *American Journal of Psychiatry, 159*, 1354–1360.

Cassileth, B. R., Vickers, A. J., & Magill, L. A. (2003). Music therapy for mood disturbance during hospitalization for autologous stem cell transplantation: A randomized controlled trial. *Cancer, 98*(12), 2723–2729.

Chengappa, K. N., Levine, J., Gershon, S., Mallinger, A. G., Hardan, A., Vagnucci, A., Pollock, B., Luther, J., Buttenfield, J., Verfaille, S., & Kupfer, D. J. (2000). Inositol as an add-on treatment for bipolar depression. *Bipolar Disorders, 2*, 47–55.

Chouinard, G., Young, S. N., Annable, L., & Sourkes, T. L. (1979). Tryptophan-nicotinamide, imipramine and their combination in depression. *Acta Psychiatrica Scandinavica, 59*, 395–414.

Christensen, L. (1991). The roles of caffeine and sugar in depression. *Nutrition Reports, 9*.

Cocilovo, A. (1999). Colored light therapy: Overview of its history, theory, recent developments and clinical applications combined with acupuncture. *American Journal of Acupuncture, 27*, 71–83.

Colombo, C., Lucca, A., Benedetti, F., Barbini, B., Campori, E., & Smeraldi, E. (2000). Total sleep deprivation combined with lithium and light therapy in the treatment of bipolar depression: Replication of main effects and interaction. *Psychiatry Research, 95*(1), 43–53.

Cook, I. A., Leuchter, A. F., Morgan, M., Witte, E., Stubbeman, W. F., Abrams, M., Rosenberg, S., & Uiitdehaage, S. H. (2002). Early changes in prefrontal activity characterize clinical responders to antidepressants. *Neuropsychopharmacology, 27*(1), 120–131.

Cooper, A. J., & Datta, S. R. (1980). A placebo-controlled evaluation of L-tryptophan in depression in the elderly. *Canadian Journal of Psychiatry, 25*(5), 386–390.

Coppen, A., Coppen, A., Shaw, D. M., & Farrell, J. P. (1963). Potentiation of the antidepressive effect of a monoamine-oxidase inhibitor by tryptophan. *Lancet, 1*, 79–81.

Coppen, A., Whybrow, P. C., Noguera, R., et al. (1972). The comparative antidepressant value of L-tryptophan and imipramine with and without attempted potentiation by liothyronine. *Archives of General Psychiatry, 26*(3), 234–241.

Cott, J. M. (1997). In vitro receptor binding and enzyme inhibition by *Hypericum perforatum* extract. *Pharmacopsychiatry, 30*, 108–112.

Crellin, R., Bottiglieri, T., & Reynolds, E. H. (1993). Folates and psychiatric disorders: Their clinical potential. *Drugs, 45*(5), 623–636.

Criconia, A., Araquistain, J., Daffina, N., et al. (1994). Results of treatment with S-adenosyl-L-methionine (SAMe) in patients with major depression and internal illnesses. *Current Therapeutic Research, 55*, 666–674.

Crown, W. H., Finkelstein, S., Berndt, E. R., Ling, D., Poret, A., Rush, J., & Russell, J. (2002). The impact of treatment-resistant depression on health care utilization and costs. *Journal of Clinical Psychiatry, 63*, 963–971.

Davidson, J., & the Hypericum Depression Trial Study Group. (2002). Effect of *Hypericum perforatum* (St John's wort) in major depressive disorder: A randomized controlled trial. *Journal of the American Medical Asscociation, 287*, 1807–1814.

Davidson, J. R., & Gaylord, S. (1998). Homeopathic and psychiatric perspectives on grief. *Alternative Therapies in Health Medicine, 4*(5), 30–35.

Davidson, J. R., Morrison, R. M., Shore, J., Davidson, R. T., & Bedayn, G. (1997). Homeopathic treatment of depression and anxiety. *Alternative Therapies in Health Medicine, 3*(1), 46–49.

Delgado, P. L., & Moreno, F. A. (2000). Role of norepinephrine in depression. *Journal of Clinical Psychiarty, 61*, Suppl. 1, 5–12.

Delle Chiale, R., Panccheri, P., & Scapicchio, P. (2000, July). *MC4: Multicenter controlled efficacy and safety trial of intramuscular S-adenosyl-methionine (SAMe) versus oral imipramine in the treatment of depression.* Paper preresented at the Collegium Internationale Neuro-psychopharmacologisum, Brussels.

Demott, K. (2002). The ideal antidepressant may be an EEG away. *Clinical Psychiatry News*, p. 17.

De Smet, P. A., & Nolen, W. A. (1996). St John's wort as an antidepressant [see Comments]. *British Medical Journal, 313*, 241–242.

De Vanna, M., & Rigamonti, R. (1992). Oral S-adenosyl-L-methionine in depression. *Current Therapeutic Research, 52*(3), 478–485.

Dressen, L., & Singg, S. (1998). Effects of Reiki on pain and selected affective and personality variables of chronically ill patients. *Subtle Energies, 9*(1), 51–82.

Drohan, M. (1999). From myth to reality: How music changes matter. *Alternative Health Practitioner, 5*(1), 25–33.

Druss, B., & Rosenheck, R. (2000). Use of practitioner-based complementary therapies by persons reporting mental conditions in the United States. *Archives of General Psychiatry, 57*, 708–714.

Dunn, A., Trivedi, M., Kampert, J., et al. (2002). The DOSE study: A clinical trial to examine efficacy and dose response of exercise as treatment for depression. *Controlled Clinical Trials, 23*, 584–603.

Edwards, R., Peet, M., Shay, J., & Horrobin, D. (1998). Omega-3 polyunsaturated fatty acid levels in the diet and in red blood cell membranes of depressed patients. *Journal of Affective Disorders, 48*, 149–155.

Einat, H., Shaldubina, A., & Belmaker, R. H. (2000). Epi-inositol: A potential antidepressant. *Drug Development Research, 50*(3), 309–315.

Elkin, I., Shea, M., Watkins, J., et al. (1989). National Institutes of Mental Health treatment of depression collaborative research program: General effectiveness of treatments. *Archives of General Psychiatry, 46*, 971–982.

Elkis, H., Friedman, L., Wise, A., & Meltzer, H. (1995). Meta-analysis of studies of ventricular enlargement and cortical sulcal prominence in mood disorders: Comparisons with controls or patients with schizophrenia. *Archives of General Psychiatry, 52*, 735–746.

Epperson, C., Terman, M., Terman, J., Hanusa, B., Oren, D., Peindl, K., & Wisner, K. (2004). Randomized clinical trial of bright light therapy for antepartum depression: Preliminary findings. *Journal of Clinical Psychiatry, 65*, 421–425.

Ernst, E. (1995a). St. John's wort, an anti-depressant? A systematic, criteria-based review. *Phytomedicine, 2*(1), 67–71.

Ernst, E. (1995b). The safety of homeopathy [Editorial]. *British Homeopathic Journal, 84*, 193–194.

Ernst, E., Rand, J. I., & Stevinson, C. (1998). Complementary therapies for depression: An overview. *Archives of General Psychiatry, 55*(11), 1026–1032.

Ernst, E., & White, A. (1997). Life-threatening adverse reactions after acupuncture? A systematic review. *Pain, 71*, 123–126.

Fanqiang, M., et al. (1994). Plasma NE concentration and 24 hour urinary MHPG-Sov excretion changes after electro-acupuncture treatment in endogenous depression. *World Journal of Acupuncture and Moxibustion, 4*(2), 45–52.

Fava, G. (2003). Can long-term treatment with antidepressant drugs worsen the course of depression? *Journal of Clinical Psychiatry, 64*, 123–133.

Fava, M., Borus, J. S., Alpert, J. E., et al. (1997). Folate, vitamin B$_{12}$ and homocysteine in major depressive disorder. *American Journal of Psychiatry, 154*(3), 426–428.

FDA black box warning on antidepressants creates concerns for clinicians. (2004). *Neuropsychiatry Review, 5*(9), 25–28.

Fetrow, C. W., & Avila, J. R. (2001). Efficacy of the dietary supplement S-adenosyl-L-methionine. *Annals of Pharmacotherapy, 35*(11), 1414–1425.

Field, T., Sunshine, W., Hernandez-Reif, M., et al. (1997). Chronic fatigue syndrome: Massage therapy effects on depression and somatic symptoms in chronic fatigue syndrome. *Journal of Chronic Fatigue Syndrome, 3*, 43–51.

Fisher, S., & Greenberg, R. (Eds.). (1997). *From placebo to panacea: Putting psychiatric drugs to the test.* New York: John Wiley & Sons.

Flaws, B., & Lake, J. (2001). *Chinese medical psychiatry: A textbook and clinical manual.* Boulder, CO: Blue Poppy Press.

Frei, R. (2004). Dearth of depression diagnoses seen among antidepressant users. *CNS News, 8*(1), 11.

Fremont, J., & Craighead, L. (1987). Aerobic exercise and cognitive therapy in the treatment of dysphoric moods. *Cognitive Therapy and Research, 11*(2), 241–251.

Friedel, H., Goa, K., & Benfield, P. (1989). S-adenosyl-L-methionine: A review of its pharmacological properties and therapeutic potential in liver dysfunction and affective disorders in relation to its physiological role in cell metabolism. *Drugs, 38*, 389–416.

Fujiwara, J., & Otsuki, S. (1974). Subtype of affective psychosis classified by response on amine precursors and monoamine metabolism. *Folia Psychiatrica et Neurologica Japonica, 28*(2), 93–100.

Gaik, F. (2003). Merging East and West: A preliminary study applying spring forest qigong to depression as an alternative and complementary treatment. *Dissertation Abstracts International B, 63*(12-B), 6093. (UMI No. 0419-4217)

Gallinat, J., Bottlender, R., Juckel, G., Juckel, G., Munke-Puchner, A., Stotz, G., Kuss, H. J., Mavrogiorgou, P., & Hegerl, U. (2000). The loudness dependency of the auditory evoked N1/P2-component as a predictor of the acute SSRI response in depression. *Psychopharmacology (Berlin), 148*(4), 404–411.

Garzya, G., Corallo, D., Fiore, A., Lecciso, G., Petrelli, G., & Zotti, C. (1990). Evaluation of the effects of L-acetylcarnitine on senile patients suffering from depression. *Drugs Under Experimental and Clinical Research, 16*(2), 101–106.

Gaylord, S., & Davidson, J. (1998). The constitution: Views from homeopathy and psychiatry. *British Homeopathic Journal, 87*, 148–153.

Gelenberg, A. J. (2000). St. John's wort update. *Biological Therapies in Psychiatry, 23*, 22–24.

Gelenberg, A. J., Shelton, R. C., Crits-Christoph, P., Keller, M., Dunner, D., Hirschfeld, R., et al. (2004). The effectiveness of St. John's wort in major depressive disorder: A naturalistic Phase 2 follow-up in which nonresponders were provided alternate medication. *Journal of Clinical Psychiatry, 65*, 1114–1119.

Ghadirian, A. M., Murphy, B. E., & Gendron, M. J. (1998). Efficacy of light versus tryptophan therapy in seasonal affective disorder. *Journal of Affective Disorders, 50*(1), 23–27.

Gibbons, R., Hur, K., Bhaumik, D., & Mann, J. (2005). The relationship between antidepressant medication use and rate of suicide. *Archives of General Psychiatry, 62*(2), 165–172.

Girolamo, G., Pepoli, V., Alonso, J., Gasquet, I., Russo, L., Vilagut, G., et al. (2004). *Psychotropic drug utilization in six European countries* (Abstract 81). Paper presented at the annual meeting of the American Psychiatric Association, New York.

Glassman, A. H., & Platman, S. R. (1969). Potentiation of a monoamine oxidase inhibitor by tryptophan. *Journal of Psychiatric Research, 7*(2), 83–88.

Glauber, H., Wallace, P., Griver, K., & Brechtel, G. (1988). Dverse metabolic effect of omega-3 fatty acids in non-insulin dependent diabetes mellitus. *Annuals of Internal Medicine, 108*(5), 663–668.

Glickman, G., Byrne, B., Pineda, C., & Brainard, G. C. (2004, June). *Light therapy for seasonal affective disorder with 470 nm narrow-band light-emitting diodes (LEDs)* (Abstract 16). Paper presented at the annual meeting of the Society for Light Treatment and Biological Rhythms, Toronto.

Gloth, F., & Hollis, A. (1999). Vitamin D vs broad spectrum phototherapy in the treatmentof seasonal affective disorder. *Journal of Nutrition, Health and Aging, 3*(1), 5–7.

Goel, N. (2004). *Bright light and negative ion treatment for chronic depression* (Abstract 90C). Paper presented at the annual meeting of the American Psychiatric Association, New York.

Golden, R., Gaynes, B., Ekstrom, R., Hamer, R., Jacobsen, F., et al. (2005). The efficacy of light therapy in the treatment of mood disorders: A review and meta-analysis of the evidence. *American Journal of Psychiatry, 162*(4), 656–662.

Greenberg, P. E., Kessler, R. C., Birnbaum, H. G., Leong, S., Lowe, S., Berglund, P., & Corey-Lisle, P. (2003). The economic burden of depression in the United States: How did it change between 1990 and 2000? *Journal of Clinical Psychiatry, 64*(12), 1465–1475.

Grevet, E. H., Tietzmann, M. R., Shansis, F. M., Hastenpflugl, C., Santana, L. C., Forster, L., Kapczinskil, F., Izquierdo, I. (2002). Behavioural effects of acute phenylalanine and tyrosine depletion in healthy male volunteers. *Journal of Psychopharmacology, 16*(1), 51–55.

Greyson, B. (1996). Distance healing of patients with major depression. *Journal of Scientific Exploration, 10*(40), 1–18.

Grinberg-Zylberbaum, J., Delaflor, M., Attie, L., & Goswami, L. (1994). The Einstein-Podolsky-Rosen paradox in the brain: The transferred potential. *Physics Essays, 7*, 422–428.

Gupta, S. K., & Singh, R. H. (2002). A clinical study on depressive illness and its Ayurvedic management. *Journal of Research in Ayurveda and Siddha, 23*(3/4), 82–93.

Hammer, L. (2001). Qualities as signs of psychological disharmony. In *Chinese Pulse* (pp. 539–594). Seattle: Eastland Press.

Harinath, K., Malhotra, A., Pal, K., Prasad, R., Kumar, R., et al. (2004). Effects of hatha yoga and omkar meditation on cardiorespiratory performance, psychologic profile and melatonin secretion. *Journal of Alternative Complementary Medicine, 10*(2), 261–268.

Harvie, M. N., Campbell, I. T., Howell, A., & Thatcher, N. (2002). Acceptability and tolerance of a low tyrosine and phenylalanine diet in patients with advanced cancer: A pilot study. *Journal of Human Nutriton and Dietics, 15*(3), 193–202.

Hasin, D., Tsai, W., Endicott, J., Meuller, T., Coryell, W., Keller, M. (1996). Five-year course of major depression: Effects of comorbid alcoholism. *Journal of Affective Disorders, 41*, 63–70.

Hechun, L., et al. (1990). Electro-acupuncture in the treatment of depressive psychosis: A controlled prospective randomized trial using electro-acupuncture and amitriptyline in 241 patients. *International Journal of Clinical Acupuncture, 1*(1), 7–13.

Hechun, L., et al. (1993). A control observation on therapeutic effects of intelligent (computerized) electro-acupuncture and common electro-acupuncture treating 77 cases of neurosis. *World Journal of Acupuncture and Moxibustion, 3*(2), 25–28.

Hechun, L., et al. (1995). Advances in clinical research on common mental disorders with computer controlled electro-acupuncture treatment. L. Tang and S. Tang, eds. Neurochemistry in Clinical Applications. Plenum Press, New York , 109–122.

Hein, O. (1991). A case of depression: Man, 40 years old. *Small Remedies Seminar Hechtel*, 160–179.

Hernandez-Reif, M., Martinez, A., Field, T., et al. (2000). Premenstrual symptoms are relieved by massage therapy. *Journal of Psychosomatic Obstetrics and Gynaecology, 21*(1), 9–15.

Hibbeln, J. (1995). Dietary polyunsaturated fatty acids and depression: When cholesterol does not satisfy. *American Journal of Clinical Nutrition, 62*, 1–9.

Hibbeln, J. R., Linnoila, M., Umhau, J. C., Rawlings, R., George, D. T., & Salem, N., Jr. (1998). Essential fatty acids predict metabolites of serotonin and dopamine in cerebrospinal fluid among healthy control subjects, and early- and late-onset alcoholics. *Biological Psychiatry, 44*, 235–242.

Hintikka, J., Tolmunen, T., Tanskanen, A., & Viinamäki, H. (2003). High vitamin B_{12} level and good treatment outcome may be associated in major depressive disorder. *BMC Psychiatry, 3*, 17.

Hinton, M., & Melonas, J. (2004). Limiting your risks when prescribing SSRIs. *Psychiatric News*, p. 28.

Hollon, S., DeRubeis, R., Shelton, R., & Weiss, B. (2002). The emperor's new drugs: Effect size and moderation effects. *Prevention and Treatment, 5*(28). Available at journals.apa.org/prevention/volume5/toc-jul15–02.html

Horrobin, D. F., & Peet, M. (2002). A dose-ranging study of the effects of ethyl-eicosapentaenoate in patients with ongoing depression despite apparently adequate treatment with standard drugs. *Archives of General Psychiatry, 59*(10), 913–919.

Isacsson, G., Holmgren, P., & Ahlner, J. (2005). Selective serotonin reuptake inhibitor antidepressants and the risk of suicide: A controlled forensic database study of 14,857 suicides. *Acta Psychiatrica Scandinavica, 111*(4), 286–290.

Jacobs, B., van Praag, H., & Gage, F. (2000). Adult brain neurogenesis and psychiatry: A novel theory of depression. *Molecular Psychiatry, 5*, 262–269.

Jacobson, N., Roberts, L., Berns, S., & McGlinchey, J. (1999). Methods for defining and determining the clinical significance of treatment effectsw: Description, application, and alternatives. *Journal of Consulting and Clinical Psychology, 67*(3), 300–307.

Janakiramaiah, N., Gangadhar, B. N., Naga Venkatesha Murthy, P. J, et al. (2000). Antidepressant efficacy of Sudarshan Kriya Yoga (SKY) in melancholia: A randomized comparison with electroconvulsive therapy (ECT) and imipramine. *Journal of Affective Disorders, 57*, 255–259.

Janicak, P. G., Dowd, S. M., Martis, B., Alam, D., Beedle, D., Krasuski, J., Strong, M. J., Sharma, R., Rosen, C., & Viana, M. (2002). Repetitive transcranial magnetic stimulation versus electroconvulsive therapy for major depression: Preliminary results of a randomized trial. *Biological Psychiatry, 51*(8), 659–667.

Janicak, P. G., Lipinski, J., Davis, J. M., Comaty, J. E., Waternaux, C., Cohen, B., Altman, E., & Sharma, R. P. (1988). S-adenosylmethionine in depression: A literature review and preliminary report. *Alabama Journal of Medical Sciences, 25*(3), 306–313.

Jensen, K., Fruensgaard, K., Ahlfors, U. G., et al. (1975). Tryptophan/imipramine in depression [Letter]. *Lancet, 2*(7942), 920.

John, E.R., Prichep, L.S. (1993). Principles of neurometric analysis of EEG and evoked potentials. In E. Niedermeyer & F. Lopes da Silva (Eds.), *Electroencephalography: Basic principles, clinical applications, and related fields.* Balitmore: Williams & Wilkins, 989–1003.

Jorm, A. F., Christensen, H., Griffiths, K. M., & Rodgers, B. (2002). Effectiveness of complementary and self-help treatments for depression. *Medical Journal of Australia, 176*(Suppl.), S84–S96.

Judd, L. (2004, May). *MDD: A new paradigm of understanding and treatment* (Abstract 58A). Paper presented at the annual meeting of the American Psychiatric Association, New York.

Keitner, G. (2004, May). Limits to the treatment of major depression (Abstract 34). Paper presented at the annual meeting of the American Psychiatric Association, New York.

Kempson, D. (2000–2001). Effects of intentional touch on complicated grief of bereaved mothers. *Omega, 42*(4), 341–353.

Kendler, K. S., Liu, X. Q., Gardner, C. O., McCullough, M. E., Larson, D., & Prescott, C. A. (2003). Dimensions of religiosity and their relationship of lifetime psychiatric and substance use disorders. *American Journal of Psychiatry, 160*, 496–503.

Kilbourne, E. M., Philen, R. M., Kamb, M. L., et al. (1996). Tryptophan produced by Showa Denko and epidemic eosinophilia-myalgia syndrome. *Journal of Rheumatology, 46*(Suppl.), 81–88.

Kim, H. L., Streltzer, J., & Goebert, D. (1999). St. John's wort for depression: A meta-analysis of well-defined clinical trials. *Journal of Nervous and Mental Disorders, 187*(9), 532–538.

Kim, Y. K., & Myint, A. M. (2004). Clinical application of low serum cholesterol as an indicator for suicide risk in major depression. *Journal of Affected Disorders, 81*, 161–166.

King, D., & Bushwick, B. (1994). Beliefs and attitudes of hospital inpatients about faith-healing and prayer. *Journal of Family Practice, 39*, 349–352.

Kinsella, J. E. (1990). Lipids, membrane receptors, and enzymes: Effects of dietary fatty acids. *Journal of Parenteral and Enteral Nutrition, 14*, 200S–217S.

Kirov, G. K., Birch, N. J., Steadman, P., & Ramsey, R. G. (1994). Plasma magnesium levels in a population of psychiatric patients: Correlation with symptoms. *Neuropsychobiology, 30*(2–3), 73–78.

Kirsch, I., Moore, T., Scoboria, A., & Nicholls, S. (2002). The emperor's new drugs: An analysis of antidepressant medication data submitted to the U.S. Food and Drug Administration. *Prevention and Treatment, 5*(23). Available at journals.apa.org/prevention/volume5/toc-jul15-02.html

Kline, N., & Sacks, W. (1980). Treatment of depression with an MAO inhibitor followed by 5-HTtp: An unfinished research project. *Acta Psychiatrica Scandinavica, 280*(Suppl.), 233–241.

Knott, V. J., Howson, A. L., Perugini, M., Ravindran, A. V., & Young, S. N. (1999). The effect of acute tryptophan depletion and fenfluramine on quantitative EEG and mood in healthy male subjects. *Biological Psychiatry, 46*(2), 229–238.

Koirala, R. R. (1992). *Clinical and behavioural study of medhya drugs on brain functions.* Unpublished doctoral dissertation, Banaras Hindu University, Varanasi, India.

Kuhs, H., Farber, D., Borgstadt, S., Mrosek, S., & Tolle, R. (1996). Amitriptyline in combination with repeated late sleep deprivation versus amitriptyline alone in major depression: A randomised study. *Journal of Affective Disorders, 37*(1), 31–41.

Kumano, H., Horie, H., Shidara, T., Kuboki, T., Suematsu, H., & Yasushi, M. (1996). Treatment of a depressive disorder patient with EEG-driven photic stimulation. *Biofeedback and Self-Regulation, 21*(4), 323–334.

Kushwaha, H. K., & Sharma, K. P. (1992). Clinical evaluation of shankhpushpi syrup in the management of depressive illness. *Sachitra Ayurved, 45*(1), 45–50.

Laakmann, G., Dienel, A., & Kieser, M. (1998). Clinical significance of hyperforin for the efficacy of *Hypericum* extracts on depressive disorders of different severities. *Phytomedicine, 5*(6), 435–442.

Labbate, L. A., Lafer, B., Thibault, A., & Sachs, G. S. (1994). Side effects induced by bright light treatment for seasonal affective disorder. *Journal of Clinical Psychiatry, 55*(5), 189–191.

Lafreniere, K. D., Mutus, B., Cameron, S., Tannous, M., Giannotti, M., & Laukkanen, E. (1999). Effects of therapeutic touch on biochemical and mood indicators in women. *Journal of Alternative and Complementary Medicine, 5*(4), 367–370.

Lai, Y. M. (1999). Effects of music listening on depressed women in Taiwan. *Issues in Mental Health Nursing, 20*(3), 229–246.

Lake, J. (2001). *Alternative and complementary therapies in mental health: Innovation and integration.* New York: Academic Press.

Lalovic, A., Merkens, L., Russell, L., Arsenault-Lapierre, G., Nowaczyk, M., et al. (2004). Cholesterol metabolism and suicidality in Smith-Lemli-Opitz syndrome carriers. *American Journal of Psychiatry, 161*, 2123–2126.

Lam, R., Wan, D., Cohen, N., & Kennedy, S. (2002). Combining antidepressants for treatment-resistant depression: A review. *Journal of Clinical Psychiatry, 63*, 685–693.

Lam, R. W., Levitan, R. D., Tam, E. M., et al. (1997). L-tryptophan augmentation of light therapy in patients with seasonal affective disorder. *Canadian Journal of Psychiatry, 42*(4), 303–306.

Lane, J. D., Kasian, S. J., Owens, J. E., & Marsh, G. R. (1998). Binaural auditory beats affect vigilance performance and mood. *Physiology and Behavior, 63*(2), 249–252.

Lansdowne, A. T., & Provost, S. C. (1998). Vitamin D_3 enhances mood in healthy subjects during winter. *Psychopharmacology (Berlin), 135*(4), 319–323.

Lantz, M. S., Buchalter, E., & Giambanco, V. (1999). St. John's wort and antidepressant drug interactions in the elderly. *Journal of Geriatric Psychiatry and Neurology, 12*(1), 7–10.

Larson, D., & Milano, M. (1996). Religion and mental health: Should they work together? *Alternative and Complementary Therapies,* 91–98.

Lawlor, D. A., & Hopker, S. W. (2001). The effectiveness of exercise as an intervention in the management of depression: Systematic review and meta-regression analysis of randomized controlled trials. *British Medical Journal, 322,* 763–767.

Leibenluft, E., Moul, D. E., Schwartz, P. J., Madden, P. A., & Wehr, T. A. (1993). A clinical trial of sleep deprivation in combination with antidepressant medication. *Psychiatry Research, 46*(3), 213–227.

Leng, G. C., Smith, F. B., Fowkes, F. G., Horrobin, D. F., Ells, K., Morse-Fisher, N., & Lowe, G. D. (1994). Relationship between plasma essential fatty acids and smoking, serum lipids, blood pressure and haemostatic and rheological factors. *Prostaglandins Leukotrienes and Essential Fatty Acids, 51,* 101–108.

Levine, J., Barak, Y., Gonzalves, M., Szor, H., Elizur, A., Kofman, O., & Belmaker, R. H. (1995). Double-blind, controlled trial of inositol treatment of depression. *American Journal of Psychiatry, 152*(5), 792–794.

Levine, J., Barak, Y., Kofman, O., & Belmaker, R. H. (1995). Follow-up and relapse analysis of an inositol study of depression. *Israeli Journal of Psychiatry and Related Sciences, 32,* 14–21.

Levitan, R. D., Shen, J. H., Jindal, R., Driver, H. S., Kennedy, S. H., & Shapiro, C. M. (2000). Preliminary randomized double-blind placebo-controlled trial of tryptophan combined with fluoxetine to treat major depressive disorder: Antidepressant and hypnotic effects. *Journal of Psychiatry Neurosciences, 25,* 337–346.

Levitt, A. J., Joffe, R. T., & Kennedy, S. H. (1991). Bright light augmentation in antidepressant nonresponders. *Journal of Clinical Psychiatry, 52*(8), 336–337.

Linde, K., Clausius, N., Ramirez, G., Melchart, D., Eitel, F., Hedges, L., & Jonas, W. (1997). Are the clinical effects of homeopathy placebo effects? A meta-analysis of placebo-controlled trials. *Lancet, 350,* 834–843.

Linde, K., & Mulrow, C. D. (2004). St John's wort for depression (Cochrane Review). In: *The Cochrane Library* (Issue 2). Chichester, UK: John Wiley & Sons.

Linde, K., Ramirez, G., Mulrow, C., Pauls, A., Weidenhammer, W., & Melchart, D. (1996). St. John's wort for depression—an overview and meta-analysis of randomized clinical trials. *British Medical Journal, 313*(7052), 253–258.

Lopez-Ibor Alino, J. J., et al. (1973). *International Pharmacopsychiatry, 8,* 145–151.

Luchins, D. (1976). Biogenic amines and affective disorders: a clinical analysis. *International Pharmacopsychiatry, 11*(3), 135–149.

Luo, H., Meng, F., Jia, Y., & Zhao, X. (1998). Clinical research on the therapeutic effect of the electro-acupuncture treatment in patients with depression. *Psychiatry and Clinical Neuroscience, 52*(Suppl.), S338–S340.

Lutz (1986). *International Journal of Mental Health, 13,* 148–177.

MacPherson, H., Thorpe, L., Thomas, K., & Geddes, D. (2004). Acupuncture for depression: First steps toward a clinical evaluation. *Journal of Alternative and Complementary Medicine, 10*(6), 1083–1091.

Maes, M., et al. (1998). Increased serum IL-6 and IL-1 receptor antagonist concentrations in major depression and treatment resistant depression. *Cytokine.*

Maes, M., Smith, R. S., Christophe, A., Cosyns, P., Desnyder, R., & Meltzer, H. Y. (1996). Fatty acid composition in major depression: Decreased omega 3 fractions in cholesteryl esters and increased C20:4 omega-6/C20:5 omega-3 ratio in cholesteryl esters and phospholipids. *Journal of Affective Disorders, 38,* 35–46.

Manji, H. K., Moore, G. J., Rajkowska, G., & Chen, G. (2000). Neuroplasticity and cellular resilience in mood disorders. *Molecular Psychiatry, 5,* 578–593.

Mantle, F. (2002). The role of alternative medicine in treating postnatal depression. *Complementary Therapies in Nursing and Midwifery, 8*(4), 197–203.

Marangell, L. B., Martinez, J. M., Zboyan, H. A., et al. (2003). A double-blind placebo-controlled study of the omega-3 fatty acid docosahexaenoic acid in the treatment of major depression. *American Journal of Psychiatry, 160*(5), 996–998.

Martin, J. L. R., Barbanoj, M. J., Schlaepfer, T. E., Clos, S., Perez, V., Kulisevsky, J., & Gironell, A. (2004). Transcranial magnetic stimulation for treating depression (Cochrane Review). In *The Cochrane Library* (Issue 2). Chichester, UK: John Wiley & Sons.

Martinez, C., Rietbrock, S., Wise, L., Ashby, D., Chick, J., Moseley, J., Evans, S., & Gunnell, D. (2005). Antidepressant treatment and the risk of fatal and nonfatal self harm in first episode depression: Nested case-control study. *British Medical Journal, 330*(7488), 389.

Mason, O., & Hargreaves, I. (2001). A qualitative study of mindfulness-based cognitive therapy for depression. *Brritish Journal of Medical Psychology, 74*(Pt. 2), 197–212.

McCraty, R., & Atkinson, M. (1999). *Cardiac influence of afferent cardiovascular input on cognitive performance and alpha activity.* Paper presented at the annual meeting of the Pavlovian Society, Tarrytown, NY.

McCraty, R., Atkinson, M., & Tomasino, D. (2001). *Science of the heart: Exploring the role of the heart in human performance.* Boulder Creek, CA: Heart Math Research Center, Institute of Heart Math.

McIntyre, M. (2000). A review of the benefits, adverse events, drug interactions and safety of St. John's wort (*Hypericum perforatum*): The implications with regard to the regulation of herbal medicines. *Journal of Alternative and Complementary Medicine, 6*(2), 115–124.

Mechcatie, E. (2004). Manufacturer halts shipments of Nefazodone: Bristol-Myers Squibb says the move is based on declining sales—not reports of liver toxicity. *Clinical Psychiatry News,* 7.

Meesters, Y., Jansen, J., Lambers, P., Bouhuys, A., Beersma, D., & Van den Hoofdakker, R. (1993). Morning and evening light treatment of seasonal affective disorder: Response, relapse and prediction. *Journal of Affective Disorders, 28*(3), 165–177.

Mendels, J., Stinnett, J. L., Burns, D., et al. (1975). Amine precursors and depression. *Archives of General Psychiatry, 32*(1), 22–30.

Mendlewicz, J., & Youdim, M. B. (1980). Antidepressant potentiation of 5-hydroxytryptophan y L-deprenil in affective illness. *Journal of Affective Disorders, 2,* 137–146.

Milligan, J., & Waldkoetter, R. (2000). Use of hemi-sync audiotapes to reduce levels of depression for alcohol-dependent patients. *Hemi-Sync Journal, 18*(1), i–iii.

Moncrieff, J., Wessely, S., & Hardy, R. (2004). Active placebos versus antidepressants for depression (Cochrane Review). In: *The Cochrane Library,* Issue 2, Chichester, United Kingdom: John Wiley & Sons.

Muller, W. E., Singer, A., Wonnemann, M., et al. (1998). Hyperforin represents the neurotransmitter reuptake inhibiting constituent of hypericum extract. *Pharmacopsychiatry, 31*(Suppl. 1), 16–21.

Murphy, G. E., Carney, R. M., Knesevich, M. A., Wetzel, R. D., & Whitworth, P. (1995). Cognitive behavior therapy, relaxation training, and tricyclic antidepressant medication in the treatment of depression. *Psychological Report, 77*(2), 403–420.

Nahas, Z., Kozel, F. A., Li, X., Anderson, B., & George, M. S. (2003). Left prefrontal transcranial magnetic stimulation (TMS) treatment of depression in bipolar affective disorder: A pilot study of acute safety and efficacy. *Bipolar Disorders, 5*, 40–47.

Nardini, M., De Stefano, R., Iannuccelli, M., et al. (1983). Treatment of depression with L-5-hydroxytryptophan combined with chlorimipramine, a double-blind study. *International Journal of Clininical Pharmacology Research, 3*(4), 239–250.

National Institutes of Health. (1991). *The National Institutes of Health (NIH) consensus statement on the diagnosis and treatment of depression in late life.* Bethesda, MD Author.

Nemets, B., Stahl, Z., & Belmaker, R. H. (2002). Addition of omega-3 fatty acids to maintenance medication treatment for recurrent unipolar depressive disorder. *American Journal of Psychiatry, 159*, 477–479.

Ness, A. R., Gallacher, J. E., Bennett, P. D., Gunnell, D. J., Rogers, P. J., Kessler, D., & Burr, M. L. (2003). Advice to eat fish and mood: A randomised controlled trial in men with angina. *Nutritional Neurosciences, 6*, 63–65.

Neumeister, A. (2004). Neurotransmitter depletion and seasonal affective disorder: Relevance for the biologic effects of light therapy. *Primary Psychiatry, 11*(6), 44–48.

Neumeister, A., Nugent, A., Waldeck, T., Geraci, M., Schwarz, M., et al. (2004). Neural and behavioral responses to tryptophan depletion in unmedicated patients with remitted major depressive disorder and controls. *Archives of General Psychiatry, 61*, 765–773.

Nieber, D., & Schlegel, S. (1992). Relationships between psychomotor retardation and EEG power spectrum in major depression. *Neuropsychobiology, 25*, 20–23.

O'Laoire, S. (1997). An experimental study of the effects of distant, intercessory prayer on self-esteem, anxiety and depression. *Alternative Therapies in Health Medicine, 3*(6), 38–53.

Osuch, E. A., Cora-Locatelli, G., Frye, M. A., Huggins, T., Kimbrell, T. A., Ketter, T. A., Callahan, A. M., & Post, R. M. (2001). Post-dexamethasone cortisol correlates with severity of depression before and during carbamazepine treatment in women but not men. *Acta Psychiatrica Scandinavica, 104*(5), 397–401.

Pampallona, S., Bollini, P., Tibaldi, G., Kupelnick, B., & Munizza, C. (2004). Combined pharmacotherapy and psychological treatment for depression: A systematic review. *Archives of General Psychiatry, 61*, 714–719.

Papakostas, G., Petersen, T., Mischoulon, D., Green, C., Nierenberg, A., Bottiglieri, T., et al. (2004a). Serum folate, vitamin B-12 and homocysteine in major depressive disorder. 2: Predictors of relapse during the continuation phase of pharmacotherapy. *Journal of Clinical Psychiatry, 65*(8), 1096–1098.

Papakostas, G., Petersen, T., Mischoulon, D., Ryan, J., Nierenberg, A., Bottiglieri, T., et al. (2004b). Serum folate, vitamin B-12, and homocysteine in major depressive disorder. 1: Predictors of clinical response in fluoxetine-resistant depression. *Journal of Clinical Psychiatry, 65*(8), 1090–1095.

Partonen, T., Leppamaki, S., Hurme, J., & Lonnqvist, J. (1998). Randomized trial of physical exercise alone or combined with bright light on mood and health-related quality of life. *Psychological Medicine, 28*(6), 1359–1364.

Peet, M., & Horrobin, D. F. (2002). A dose-ranging study of the effects of ethyl-eicosapentaenoate in patients with ongoing depression despite apparently adequate treatment with standard drugs. *Archives of General Psychiatry, 59*(10), 913–919.

Peet, M., Murphy, B., Shay, J., & Horrobin D. (1998). Depletion of omega-3 fatty acid levels in red blood cell membranes of depressive patients. *Biological Psychiatry, 43*, 315–319.

Peniston, E. G., & Kulkosky, P. J. (1989). Alpha-theta brainwave training and beta-endorphin levels in alcoholics. *Alcoholism, Clinical and Experimental Research, 13*(2), 271–279.

Pettegrew, J. W., Levine, J., & McClure, R. J. (2000). Acetyl-L-carnitine physical-chemical, metabolic, and therapeutic properties: Relevance for its mode of action in Alzheimer's disease and geriatric depression. *Molecular Psychiatry, 5*, 616–632.

Peveler, R., Kendrick, A., Thompson, C., & Buxton, M. (2004, May). Cost-effectiveness of antidepressants in primary care (Abstract 9D). Paper presented at the annual meeting of the American Psychiatric Association, New York.

Piscitelli, S. C., Burstein, A. H., Chaitt, D., et al. (2000). Indinavir concentrations and St John's wort. *Lancet, 355*, 547–548.

Poldinger, W., Calanchini, B., & Schwarz, W. (1991). A functional-dimensional approach to depression: Serotonin deficiency as a target syndrome in a comparison of 5-hydroxytryptophan and fluvoxamine. *Psychopathology, 24*, 53–81.

Pope, H. G., Jones, J. M., Hudson, J. I., et al. (1985). Toxic reactions to the combination of monoamine oxidase inhibitors and tryptophan. *Americal Journal of Psychiatry, 142*(4), 491–492.

Princhep, L., John, E., Essig-Peppard, T., et al. (1990). Neurometric sub-typing of depressive disorders. In C. Cazzullo, G. Invernizzi, E. Sacchetti, et al. (Eds.), *Plasticity and morphology of the CNS.* London: MTP Press.

Puri, B. K., Counsell, S. J., Richardson, J., & Richardson, A. J. (2002). Eicoaspentaenoic acid in treatment-resistant depression. *Archives of Psychiatry, 59*(1), 91–92.

Quattrocki, E., Baird, A., & Yurgelun-Todd, D. (2000). Biological aspects of the link between smoking and depression. *Harvard Review of Psychiatry, 8*, 99–110.

Quitkin, F., Rabkin, J., Gerald, J., Davis, J., & Klein, D. (2000). Validity of clinical trials of antidepressants. *American Journal of Psychiatry, 157*, 327–337.

Rabkin, J., Ferrando, S., Wagner, G., & Rabkin, R. (2000). DHEA treatment for HIV+ patients: Effects on mood, androgenic and anabolic parameters. *Psychoneuroendocrinology, 25*(1), 53–68.

Rao, B., & Broadhurst, A. D. (1976). Tryptophan and depression [Letter]. *British Medical Journal;1*(6007), 460.

Rees, B. L. (1995). Effect of relaxation with guided imagery on anxiety, depression, and self-esteem in primiparas. *Journal of Holistic Nursing, 13*, 255–267.

Reiser, L., & Reiser, M. (1985). Endocrine disorders. In H. I. Kaplan & B. J. Sadock (Eds.), *Comprehensive textbook of psychiatry* (pp. 1167–1178). Baltimore: Williams & Wilkins.

Remick, R. A. (2002). Diagnosis and management of depression in primary care: A clinical update and review. *Canadian Medical Association Journal, 167*, 1253–1260.

Reynolds, E. H., Preece, J. M., Bailey, J., & Coppen, A. (1970). Folate deficiency in depressive illness. *British Journal of Psychiatry, 117*(538), 287–292.

Riederer, P., Tenk, H., Werner, H., Bischko, J., Rett, A., & Krisper, H. (1975). Manipulation of neurotransmitters by acupuncture (a preliminary communication). *Journal of Neural Transmission, 37*, 81–84.

Riemann, D., Konig, A., & Hohagen, F., Kiemen, A., Voderholzer, U., Backhaus, J., Bunz, J., Wesiack, B., Hermle, L., & Berger, M. (1999). How to preserve the antidepressive effect of sleep deprivation: A comparison of sleep phase advance and sleep phase delay. *European Archives of Psychiatry and Clinical Neuroscience, 249*(5), 231–237.

Robinson, L. (1996). *The effects of therapeutic touch on the grief experience.* Unpublished doctoral dissertation, University of Alabama, Birmingham.

Rosenbaum, J., Fava, M., Falk, W. E., et al. (1990). The antidepressant potential of oral S-adenosyl-L-methionine. *Acta Psychiatrica Scandinavica, 81*(5), 432–436.

Rosenfeld, J. P. (2000). An EEG biofeedback protocol for affective disorders. *Clinical Electroencephalography, 31*, 7–12.

Sabelli, H. C., Fawcett, J., Gusovsky, F., et al. (1986). Clinical studies on the phenylethylamine hypothesis of affective disorder: Urine and blood phenylacetic acid and phenylalanine dietary supplements. *Journal of Clinical Psychiatry, 47*(2), 66–70.

Sageman, S. (2004). Breaking through the despair: Spiritually oriented group therapy as a means of healing women with severe mental illness. *Journal of the American Academy of Psychoanalysis and Dynamic Psychiatry, 32*(1), 125–141.

Sano, I. (1972). L-5-hydroxytryptophan-(L-5-HTP) therapie (German). *Folia Psychiatrica et Neurologica Japonica, 26*(1), 7–17.

Saratikov, A. S., & Krasnov, E. A. (1987). Clinical studies of Rhodiola. In A. S. Saratikov & E. A. Krasnov (Eds.), *Rhodiola rosea is a valuable medicinal plant (Golden Root)* (pp. 216–227). Tomsk, Russia: Tomsk State University.

Sarchiapone, M., Camardese, G., Roy, A., et al. (2001). Cholesterol and serotonin indices in depressed and suicidal patients. *Journal of Affective Disorders, 62*(3), 217–219.

Sargent, P. A., Williamson, D. J., & Cowen, P. J. (1998). Brain 5-HT neurotransmission during paroxetine treatment. *British Journal of Psychiatry, 172*, 49–52.

Saxby, E., & Peniston, E. G. (1995). Alpha-theta brainwave neurofeedback training: An effective treatment for male and female alcoholics with depressive symptoms. *Journal of Clinical Psychology, 51*(5), 685–693.

Schatzberg A. (2002). Major depression: Causes or effects? [Editorial]. *American Journal of Psychiatry, 159*(7), 1077–1079.

Schmidt, P., Daly, R., Bloch, M., Smith, M., Danaceau, M., et al. (2005). Dehydroepiandrosterone monotherapy in midlife-onset major and minor depression. *Archives of General Psychiatry, 62*, 154–162.

Schnyer, R., & Allen, J. (2001). Acupuncture in the treatment of depression: A manual for practice and research. New York: Churchill Livingstone.

Schrader, E. (2000). Equivalence of St John's wort extract (Ze 117) and fluoxetine: A randomized, controlled study in mild-moderate depression. *International Clinical Psychopharmacology, 15*(2), 61–68.

Schrader, G. (1994). Natural history of chronic depression: Predictors of change in severity over time. *Journal of Affective Disorders, 32*(3), 219–222.

Schubert, H., & Halama, P. (1993). Depressive episode primarily unresponsive to therapy in elderly patients: Efficacy of Ginkgo biloba extract (EGb 761) in combination with antidepressants. *Geriatr Forschung, 3*, 45–53.

Schwartz, G., & Russek, L. (1996). Neurotherapy and the heart: The challenge of energy cardiology. *Journal of Neurotherapy*, 1–8.

Schwartzman, L. (1998). *Tai chi and Parkinson's disease.* Paper presented at the Second World Congress on Qigong.

Sevar, R. (1995). Cyclical depression: A preliminary report. *SIMILE, 5*(1), 17–19.

Shannahoff-Khalsa, D. (2004). An introduction to Kundalini Yoga meditation techniques that are specific for the treatment of psychiatric disorders. *Journal of Alternative and Complementary Medicine, 10*(1), 91–101.

Shannahoff-Khalsa, D. S., Ray, L. E., Levine, S., et al. (1999). Randomized controlled trial of yogic meditation techniques for patients with obsessive-compulsive disorder. *CNS Spectrums, 4*, 34–47.

Sharma, K. P., Kushwaha, H. K., & Sharma, S. S. (1993). A placebo-controlled trial on the efficacy of Mentat in managing depressive disorders. *Probe, 1*(33), 26.

Shaw, D. M., Johnson, A. L., & MacSweeney, D. A. (1972). Tricyclic antidepressants and tryptophan in unipolar affective disorder. *Lancet, 2*(7789), 1245.

Shaw, K., Turner, J., & Del Mar, C. (2004). Tryptophan and 5-hydroxytryptophan for depression (Cochrane Review). In *The Cochrane Library* (Issue 2). Chichester, UK: John Wiley & Sons.

Shealy, C., Cacy, R., Culver, D., et al. (1993). Non-pharmaceutical treatment of depression using a multimodal approach. *Subtle Energies, 4*(2), 125–134.

Shore, A. G. (2004). Long-term effects of energetic healing on symptoms of psychological depression and self-perceived stress. *Alternative Therapies in Health Medicine, 10*(3), 42–48.

Silva de Lima, M., & Hotopf, M. (2003). A comparison of active drugs for the treatment of dyymia. *Cochrane Database Systematic Reviews,* (3), CD047.

Silvers, K. M., & Scott, K. M. (2002). Fish consumption and self-reported physical and mental health status. *Public Health Nutrition, 5*(3), 427–431.

Simon, G., Fleck, M., Lucas, R., & Bushnell, D. (2004). Prevalence and predictors of depression treatment in an international primary care study. *American Journal of Psychiatry, 161*, 1626–1634.

Small, J. (1993). Psychiatric disorders and EEG. In E. Niedermeyer & F. Lopes da Silva (Eds.), *Electroencephalography: Basic principles, clinical applications, and related fields* (pp. 581–596). Baltimore: Williams & Wilkins.

Smith, J. L., & Noon, J. (1998). Objective measurement of mood change induced by contemporary music. *Journal of Psychiatric and Mental Health Nursing, 5*(5), 403–408.

Smith, R., Tiberi, A., & Marshall, J. (1994). The use of cranial electrotherapy stimulation in treatment of closed-head-injured patients. *Brain Injury, 8*(4), 357–361.

Smith, T. B., McCullough, M. E.,& Poll, J. (2004). Religiousness and depression: evidence for a main effect and the moderating influence of stressful life events. *Psychology Bulletin, 129*(4), 614–636.

Speer, A. M., Kimbrell, T. A., Wassermann, E. M., Repella, J., Willis, M. W., Herscovitch, P., & Post, R. M. (2000). Opposite effects of high and low frequency rTMS on regional brain activity in depressed patients. *Biological Psychiatry, 48*(12), 1133–1141.

Spence, D. (1990). Day to day management of anxiety and depression. *British Homeopathic Journal, 79*, 39–44.

Steegmans, P. H., Fekkes, D., Hoes, A. W., Bak, A. A., Van der Does, E., & Grobbe, D. E. (1996). Low serum cholesterol concentration and serotonin metabolism in men. *British Medical Journal, 312*, 221.

Stimpson, N., Agrawal, N., & Lewis, G. (2002). Randomised controlled trials investigating pharmacological and psychological interventions for treatment-refractory depression. *British Journal of Psychiatry, 181*, 284–294.

Stoll, A. L., Severus, W. E., Freeman, M. P., Rueter, S., Zboyan, H. A., Diamond, E., Cress, K. K., & Marangell, L. B. (1999). Omega 3 fatty acids in bipolar disorder: A preliminary double-blind, placebo-controlled trial. *Archives of General Psychiatry, 56*(5), 407–412.

Strous, R. D., Maayan, R., Lapidus, R., Stryjer, R., Lustig, M., Kotler, M., & Weizman, A. (2003). Dehydroepiandrosterone augmentation in the management of negative, depressive, and anxiety symptoms in schizophrenia. *Archives of General Psychiatry, 60*(2), 133–141.

Su, K. P., Huang, S. Y., Chiu, C. C., & Shen, W. W. (2003). Omega-3 fatty acids in major depressive disorder: A preliminary double-blind, placebo-controlled trial. *European Neuropsychopharmacology, 13*(4), 267–271.

Suffin, S. C., Gutierrez, N. M., Karan, S., Aurua, D., Emory, W. H., & Kling, A. (1997, May). *Neurometric EEG predicts pharmacotherapeutic outcome in depressed outpatients: A prospective trial.* Paper presented at the annual meeting of the American Psychiatric Association, San Diego, CA.

Sussman, N. (2004). The "file-drawer" effect: Assessing efficacy and safety of antidepressants. *Primary Psychiatry*, p.12.

Szegedi, A., Kohnen, R., Dienel, A., & Kieser, M. (2005). Acute treatment of moderate to severe depression with Hypericum extract WS 5570 (St John's wort): Randomised controlled double blind non-inferiority trial versus

paroxetine. *British Medical Journal, 330*(7490), 503. Erratum in *British Medical Journal, 330*(7494), 759 (dosage error in text).

Tang, C., et al. (1990). *Effects of qigong and Taijiquan on reversal of aging process and some psychological functions.* Paper presented at the Third National Academic Conference on Qigong Science.

Tanskanen, A., Hibbeln, J. R., Hintikka, J., Haatainen, K., Honkalampi, K., & Viinamäki, H. (2001). Fish consumption, depression and suicidality in a general population. *Archives of General Psychiatry, 58*, 512–513.

Taylor, M. J., Carney, S., Geddes, J., & Goodwin, G. (2004). Folate for depressive disorders (Cochrane Review). In *The Cochrane Library* (Issue 2). Chichester, UK: John Wiley & Sons.

Taylor, M. J., Wilder, H., Bhagwagar, Z., & Geddes, J. (2004). Inositol for depressive disorders (Cochrane Review). In *The Cochrane Library* (Issue 2). Chichester, UK: John Wiley & Sons.

Tempesta, E., Casella, L., Pirrongelli, C., Janiri, L., Calvani, M., & Ancona, L. (1987). L-acetylcarnitine in depressed elderly subjects: A cross-over study vs placebo. *Drugs Under Experimental and Clinical Research, 13*(7), 417–423.

Terman, M., & Terman, J. (1995). Treatment of seasonal affective disorder with a high-output negative ionizer. *Journal of Alternative and Complementary Medicine, 1*(1), 87–92.

Terman, M., & Terman, J. S. (1999). Bright light therapy: Side effects and benefits across the symptom spectrum. *Journal of Clinical Psychiatry, 60*(11), 799–809.

Terman, M., Terman, J. S., & Ross, D. C. (1998). A controlled trial of timed bright light and negative air ionization for treatment of winter depression. *Archives of General Psychiatry, 55*(10), 875–882.

Thase, M. (2002). Antidepressant effects: The suit may be small, but the fabric is real. *Prevention and Treatment, 5.* Available at journals.apa.org/prevention/ volume5/toc-jul15–02.html

Thatcher, R. (1998, Spring). Normative EEG databases and EEG biofeedback. *Journal of Neurotherapy*, 8–36.

Tiemeier, H., van Tuijl, H., Hofman, A., Kiliaan, A., & Breteler, M. (2003). Plasma fatty acid composition and depression are associated in the elderly: The Rotterdam study. *American Journal of Clinical Nutrition, 78*(1), 40–46.

Tkachuk, G., & Martin, G. (1999). Exercise therapy for patients with psychiatric disorders: Research and clinical implications. *Professional Psychology, Research and Practice, 30*, 275–282.

Torta, R., Zanalda, F., Rocca, P., et al. (1988). Inhibitory activity of *S*-adenosyl-*L*-methionine on serum gamma-glutamyl-transpeptidase increase induced by psychodrugs and anticonvulsants. *Current Therapeutic Research, 44*, 144–159.

Trivedi, M. H., & Kleiber, B. A. (2001). Algorithm for the treatment of chronic depression. *Journal of Clinical Psychiatry, 62*(Suppl. 6), 22–29.

Upton, R. (1997). St. John's wort (*Hypericum perforatum*). In R. Upton (Ed.), *American herbal pharmacopoeia and therapeutic compendium.* Santa Cruz, CA: American Herbal Pharmacopoeia.

van Hiele, L. J. (1980). l-5-hydroxytryptophan in depression: The first substitution therapy in psychiatry? The treatment of 99 out-patients with "therapy-resistant" depressions. *Neuropsychobiology, 6*(4), 230–240.

Van Praag, H. M. (1984). In search of the mode of action of antidepressants: 5-HTP/tyrosine mixtures in depression. In *Frontiers of biochemistry and pharmacological research in depression* (pp. 301–314). New York: Raven Press.

Van Praag, H. M., van den Burg, W., Bos, E. R., & Dols, L. C. (1974). 5-hydroxytryptophan in combination with clomipramine in "therapy-resistant" depression. *Psychopharmacologia, 38*(3), 267–269.

Viguera, A., Baldessarini, R., & Friedberg, J. (1998). Discontinuing antidepressant treatment in major depression. *Harvard Review of Psychiatry, 5*, 293–306.

Villa, B., Calabresi, L., Chiesa, G., Rise, P., Galli, C., & Sirtori, C. R. (2002). Omega-3 fatty acid ethyl esters increase heart rate variability in patients with coronary disease. *Pharmacological Research, 45*(6), 475.

Vorbach, E. U., Arnoldt, K. H., & Hubner, W. D. (1997). Efficacy and tolerability of St. John's wort extract LI 160 versus imipramine in patients with severe depressive episodes according to ICD-10. *Pharmacopsychiatry, 30*(Suppl. 2), 81–85.

Waite ,W., & Holder, M. (2003). Assessment of the Emotional Freedom Technique. *Scientific Review of Mental Health Practice, 2*(1), 20–26.

Waldkoetter, R. O., & Sanders, G. O. (1997). Auditory brainwave stimulation in treating alcoholic depression. *Perceptual and Motor Skills, 84*(1), 226.

Walton, K., Pugh, N., Gelderloos, P., & Macrae, P. (1995). Stress reduction and preventing hypertension: Preliminary support for a psychoneuroendocrine mechanism. *Journal of Alternative and Complementary Medicine, 1*, 263–283.

Wang, J. (1993). *Role of qigong on mental health.* Paper presented at the Second World Conference Acad Exch Med. Qigong.

Warman, V. L., Dijk, D. J., Warman, G. R., Arendt, J., & Skene, D. J. (2003). Phase advancing human circadian rhythms with short wavelength light. *Neuroscience Letters, 342*, 37–40.

Webb, W., & Gehi, M. (1981). Electrolyte and fluid imbalance: Neuropsychiatric manifestations. *Psychosomatics, 22*(3), 199–203.

Weller, E., Kang, J., & Weller, R. (2004). Clinical perspective on pediatric depression: How the evidence tipped SSRIs' risk-benefit balance. *Current Psychiatry, 3*(10), 15–18.

Werneke, U., Horn, O., & Taylor, D. (2004). How effective is St. John's wort? The evidence revisited. *Journal of Clinical Psychiatry, 65*(5), 611–627.

Wileman, S. M., Eagles, J. M., Andrew, J. E., Howie, F. L., Cameron, I. M., McCormack, K., & Naji, S. A. (2001). Light therapy for seasonal affective disorder in primary care: Randomized controlled trial. *British Journal of Psychiatry, 178,* 311–316.

Williams, R., Maturen, A., & Sky-Peck, H. (1987). Pharmacologic role of rubidium in psychiatric research. *Comprehensive Therapy, 13*(9), 46–54.

Wolkowitz, O. M., Reua, V. I., Keebler, A., et al. (1999). Double-blind treatment of major depression with dehydroepiandrosterone. *American Journal of Psychiatry, 156*(4), 646–649.

Wolkowitz, O. M., Reus, V. I., Roberts, E., Manfredi, F., Chan, T., Raum, W. J., Ormiston, S., Johnson, R., Canick, J., Brizendine, L., & Weingartner, H. (1997). Dehydroepiandrosterone (DHEA) treatment of depression. *Biological Psychiatry, 41*(3), 311–318.

Woolery, A., Myers, H., Sternlieb, B., & Zeltzer, L. (2004). A yoga intervention for young adults with elevated symptoms of depression. *Alternative Therapies in Health Medicine, 10*(1), 60–63.

Yong-Ku, K. (2003). Serum lipid levels and suicide attempts. *Acta Psychiatrica Scandinavica, 108,* 215–221.

Zaren, A. (1995). A case of fatigue and depression. *Homeopathic Links, 4,* 21–24.

General Referenes

Bell, I., Baldwin, C., Schwartz, G., Russek, L. (1998). Integrating belief systems and therapies in medicine: Application of the eight world hypotheses to classical homeopathy. *Integrative Medicine: Integrating Conventional and Alternative Medicine, 1,* 95–105.

Borg, H. (2003). Alternative method of gifted identification using the AMI: An apparatus for measuring for measuring internal meridians and their corresponding organs. *Journal of Alternative and Complementary Medicine, 9*(6), 861–867.

Bottiglieri, T. (1997). Ademetionine (*S*-adenosylmethionine) neuropharmacology: Implications for drug therapies in psychiatric and neurological disorders. *Expert Opinion on Investigational Drugs, 6,* 417–426.

Bottiglieri, T., & Hyland, K. (1994). *S*-adenosylmethionine levels in psychiatric and neurological disorders: A review. *Acta Neurologica Scandinavica Supplementum, 54,* 19–26.

Crismon, M., Trivedi, M., & Pigott, T. (1999). The Texas Medication Algorithm Project: Report of the Texas Consensus Conference Panel on Medication Treatment of Major Depressive Disorder. *Clinical Psychiatry, 60*(3), 142–146.

Ernst, E., & Resch, K. (1996). Clinical Trials of Homeopathy: A re-analysis of a published review. *Forschende Komplementarmedizin, 3,* 85–90.

Fugh-Berman, A., & Cott, J. M. (1999). Dietary supplements and natural products as psychotherapeutic agents. *Psychosomatic Medicine, 61*(5), 712–728

Goldman, A. (2002). *Long-term effects of energetic healing on symptoms of psychological depression and self-perceived stress.* Unpublished doctoral dissertation, Institute Of Transpersonal Psychology.

Hein, O. (1993). A case of depression: Man 24 years old. *Small Remedies Seminar Hechtel,* 39–50.

Kagan, B. L., Sultzer, D. L., Rosenlicht, N., & Gerner, R. H. (1990). Oral *S*-adenosylmethionine in depression: A randomized double-blind, placebo-controlled trial. *American Journal of Psychiatry, 147*(5), 591–595.

Kessler, R., & Soukup, J. (2001). The use of complementary and alternative therapies to treat anxiety and depression in the United States. *American Journal of Psychiatry, 158*(2), 289–294.

Kleijnen, J., Knipschild, P., & ter Riet, G. (1991). Clinical trials of homeopathy. *British Medical Journal, 302,* 316–323.

Koenig, H., & Futterman, A. (1995, March). *Religion and health outcomes: A review and synthesis of the literature.* Paper presented at the Conference on Methodological Advances in the Study of Religion, Health and Aging, Kalamazoo, MI.

Levin, J. S. (1996). How religion influences morbidity and health: Reflections on natural history, salutogenesis and host resistance. *Social Sciences Medicine, 43,* 849–864.

McCaffrey, A., Eisenberg, D., Legedza, A., Davis, R., & Phillips, R. (2004). Prayer for health concerns: Results of a national survey on prevalence and patterns of use. *Archives of Internal Medicine, 164,* 858–862.

Princhep, J., Ahn, H., et al. (1988). Neurometrics: Computer assisted differential diagnosis of brain dysfunctions. *Science, 293,* 162–169.

Radin, D. I. (2004). Event-related electroencephalographic correlations between isolated human subjects. *Journal of Alternative and Complementary Medicine, 10*(2), 315–323.

Ruschitzka, F., Meier, P. J., Turina, M., et al. (2000). Acute heart transplant rejection due to Saint John's wort. *Lancet, 355,* 548–549.

Schellenberg, R., Sauer, S., & Dimpfel, W. (1998). Pharmacodynamic effects of two different hypericum extracts in healthy volunteers measured by quantitative EEG. *Pharmacopsychiatry, 31*(Suppl. 1), 44–53.

Schwartz, G., & Russek, L. (1998). The plausibility of homeopathy: The systemic memory mechanism. *Integrative Medicine: Integrating Conventional and Alternative Medicine, 1*(2), 53–59.

Smith, T. B., McCullough, M. E., & Poll, J. (2003). Religiousness and depression: Evidence for a main effect and the moderating influence of stressful life events. *Psychological Bulletin, 129*(4), 614–636. Erratum in *Psychological Bulletin, 130*(1), 65.

Van Londen, L., Molenaar, R., Goekoop, J., Zwinderman, A., & Rooijmans, H. G. M. (1998). Three- to 5-year prospective follow-up of outcome in major depression. *Psychological Medicine, 28*(3), 731–735.

Vorbach, E. U., Hubner, W. D., & Arnoldt, K. H. (1994). Effectiveness and tolerance of the hypericum extract LI 160 in comparison with imipramine: Randomized double-blind study with 135 outpatients. *Journal of Geriatric Psychiatry and Neurology* (Suppl. 1), S19–S23.

9

The Integrative Management of Mania and Cyclic Mood Changes

This chapter covers the integrative management of mania and cyclic mood changes. The integrative management of single or recurring episodes of depressed mood is reviewed in Chapter 8.

◆ Background

Mania and Cyclic Mood Changes Are Present in Many Symptom Patterns

Mania and cyclic mood changes may occur alone or in the context of other symptom patterns. In Western psychiatry, bipolar disorder is diagnosed on the basis of one or more episodes of mania. Many symptom patterns involving cyclic mood changes are regarded as variant forms of bipolar disorder. Bipolar I disorder is the most severe form of the syndrome. Bipolar II disorder and cyclothymic disorder are regarded as milder variants. Neurobiological, psychodynamic, energetic, or other causes of cyclic mood changes probably vary depending on whether the broader symptom pattern includes persisting depressed mood, recurring episodes of depression or mania, or cyclic mood changes alternating between mania and depression. In other words, symptom patterns involving depression, mania, or cyclic changes in mood are best understood in the context of the broader narrative history of each patient. These differences translate into disparate assessment approaches that will most likely yield useful information about the causes or underlying psychological or energetic meanings that correspond to a symptom pattern of cyclic mood changes and, in a parallel fashion, the selection of treatments that most effectively address the identified causes or meanings.

The integrative management of fluctuating mood states takes into account the characteristics and time course of mood symptoms on a case-by-case basis, including the temporal pattern of mood changes, the severity symptoms, the co-occurrence of depressed mood and mania, and the presence of other symptoms, including anxiety, psychosis, etc.

Bipolar Disorder Causes an Enormous Economic and Social Burden

It is estimated that 1% of the adult population in the United States experiences persisting mood swings and fulfills criteria for the diagnosis of bipolar disorder as given in the fourth edition of the *Diagnostic and Statistical Manual of Mental Disorders* (*DSM-IV*; Robins & Regier, 1991). Bipolar disorder is a heritable mental illness. Dysregulations in circadian rhythms probably cause the affective and behavioral symptom patterns that are described in current Western psychiatric nosology as bipolar disorders I and II. Recent findings from genetic studies suggest that decreased expression of ribonucleic acid (RNA) coding for mitochondrial proteins results in dysregulations of energy metabolism in the brain, especially in the hippocampus (Konradi, Eaton, MacDonald, Walsh, Benes, & Heckers, 2004). First-degree relatives of bipolar individuals are much more likely to develop the disorder than the population at large. Bipolar illness in one identical twin corresponds to a 70% risk that the other twin will also have the disorder. This risk is estimated at 15% in dizygotic twins (Gurling et al., 1995). Recurrent episodes of mania are associated with progressive deterioration in social and occupational functioning, and often lead to job loss and divorce (Prien & Gelenberg, 1989). Approximately two thirds of individuals diagnosed with bipolar disorder are unemployed, although most have attended college ("WHO Report," 2001). One fourth of bipolar I patients attempt suicide, and 15% eventually succeed.

Manic Episodes Are Associated with Many Disparate Symptoms

In conventional Western psychiatry, mania is a symptom pattern that may encompass many disparate affective, behavioral, and cognitive symptoms, including pressured speech, racing thoughts, euphoric or irritable mood, agitation, inflated self-esteem, distractibility, excessive or inappropriate involvement in pleasurable activities, increased goal-directed activity, diminished need for sleep, and, in severe cases, psychosis. According to the *DSM-IV*, criteria for a *manic episode* are fulfilled when elevated or irritable mood lasts at least 1 week, is accompanied by at least three of the above symptoms, significant social or occupational impairment is present, and symptoms cannot be explained by substance abuse or a medical condition. In contrast, criteria for a *hypomanic episode* are fulfilled when elevated or irritable mood persists at least 4 days, together with three or more of the above symptoms, medical problems and substance abuse are ruled out as causes, but functioning is not severely impaired. In conventional Western psychiatry, an individual who has experienced one or more manic episodes is diagnosed with *bipolar I disorder,* while an individual who has experienced one or more hypomanic episodes is diagnosed with *bipolar II disorder.* The typical bipolar I patient has had many manic episodes, although the diagnosis of bipolar I can be made after only one manic episode. Eighty percent or more of patients who experience mania will have subsequent manic episodes (Winokur, Clayton, & Reich, 1969). According to the *DSM-IV*, a history of a previous depressive episode is not required for a formal diagnosis of bipolar I disorder. In contrast, bipolar II disorder can be diagnosed only after an individual has experienced at least one hypomanic episode and at least one depressive episode. Moderate or severe depressive episodes typically alternate with manic symptoms in both syndromes. However, in a variant of the syndrome called *mixed mania,* symptoms of mania and depressed mood occur during the same period of time. Rapid cycling is another variant of the syndrome in which at least four complete mood episodes take place during any 12-month period. Another milder variant, *cyclothymic disorder,* is diagnosed when multiple hypomanic and depressive episodes take place over a 2-year period, but there are no manic, mixed, or severe depressive episodes. Patients diagnosed with bipolar I disorder are symptomatic ~50% of the time. Depressive symptoms are reported 3 times more often than mania and 5 times more often than rapid cycling or mixed episodes (Judd et al., 2002).

◆ The Integrative Assessment of Mania and Cyclic Mood Symptoms

Overview of Conventional Approaches Used to Assess Mania and Cyclic Mood Changes

Western trained psychiatrists establish a diagnosis of bipolar disorder on the basis of history and mental status examination. There is often a clear family history of cyclic mood changes, especially in first-degree relatives. When taking the history, it is sometimes difficult to differentiate between transient periods of mania or hypomania and acute agitation related to other causes. A careful longitudinal history usually establishes a persisting pattern of cyclic mood changes. Laboratory studies and functional brain imaging studies are performed to rule out a possible underlying medical problem. Thyroid disease, strokes (especially in the right frontal area of the brain), multiple sclerosis, rarely seizure disorders, and other neurological disorders can manifest as manic or cyclic mood changes. Chronic drug abuse, especially of stimulants, can result in alternating periods of euphoria or irritability and depression. Many conventional drugs, or interactions between drugs, can also result in manic or depressive mood changes.

Even when possible medical or other so-called organic causes have been ruled out, a primary diagnosis of bipolar I disorder is often difficult to establish because of the heterogeneity of symptoms included in conventional diagnostic criteria. For example, the patient may display euphoric, agitated, or irritable mood, and may fail to disclose a history of psychotic episodes or mood changes related to chronic drug abuse. Symptom patterns of severe emotional dysregulation associated with severe personality disorders, especially borderline personality disorder, often resemble the symptom patterns diagnosed as variants of bipolar disorder. In this context there is ongoing debate over the validity of the bipolar variant called rapid cycling, which can be interpreted both as a primary mood disorder and as a severe personality disorder, depending on the training and philosophical outlook of the clinician. Establishing a definitive diagnosis of bipolar II,

cyclothymic disorder, and bipolar disorder not otherwise specified (NOS) is equally problematic in view of overlapping criteria between these and other *DSM-IV* disorders, including major depressive disorder, schizoaffective disorder, personality disorders, and others.

Overview of Nonconventional Approaches Used to Assess Mania and Cyclic Mood Changes

At the time of writing, nonconventional approaches used to assess the causes of mania or cyclic mood changes have not been substantiated by compelling research findings. However, provisional research findings suggest that two assessment approaches probably provide accurate and reliable information about the causes of this symptom pattern. Red blood cell (RBC) folate levels are consistently low in bipolar patients, and supplementation may therefore prove to be a reasonable and effective adjunct to many conventional and nonconventional treatments. Another emerging assessment approach is the use of quantitative electroencephalography (qEEG) in acutely manic patients who have not yet been treated with conventional medications. Abnormal qEEG findings in left frontal brain regions predict improved response to conventional mood-stabilizing medications.

Four emerging biological approaches reviewed below possibly provide accurate and reliable information about the causes of mania or cyclic mood changes. These are serologic assays of lithium (i.e., in non-lithium-treated patients), γ-aminobutyric acid (GABA, the principle inhibitory neurotransmitter), *N*-acetylaspartate (in children predisposed to bipolar disorder), and homovanillic acid (HVA). High pretreatment serum HVA levels may correspond to lower effective doses of certain conventional or nonconventional treatments of mania or cyclic mood changes. **Table 9–1** lists provisional nonconventional approaches used to assess mania and cyclic mood changes. **Table 9–2** shows assessment approaches that possibly provide accurate diagnostic information about the causes of mania or cyclic mood changes.

Table 9–1   Provisional Nonconventional Approaches Used to Assess Mania and Cyclic Mood Changes

Category	Assessment Approach	Evidence for Specific Diagnostic Information	Positive Findings Suggest Efficacy of This Treatment
Biological	RBC folate level	Abnormally low RBC folate levels (but normal serum folate levels) are common in bipolar patients	Supplementation with folate may reduce severity of both manic and depressive symptoms in bipolar patients
Somatic	None at time of writing		
Energy-information approaches validated by Western science		Left-sided qEEG abnormalities in acute mania may correlate with improved response to conventional treatments	Pretreatment qEEG may facilitate selection of the most effective conventional treatment
Energy-information approaches not validated by Western science	None at time of writing		

qEEG, quantitative electroencephalography; RBC, red blood cell (count)

Table 9–2 Assessment Approaches That May Yield Specific Information about Causes of Mania or Cyclic Mood Changes

Category	Assessment Approach	Evidence for Specific Diagnostic Information	Comments
Biological	Serum lithium level	Low trace lithium levels (i.e., from low nutritional intake) are common in acute mania	Supplementation with trace lithium in the diet may reduce the risk of acute mania in predisposed individuals
	Serum GABA level	Pretreatment serum GABA levels (need levels) might predict improved response to divalproex but not other mood stabilizers	Manic patients with low pretreatment serum GABA levels should be preferentially started on divalproex (Depakote). A possible beneficial role of supplementation remains unclear
	CNS N-acetylaspartate	Children with low brain levels of N-acetylaspartate by MRS may be at increased risk of developing bipolar disorder	MRS is not indicated as a routine screening approach for at-risk children
	Serum HVA	High pretreatment serum HVA levels predict improved response to lower doses of conventional antipsychotics in acute mania	Check serum homovanillic acid level to estimate effective dose range when treating an acute manic episode to achieve optimum antipsychotic dosing strategy and minimize risk of adverse effects
Somatic	None at time of writing		
Energy-information assessment approaches validated by Western science	None at time of writing		
Energy-information assessment approaches not (yet) validated by Western science	VAS analysis	The VAS reflex may provide specific information about conventional or nonconventional treatments in difficult cases of rapid mood cycling	Measuring the VAS reflex is an easy and inexpensive method that can be used adjunctively in integrative treatment planning

CNS, central nervous system; GABA, γ-aminobutyric acid; HVA, homovanillic acid; MRS, magnetic resonance spectroscopy; VAS, vascular autonomic signal.

Substantiated Approaches Used to Assess Mania and Cyclic Mood Changes

At the time of writing, there are no substantiated nonconventional assessment approaches in any category (i.e., biological, somatic, and energy-information approaches).

Provisional Approaches Used to Assess Mania and Cyclic Mood Changes

Biological Approaches

◆ **Low RBC folic acid levels but normal serum levels are common in bipolar patients** Folic acid deficiency may be a common nutritional factor in manic patients diagnosed with bipolar disorder (Coppen, Chaudhry, & Swade, 1986). Chronic folate deficiency is believed to interfere with normal synthesis of serotonin. Manic patients often have abnormally low red blood cell folic acid levels but normal serum folic acid levels (Hasanah, Khan, Musalmah, & Razali, 1997; Lee, Chow, Shek, Wing, & Chen, 1992). Chronic folate deficiency is associated with both phases of bipolar illness; however, bipolar patients who are taking lithium often have normal RBC folate levels (McKeon, Shelley, O'Regan, & O'Brian, 1991).

Somatic Approaches

At the time of writing, there are no assessment approaches in this category.

Assessment Approaches Based on Forms of Energy-Information Validated by Western Science

Left-Sided qEEG Abnormalities May Predict Improved Response to Conventional Treatments of Mania

Abnormal EEG findings are more common in mania than depressed mood (Hughes & Roy, 1999). Depressed mood, psychosis, and acute mania are associated with distinctive patterns of brain electrical activity on qEEG mapping. Global disturbances in EEG synchronization are similar in schizophrenia and bipolar disorder. However, in contrast to schizophrenics, bipolar patients do not show disorganization in the superior temporal lobes. Nonmedicated manic patients have lower EEG amplitudes in the left anterior and temporal brain regions (Small, Milstein, Malloy, Klapper, Golay, & Medlock, 1998). Additionally, qEEG findings may predict differential response rates to conventional treatments (Small, Milstein, Malloy, Medlock, & Klapper, 1999). Specific abnormal findings may predict differential response rates to different classes of conventional mood-stabilizing or antipsychotic medications (Small et al., 1998). Nonresponders to conventional medications are more likely to have diffuse theta activity at baseline, as well as higher amplitudes in the left temporoparietal regions during treatment. Acutely manic inpatients who responded to subsequent conventional treatments were more likely to have left-sided abnormalities. The significance of these findings is limited by the low rate of cooperation of acutely manic inpatients in studies completed to date.

Assessment Approaches Based on Forms of Energy Information Not Validated by Western Science

At the time of writing, there are no provisional assessment approaches in this category.

Assessment Approaches That May Yield Specific Diagnostic Information about Causes of Mania and Cyclic Mood Changes

Biological Treatments

◆ **Low trace levels of lithium are common in acute mania** Lithium is generally obtained in trace amounts from drinking water. The findings of a few small studies suggest that psychiatric hospital admissions of acutely manic or psychotic patients are inversely correlated with nutritional lithium intake (Dawson, 1991).

◆ **Elevated serum GABA levels predict improved response of mania to divalproex** High serum GABA levels may predict improved response of manic symptoms to divalproex (Depakote), an important conventional treatment of bipolar manic episodes. However, pretreatment GABA levels do not predict improved response to lithium. In a large placebo-controlled double-blind trial, acutely manic patients found to have abnormally high serum GABA levels responded differentially to divalproex (Petty et al., 1996). GABA levels normalized with clinical response to treatment. There was no correlation between pretreatment serum GABA levels and the severity of manic symptoms. Serum GABA levels may help to clarify treatment planning in manic patients who fail to respond to lithium or other conventional mood-stabilizing agents.

◆ **Children with low brain N-acetylaspartate levels may be at increased risk of developing bipolar disorder** Findings from a functional brain-imaging study using proton magnetic resonance spectroscopy suggest that children at risk of developing bipolar disorder have abnormally low brain levels of N-acetylaspartate (Chang, Adleman, Dienes, Barnea-Goraly, Reiss, & Ketter, 2003). The relationship between low levels of N-acetylalspartate and the progression of bipolar disorder is unclear. Children with low brain levels of this amino acid may be at increased risk of developing bipolar disorder at an early age.

◆ **High serum HVA levels suggest lower effective doses of typical antipsychotics** Pretreatment serum homovanillic acid levels may predict improved response to conventional antipsychotic medications in acute mania or psychosis (Chou et al., 2000). Higher serum HVA levels predict improved response to low doses of typical antipsychotics, including haloperidol (e.g., 5 mg/day). Abnormally low pretreatment HVA levels suggest the need for higher dosing strategies of typical antipsychotics (e.g., up to 25 mg/day). High levels may reflect higher turnover of dopamine in the brain and therefore lower effective doses of conventional dopamine-blocking antipsychotics. It is unclear whether these findings generalize to treatment strategies using atypical antipsychotics or other conventional medications.

Somatic Approaches

At the time of writing, there are no assessment approaches in this category.

Approaches Based on Forms of Energy Information Validated by Western Science

At the time of writing, there are no assessment approaches in this category.

Approaches Based on Forms of Energy Information Not Validated by Western Science

◆ **Analysis of the VAS reflex may help to identify effective treatment choices** A case report suggests that the VAS reflex may provide useful information when approaching rapidly cycling mood changes that are poorly responsive to conventional treatments. The VAS reflex was used to identify a regimen of L-tryptophan 22 g/day, vitamin C 10 g/day, and B vitamins as appropriate treatments of the energetic imbalance underlying poorly controlled rapid cycling mood changes in a 30-year-old man. A specific auricular acupuncture protocol was started on the basis of these findings, and the patient's previously nonresponsive mood symptoms soon normalized. The author suggests that using VAS to identify treatments that effectively restored energetic balance in this case resulted in substantial cost savings (Ackerman, 1989).

◆ The Integrative Treatment of Mania and Cyclic Mood Symptoms

Limited Efficacy and Noncompliance Interfere with Conventional Treatments of Bipolar Disorder

Many conventional drugs are used to treat mania and cyclic mood changes, including mood stabilizers such as lithium carbonate and divalproex, antidepressants, antipsychotics, and sedative-hypnotics. Available conventional treatments of both the depressive and manic phases of bipolar disorder have only a moderate record of success. This is due in part to a high rate of noncompliance with conventional pharmacological treatments among bipolar patients, and due in part to limited efficacy of available conventional treatments addressing both the depressive and manic phases of the illness. Less than one third of all bipolar patients receive any treatment for manic or depressive symptoms during the active phase of their illness (Goodwin & Jamison, 1990). Because less severe symptoms of mania often go unreported, and because many symptoms of hypomania resemble agitation or anxiety, there is ongoing debate over the prevalence of bipolar disorder compared with major depressive disorder. Failure to confirm a history of mania or hypomania often leads to an erroneous diagnosis of unipolar depression, as well as inappropriate conventional or nonconventional treatment (Benazzi, 1997). Only half of conventional medications prescribed for the treatment of bipolar mood symptoms are based on good evidence of clinical efficacy (Boschert, 2004). Findings from two large controlled studies show that a significant percentage of bipolar patients who take conventional antidepressants not only fail to improve but become worse. Fewer than half of patients who take conventional maintenance treatments following an initial manic episode report sustained control of their symptoms (Tohen, Waternaux, & Tsuang, 1990). However, the relapse rate among bipolar patients who adhere to lithium carbonate or other conventional mood stabilizers is also very high at ~40% (Strober, Morrell, Lampert, & Burroughs, 1990). Further, the use of conventional antidepressants does not reduce the frequency of depressive symptoms in bipolar patients over the long term and does not lead to increased time spent in remission.

As many as one half of patients who are treated for bipolar disorder fail to adhere to their recommended regimens of conventional mood stabilizers, often because of adverse effects (Goodwin & Jamison, 1990). Bipolar patients who discontinue lithium carbonate or other conventional mood stabilizers are almost certain to relapse. There is evidence that discontinuation of lithium carbonate and other conventional treatments is associated with reduced efficacy if these medications are resumed in the future (Post, 1993).

The findings of a systematic review demonstrate that combining different conventional drug treatments, an accepted approach in Western psychiatry, does not significantly improve outcomes compared with individual mood stabilizers. A structured Cochrane review of seven studies (four of which were randomized) involving 358 patients concluded that adding an antidepressant to lithium therapy does not substantially increase protection against bipolar depressive recurrences (Ghaemi, Lenox, & Baldessarini, 2001).

Transcranial magnetic stimulation (TMS) is an evolving treatment that may have beneficial therapeutic effects similar to those of conventional electroconvulsive therapy (ECT) and is associated with a markedly lower risk of adverse effects. Repetitive TMS of the left prefrontal cortex may be an effective treatment of the depressive phase of bipolar illness, and there have been no reports of mania induction in patients who are stable on medications (Nahas, Kozel, Li, Anderson, & George, 2003). Preliminary results of TMS for mania are promising, especially when the right prefrontal region of the brain is stimulated (Grisaru, Chudakov, Yaroslavsky, & Belmaker, 1998). However, findings of controlled trials using sham TMS have been inconsistent (Kaptsan, Yaroslavsky, Applebaum, Belmaker, & Grisaru, 2003).

The Integrative Management of Mania and Cyclic Mood Symptoms: A Review of Basic Concepts

In contrast to conventional Western psychiatry, the integrative management of mania and cyclic mood changes is not based on the assumption that disparate patterns of changing mood symptoms are variants of a single diagnostic entity or disorder. In fact, in the routine clinical practice of conventional Western psychiatry, all symptoms required to diagnose a manic, hypomanic, or mixed episode are rarely encountered. More often discrete symptoms of mania take place in isolation or in combination with disparate cognitive, affective, or behavioral symptoms, and the mix and severity of symptoms generally change in complex ways over time. For example, the most prominent or most impairing symptom during a manic episode may be euphoric or irritable mood, agitation, grandiose delusions, racing thoughts, or pressured speech. In clinical practice each of these symptoms may be experienced alone, together with other symptoms of mania,

or together with unrelated symptoms, including anxiety, depression, psychosis, and varying degrees of cognitive impairment. The symptom pattern that is called a manic episode in Western psychiatry typically evolves over time, such that different symptoms are more prominent at different times during the course of a given episode, and the primary symptom pattern (i.e., if any primary or core pattern can be ascertained) continues to change over the course of the illness. For practical purposes, in the day-to-day clinical practice of Western psychiatry, the most prominent or impairing symptom or symptom pattern becomes the immediate focus of clinical attention. The bipolar patient is therefore treated symptomatically on an ongoing basis because a clear persisting symptom pattern is seldom if ever present during the course of illness. Like conventional Western psychiatry, the integrative management of mania and cyclic mood changes focuses on the core symptom or core symptom pattern of greatest clinical concern during a particular period in of the patient's illness while taking into account the dynamic course of cyclic mood changes over time.

In contrast to the conventional Western management of bipolar disorder, the integrative management of mania and cyclic mood changes is based on a multidimensional treatment plan that take into account psychological, medical, social, family, and possibly energetic or spiritual factors, together with pertinent assessment findings of biological, somatic, or energetic causes or meanings associated with the symptom pattern. When anxiety, depressed mood, or cognitive impairment occurs in the context of a broader pattern of mania or cyclic mood changes, it is appropriate to use integrative approaches addressing those core symptoms. A significant percentage of patients diagnosed with bipolar disorder use complementary, alternative, or integrative approaches in addition to conventional pharmacological treatments (Dennehy, Gonzale, & Suppes, 2004). It is important for psychiatrists, other mental health professionals, and nonconventionally trained practitioners who treat patients complaining of cyclic mood changes to be aware of current evidence for the various treatment modalities before making specific recommendations to patients.

Substantiated and Provisional Nonconventional Treatments of Mania and Cyclic Mood Changes

At the time of writing, nonconventional treatments of mania and cyclic mood changes have not been substantiated by compelling research evidence. Provisional nonconventional treatments of mania and cyclic mood changes include omega-3 fatty acids, EMPowerPlus (TrueHope, Shelby, MT), L-tryptophan, and phosphatidylcholine alone or adjunctively with conventional mood stabilizers. EMPowerPlus™ represents a unique approach to the management of bipolar symptoms and will probably become a significant adjunctive and possibly stand-alone treatment. The adjunctive use of omega-3 fatty acids will likely also become a standard adjunctive therapy in the near future. Acute tyrosine depletion may be an effective approach for reducing acute symptoms of mania in some cases. Provisional maintenance therapies include trace lithium supplementation, folinic acid (a form of folate), and regular early morning bright light exposure. **Table 9–3** lists provisional nonconventional treatments of mania or cyclic mood changes.

Table 9–3　Provisional Nonconventional Treatments of Mania and Cyclic Mood Changes

	Treatment Approach	Evidence for Modality or Integrative Approaches	Comments (Including Safety Issues or Contraindications)
Biological	EMPowerPlus acute tyrosine depletion	EMPowerPlus may be an effective adjunctive or stand-alone treatment of depressive and manic symptoms.	*Caution:* Titrating patients on EMPowerPlus requires careful monitoring, and there is a risk of toxicity when combined with conventional medications
		Some bipolar patients were able to reduce conventional medications by one half when taking EMPowerPlus.	
		Some bipolar patients remain stable off all conventional medications when taking EMPowerPlus.	
		A branched-chain amino acid drink that excludes tyrosine may be an effective treatment in some cases of acute mania	Specialized preparations of branched-chain amino acids should be administered under medical supervision
	L-tryptophan	L-tryptophan may reduce the frequency of depressive mood swings and reduce the severity of mania in bipolar patients.	*Caution:* Dietary restriction of L-tryptophan can precipitate depressed mood in bipolar patients
		L-tryptophan 3 g tid added to lithium may improve symptoms of mania more than lithium alone	
	Omega-3 fatty acids	EPA (1–2 g/day) in combination with conventional mood stabilizers may reduce severity and frequency of manic episodes	High doses of omega-3s may cause GI side effects. There is one case report of EPA-induced hypomania
	Choline and phosphatidylcholine	Adding choline (2–7 g/day) to therapeutic doses of lithium may improve response in rapid-cycling episodes.	*Note:* Check thyroid levels in nonresponders to choline or phosphatidylcholine supplementation
		Adding phosphatidylcholine (15–30 g/day) improves both depression and mania in bipolar patients	
	Folic acid 200 μg/day	Folic acid 200 μg/day may augment the effects of lithium in mania	Combining folic acid with lithium does not pose potential safety issues
	Trace lithium supplementation	Lithium in trace amounts (50 μg with meals) may reduce the frequency and severity of both depressive and manic symptoms	There are no contraindications to the use of lithium in trace amounts
	Magnesium supplementation	Magnesium supplementation 40 mEq/day may be an effective treatment of rapid-cycling episodes	Patients should consult with their primary care physician before starting magnesium supplementation
Somatic and mind–body approaches	None at time of writing		
Energy-information approaches validated by Western science	None at time of writing		
Energy-information approaches not (yet) validated by Western science	None at time of writing		

EPA, ecosapentanoic acid; GI, gastrointestinal

Substantiated Nonconventional Treatments of Mania and Cyclic Mood Changes

At the time of writing, there are no rigorously substantiated nonconventional treatments of mania or cyclic mood changes. It is important to remark that some provisional treatments are probably as effective as widely used conventional pharmacological treatments of bipolar disorder.

Provisional Nonconventional Treatments of Mania and Cyclic Mood Changes

Biological Approaches

◆ **EMPowerPlus, a proprietary nutrient formula, is probably an effective adjunctive or stand-alone treatment of both depressive and manic symptoms in bipolar disorder** The findings of four cases series and two cases studies suggest that EMPowerPlus™, a proprietary nutrient formula containing 36 separate constituents including chelated minerals, vitamins, and trace elements, may significantly reduce symptoms of mania and depressed mood (Kaplan, Crawford, Gardner, & Farrelly, 2002; Kaplan, Fisher, Crawford, Field, & Kolb, 2004; Kaplan et al., 2001; Popper, 2001; Simmons, 2002). The mechanism of action may involve correction of in-born metabolic errors that predispose some individuals to become symptomatic when certain micronutrients are deficient in the diet (Kaplan et al., 2001). Bipolar patients may be genetically predisposed to develop manic or depressive mood symptoms related to different micronutrient deficiencies. Patients described in all five of these publications took an early version of EMPowerPlus™, consisting of 32 capsules daily in four divided doses. The 11 adult patients who completed the 6-month protocol in one series were able to reduce their conventional mood stabilizing medications by half while improving clinically according to standardized symptom rating scales (Kaplan et al., 2001). In another case series, 13 out of 19 Bipolar patients who continued to take EMPowerPlus™ reportedly remained stable after discontinuing conventional mood stabilizing medications (Simmons, 2002). Four patients stopped taking the nutrient formula because of gastrointestinal side effects including nausea and diarrhea; the currently-marketed version of EMPowerPlus™ is reported to have solved the problem of gastrointestinal side-effects, which were significant with this earlier version. Three other patients resumed conventional mood stabilizers while taking EMPowerPlus™ because of recurring manic symptoms Significantly, at the time of writing 11 of the 19 patients in the case series who elected to discontinue conventional mood stabilizers while continuing EMPowerPlus™ have remained stable for more than one year, and one child has reportedly remained stable on EMPowerPlus™ alone for more than four years (Kaplan et al., 2002). The other publications present similar success rates in both adults (Popper, 2001) and children (Kaplan et al., 2004). A randomized placebo-controlled double-blind study in adults with bipolar disorder is on-going at this time in Canada. Participants are required to be medication-free prior to screening and for the duration of the trial. Findings to date suggest that EMPowerPlus™ is probably beneficial alone and possibly also in combination with small doses of conventional mood stabilizers (see *safety concerns*). More studies are needed to clarify whether a micronutrient formula alone is sufficient to stabilize Bipolar patients, and to determine whether particular micronutrient formulas are more efficacious than others.

Safety concerns The micronutrients reportedly potentiate the effects of mood stabilizers and necessitate gradual dose reductions as EMPowerPlus™ is started (Popper 2001). The current version consists of 15 capsules per day, usually divided into three doses. Researchers caution clinicians who are considering recommending EMPowerPlus™ to proceed gradually while carefully monitoring for adverse effects when transitioning Bipolar patients to the micronutrient formula in order to minimize the risk of toxicity. Lowering the doses of conventional mood stabilizing medications too rapidly after starting a patient on EMPowerPlus™ (or another nutrient formula) entails the risk of worsening symptoms, while maintaining conventional medications at their usual doses may result in significant toxicity.

◆ **A Branched-chain amino acid drink resulting in acute depletion of tyrosine and phenylalanine may reduce symptoms of acute mania** Oral administration of certain branched-chain amino acids may rapidly improve acute manic symptoms by interfering with the synthesis of the catecholamine neurotransmitters norepinephrine and dopamine (Barrett & Leyton, 2004). A mixture of bioavailable amino acids excluding tyrosine and phenylalanine (the precursor of tyrosine) is believed to reduce brain dopamine in bipolar patients, resulting in diminished manic symptoms and improved overall cognitive functioning (Gijsman et al., 2002). Twenty adult inpatients diagnosed with mania were randomized to receive the tyrosine-free mixture or placebo 4 hours before methamphetamine, which stimulates dopamine release, resulting in a manic-like state (McTavish et al., 2001). Significant improvements in objective and subjective indicators of mania were noted in patients taking the tyrosine-free mixture of amino acids. The researchers speculated that restricting tyrosine in manic patients would result in diminished brain dopamine and attenuation of non-stimulant-induced manic symptoms. In another 7-day double-blind, placebo-controlled study, 25 bipolar patients were randomized to receive a special tyrosine-free amino acid drink (60 g/day) versus placebo (Scarna, Gijsman, McTavish, Harmer, Cowen, & Goodwin, 2003). Severity ratings of manic symptoms were significantly reduced within 6 hours of treatment. Improvements were sustained with repeated administration, and this effect persisted 1 week following the end of the study. These findings suggest that ingestion of an amino acid drink that results in acute depletion of the tyrosine may be a beneficial treatment of acute mania.

◆ **Susceptible individuals should consume adequate amounts of L-tryptophan** Bipolar patients may be genetically susceptible to mood swings when certain amino acids are unavailable in the diet. When L-tryptophan is restricted or excluded from the diet, bipolar patients are more susceptible to depressive mood swings than healthy adults. Bipolar patients who were stable on lithium and subsequently subjected to acute tryptophan depletion had reduced brain serotonin as shown by significant reductions in auditory evoked potentials (Hughes, Dunne, & Young, 2000; Young, Hughes, & Ashton, 2000). However, these patients did not report transient depressed mood (Johnson, El-Khoury, Aberg-Wistedt, Stain-Malmgren, & Mathe, 2001). Acute dietary depletion of L-tryptophan may also result in depressed mood in genetically susceptible relatives of bipolar patients. Findings of double-blind, placebo-controlled studies show that unaffected first-degree relatives of patients diagnosed with bipolar disorder experienced clinically significant depressed mood, impulsive behavior, impaired long-term memory, and slowed information processing when subjected to acute dietary restriction of L-tryptophan (Quintin et al., 2001; Sobczak, Riedel, Booij, Aan Het Rot, Deutz, & Honig, 2002). All of these symptoms were reported within 5 hours following L-tryptophan depletion. Susceptible healthy adults (i.e., first-degree relatives of bipolar patients) had lower platelet serotonin levels and fewer imipramine binding sites, suggesting that increased susceptibility to depressed mood in this population is related to a heritable difference in serotonergic activity.

Acute dietary depletion of L-tryptophan in bipolar patients has been reported to result in depressed mood but does not impair cognitive functioning (Hughes, Gallagher, & Young, 2002). These findings suggest that L-tryptophan supplementation may be an effective treatment of mania. However, research findings on L-tryptophan in mania are inconsistent because of small study sizes, methodological differences, and the fact that L-tryptophan is principally used as an adjunctive treatment of bipolar mania but seldom as a monotherapy. Some studies have found clinically significant reductions in acute mania with L-tryptophan at 6 to 12 g/day (Chouinard, Young, & Annable, 1985), whereas others report no evidence of beneficial effects (Chambers & Naylor, 1978). In one small double-blind trial, bipolar manic patients treated with L-tryptophan at 3 g 3 times a day and conventional lithium therapy improved more than patients taking lithium alone (Brewerton & Reus, 1983).

Omega-3 Fatty Acids, Choline, and Phosphatidylcholine

◆ **EPA, an omega-3 fatty acid, may be an effective adjunctive treatment of bipolar disorder**   Findings from case reports and two small double-blind studies suggest that omega-3 fatty acids improve manic symptoms in bipolar patients who continue to take conventional mood stabilizers. In a 4-month double-blind, placebo-controlled study (Stoll et al., 1999), 30 patients were treated with omega-3 fatty acids (9.6 g/day) versus placebo while continuing their conventional mood-stabilizing medications (including lithium, valproic acid, carbamazepine, among others). Patients who took omega-3 fatty acids alone remained in remission significantly longer than matched patients receiving a placebo. Significantly, patients who took only omega-3 fatty acids remained in remission significantly longer than patients who were treated with placebo only. The researchers postulated that conventional mood-stabilizing medications including lithium, dopamine antagonists, and serotonin-blocking agents are effective in the treatment of mania through a mechanism of action that is similar to that proposed for fatty acids. In a 4-month study (Keck et al., 2002), 121 rapid cycling or depressed bipolar patients were treated with ecosapentanoic acid (EPA; 6 g/day) in combination with a conventional mood stabilizer. Outcomes were not significantly different for patients treated with EPA or placebo. However, depressed bipolar patients randomized to adjunctive EPA (1 or 2 gm/day) reported significant improvements in mood compared to the placebo group and patients taking 1 or 2 gm experienced equivalent improvements (Frangou, Lewis, McCrone, 2000). In addition to general health benefits, cardiovascular benefits (Schmidt & Dyerberg, 1994), and psychiatric treatment benefits of omega-3 fatty acids, some patients taking EPA supplements in combination with lithium carbonate have reported improvements in symptoms

of psoriasis presumably caused by a general deficiency in omega-3s or a side effect of lithium (Akkerhuis & Nolen, 2003).

To date, no large double-blind studies have been done to determine the efficacy of omega-3 fatty acids as a stand-alone treatment of mania. However, a double-blind study still in the recruitment phase at the time of writing is being sponsored by the National Center for Complementary and Alternative Medicine, National Institutes of Health. The study will examine the efficacy of omega-3 fatty acids as a maintenance therapy in 120 bipolar I patients over a 12-month period. Patients will be randomized to receive omega-3s versus placebo in combination with their ongoing mood-stabilizing medication. Results of this study will help to clarify the potential role of omega-3 fatty acids as a maintenance treatment of bipolar I disorder, and may also provide useful insights about safe and appropriate ways to combine mood-stabilizing agents with omega-3s in different patient populations.

Omega-3 fatty acids pose few safety issues. There is one case report of apparent hypomania induced by high doses of omega-3 fatty acids (Kinrys, 2000). Rare cases of increased bleeding times, but not increased risk of bleeding, in patients taking aspirin or anticoagulants have been reported. On the basis of promising case reports and inconclusive research findings to date, omega-3 fatty acids can be regarded as an important provisional treatment of mania and bipolar illness.

◆ **Adding choline to lithium may reduce the severity of manic symptoms**   Many case reports and case series suggest that choline, a B complex vitamin, reduces the severity of mania. Choline is a necessary constituent for the biosynthesis of acetylcholine (Ach). It has been postulated that abnormally low brain levels of Ach are a primary cause of mania (Leiva, 1990). In a small case study of treatment-refractory, rapid-cycling bipolars who were taking lithium, 4 out of 6 patients responded to the addition of 2000 to 7200 mg a day of free choline. The two nonresponders were also taking hypermetabolic doses of thyroid medication. Clinical improvement correlated with increased intensity of the basal ganglia choline signal as measured on proton magnetic resonance imaging (MRI). The effect of choline on depressive symptoms was variable (Stoll, Sachs, Cohen, Lafer, Christensen, & Renshaw, 1996). Case reports, open trials, and one small double-blind study suggest that supplementation with phosphatidylcholine at 15 to 30 g/day reduces the severity of both mania and depressed mood in bipolar patients, and that symptoms recur when phosphatidylcholine is discontinued (Leiva, 1990; Stoll et al., 1996).

◆ **Folic acid supplementation may improve response to lithium**   Findings of a double-blind study suggest that folic acid (200 μg/day) may enhance the beneficial effects of lithium carbonate in acutely manic patients (Coppen et al., 1986; Hasanah et al., 1997).

Minerals (Lithium, Magnesium, and Potassium)

Supplementation with trace amounts of natural lithium may reduce the severity of both depressive and manic symptoms.

Findings of a small open study suggest that patients diagnosed with bipolar disorder who exhibit mania or depressed mood respond to low doses (50 μg with each meal) of a natural lithium preparation (Fierro, 1988). Post-treatment serum lithium levels were undetectable in patients who responded to trace lithium supplementation. Findings of a small pilot study suggest that magnesium supplementation at 40 mEq/day may be as effective as lithium in the treatment of rapidly cycling bipolar patients (Chouinard, Beauclair, Geiser, & Etienne, 1990).

Treatments Based on Forms of Energy or Information That Are Validated by Western Science

At the time of writing, there are no treatment approaches in this category.

Treatments Based on Forms of Energy or Information That Are Not Validated by Western Science

At the time of writing, there are no treatment approaches in this category.

Possibly Effective Nonconventional Treatments of Mania and Cyclic Mood Changes

At the time of writing, possibly effective herbal treatments of mania and cyclic mood changes include St. John's wort (especially when there are seasonal mood swings) and *Rauwolfia serpentina,* which may prove beneficial as an augmenter of conventional lithium therapy. Monthly vitamin B_{12} injections may reduce the risk of recurring manic episodes, and there is preliminary evidence that potassium supplementation reduces lithium-induced tremor, potentially increasing compliance. The regular practice of meditation or yoga promotes calmness and may be beneficial in general for patients who experience mania and cyclic mood changes. Possibly effective treatments of mania and cyclic mood changes are summarized in **Table 9–4**.

Biological Treatments

◆ **Medicinal herbs**

St. John's wort (Hypericum perforatum) combined with bright light exposure may be an effective treatment of seasonal depressed mood St. John's wort may prove to be an effective adjunctive treatment of the cyclic mood changes observed in a pattern of recurring cyclic mood changes known as seasonal affective disorder (SAD). In an open study, 169 self-referred patients

Table 9–4   Possibly Effective Nonconventional Treatments of Mania and Cyclic Mood Changes.

Category	Treatment Approach	Evidence for Claimed Treatment Effect	Comments
Biological	St. John's wort (*Hypericum perforatum*)	St John's wort may be an effective treatment of SAD. Combining St. John's wort with bright light exposure may be more effective in SAD than either approach alone	*Caution:* Patients should use St. John's wort under medical supervision. St. John's wort interacts with many conventional drugs, including protease inhibitors, oral contraceptives, and warfarin
	Rauwolfia serpentina	*Rauwolfia serpentina* may be beneficial in mania that does not respond to conventional mood stabilizers. *R. serpentina* may augment the mood-stabilizing effects of lithium.	Rauwolfia serpentina may be safely combined with lithium but should be used only under the supervision of a trained Ayurvedic practitioner
	B_{12} supplementation	Monthly B_{12} injections may reduce the risk of recurring manic episodes	Check serum level before giving B_{12} injections (patients who are not deficient will probably not benefit)
	Potassium supplementation	Potassium 20 mEq bid may reduce lithium-induced tremor and improve compliance	*Caution:* Patients who have cardiac arrhythmias or take antiarrhythmic drugs should consult with their physicians before taking potassium
Somatic and mind–body approaches	Meditation and mindfulness training	Certain meditation practices promote calmness and may be beneficial in mania or hypomania	*Caution:* Rare cases of hypomania have been reported following meditation. Bipolar patients should avoid activating meditation practices
	Yoga	Certain Yogic breathing practices and postures probably promote calmness in general and may be beneficial in mania or hypomania	*Caution:* Bipolar patients should avoid yoga practices that are stimulating
Energy-information approaches validated by Western science	None at time of writing		
Energy-information approaches not (yet) validated by Western science	None at time of writing		

SAD, seasonal affective disorder

complaining of seasonal mood changes were treated with St. John's wort versus St. John's wort combined with bright light exposure (Wheatley, 1999). Patients in both treatment groups experienced significant improvements in symptoms of anxiety and insomnia. Patients in the combined treatment group reported greater improvement in insomnia compared with patients taking only St. John's wort. St. John's wort alone or in combination with bright light exposure may be an effective treatment of patients complaining of seasonal mood changes.

Rauwolfia serpentina may be beneficial in cases of mania that are not responsive to conventional drugs Rauwolfia serpentina is used in Ayurvedic medicine to treat symptoms of mania and cyclic mood changes that resemble the Western diagnosis of bipolar disorder. Findings from early studies suggest that this herbal medicine may be especially effective in cases where manic episodes do not respond to lithium or other conventional mood stabilizers (Bacher & Lewis, 1979). *R. serpentina* may be safely combined with lithium, and reportedly augments the mood-stabilizing effects of lithium, permitting a reduction in the therapeutic dose of lithium in some cases. This is a potentially significant integrative strategy because reducing the effective lithium dose may diminish adverse effects and improve compliance (Berlant, 1986).

◆ **Vitamins and minerals**

B_{12} supplementation may lower risk of recurring manic episodes Case reports suggest that mania is sometimes related to vitamin B_{12} deficiency, and that monthly B_{12} injections reduce the risk of recurring manic episodes (Goggans, 1984).

Potassium supplementation may reduce lithium side effects Findings from animal research and a small open study suggest that bipolar patients who take potassium 20 mEq twice daily with their conventional lithium therapy experience fewer side effects, including tremor, compared with patients who take lithium alone (Tripuraneni, 1990). No changes in serum lithium levels were reported in patients taking potassium. Pending confirmation of these findings by a larger double-blind trial, potassium supplementation may provide a safe, cost-effective integrative approach for the management of bipolar patients who are unable to tolerate therapeutic doses of lithium due to tremor and other adverse effects. Patients who have cardiac arrhythmias or are taking antiarrhythmic medications should consult with their physicians before considering taking a potassium supplementation.

Somatic and Mind–Body Approaches

◆ **Meditation and mindfulness training** Meditation and other mindfulness training techniques are widely used to self-treat symptoms of mania. Anecdotal reports suggest beneficial moderating effects in bipolar disorder; however, formal studies have not been done. Rare case reports suggest that mania can be precipitated by intensive meditation practice, and bipolar patients who pursue meditation or mindfulness training should be encouraged to use moderation, avoid activating techniques, and practice under the supervision of a skilled instructor (Yorston, 2001).

◆ **Regular yoga practice** Bipolar patients sometimes practice yoga in efforts to improve symptoms of both mania and depressed mood. There is a growing research literature on yoga in depression; however, studies examining possible protective effects of yoga in mania have not been done. As is true of meditation, certain yoga practices are probably associated with general calming effects, whereas others tend to be stimulating. It is suggested that patients who are experiencing manic symptoms should use only relaxing yoga postures, and avoid vigorous Yogic breathing practices that can cause agitation and potentially induce hypomania or mania by lowering the serum lithium level (Gerbarg & Brown, 2006)

Treatments Based on Forms of Energy or Information Approaches That Are Validated by Western Science

At the time of writing, there are no treatment approaches in this category.

Treatments Based on Forms of Energy or Information Approaches That Are Not Validated by Western Science

At the time of writing, there are no treatment approaches in this category.

◆ The Integrative Management Algorithm for Mania and Cyclic Mood Symptoms

Figure 9–1 Is the integrative management step-by-step approach to evaluation and treatment of mania and cyclic mood symptoms. Note that specific assessment and treatment approaches are representative examples of reasonable choices. Moderate symptoms often respond to exercise, dietary modification, mind–body practices, and energy-information therapies. When managing severe symptoms, emphasize biological therapies. Encourage exercise and other lifestyle changes in motivated patients. Consider conventional, nonconventional, and integrative approaches that have not been tried.

See evidence tables and text for complete reviews of evidence-based options.

Before implementing any treatment plan, always check evidence tables and Web site updates at www.thieme.com/mentalhealth for specific assessment and treatment protocols, and obtain patient informed consent.

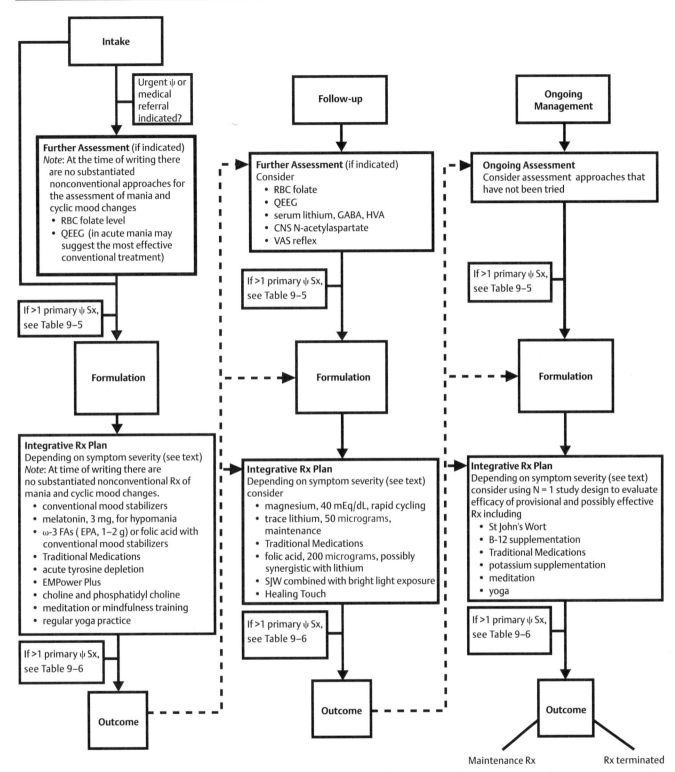

Figure 9–1 Integrative management step-by-step approach to evaluation and treatment of mania and cyclic mood changes. Note that specific assessment and treatment approaches are representative examples of reasonable choices. Moderate symptoms often respond to exercise, dietary modification, mind–body practices, and energy-information therapies. Rx, treatment; Sx, symptoms

◆ Integrated Approaches to Consider When Two or More Core Symptoms Are Present

Table 9–5 shows the assessment approaches to consider using when mania or cyclic mood changes are the focus of clinical attention and one or more other symptoms are being assessed concurrently.

Table 9–6 outlines the treatment approaches to consider using when mania or cyclic mood changes are the focus of clinical attention and one or more other symptoms are being treated concurrently.

Table 9–5 Assessment Approaches to Mania or Cyclic Mood Changes When Other Symptoms Are Being Assessed Concurrently

Other Symptom(s) Being Assessed Concurrently	Assessment Approach	Comments
Depressed mood	Serologic studies	Low trace lithium levels (i.e., from low nutritional intake) are common in acutely manic patients.
		Limited evidence suggests that pretreatment serum GABA levels predict improved response of mania and cyclic mood changes to divalproex (Depakote) but not other mood stabilizers.
		Low serum folate predicts nonresponse to conventional and nonconventional treatments of depressed mood but not mania
	qEEG brain mapping	Abnormal qEEG findings suggest specific treatment strategies and differentiate unipolar from bipolar depressed mood.
		Limited evidence suggests that pretreatment qEEG findings in manic or cycling patients facilitates selection of the most effective conventional drug treatment.
		Limited evidence suggests that specific qEEG findings predict differential response rates to some conventional antidepressants, including SSRIs, and some nonconventional antidepressants
	Chinese medical pulse diagnosis and VAS reflex	Limited evidence suggests that Chinese pulse diagnosis and analysis of VAS provide specific information about energetic imbalances when evaluating mania, cyclic mood changes, and depressed mood. Analysis of VAS may facilitate selection of conventional and nonconventional treatments of mania and depressed mood
Anxiety	Serologic studies	Limited evidence suggests that deficiencies of niacin and vitamins B_6, C, and E are associated with generalized anxiety.
		Limited evidence suggests that total serum cholesterol is elevated in chronically anxious patients.
		Limited evidence suggests that deficiencies of magnesium, selenium, and phosphorus are associated with chronic anxiety
	qEEG brain mapping	Emerging evidence suggests that specific qEEG findings can be used to guide treatment selection in anxious patients, including conventional drugs and EEG-biofeedback training
Psychosis	Serologic studies	Abnormally low RBC folate levels (but normal serum folate levels) are common in bipolar patients.
		Limited evidence suggests that high pretreatment serum HVA levels predict improved response to lower doses of conventional antipsychotics in acutely manic patients with psychotic symptoms.
		Limited evidence suggests that abnormally low serum and RBC folate levels correlate with increased risk of schizophrenia and other psychotic syndromes
	qEEG brain mapping	Limited evidence suggests that specific qEEG findings correlate with differential response rates of acutely manic or psychotic patients to both conventional and nonconventional treatments
	Analysis of VAS reflex	Limited evidence suggests that the VAS reflex provides useful information when identifying conventional treatments and doses that will be effective in previously nonresponsive psychotic patients
Cognitive impairment	Serologic studies	Limited evidence suggests that abnormally low levels of zinc and magnesium correlate with the risk of developing Alzheimer's disease; however, findings are inconsistent

Table 9–5 Assessment Approaches to Mania or Cyclic Mood Changes When Other Symptoms Are Being Assessed Concurrently *(Continued)*

Other Symptom(s) Being Assessed Concurrently	Assessment Approach	Comments
	qEEG brain mapping	qEEG mapping, VEP, and AER studies facilitate early diagnosis and more aggressive treatment of early Alzheimer's and mild cognitive impairment.
		qEEG mapping provides useful information when planning EEG-biofeedback protocols addressing cognitive impairment in general.
		qEEG mapping can be used to evaluate response to conventional and nonconventional cognitive enhancing treatments
Substance abuse or dependence	Serologic studies	In alcohol abuse the magnitude of serum deficiencies of vitiamins A and C and some B vitamins, as well as zinc, magnesium, and essential fatty acids, is an indicator of the severity of malnutrition.
		Elevated serum homocysteine is an indicator of chronic alcohol abuse and returns to normal levels soon after cessation of alcohol abuse
	qEEG brain mapping	Limited evidence suggests that qEEG brain mapping provides useful information when planning specific EEG-biofeedback protocols for relapsing alcoholics or narcotics abusers
	AER	Conventional treatments of heroin detoxification normalize AER findings
	Chinese medical pulse diagnosis and VAS reflex	Limited evidence suggests that VAS analysis provides useful information when planning detoxification protocols based on acupuncture and conventional medications
Disturbance of sleep or wakefulness	Serologic studies	Deficiencies in folic acid and vitamins C, E, and B_{12} are correlated with increased daytime sleepiness and insomnia.
		Abnormally low serum levels of magnesium and zinc are often associated with increased daytime sleepiness
	Chinese pulse diagnosis	Limited evidence suggests that Chinese pulse diagnosis provides clinically useful information about energetic imbalances that manifest as daytime sleepiness or nighttime wakefulness

AER, auditory evoked response; EEG, electroencephalography; GABA, γ-aminobutyric acid; HVA, homovanillic acid; qEEG, quantitative electroencephalography; RBC, red blood cell (count); SSRI, selective serotonin reuptake inhibitor; VAS, vascular autonomic signal; VEP, visual evoked potential

Table 9–6 Treatment Approaches to Mania or Cyclic Mood Changes When Other Symptoms Are Being Treated Concurrently

Other Symptom(s) Being Treated Concurrently	Treatment Approach	Comments
Depressed mood	Folate	Folic acid 200 μg/day may augment the effects of lithium in mania.
		Folate 0.5 to 1 mg/day augments the effects of conventional antidepressants and SAMe
	Omega-3 essential fatty acids	EPA 1 to 2 g/day in combination with conventional mood stabilizers may reduce severity and frequency of manic episodes.
		Combining omega-3 fatty acids (especially EPA) 1 to 2 g/day with conventional antidepressants improves response and may accelerate response rate.
		Limited evidence suggests that EPA alone is an effective treatment of severe depressed mood
	L-tryptophan	Limited evidence suggests that L-tryptophan reduces the frequency of depressive mood swings and reduces the severity of mania in bipolar patients.
		L-tryptophan 3 g tid added to lithium may improve symptoms of mania more than lithium alone.
		L-tryptophan 2 g augments fluoxetine 20 mg and improves sleep quality in depressed individuals.
		L-tryptophan 1 to 2 g combined with bright light therapy is more effective than either approach alone in seasonal depressed mood.
		Limited evidence suggests that L-tryptophan 1 to 2 g is equivalent to imipramine 150 mg and other conventional antidepressants

(Continued)

Table 9–6 Treatment Approaches to Mania or Cyclic Mood Changes When Other Symptoms Are Being Treated Concurrently *(Continued)*

Other Symptom(s) Being Treated Concurrently	Treatment Approach	Comments
	B_{12} supplementation	Monthly B_{12} injections may reduce the risk of recurring manic episodes. (*Note:* Patients who are not B_{12} deficient will probably not benefit.)
		Patients with normal B_{12} serum levels respond better to conventional antidepressants than patients who are B_{12} deficient
	St. John's wort	St. John's wort may be an effective treatment of SAD.
		Combining St. John's wort with bright light exposure may be more effective against SAD than either approach alone.
		Standardized preparations of St. John's wort (300 mg tid) have comparable efficacy to conventional antidepressants for moderate depressed mood.
		Limited evidence suggests that St. John's wort at higher doses (up to 1800 mg/day) is effective against severe depressed mood.
		Caution: St. John's wort is contraindicated in patients taking protease inhibitors, immunosuppressive agents, theophylline, and oral contraceptives. It should be avoided in pregnancy and in patients taking MAOI antidepressants
	Mindfulness training	Limited evidence suggests that certain meditation practices promote calmness and are beneficial in mania or hypomania.
		Mindfulness training is probably as effective as cognitive therapy in moderate depressed mood
Anxiety	L-tryptophan and 5-HTP	L-tryptophan (2–3 g/day) or 5-HTP (25–100 mg up to 3 times a day) is probably an effective treatment of generalized anxiety.
		5-HTP may prevent panic attacks
	Music and binaural sound	Regular listening to soothing music or certain binaural sounds can significantly reduce generalized anxiety
Psychosis	Omega-3 essential fatty acids	Limited evidence suggests that the omega-3 essential fatty acid EPA (1–4 g) alone or in combination with conventional antipsychotics (and especially clozapine) improves psychotic symptoms. Beneficial effects may be more robust in the early acute phase of psychotic illnesses
Cognitive impairment	Dietary changes	Moderate wine consumption, reduced saturated fats, and reduced total caloric intake are correlated with reduced risk of developing Alzheimer's disease.
		Limited evidence suggests that diets high in fish or other sources of omega-3 fatty acids and low in omega-6 fatty acids are associated with a reduced risk of developing dementia
	Folate and vitamin B_{12}	Daily folate, vitamin B_{12}, or thiamine supplementation may be beneficial in some cases of age-related cognitive decline and Alzheimer's disease
Substance abuse or dependence	Dietary changes	Alcoholics who improve their diets, including reduced intake of refined sugar and caffeine and increased intake of omega-3 fatty acids and protein, probably have an increased chance for maintaining sobriety
	Mindfulness training	Abstinent alcoholics and addicts who engage in a regular mindfulness practice or meditation probably have a reduced risk of relapse
		Spiritually focused support groups probably reduce relapse risk
Disturbance of sleep or wakefulness	L-tryptophan and 5-HTP	Combining L-tryptophan 2 g with a conventional antidepressant probably enhances antidepressant response and improves sleep quality.
		5-HTP and L-tryptophan probably reduce symptoms of mild or situational insomnia.
		5-HTP increases sleep duration in obstructive sleep apnea and narcolepsy

PA, ecosapentanoic acid; 5-HTP, 5-hydroxytryptophan; MAOI, monoamine oxidase inhibitor; SAD, seasonal affective disorder; SAMe, *S*-adenosylmethionine

Case Vignette

History and Initial Presentation

Lisa is a divorced 33-year-old lawyer who was diagnosed with major depressive disorder 10 years ago because of recurring severe depressive episodes starting in adolescence. She was first treated for depressed mood at the age of 24 with fluoxetine (Prozac) and has subsequently been tried on many different antidepressants over the years, including selective serotonin reuptake inhibitors (SSRIs), tricyclics, and atypical agents, both singly and in various combinations, all with limited benefit for her mood symptoms. Lisa exercises to keep her mood stable and has no medical problems. At the time of her first manic episode, she had been taking venlafaxine (Effexor) at 300 mg, and bupripion (Wellbutrin) at 150 mg for about 2 years with intermittent compliance because of adverse effects.

Lisa had begun to educate herself about nonconventional treatments for depression around the time she became acutely manic with pressured speech, an almost complete absence of the need for sleep, racing thoughts, and grandiose delusions, all of which lasted more than 1 week. She agreed to voluntary psychiatric hospitalization and was started on a conventional mood stabilizer (divalproex) together with an atypical antipsychotic at bedtime, and a strong sedative–hypnotic at night to help with sleep and as needed during the day for agitation. The Effexor and Wellbutrin were initially held, then restarted at lower doses on the second day of hospitalization. On the new regimen Lisa experienced some nausea and feelings of sedation that lasted through the late morning, but she tolerated conventional medications without severe adverse effects and improved rapidly. After 3 days of hospitalization, she was discharged with a 2-week supply of medications, referred to a local bipolar support group, and scheduled for 2-week follow-up with a psychiatrist in the community.

The antipsychotic was discontinued on the initial follow-up appointment, and Lisa was advised to take it for any recurring psychotic symptoms. Lisa continued on the other prescribed medications, attended the support group, and worked on stress management. Over the ensuing 2 months, both antidepressants were gradually increased to the doses she had been on before her manic episode. Loss of libido was the only significant adverse effect. During the subsequent 6 months there were no further manic episodes, but Lisa complained of feeling down too much of the time. Monthly blood work confirmed that her serum divalproex level was in a therapeutic range and liver enzymes were not elevated. Lisa continued to see her psychiatrist for routine 20-minute appointments every 6 weeks. Follow-up appointments focused on medication management and stress reduction skills.

Assessment, Formulation, and Integrative Treatment Plan

After 3 months on divalproex 1500 mg at bedtime, Lisa became concerned about weight gain, hair loss, and a noticeable tremor in both hands. At her routine physical exam, Lisa learned that her blood pressure was elevated, was started on an antihypertensive, and was encouraged to begin a weight loss and exercise program. A friend recommended Dr. Evans, an integrative psychiatrist. Dr. Evans confirmed a probable diagnosis of bipolar I disorder and reviewed likely causes of adverse effects (divalproex: weight gain, hair loss, and tremor; and venlafaxine: elevated blood pressure and loss of libido). In view of Lisa's history of poor response to conventional antidepressants, Dr. Evans ordered a red blood cell (count) (RBC) folate level and reviewed alternative conventional and nonconventional treatment options that had not previously been tried. Lisa was instructed to taper and discontinue venlafaxine over 2 weeks while staying on her current dose of Wellbutrin. She was started on an omega-3 fatty acid supplement containing 2 g/day of EPA as an adjunctive treatment and instructed to continue taking divalproex. Lisa was encouraged to take a high-potency vitamin B complex formula that included folic acid and B$_{12}$, and to continue a regular exercise program. Dr. Evans told Lisa about EMPower-Plus, which he had successfully used to treat other patients with similar histories of mania and cyclic mood changes. He informed Lisa that findings supporting use of EMPowerPlus for bipolar disorder were still preliminary and summarized unresolved safety issues. Dr. Evans provided Lisa with a case report that included a review of the risk of toxic interactions between micronutrients in the formula and conventional mood stabilizers. He informed Lisa that she would be asked to sign an informed consent indicating that she understood that EMPowerPlus was an experimental treatment if she elected to begin a trial on EMPowerPlus after reviewing the written materials.

Three-Week Follow-Up

At the 3-week follow-up session, Lisa appeared brighter than at her initial appointment. Going off the venlafaxine had been difficult, but her libido and energy level had improved noticeably. Her blood pressure had normalized within a few days of discontinuing venlafaxine, and her family physician had discontinued the antihypertensive medication. Lisa's RBC folic acid level had returned to the normal range, and she had started the omega-3 fatty acid supplements and vitamin B complex as instructed. She had continued to exercise, and her weight had remained stable. After carefully reviewing the information on EMPowerPlus, Lisa had decided to try this nutrient formula, and signed a consent form after going over possible adverse effects in detail with Dr. Evans. She agreed to gradually taper her dose of divalproex to 750 mg/day over 1 month while gradually increasing her EMPowerPlus supplement over the same period. Biweekly sessions were scheduled, and Lisa was instructed to call in the event of adverse effects or recurring manic or depressive symptoms.

Follow-Up and Subsequent Course of Treatment

Two weeks after starting EMPowerPlus, Lisa had reduced her nighttime valproex dose to 1000 mg. The tremor had noticeably diminished, but there had been no change in weight. Her mood remained stable, and there were no adverse effects. Two weeks later, Lisa further reduced her dose on divalproex to 750 mg, while gradually increasing the EMPowerPlus as instructed. She continued to tolerate this regimen and lost 2 pounds without dieting. Lisa's mood remained stable, and there were no warning signs of recurring mania or depression. She continued to exercise regularly and remained on a combined regimen of divalproex 750 mg at bedtime, Wellbutrin 150 mg, a high-potency B complex, a recommended brand and dose of omega-3s, and EMPowerPlus, and followed a daily stress reduction program that included deep breathing, guided imagery, and calming music. Six months after her initial appointment with Dr. Evans, Lisa had returned to her previous weight, her mood remained stable, and she continued to tolerate her integrative regimen without adverse effects.

References

Ackerman, J. (1989). VAS analysis in determining auriculotherapy protocol in 30 year unresponsive bipolar male. In *Proceedings from Energy Fields in Medicine Conference: A study of device technology based on acupuncture meridians and chi energy* (pp. 124–189).

Akkerhuis, G. W., & Nolen, W. A. (2003). Lithium-associated psoriasis and omega-3 fatty acids. *American Journal of Psychiatry, 160*(7), 1355.

American Psychiatric Association. (1994). Practice guidelines for treatment of patients with bipolar disorder. *American Journal of Psychiatry, 151*(Suppl. 12), 1–36.

Bacher, N. M., & Lewis, H. A. (1979). Lithium plus reserpine in refractory manic patients. *American Journal of Psychiatry, 136*(6), 811–814.

Barrett, S., & Leyton, M. (2004). Acute phenylalanine/tyrosine depletion: A new method to study the role of catecholamines in psychiatric disorders. *Primary Psychiatry, 11*(6), 37–41.

Benazzi, F. (1997). Prevalence of bipolar II disorder in outpatient depression: A 203-case study in private practice. *Journal of Affective Disorders, 43*(2), 163–166.

Berlant, J. L. (1986). Neuroleptics and reserpine in refractory psychoses. *Journal of Clinical Psychopharmacology, 6*(3), 180–184.

Boschert, S. (2004, June). Evidence-based treatment largely ignored in bipolar disorder. *Clinical Psychiatry News*, p. 1.

Brewerton, T., & Reus, V.(1983). Lithium carbonate and L-tryptophan in the treatment of bipolar and schizoaffective disorders. *American Journal of Psychiatry, 140*, 757–760.

Chambers, C., & Naylor, G. (1978). A controlled trial of L-tryptophan in mania. *British Journal of Psychiatry, 132*, 555–559.

Chang, K., Adleman, N., Dienes, K., Barnea-Goraly, N., Reiss, A., & Ketter, T. (2003). Decreased *N*-acetylaspartate in children with familial bipolar disorder. *Biological Psychiatry, 53*(11), 1059–1065.

Chou, J. C., Czobor, P., Tuma, I., Charles, O., Bebe, R., Cooper, T. B., Chang, W. H., Lane, H. Y., & Stone, D. L. (2000). Pretreatment plasma HVA and haloperidol response in acute mania. *Journal of Affective Disorders, 59*(1), 55–59.

Chouinard, G., Beauclair, L., Geiser, R., & Etienne, P. (1990). A pilot study of magnesium aspartate hydrochloride (Magnesiocard) as a mood stabilizer for rapid cycling bipolar affective disorder patients. *Progress in Neuropsychopharmacology and Biological Psychiatry, 14*(2), 171–180.

Chouinard, G., Young, S., & Annable, L. (1985). A controlled clinical trial of L-tryptophan in acute mania. *Biological Psychiatry, 20*(5), 546–557.

Coppen, A., Chaudhry, S., & Swade, C. (1986). Folic acid enhances lithium prophylaxis. *Journal of Affective Disorders, 10*(1), 9–13.

Dawson, E. (1991). The relationship of tap water and physiological levels of lithium to mental hospital admission and homicide in Texas. In Schrauzer, G. N. & Klippel, K. F. (Eds.), *Lithium in biology and medicine* (pp. 169–188). Cambridge: VCH.

Dennehy, E. B., Gonzalez, R., & Suppes, T. (2004). Self-reported participation in nonpharmacologic treatments for bipolar disorder. *Journal of Clinical Psychiatry, 65*(2), 278.

Fierro, A. (1988, January). Natural low dose lithium supplementation in manic-depressive disease. *Nutrition Perspectives*, pp. 10–11.

Frangou, S., Lewis, M., McCrone, P. (2006) Efficacy of ethyl-eicosapentaenoic acid in bipolar depression: randomised double-blind placebo-controlled study. *British Journal of Psychiatry, 188*, 46–50.

Gerbarg, P., & Brown, D. (2006). Yoga in psychiatry. In: Lake & Spiegel (Eds.), *A clinical manual of complementary and alternative treatments in mental health*. Washington, DC: American Psychiatric Press.

Ghaemi, S. N., Lenox, M. S., & Baldessarini, R. J. (2001). Effectiveness and safety of long-term antidepressant treatment in bipolar disorder. *Journal of Clinical Psychiatry, 62*(7), 565–569.

Gijsman, H. J., Scarna, A., Harmer, C. J., McTavish, S. B., Odontiadis, J., Cowen, P. J., & Goodwin, G. M. (2002). A dose-finding study on the effects of branch chain amino acids on surrogate markers of brain dopamine function. *Psychopharmacology (Berlin), 160*(2), 192–197.

Goggans, F. C. (1984). A case of mania secondary to vitamin B$_{12}$ deficiency. *American Journal of Psychiatry, 141*(2), 300–301.

Goodwin, F., & Jamison, K. (1990). *Manic-depressive illness*. New York: Oxford University Press.

Grisaru, N., Chudakov, B., Yaroslavsky, Y., & Belmaker, R. H. (1998). Transcranial magnetic stimulation in mania: A controlled study. *American Journal of Psychiatry, 155*(11), 1608–1610.

Gurling, H., Smyth, C., Kalsi, G., et al. (1995). Linkage findings in bipolar disorder. *Nature Genetics, 10*, 8–9.

Hasanah, C. I., Khan, U. A., Musalmah, M., & Razali, S. M. (1997). Reduced red-cell folate in mania. *Journal of Affective Disorders, 46*, 95–99.

Hughes, J. H., Dunne, F., & Young, A. H. (2000). Effects of acute tryptophan depletion on mood and suicidal ideation in bipolar patients symptomatically stable on lithium. *British Journal of Psychiatry, 177*, 447–451.

Hughes, J. H., Gallagher, P., & Young, A. (2002). Effects of acute tryptophan depletion on cognitive function in euthymic bipolar patients. *European Neuropsychopharmacology, 12*(2),1 23–128.

Hughes, J., & Roy, E. (1999). Conventional and quantitative electroencephalography in psychiatry. *Journal of Neuropsychiatry and Clinical Neurosciences, 11*, 190–208.

Johnson, L., El-Khoury, A., Aberg-Wistedt, A., Stain-Malmgren, R., & Mathe, A. A. (2001). Tryptophan depletion in lithium-stabilized patients with affective disorder. *International Journal of Neuropsychopharmacology, 4*(4), 329–336.

Judd, L. L., Akiskal, H. S., Schettler, P. J., et al. (2002). The long-term natural history of the weekly symptomatic status of bipolar I disorder. *Archives of General Psychiatry, 59*(6), 530–537.

Kaplan, B. J., Crawford, S. G., Gardner, B., & Farrelly, G. (2002). Treatment of mood lability and explosive rage with minerals and vitamins: Two case studies in children. *Journal of Child and Adolescent Psychopharmacology, 12*(3), 203–218.

Kaplan, B. J., Fisher, J. E., Crawford, S. G., Field, C. J., & Kolb, B. (2004). Improved mood and behavior during treatment with a mineral-vitamin supplement: An open-label case series. *Journal of Child and Adolescent Psychopharmacology, 14*(1), 115–122.

Kaplan, B. J., Simpson, J. S., Ferre, R. C., et al. (2001). Effective mood stabilization with a chelated mineral supplement: An open-label trial in bipolar disorder. *Journal of Clinical Psychiatry, 62*, 936–944.

Kaptsan, A., Yaroslavsky, Y., Applebaum, J., Belmaker, R. H., Grisaru, N. (2003). Right prefrontal TMS versus sham treatment of mania: A controlled study. *Bipolar Disorders, 5*(1), 36–39.

Keck, P. E., Jr., Freeman, M. P., McElroy, S. L., Altshuler, L. L., Denicoff, K. D., Nolen, W. A., Suppes, T., Frye, M., Kupka, R., Leverich, G. S., Grunze, H., Walden, J., & Post, R. M. (2002). A double-blind, placebo-controlled trial of eicosapentanoic acid in rapid cycling bipolar disorder [Abstract]. *Bipolar Disorders, 4*(Suppl. 1), 26–27.

Kinrys, G. (2000). Hypomania associated with omega-3 fatty acids. *Archives of General Psychiatry, 57*(7), 715–716.

Konradi, C., Eaton, M., MacDonald, M. L., Walsh, J., Benes, F. M., & Heckers, S. (2004). Molecular evidence for mitochondrial dysfunction in bipolar disorder. *Archives of General Psychiatry, 61*, 300–308.

Lee, S., Chow, C. C., Shek, C. C., Wing, Y. K., & Chen, C. N. (1992). Folate concentration in Chinese psychiatric outpatients on long-term lithium treatment. *Journal of Affective Disorders; 24*(4), 265–270.

Leiva, D. B. (1990). The neurochemistry of mania: A hypothesis of etiology and rationale for treatment. *Progress in Neuropsychopharmacology and Biological Psychiatry, 14*(3), 423–429.

McKeon, P., Shelley, R., O'Regan, S., & O'Brian, J. (1991). Serum and red cell folate and affective morbidity in lithium prophylaxis. *Acta Psychiatrica Scandinavica, 83*(3), 199–201.

McTavish, S. F., McPherson, M. H., Harmer, C. J., Clark, L., Sharp, T., Goodwin, G., & Cowen, P. (2001). Antidopaminergic effects of dietary tyrosine depletion in healthy subjects and patients with manic illness. *British Journal of Psychiatry, 179*, 356–360.

Nahas, Z., Kozel, F. A., Li, X., Anderson, B., & George, M. S. (2003). Left prefrontal transcranial magnetic stimulation (TMS) treatment of depression in bipolar affective disorder: A pilot study of acute safety and efficacy. *Bipolar Disorders, 5*(1), 40–47.

Petty, F., Rush, A. J., Davis, J. M., Calabrese, J., Kimmel, S., Kramer, G., Small, J., Miller, M., Swann, A., Orsulak, P., Blake, M., & Bowden, C. (1996). Plasma GABA predicts acute response to divalproex in mania. *Biological Psychiatry, 39*(4), 278–284.

Popper, C. W. (2001). Do vitamins or minerals (apart from lithium) have mood-stabilizing effects? *Journal of Clinical Psychiatry, 62*, 933–935.

Post, R. (1993). Issues in the long-term management of bipolar affective illness. *Psychiatric Annals, 23*, 86–93.

Prien, R. F., Gelenberg, A. J. (1989). Alternatives to lithium for preventative treatment of bipolar disorder. *American Journal of Psychiatry, 146,* 840–848.

Quintin, P., Benkelfat, C., Launay, J. M., Arnulf, I., Pointereau-Bellenger, A., Barbault, S., Alvarez, J. C., Varoquaux, O., Perez-Diaz, F., Jouvent, R., & Leboyer, M. (2001). Clinical and neurochemical effect of acute tryptophan depletion in unaffected relatives of patients with bipolar affective disorder. *Biological Psychiatry, 50*(3), 184–190.

Robins, L., & Regier, D. (Eds.). (1991). *Psychiatric disorders in America: The epidemiologic catchment area study.* New York: Free Press.

Scarna, A., Gijsman, H. J., McTavish, S. F., Harmer, C. J., Cowen, P. J., & Goodwin, G. M. (2003). Effects of a branched-chain amino acid drink in mania. *British Journal of Psychiatry, 182,* 210–213.

Schmidt, E. B., & Dyerberg, J. (1994). Omega-3 fatty acids: Current status in cardiovascular medicine. *Drugs, 47*(3), 405–424.

Simmons, M. (2003). Nutritional approach to bipolar disorder. *Journal of Clinical Psychiatry, 64*(3), 338.

Small, J. G., Milstein, V., Malloy, F. W., Klapper, M. H., Golay, S. J., & Medlock, C. E. (1998). Topographic EEG studies of mania. *Clinical EEG, 29*(2), 59–66.

Small, J. G., Milstein, V., Malloy, F. W., Medlock, C. E., & Klapper, M. H. (1999). Clinical and quantitative EEG studies of mania. *Journal of Affective Disorders, 53*(3), 217–224.

Sobczak, S., Riedel, W. J., Booij, I., Aan Het Rot, M., Deutz, N. E., & Honig, A. (2002). Cognition following acute tryptophan depletion: Difference between first-degree relatives of bipolar disorder patients and matched healthy control volunteers. *Psychological Medicine, 32*(3), 503–515.

Stoll, A. L., Sachs, G. S., Cohen, B. M., Lafer, B., Christensen, J. D., & Renshaw, P. F. (1996). Choline in the treatment of rapid-cycling bipolar disorder: Clinical and neurochemical findings in lithium-treated patients. *Biological Psychiatry, 40,* 382–388.

Stoll, A. L., Severus, W .E., Freeman, M .P., et al. (1999). Omega-3 fatty acids in bipolar disorder. *Archives of General Psychiatry, 56,* 407–412.

Strober, M., Morrell, W., Lampert, C., & Burroughs, J. (1990). Relapse following discontinuation of lithium maintenance therapy in adolescents with bipolar I illness: A naturalistic study. *American Journal of Psychiatry, 147,* 457–461.

Tohen, M., Waternaux, C. M., & Tsuang, M. T. (1990). Outcome in mania: A 4-year prospective follow-up on 75 patients utilizing survival analysis. *Archives of General Psychiatry, 47,* 1106–1111.

Tripuraneni, B. (1990, May). (Abstracts NR 100, 210). Paper presented at the annual meeting of the American Psychiatric Association.

Wheatley, D. (1999). Hypericum in seasonal affective disorder (SAD). *Current Medical Research and Opinion, 15*(1), 33–37.

Winokur, G., Clayton, P., & Reich, T. (1969). *Manic depressive illness.* St. Louis, MO: C. V. Mosby.

Yorston, G. A. (2001). Mania precipitated by meditation: A case report and literature review. *Mental Health, Religion and Culture, 4*(2), 209–213.

Young, A. H., Huges, J. H., & Ashton, C. H. (2000). Brain 5-HT function in bipolar affective disorder. *Acta Neuropsychiatrica, 12*(3), 91–95.

10

Integrative Management of Anxiety

◆ Background

Anxiety Syndromes Are an Important Unmet Challenge in Mental Health Care

Western psychiatry currently describes five major groups of disorders in which anxiety symptoms play a central role: generalized anxiety disorder (GAD), panic disorder, social phobia and specific phobias, obsessive-compulsive disorder (OCD), and post-traumatic stress disorder (PTSD). Specific criteria in the fourth edition of the *Diagnostic and Statistical Manual of Mental Disorders* (*DSM-IV*) are used to define generalized anxiety due to medical conditions, as well as generalized anxiety due to drug abuse. In the United States, an estimated 23 million individuals suffer from severe anxiety symptoms, including panic attacks, social anxiety, agoraphobia, fear of heights, and other specific phobias, obsessions, and compulsions (Kessler et al., 2005; Robins et al., 1984). The 6-month prevalence rate of *DSM-IV* anxiety disorders has been estimated at 8.9%, making them the third most common mental disorders, behind depression and substance abuse (Burke & Regier, 1988). Estimates of prevalence rates of *DSM-IV* anxiety disorders vary significantly,

depending on the instruments used to obtain clinical data. For example, phobias, PTSD, and panic disorder are diagnosed much less frequently by clinical psychiatrists than predicted based on prevalence rates from large epidemiologic studies using detailed structured clinical interviews (Moran, 2004). Almost one third of total U.S. mental health care costs (approximately US$50 billion) goes to the treatment of anxiety disorders (DeBartolo, Hofmann, & Barlow, 1995). This situation is complicated by risks of serious adverse effects or addiction associated with many conventional drugs used to treat anxiety.

The five major anxiety disorders in Western psychiatric nosology do not adequately reflect the complexity and individuality of anxiety symptom patterns reported by patients. Chronically anxious patients typically experience a range of symptoms, including depressed or labile mood, transient or chronic cognitive impairment, subjective feelings of distress, dissociative symptoms, and behavioral disturbances. There is considerable overlap between the phenomenology of anxiety disorders and other *DSM-IV* disorders. In clinical practice the artificial boundaries between formally described disorders in *DSM-IV* are seldom recognized, and Western-trained mental health professionals generally focus on the most impairing psychological and behavioral symptoms described by the anxious patient at any given time in the course of his or her illness. The resulting approach to patient care is highly individualized and resembles methods employed by the integrative practitioner.

Generalized Anxiety

DSM-IV criteria for generalized anxiety disorder have changed substantially since the disorder was initially formulated in 1980. With the introduction of the revised version of the third edition of the *DSM* (*DSM-III-R*) in the late 1980s, GAD was elevated from the status of a diagnosis of exclusion associated with many vague or transient anxiety symptoms, to a discrete diagnostic entity associated with a more specific symptom pattern of longer duration. At present, criteria required to diagnose GAD include excessive or unrealistic worry that persists at least 6 months and the presence of six or more physical or psychological symptoms associated with general feelings of anxiety. The *DSM-IV* criteria include three major symptom categories: motor tension, autonomic hyperactivity, and vigilance or "scanning." As is true for the other *DSM* anxiety disorders, core symptoms of GAD cannot be explained by a medical disorder, substance abuse, or another major psychiatric disorder, and must be associated with significant social or occupational impairment. Depending on which criteria are used to diagnose GAD, between 2.5 and 6.0% of the general population fulfill criteria for this disorder (Weissman & Merikangas, 1986). Social, psychodynamic, and neurobiological models have been put forward in efforts to explain generalized anxiety. The current dominant model in conventional psychiatry ascribes persisting feelings of generalized anxiety to a cybernetic-like process in which chronic stress results in neurobiological and endocrinological changes that in turn manifest as chronic anxiety (Barlow, 1988).

In biomedical psychiatry, there is ongoing controversy over the legitimacy of GAD as a discrete diagnostic entity because of the heterogeneity of symptom patterns that qualify as this disorder (Barlow, 1988). Furthermore, symptoms of generalized anxiety vary widely in relation to differences in cultural and socioeconomic background, and the generally anxious patient typically experiences a changing pattern of core symptoms over time, including depressed mood, obsessions, sleep disturbances, panic attacks, and other symptoms that are not regarded as core symptoms of GAD. For these reasons it has been argued that GAD provides a "wastebasket" category for chronically anxious patients who do not fulfill more specific criteria for other *DSM-IV* disorders.

Panic Attacks

Panic attacks may be triggered by an unexpected or frightening situation or object, but in many cases there is no identifiable trigger or cue. Panic attacks encompass many physical and psychological symptoms, including dizziness, perspiration, hyperventilation or shortness of breath, elevated heart rate or palpitations, feelings of intense dread, fear of dying, and sometimes depersonalization, derealization, or other dissociative symptoms. There is considerable variation in the duration and severity of symptoms that take place during panic attacks, and the same individual may experience different symptoms during successive panic attacks. The *DSM-IV*

defines **panic disorder** as a recurring pattern of at least four untriggered panic attacks involving at least four characteristic symptoms within a 4-week period. Using these criteria, the prevalence of panic disorder in the general U.S. population has been estimated at 3.5%, and symptoms usually begin in the second or third decade of life (Eaton, Kessler, Wittchen, & Magee, 1994). A much larger percentage of the population experiences panic attacks alone or together with other cognitive or affective symptoms without fulfilling strict *DSM-IV* criteria for panic disorder. These individuals nevertheless suffer from significant social and occupational impairment.

Biological, social, and psychodynamic theories have been advanced in attempts to explain different anxiety syndromes. Panic attacks and generalized anxiety are probably associated with separate underlying mechanisms of action. Hereditary factors probably play a role in the development of panic disorder, and individuals prone to developing this syndrome typically exhibit panic symptoms when challenged with 35% CO_2, consistent with the theory that recurring panic symptoms are related to abnormal functioning in brainstem areas that regulate respiration (Bussi, Perna, Allevi, Caldirola, & Bellodi, 1997). In contrast, generally anxious individuals are not sensitive to CO_2, but become symptomatic when dietary or metabolic factors result in decreases in central nervous system (CNS) serotonin (Klaassen, Klumperbeek, Deutz, van Praag, & Griez, 1998). The majority of individuals who suffer from panic attacks eventually develop phobic avoidance of large open spaces (**agoraphobia**) or avoidance of specific situations or objects they associate with previous panic attacks. As many as one half of individuals who experience frequent panic attacks become depressed, and 10% eventually attempt suicide (Weissman et al., 1990). Thus, a pattern of recurring panic attacks often evolves into a complex symptom pattern involving general social avoidance and isolation, avoidance of feared situations or objects, and depressed mood.

Phobias

Western psychiatry defines three distinct phobic syndromes: social phobia, specific phobias, and agoraphobia. The symptom patterns of phobic disorders are overlapping, and in the absence of a careful history it is often difficult to differentiate one phobia from another or from panic attacks. Important distinctions are made on the basis of the situation or object that precipitates feelings of intense anxiety.

The social phobic typically experiences intense anxiety in most social situations. Social phobia is believed to be one of the most common psychiatric disorders, with an estimated lifetime prevalence of over 13% (Kessler et al., 1994). Social anxiety is frequently associated with chronic psychosis, depressed mood, substance abuse, and other cognitive or affective symptoms. Social phobia causes considerable impairment in social, occupational, and academic performance.

In contrast to social phobia, the *DSM-IV* diagnosis of specific phobia stipulates that "excessive or unreasonable" anxiety takes place in response to a specific object or situation. The *DSM-IV* defines five subtypes of specific phobias: animal type, natural environmental type, blood–injection–injury type, situational type, and a catchall subtype for all other specific phobias. Fear of flying is considered to be a specific kind of situational phobia, and fear of spiders (**arachnophobia**) is considered to be a specific kind of animal phobia. It is estimated that 11% of the population will fulfill criteria for a phobic disorder at some point in the lifespan (Kessler et al., 1994). Specific phobias seldom occur in isolation. Phobic individuals often have two, three, or four specific phobias, and specific phobias often co-occur with panic attacks and agoraphobia.

In agoraphobia, the individual experiences intense anxiety in anticipation of having a panic attack, typically in places where it is difficult or impossible to obtain help. The lifetime prevalence of agoraphobia with or without a history of panic attacks is estimated at between 3.5 and 5.0% (Kessler et al., 1994).

In social phobia, specific phobias, and agoraphobia, intense anxiety associated with avoidant behavior causes significant social or occupational impairment, and cannot be explained by a medical condition, another major psychiatric disorder (including other anxiety disorders), or the effects of medications, alcohol, or illicit drugs. Agoraphobia is almost always associated with a history of panic attacks, but patients with specific phobias and social phobia often experience panic attacks also. Phobic patients often have complicated psychiatric histories, including comorbid depressed mood and alcohol or substance abuse. Using DSM-IV criteria, social phobia is often difficult to distinguish from avoidant personality disorder or schizoid personality disorder because of many overlapping symptoms.

Obsessions and Compulsions

Obsessive-compulsive disorder is characterized by intrusive irrational thoughts and repeated ritualized behaviors that are typically associated with significant social, academic, and occupational impairment. It is estimated that 3% of the general population fulfills DSM-IV criteria for OCD (Angst, 1994). Irrational preoccupations with fears of contamination or infection are common obsessions. Repetitive counting, washing, and locking doors are common compulsions. Hoarding is regarded as a special kind of compulsive behavior.

The dominant symptom pattern can be obsessions, compulsions, or both kinds of symptoms. By definition, **obsessions** are mental symptoms. **Compulsions** can be complex mental rituals like counting pages or mentally repeating specific sequences of numbers, or they can manifest as repetitive or ritualized external behaviors. The symptom pattern of obsessions and compulsions typically evolves over time, with quiescent periods separating periods of greater or lesser symptom severity.

A diagnosis of OCD can only be made when possible medical causes have been ruled out. An OCD-like symptom pattern sometimes takes place following streptococcal infection in early childhood, and rare cases of OCD have been reported following hemorrhagic stroke in the caudate or other limbic areas of the brain. When OCD symptoms have an identifiable neurological cause, they are often associated with a tic disorder. There is some evidence that the risk of developing OCD may be affected by heritable factors. The symptoms of OCD often occur together with trichotillomania, body dysmorphic disorder, depression, and other anxiety disorders. Finally, overlapping features exist between obsessive-compulsive personality disorder (OCPD) and OCD, and many patients who are diagnosed with one disorder are also eventually diagnosed with the other disorder.

In practice it is often difficult for Western-trained psychiatrists to accurately differentiate obsessions from **ruminations**

(intrusive self-critical thoughts in severe depression), delusions, racing thoughts, and somatic preoccupations. Anxious or psychotic patients often experience recurring intrusive thoughts that do not fulfill all DSM-IV criteria for obsessions but are nevertheless associated with significant social or occupational impairment. Compulsive thoughts or ritualized behaviors also take place outside of the complex symptom pattern required for a formal diagnosis of OCD. Examples include compulsive hair pulling and picking at the skin, compulsive eating behavior, and the repetitive ritualized or self-injurious behaviors that are characteristic of autism. Most individuals who experience recurring obsessions or compulsions do not fulfill the formal DSM-IV criteria required to diagnose OCD, and typically exhibit a changing pattern of milder or more severe symptoms over time. Therefore, as is also true for the other DSM-IV anxiety disorders, Western-trained psychiatrists and other mental health professionals treat particular obsessions and compulsions that cause significant distress or impairment at any given time in the course of the patient's illness.

Post-Traumatic Stress Disorder

Post-traumatic stress disorder is the Western psychiatric designation of a complex symptom pattern that often follows exposure to severe physical or psychological trauma. One percent of women in the United States will fulfill criteria for a DSM-IV diagnosis of PTSD at some point during their lives (Helzer, Robins, & McEvoy, 1987). One third of Vietnam combat veterans may have PTSD (Kulka et al., 1990). DSM-IV criteria permit the diagnosis of PTSD when the trauma is experienced directly or witnessed. The trauma may be a single repeated event or a prolonged situation that causes severe stress and is outside the range of ordinary human experience. A period of psychic numbing often follows the immediate trauma. This is often followed by repetitive intrusive memories of the traumatic experience (**flashbacks**) sometimes associated with symptoms of autonomic arousal (sweating, elevated heart rate), nightmares, and hypervigilance. The patient may experience profound feelings of detachment and loss, and actively avoid situations that remind him or her of the traumatic event. There may be amnesia for events or individuals associated with the trauma. Depressed mood, anxiety, anger, intense shame or guilt feelings, distractibility, irritability, and an exaggerated startle response are common even years after the traumatic episode. The patient may experience psychotic symptoms, including full-blown dissociative episodes and auditory or visual hallucinations, is often profoundly impaired by his or her symptoms, and is unable to hold a job or stay in a relationship. It has been estimated that 20 to 80% of individuals diagnosed with PTSD abuse alcohol or drugs in efforts to self-treat their symptoms. A significant percentage of individuals diagnosed with PTSD also fulfill DSM-IV criteria for generalized anxiety disorder, panic disorder, phobic disorders, major depressive disorder, obsessive-compulsive disorder, and antisocial personality disorder (Sierles, Chen, McFarland, & Taylor, 1983). Individuals who were severely traumatized during childhood have a greater likelihood of developing a personality disorder, including narcissistic and antisocial personality, compared with the population at large. In conventional Western psychiatric diagnosis, it is often difficult to distinguish causative factors of PTSD from symptoms that were present prior to the traumatic experience. As is the case for the other major *DSM-IV* categories of anxiety disorders, relatively few individuals who become symptomatic following traumatic exposure fulfill criteria required for a diagnosis of PTSD. The symptom pattern typically includes many different kinds of affective and behavioral symptoms, continues to evolve, and overlaps significantly with other *DSM-IV* disorders. For these reasons, after diagnosing a patient with PTSD, Western-trained mental health professionals generally identify and treat symptoms that cause the greatest degree of social or occupational impairment. Depending on the patient's progress, the focus of clinical attention can shift from severe depressed mood to panic attacks to psychotic symptoms to disturbed sleep to drug abuse or any combination of these.

◆ The Integrative Assessment of Anxiety

Overview of Conventional Approaches Used to Assess Anxiety

Western-trained psychiatrists diagnose anxiety disorders on the basis of history and specialized diagnostic instruments, including the Hamilton Rating Scale for Anxiety (Ham-A). Laboratory studies are performed when there is a concern about possible underlying medical causes. Medical problems that are sometimes associated with anxiety include abnormal heart rhythms, certain tumors, respiratory illnesses, seizure disorders, diseases of the thyroid, and other endocrinological disorders.

Overview of Nonconventional Approaches Used to Assess Anxiety

At the time of writing, nonconventional approaches used to assess anxiety are not substantiated by compelling research evidence.

Quantitative electroencephalography (qEEG) analysis is a significant emerging clinical method that may prove useful for predicting the response of obsessions and compulsions to conventional medications. Increased α (alpha) power on qEEG may correspond to an increased likelihood of responding to selective serotonin reuptake inhibitors (SSRIs) or possibly EEG biofeedback. In contrast, increased θ (theta) activity may predict decreased response rates to conventional antiobsessional medications.

Case reports and the findings of a few studies suggest that serological analysis may yield accurate information about the causes of anxiety. Useful indicators of biological causes of anxiety include total serum cholesterol (elevated in chronically anxious patients), serum vitamin levels (deficiencies in B_6, C, and E may correlate with generalized anxiety), and serum mineral levels (deficiencies in selenium, magnesium, and phosphorus may correlate with an increased risk of generalized anxiety). Assessment approaches that possibly yield useful diagnostic information about the causes of anxiety include constitutional assessment and electrodermal skin testing (EST). Constitutional assessment by a homeopathic physician may provide useful information when selecting the most appropriate homeopathic remedies addressing putative energetic imbalances believed to manifest as anxiety. EST may provide useful information about the efficacy of Healing Touch or Reiki in the treatment of anxiety. **Table 10–1** lists substantiated and provisional nonconventional approaches used to assess anxiety. **Table 10–2** lists approaches that possibly yield useful information in the assessment of anxiety.

Substantiated Approaches Used to Assess Anxiety

At the time of writing, nonconventional approaches used to assess anxiety have not been substantiated by compelling research evidence.

Table 10–1 Provisional Nonconventional Approaches Used to Assess Anxiety

	Provisional Assessment Approach	Evidence for Specific Diagnostic Information	Positive Finding Suggests Efficacy of This Treatment
Biological	None at time of writing		
Somatic	None at time of writing		
Energy-information assessment approaches validated by Western science	qEEG and HRV analysis	Specific qEEG changes may correspond to disparate anxiety symptoms.	Specific qEEG findings may guide treatment selection, including conventional drugs and EEG biofeedback training.
		In OCD increased α power predicts response to SSRIs, increased θ power predicts nonresponse to SSRIs.	SSRIs or other treatments directed at serotonin are probably effective in OCD patients with increased α activity, but less effective where there is increased θ activity.
		Measures of HRV are useful indicators of the intensity of anxiety	HRV is sometimes useful when assessing the effectiveness of conventional and nonconventional treatments
Energy-information assessment approaches not validated by Western science	None at time of writing		

EEG, electroencephalography; HRV, heart rate variability; OCD, obsessive-compulsive disorder; qEEG, quantitative electroencephalography; SSRI, selective serotonin reuptake inhibitor

Table 10–2 Nonconventional Assessment Approaches That May Provide Specific Diagnostic Information about Causes of Anxiety

Category	Assessment Approach	Evidence for Specific Diagnostic Information	Comments
Biological	Total serum cholesterol	Total serum cholesterol may be elevated in chronically anxious patients	Cholesterol levels normalize when conventional treatments are successful (**Note:** Chronically depressed patients may have low cholesterol levels.)
	Serum vitamin levels	Deficiencies of niacin and vitamins B₆, C, and E may be associated with generalized anxiety	Vitamin supplementation may reduce symptoms of generalized anxiety in deficient individuals
	Serum mineral levels	Deficiencies of magnesium, selenium, and phosphorus may be associated with chronic anxiety	Mineral supplements and dietary changes may reduce symptoms of chronic anxiety in deficient individuals
	Urinary glutamate level	High urinary glutamate levels may correlate with general anxiety	Targeted amino acid therapies that reduce high CNS glutamate may reduce symptoms of anxiety
Somatic	None at time of writing		
Energy-information assessment approaches validated by Western science	None at time of writing		
Energy-information assessment approaches not validated by Western science	Constitutional assessment	Certain findings in homeopathic constitutional assessment may correlate with increased anxiety	Constitutional assessment findings may guide selection of effective homeopathic remedies in anxious patients
	Electrodermal skin testing (EDST)	EDST may help confirm the efficacy of both conventional treatments and Healing Touch treatments of anxiety	EDST may provide a way to measure energetic changes following Healing Touch or conventional treatments of anxiety

CNS, central nervous system

Provisional Approaches Used to Assess Anxiety

Biological Approaches

At the time of writing, there are no assessment approaches in this category.

Somatic Approaches

At the time of writing, there are no assessment approaches in this category.

Approaches Based on Forms of Energy or Information That Are Validated by Western Science

◆ **EEG changes may correlate with specific anxiety symptoms, and qEEG findings may predict differential response to conventional treatments** Anxiety symptoms frequently correlate with abnormal EEG or electrocardiogram (EKG) findings. EEG changes typically associated with anxiety include decreased α activity in generalized anxiety, increased θ activity in obsessive-compulsive patients, and paroxysmal activity in patients who experience panic attacks (Hughes & Roy, 1999). EKG findings in anxious patients typically reveal increased sympathetic activity and decreased parasympathetic activity. Quantitative electroencephalography findings may predict differential response rates of OCD patients to conventional medications. In one series, ~80% of OCD patients who exhibited increased α power responded to SSRIs, compared with 80% of OCD patients with increased θ activity who did not respond to SSRIs (Princhep et al.,

1993). Abnormal qEEG findings associated with other anxiety symptoms are highly inconsistent, and the future role of qEEG in the assessment of other anxiety symptom patterns remains unclear. Measurements of heart rate variability (HRV) are sometimes helpful when assessing the efficacy of conventional or nonconventional treatments of anxiety (McCraty, Barrios-Choplin, Rozman, Atkinson, & Watkins, 2001).

Approaches Based on Forms of Energy or Information That Are Not Validated by Western Science

At the time of writing, there are no assessment approaches in this category.

Assessment Approaches That May Provide Specific Diagnostic Information about Causes of Anxiety

Biological Approaches

◆ **Elevated serum cholesterol may be a marker for many anxiety symptoms** Elevated serum cholesterol may be a biological marker for different anxiety syndromes, including generalized anxiety, panic attacks, and possibly obsessive-compulsive disorder (Peter, Tabrizian, & Hand, 2000). In general, anxious patients diagnosed with OCD have higher serum cholesterol levels compared with individuals diagnosed with panic disorder (Peter, Tabrizian, & Hand, 1997). For unclear reasons, the successful response of anxiety symptoms to conventional medications is associated with a reduction of total serum cholesterol to normal levels. In contrast to high cholesterol levels in chronically anxious patients, chronically depressed individuals may have low serum cholesterol levels.

◆ **Vitamin deficiencies are associated with increased risk of generalized anxiety** The findings of a large observational study suggest that abnormally low serum levels of certain B vitamins (thiamine, B_6, and niacin), as well as vitamins C and E, are associated with an increased risk of generalized anxiety (Heseker, Kubler, Pudel, & Westenhoffer, 1992). Assessment of vitamin deficiency states is especially important in anxious individuals who do not take supplements or who are at risk of one or more vitamin deficiency syndromes because of chronic malnutrition or a medical problem that interferes with normal absorption or metabolism.

◆ **Chronically anxious patients are often deficient in magnesium, selenium, or phosphorus** Chronically anxious patients are often deficient in magnesium, selenium, or phosphorus (Durlach, Durlach, Bac, Bara, & Guiet-Bara, 1994; McCleane & Watters, 1990; Webb & Gehi, 1981). Mineral deficiencies often occur in patients who are malnourished in general, and many malnourished individuals experience chronic anxiety. It is always prudent to check serum chemistries of chronically anxious patients, especially those who may be malnourished and who do not take quality vitamin and mineral supplements.

◆ **Urinary glutamate levels may correlate with the severity of anxiety symptoms** Preliminary findings suggest that urinary levels of glutamate may correlate with the overall level of anxiety. Glutamate is a metabolite of glutamic acid, an important excitatory neurotransmitter. Individuals who have relatively lower brain glutamic acid levels (and correspondingly lower urinary glutamate levels) tend to be less anxious in general compared with individuals with higher levels. In one dataset reports of anxiety were 33% higher among individuals with urinary glutamate levels above 25 μm of glutamate per gram of creatinine (personal communication with Dr. Gottfried Kellerman, Neuroscience Inc., January 2005).

Somatic Approaches

At the time of writing, there are no assessment approaches in this category.

Approaches Based on Forms of Energy or Information That Are Validated by Western Science

At the time of writing, there are no assessment approaches in this category.

Approaches Based on Forms of Energy or Information That Are Not Validated by Western Science

◆ **Constitutional assessment may clarify energetic patterns associated with anxiety** Homeopathic assessment rests on a comprehensive analysis of biological, social, and psychological complaints. Presumed energetic imbalances are inferred on the basis of symptoms and history, and the homeopathic physician selects specific remedies with the goal of correcting those imbalances. Certain constitutional patterns are frequently

associated with chronic anxiety. Identification of the underlying constitutional pattern guides the homeopathic physician in the selection of a specific constitutional remedy.

◆ **EDST may help determine whether Healing Touch is helpful for stress reduction** Electrodermal skin testing (EDST) may prove to be a useful assessment approach when determining whether conventional or subtle energy treatments of anxiety will be effective for a particular patient (Forbes, Rust, & Becker, 2004). Healing Touch practitioners conducted six trials comparing the anxiety-reducing efficacy of conventional relaxation with Healing Touch. They concluded that EDST reliably measured changes in bioenergy in meridians (according to Chinese medical theory) following both conventional and subtle energy treatments of anxiety (Stouffer, Kaiser, Pitman, & Rolf, 2003).

◆ The Integrative Treatment of Anxiety

Conventional Treatments of Anxiety Are Sometimes Effective but Limited

Cognitive-behavioral therapy, supportive psychotherapy, and psychopharmacology are established conventional treatments of anxiety. Double-blind studies have verified the efficacy of benzodiazepines and SSRIs in the short-term treatment of recurring panic attacks and generalized anxiety. Certain conventional drugs are effective treatments of social phobia; however, at the time of writing, there are no conventional psychopharmacological treatments of specific phobias. Behavioral therapies including graded exposure and flooding are beneficial in social anxiety and performance anxiety. The conventional management of obsessive-compulsive disorder and PTSD typically involves combining psychotherapy and medications.

Conventional treatments of anxiety are often beneficial but have limited efficacy. A meta-analysis of high-quality studies concluded that the efficacy of conventional treatments varies widely depending on the core anxiety symptom being treated (Westen & Morrison, 2001). Panic attacks tend to improve and remain improved in response to medications like lorazepam (Ativan) and clonazepam (Klonapin), but patients who chronically use benzodiazepines to control panic symptoms are at significant risk of benzodiazepine dependence and withdrawal. Furthermore, most patients who complain of generalized anxiety have initial positive responses to conventional treatments but remain symptomatic over the long term. Phobias, obsessions and compulsions, and symptoms of post-traumatic stress are often poorly responsive to conventional Western treatments (Westen & Morrison, 2001). This is complicated by the fact that many patients who experience these symptoms chronically are too impaired to seek treatment and frequently have comorbid symptoms, including depressed mood, sleep disturbances, and substance abuse.

In sum, anxiety is difficult to accurately characterize and treat because of significant individual differences in the type and severity of symptoms and complex medical, psychological, social, and cultural factors that cause or exacerbate anxiety symptoms. Conventional standards of care for the acutely or chronically anxious patient are also difficult to define because of differences in the training, experience, and skill of conventionally trained mental health professionals.

Nonconventional Treatments of Anxiety

Extensive research has been done on nonconventional treatments of generalized anxiety, but relatively little work has been done with respect to panic attacks, phobias, obsessions, or compulsions. Kava kava (*Piper methysticum*) and L-theanine (γ-ethylamino-L-glutamic acid) are substantiated nonconventional treatments of generalized anxiety. Regular relaxation, meditation, and mindfulness practice improve many symptoms of generalized anxiety and may be safely combined with biological or energy-information therapies. Virtual reality graded exposure therapy (VRGET) is a rapidly evolving modality that will almost certainly play a significant future role in the treatment of many anxiety symptom patterns that are poorly responsive to conventional psychological and pharmacological approaches. VRGET is an effective and cost-effective treatment of generalized anxiety, social phobia, specific phobias, and panic attacks. EEG and electromyography (EMG) biofeedback are probably as effective as regular relaxation

training or mind–body practices for moderate symptoms of generalized anxiety. Substantial evidence supports the use of microcurrent stimulation of the brain in the management of generalized anxiety. At the time of writing, provisional treatments of anxiety include dietary changes, supplementation with L-tryptophan or 5-hydroxytryptophan (5-HTP), regular exercise, massage, EEG and other forms of biofeedback training, acupuncture (including electroacupuncture), and Reiki. Limited research findings, anecdotal reports, and inconsistent evidence suggest that passionflower extract, Ashwagondha *(Withania somnifera),* certain vitamins and minerals, the essential oils of lavender and rosemary, dehydroepiandrosterone (DHEA), certain Bach flower remedies, Healing Touch, qigong, certain homeopathic remedies, paraspinal electrical stimulation, thought field therapy, and intercessory prayer are possibly effective treatments in some cases of anxiety.

Table 10–3 outlines the substantiated and provisional nonconventional treatments of anxiety.

Table 10–3 Substantiated and Provisional Nonconventional Treatments of Anxiety

	Treatment Approach	Evidence for Modality or Integrative Approaches	Comments (Including Safety Issues or Contraindications)
Substantiated			
Biological	Kava	Kava 70–240 mg/day is probably as effective as conventional drugs for generalized anxiety	*Caution:* Rare cases of liver failure probably related to contamination. *Caution:* Avoid concurrent use of benzodiazepines
	L-theanine	L-theanine 50–200 mg/day is effective for moderate anxiety, and 800 mg/day in divided doses is effective for more severe anxiety	L-theanine does not cause drowsiness, and there is no evidence of adverse effects or toxic interactions with other conventional or nonconventional biological treatments
Somatic or mind–body	Relaxation and guided imagery	Relaxation is as effective as conventional treatments of moderate generalized anxiety. Guided imagery is beneficial for generalized anxiety, panic and traumatic memories	*Caution:* Panic attacks have been reported during relaxation exercises in predisposed patients
	Yoga	Regular yoga practice is beneficial for many anxiety symptoms and may permit the patient to reduce doses of conventional medications	*Caution:* Rare case reports of air embolism or basilar artery occlusion during strenuous yoga practice. Physically impaired patients should first consult their physicians
	Meditation and mindfulness-based stress reduction (MBSR)	Regular meditation or mindfulness training reduces symptoms of generalized anxiety	Mindfulness training reduces the severity of physical symptoms associated with chronic anxiety, including irritable bowel syndrome
Energy-information approaches validated by Western Science	VRGET	VRGET is as effective as conventional exposure therapies for specific phobias, social phobia, and panic disorder	Rare transient adverse effects of VRGET include mild nausea, headaches, and dizziness. *Caution:* Psychotic patients, patients with seizure disorders or other neurologic disorders, and substance abusing patients should be advised against using VRGET
	Videoconferencing	Videoconferencing permits establishment of a therapeutic alliance and is as effective as face-to-face CBT for many anxiety symptoms, including agoraphobia and panic attacks	Videoconferencing provides an effective means for severely impaired individuals to receive treatment

Table 10–3 Substantiated and Provisional Nonconventional Treatments of Anxiety *(Continued)*

Treatment Approach	Evidence for Modality or Integrative Approaches	Comments (Including Safety Issues or Contraindications)
Biofeedback	EEG, EMG, GSR, and thermal biofeedback are effective treatments of generalized anxiety and sometimes permit dose reductions of conventional drugs. Combined GSR biofeedback and relaxation is more effective than either approach alone	It is not clear how long the beneficial effects of biofeedback continue after treatment is discontinued
Microcurrent electrical stimulation (CES)	CES has comparable efficacy to conventional drug treatments of generalized anxiety and phobias, and may permit dose reductions of conventional drugs	Residual benefits of CES may continue for months following treatment
Energy-information approaches not validated by Western science — None at time of writing		
Provisional		
Biological — Dietary changes	Avoiding refined sugar and caffeine, increasing protein and foods containing tryptophan may reduce symptoms of generalized anxiety or panic	Dietary changes that are beneficial in anxious individuals should be encouraged on the basis of general health benefits
Ayurvedic herbs	Ayurvedic herbs, including *Bacopa monniera*, *Centella asiatica*, and a compound herbal formula, Geriforte, reduce symptoms of generalized anxiety	Serious adverse effects of these Ayurvedic herbs have not been reported at recommended doses. All patients using Ayurvedic herbs should be supervised by an Ayurvedic physician
L-tryptophan and 5-HTP	L-tryptophan 2–3 g/day or 5-HTP 25 to 100 mg up to 3 times a day is probably an effective treatment of generalized anxiety. 5-HTP may prevent panic attacks	*Caution:* When combining 5-HTP and a conventional medication, the risk of serotonin syndrome can be minimized by starting 5-HTP at low doses (e.g., 25 mg/day) and gradually increasing the dose while monitoring for adverse effects, including insomnia and nervousness
Inositol	Inositol (up to 20 g/day) is probably an effective treatment of panic attacks, and may reduce symptoms of agoraphobia, obsessions, and compulsions	Serious adverse effects have not been reported when inositol is used at therapeutic doses
Somatic or mind–body — Exercise	Regular aerobic or strengthening exercise reduces generalized anxiety symptoms and may reduce the frequency and severity of panic attacks	*Caution:* Patients with heart disease, chronic pain syndromes. or other serious medical illnesses should always consult their physician before starting an exercise program
Massage	Regular massage reduces the severity of chronic moderate anxiety	*Note:* Individuals with chronic pain syndromes should consult their physician before receiving massage therapy
Energy-information approaches validated by Western science — Music and binaural sound	Regular listening to soothing music or certain binaural sounds can significantly reduce generalized anxiety	*Note:* The experience of music or binaural sound is more effective when there are no distractions. Anxious patients should be encouraged to become absorbed in music or binaural sounds on a regular basis
HRV biofeedback training	Biofeedback training using HRV probably reduces symptoms of generalized anxiety	Energy cardiology combines HRV and EEG biofeedback and is probably an effective treatment of anxiety
Energy-information approaches not validated by Western science — Acupuncture and electroacupuncture	Some acupuncture and electroacupuncture protocols probably reduce symptoms of generalized anxiety	*Note:* Rare adverse effects of acupuncture include bruising, fatigue, and fainting. Very rare cases of pneumothorax have been reported.
Reiki	Regular Reiki treatments may be beneficial for anxiety related to pain or depressed mood	Both contact and noncontact Reiki may reduce anxiety symptoms

CBT, cognitive-behavioral therapy; EEG, electroencephalography; EMG, electromyography; 5-HTP, 5-hydroxytryptophan; GSR, galvanic skin response; HRT, heart rate variability; VRGET, virtual reality graded exposure therapy

Substantiated Treatments of Anxiety

Biological Treatments

◆ Medicinal herbs

Kava kava (Piper methysticum) is an effective treatment of generalized anxiety   In traditional Polynesian cultures, kava is used for ceremonial purposes and as an inebriant. In contrast to benzodiazepines, when kava is used at recommended doses (typically 60–300 mg/day), patients do not experience mental slowing or impaired cognitive functioning (Russell, Bakker, & Singh, 1987). The use of kava as a treatment of anxiety has been extensively reviewed in the biomedical and alternative medical literature. Animal studies suggest that the putative mechanism of action involves serotonin blockade in the amygdala by α-pyrones, a principle bioactive constituent of kava. Kava interferes with norepinephrine reuptake and is known to have binding affinity with both γ-aminobutyric acid (GABA) and N-methyl-D-asparate (NMDA) receptors, both of which modulate anxiety. Kava may also reduce anxiety by influencing vagal heart tone in patients with generalized anxiety (Watkins, Connor, & Davidson, 2001). A Cochrane systematic review of 11 controlled double-blind studies that included over 600 patients concluded that kava was superior to placebo for the short-term management of generalized anxiety (Pittler & Ernst, 2004). Double-blind studies and one meta-analysis (Hansel, 1996; Singh & Blumenthal, 1996) support the use of kava preparations standardized to 70% kava lactones at doses between 70 and 240 mg/day for the treatment of stress and moderate anxiety, but not severe anxiety or agitation. An early systematic review of seven quality studies involving a total of 377 patients concluded that kava at 300 mg/day is more effective than placebo in reducing nonpsychotic anxiety states (Pittler & Ernst, 2000). Daily use of standardized kava preparations at 100 to 200 mg/day effectively reduces anxiety symptoms associated with menopause (De Leo et al., 2000).

Kava compares favorably to benzodiazepines and other conventional antianxiety drugs. The findings of a small double-blind, controlled trial suggest that generally anxious patients who gradually increase their daily dose of kava (up to 300 mg/day) while tapering off a benzodiazepine do not experience worsening anxiety or benzodiazepine withdrawal (Malsch & Kieser, 2001). A randomized placebo-controlled, multicenter study enrolling 129 outpatients concluded that a standardized kava preparation was as effective as two commonly prescribed antianxiety agents (buspirone and opipramol) in the treatment of generalized anxiety (Boerner, Sommer, Berger, Kuhn, Schmidt, & Mannel, 2003). Three fourths of patients in both the kava group and the conventional drug group were classified as "treatment responders," and experienced 50% or greater reductions in Ham-A scores.

Safety Issues Associated with Kava   Kava is generally well tolerated even at doses significantly above usual therapeutic doses. Uncommon adverse effects include gastrointestinal upset, rash, headaches, and dizziness (Schulz, Hansel, & Tyler, 2001). In recent decades there have been reports of kava inebriation (Matthews et al., 1988), although this social phenomenon has not been observed in Europe, where kava preparations are used medicinally to treat anxiety. Rare case reports suggest that kava may cross-react with benzodiazepines, increasing their sedating effects (Almeida & Grimsley, 1996), but kava does not potentiate the effects of alcohol consumption in humans. Rare case reports of hepatitis (Escher et al., 2001) and fulminent liver failure (Kraft et al., 2002) have led to restrictions in the sale of kava products in many European countries and a warning by the U.S. Food and Drug Administration. However, independent experts have concluded that most reported cases of liver failure were associated with a processing mistake, resulting in toxic levels of alkaloids in a single batch of kava (Dragull, Yoshida, & Tang, 2003; Waller, 2002). Nevertheless, it is judicious to advise patients against taking kava when there is a question of alcohol abuse or concurrent use of conventional sedative-hypnotics (Bone 1993/1994). One case report suggests that kava may interfere with antiparkinsonian drugs (Izzo & Ernst, 2001).

◆ Other natural products

L-theanine is an effective treatment of moderate and severe anxiety and does not cause drowsiness   Green tea is used as a restorative in traditional Chinese medicine and contains many bioactive constituents, including the amino acid L-theanine (γ-ethyl-amino-L-glutamic acid). In recent years L-theanine has been extracted from green tea and is now widely used to treat anxiety symptoms and depressed mood in China, Japan, and other Asian countries. The calming effects of L-theanine are believed to compensate for the stimulating effects of caffeine in green tea (Kakuda et al., 2000). The antianxiety effect of L-theanine is achieved through enhanced α brain wave activity and increased synthesis of GABA (Juneja et al., 1999; Kakuda et al., 2000). Increased GABA, in turn, increases brain levels of dopamine and reduces serotonin, resulting in general feelings of calm and well-being (Mason, 2001). Changes in brain electrical activity measured by EEG are dose-dependent, and are similar to beneficial EEG changes observed in meditation, including increased α waves in the occipital and parietal regions (Ito et al., 1998). A calming effect is usually noted within 30 to 40 minutes after L-theanine is taken at a dose of 50 to 200 mg, and typically lasts 8 to 10 hours. Moderate anxiety symptoms often improve with a regimen of 200 mg once or twice daily. More severe anxiety symptoms may require doses up to 600 to 800 mg daily, taken in increments of 100 to 200 mg spaced over the day. Unlike benzodiazepines and other conventional antianxiety treatments, L-theanine does not result in increased drowsiness, slowed reflexes, or impaired concentration. There is no risk of developing tolerance or dependence, and there have been no reports of serious adverse side effects or interactions with other natural products or conventional synthetic drugs.

Somatic and Mind–Body Approaches

◆ Applied relaxation is comparable to cognitive therapy in generalized anxiety   *Applied relaxation* is a generic term for somatic or mind–body exercises that are used to diminish generalized anxiety. Relaxation techniques include sustained deep breathing (Davis, Eshelman, & McKay, 1982), progressive muscle relaxation, guided imagery, and systematic desensitization. The physiology of relaxation has been investigated for many decades. Several models have been proposed to explain its anxiety-reducing effects, including Benson's relaxation response and Selye's general adaptation syndrome, among others. One model posits that anxiety is associated with muscle tension, and is reduced by behaviors or cognitions that diminish tension and autonomic arousal. Regular relaxation is

an important mainstream treatment of anxiety, including specific phobias, social phobia, and generalized anxiety. The effectiveness of relaxation as a treatment of different anxiety symptoms has been extensively reviewed (Titlebaum, 1988).

Guided imagery is a commonly used self-directed treatment of anxiety. Applied relaxation techniques are often practiced together with mental imagery, meditation, or mindfulness training. Imagery can be individualized to the specific anxiety symptoms of each patient, and is known to have beneficial effects on the immune system, physiological stress responses, and cognitive-emotional functioning in general (Achterberg, 1985). The consistent practice of mental imagery effectively reduces many kinds of anxiety symptoms, including generalized anxiety, panic, and traumatic memories (Achterberg, Dossey, & Kolkmeier, 1994; Zahourek, 1998). Imagery and relaxation techniques are often used together to induce hypnotic trance states, resulting in a dramatic reduction in symptoms of generalized anxiety (Spiegel & Spiegel, 1978).

In a 5-month prospective study, generally anxious patients randomized to a relaxation group versus a group treated with conventional antidepressants and relaxation experienced equivalent and significant improvements in state anxiety levels by the end of the trial (Bernal, Cercos, Fuste, & Valiverdu, 1995). In a small controlled trial, 36 anxious adult outpatients randomized to 12 weekly sessions of applied relaxation or conventional cognitive therapy experienced significant and comparable reductions in anxiety (Ost & Breitholtz, 2000). Combining relaxation with guided imagery is probably more effective than either approach alone. In an open trial 60 women reporting anxiety and postpartum depressed mood experienced significant reductions in both anxiety and depressed mood using a combined relaxation-guided imagery protocol during the first 4 weeks after childbirth (Rees, 1995). In contrast to the largely beneficial effects of relaxation on generalized anxiety symptoms, panic attacks are sometimes reported by individuals diagnosed with panic disorder during applied relaxation exercises (Knott, Bakish, Lusk, & Barkely, 1997).

◆ **Regular yoga practice is beneficial in generalized anxiety, phobias, and OCD** Open studies, consistent anecdotal evidence, and a long historical tradition of use confirm that the regular practice of yoga is beneficial for individuals who are generally anxious. The regular and skillful practice of specific Yogic postures or breathing methods results in sustained changes in brain activation and possibly beneficial changes in neurotransmitter activity that manifest as a subjective state of alert calmness. Training in a particular style of Yoga called Sudarshan kriya involves a specialized breathing technique that reportedly decreases serum cortisol, the major stress hormone in humans (Gangadhar et al., 2000). Patients diagnosed with any anxiety disorder improve significantly when they combine a daily Yoga practice with relaxation and mindfulness training (Miller, Fletcher, & Kabat-Zinn, 1995). Yoga reduces anxiety in patients with hypertension and epilepsy (Chaudhary et al., 1988; Panjwani et al., 1995), and probably reduces test anxiety (Malathi & Damodaran, 1999). There is evidence that regular Yoga practice reduces the need for conventional drugs in generally anxious patients (Chaudhary et al., 1988). Findings of a small controlled study showed that the regular practice of a specific Kundalini left-nostril breathing technique significantly reduced symptom severity in patients diagnosed with obsessive-compulsive disorder (Shannahoff-Khalsa et al., 1999).

Safety issues in Yoga There are no absolute contraindications to the practice of Yogic postures or breathing exercises. There are rare case reports of fatal air embolism and basilar artery occlusion following vigorous Yogic practices. Patients with cardiovascular disease, chronic pain syndromes, or other physical impairments should consult with their physician before undertaking yoga or any mind–body training program that can potentially affect their autonomic activity. Many anxious or chronically stressed patients in my private practice have benefited greatly from the regular practice of yoga or other mind–body techniques, to the extent that some have been able to significantly reduce and in some cases discontinue conventional medications. I routinely encourage patients who are open to mind–body approaches to find a Yoga instructor and begin a regular practice.

◆ **Regular meditation or mindfulness training reduces psychological and physical symptoms of generalized anxiety** Meditation practices are used in many cultures to reduce anxiety and to maintain optimal psychological and spiritual health. Meditation has been extensively studied as a treatment of anxiety. Beneficial physiological effects of meditation include decreased oxygen consumption, respiratory rate, and blood pressure, as well as EEG changes associated with decreased autonomic arousal (Delmonte, 1985). Mindfulness-based stress reduction (MBSR) is an integrative approach pioneered by Kabat-Zinn (1990) that has been validated as highly effective for reducing the physical, emotional, and cognitive consequences of chronic stress. MBSR incorporates elements of different Eastern meditation practices and Western psychology. Increasing numbers of psychologists and psychiatrists are trained in MBSR, and its methods are now widely employed in health maintenance organizations. Research findings show that the consistent practice of mindfulness meditation, in which the patient practices detached self-observation, significantly reduces generalized anxiety and other anxiety symptoms (Kabat-Zinn et al., 1992; Miller et al., 1995). In one study 93% of patients ($N = 322$) who started a 10-week MBSR program successfully completed it, and the majority of those reported significantly decreased physical and emotional distress, improved quality of life, a greater sense of general well-being, increased optimism, and increased feelings of control (Abbey 2004). Patients diagnosed with irritable bowel syndrome (IBS), a frequent concomitant of generalized anxiety, experienced significantly fewer symptoms of both IBS and anxiety when they engaged in two brief (15-minute) daily sessions of mindfulness meditation (Keefer & Blanchard, 2001). The cultivation of increased self-awareness in the present moment through mindfulness training helps the anxious patient to make choices that permit avoidance of potentially stressful situations or engage in more effective coping when stress is unavoidable (Epstein, 1999).

Treatments Based on Forms of Energy or Information That Are Validated by Western Science

◆ **VRGET is an effective treatment of specific phobias, generalized anxiety, panic disorder, and agoraphobia** Controlled studies confirm that virtual reality graded exposure therapy (sometimes called experiential cognitive therapy, or ECT, in European countries) is more effective than conventional imaginal exposure therapy (using mental imagery to provoke the feared object or situation), and has comparable efficacy to in vivo exposure therapy (Emmelkamp, Bruynzeel, DRost, & Van de Mast, 2001; Pertaub, Slater, & Barker, 2001). Anxious or phobic patients are frequently unable to tolerate conventional kinds of exposure therapy, and remain chronically impaired because they never become desensitized to a feared object or situation. Like in vivo and imaginal exposure therapy, VRGET has the goal of desensitizing the patient to a situation or object that would normally cause anxiety or panic.

VRGET is an effective treatment of many anxiety symptom patterns, including specific phobias, generalized anxiety, panic disorder with agoraphobia (Vincelli, Choi, Molinari, Wiederhold, & Riva, 2000), and post-traumatic stress disorder (Riva et al., 2001). In a controlled study, VRGET and conventional cognitive-behavioral therapy were equally effective in the treatment of panic disorder with agoraphobia; however, patients who underwent VRGET required 33% fewer sessions (Vincelli, Anolli, Bouchard, Wiederhold, Zurloni, & Riva, 2003). Case reports and controlled studies have demonstrated the effectiveness of VRGET in many specific phobias, including fear of flying (Rothbaum, Smith, Hodges, & Lee, 2000; Wiederhold, Jang, Gevirtz, Kim, Kim, & Wiederhold, 2002), fear of heights, fear of small animals, fear of driving, and others (Glantz, Durlach, Barnett, & Aviles, 1996; Rothbaum & Hodges, 1999). In one controlled study, 65% of anxious adults (*N* = 45) diagnosed with a specific anxiety disorder according to *DSM-IV* criteria reported significant reductions in 4 of 5 anxiety measures (Maltby, Kirsch, Mayers, & Allen, 2002). VRGET is as effective as conventional exposure therapy for fear of flying, and is more cost-effective because both patient and therapist avoid significant time commitments and the need to use airplanes (Rothbaum & Hodges, 1999; Rothbaum et al., 2000). In a pilot study individuals who overcame fear of flying using VRGET combined with biofeedback, including respirations, galvanic skin response (GSR) and heart rate, were able to fly without the use of conventional medications or alcohol 3 months after treatment ended (Wiederhold et al., 2002). VRGET is also beneficial for traumatized patients who have been diagnosed with PTSD. A virtual environment that simulates the devastation that took place following the September 11, 2001, attacks of the World Trade Center in New York has been successfully used to treat individuals who suffered from severe PTSD following the attacks (Difede & Hoffman, 2002). Emerging evidence suggests that combining VRGET with D-cycloserine (see discussion below), a partial NMDA agonist, results in greater improvement in symptoms of **acrophobia** (fear of heights) compared with VRGET alone. VRGET will become more available as technology costs continue to decrease and will soon become a widely used and cost-effective approach for the outpatient treatment of panic attacks, post-traumatic stress disorder, agoraphobia, social phobia, and specific phobias.

Several VRGET tools are available over the Internet, permitting mental health professionals to guide patients in the use of these computer-based advanced exposure protocols through real-time videoconferencing anywhere high-speed Internet access is available (Botella et al., 2000). Future integrative approaches to phobias, panic attacks, and other severe anxiety syndromes will probably combine VRGET with biofeedback in outpatient settings or in the patient's home via broadband Internet connections, with conventional cognitive-behavioral therapy (CBT), mind–body practices, and conventional medications.

Safety considerations and contraindications in VRGET   Fewer than 4% of individuals experience transient symptoms of disorientation, nausea, dizziness, headache, and blurred vision when in a virtual environment. "Simulator sleepiness" is a feeling of generalized fatigue that occurs infrequently. Intense sensory stimulation during VRGET can trigger migraine headaches, seizures, or gait abnormalities in individuals who have these medical problems. VRGET is therefore contraindicated in these populations. Anxious patients who are actively abusing alcohol or narcotics should not use VRGET. Patients who have disorders of the vestibular system should be advised against trying VRGET. Psychotic patients should not use VRGET because immersion in a virtual environment can exacerbate delusions and potentially worsen reality testing (Wiederhold & Wiederhold, 2005).

◆ **Broadband videoconferencing is as effective as face-to-face consultation**   Chronically anxious patients, especially patients with panic disorder or agoraphobia, are frequently too impaired by their symptoms to seek professional care. Others are too geographically isolated to obtain conventional cognitive-behavioral therapy or pharmacological treatment for severe anxiety syndromes. Videoconferencing has been explored as a realistic alternative mode of treatment delivery to these patients. An effective therapeutic alliance can be achieved between therapist and patient when CBT is done by videoconference (Bouchard et al., 2000; Manchanda & McLaren, 1998). Although CBT can be done by telephone (*telepsychiatry*), videoconferencing has the advantage of permitting the therapist to demonstrate behavioral exercises to the patient, and both therapist and patient are able to accurately observe nonverbal behaviors during sessions. A large controlled study showed that CBT is equally effective for a range of anxiety symptoms when done face-to-face or via broadband videoconferencing (Day & Schneider, 2002). CBT delivered via videoconferencing is as effective as face-to-face CBT in patients with both panic disorder and agoraphobia (Bouchard et al., 2004). This finding is highly significant and provides a viable alternative to routine CBT for this severely impaired population who might otherwise not utilize mental health services.

◆ **EMG-, GSR-, and EEG-biofeedback training reduces symptoms of generalized anxiety**   Biofeedback has nonspecific beneficial effects on many anxiety symptoms. Electromyelography, thermal, and EEG-biofeedback training are efficacious treatments of generalized anxiety (Hurley & Meminger, 1992; Vanathy, Sharma, & Kumar, 1998; Wenck, Leu, & D'Amato, 1996). The clinical effectiveness of biofeedback training is probably equivalent to conventional relaxation techniques (Roome & Romney, 1985; Scandrett, Bean, Breeden, & Powell, 1986) for the management of generalized anxiety in both adults and children. Chronically anxious patients trained in EEG or EMG biofeedback achieve symptom reduction similar to those taking conventional antianxiety medications (Rice, Blanchard, & Purcell, 1993; Sarkar, Rathee, & Neera, 1999). GSR biofeedback in combination with a relaxation technique improves anxiety more than relaxation alone (Fehring, 1983). The long-term benefits of EEG biofeedback for anxious patients have not been clearly established. One study evaluated two EEG-biofeedback machines on patients complaining of anxiety and burnout in an addiction treatment center (Ossebaard, 2000). Although patients experienced immediate reductions in state anxiety during biofeedback training, long-term effects on burnout were not maintained following discontinuation of treatment.

◆ **Microcurrent electrical stimulation is an effective treatment of generalized anxiety** Microcurrent electrical stimulation, also called cranioelectrotherapy stimulation (CES), is an effective treatment of generalized anxiety. Studies employing qEEG have confirmed beneficial changes in brain electrical activity when this approach is used (Schroeder & Barr, 2001) A meta-analysis of double-blind controlled trials comparing CES with a sham treatment (i.e., electrodes applied but with no current) concluded that measures of generalized anxiety improved in 7 of 8 studies, and the magnitude of improvement reached statistical significance in 4 of these (Klawansky, Yeung, Berkey, Shah, Phan, & Chalmers, 1995). A larger review encompassing 34 sham-controlled trials conducted between 1963 and 1996 concluded that regular CES treatments resulted in short-term symptomatic relief of generalized anxiety symptoms mediated by direct effects on autonomic brain centers (DeFelice, 1997). In a 10-week open trial of daily self-administered CES therapy in 182 individuals diagnosed with *DSM-III* anxiety disorders, 73% of patients reported significant reductions in anxiety that were maintained at 6-month follow-up (Overcash, 1999). Significantly, one fourth of patients enrolled in this study had failed trials on conventional drugs, and 58% had received no previous treatment of any kind for their anxiety symptoms. In general, patients who receive at least 4 to 6 CES treatments experience more sustained reductions in anxiety compared with patients who receive fewer treatments. The results of a small double-blind, sham-controlled study (*N* = 20) suggest that a single CES treatment of patients who report generalized stress results in beneficial changes in autonomic arousal as measured by decreases in EMG and heart rate that are sustained at least 1 week following treatment (Heffernan, 1995). Patients diagnosed with one or more phobias using *DSM* criteria reported significant reductions in state anxiety when exposure to the anxiety-inducing stimulus was followed by 30 minutes of CES treatment (Smith & Shiromoto, 1992). Comparable anxiety reduction was achieved with CES and conventional antianxiety medications, suggesting that CES may be an effective approach for phobic patients who wish to discontinue conventional drugs. Hospitalized patients with histories of drug or alcohol abuse reported significant reductions in anxiety compared with matched patients who received sham CES (Schmitt, Capo, & Boyd, 1986). Serious adverse effects of microcurrent electrical brain stimulation have not been reported.

Treatments Based on Forms of Energy or Information That Are Not Validated by Western Science

At the time of writing, there are no substantiated treatment approaches in this category.

Provisional Treatments of Anxiety

Biological Treatments

◆ **Dietary changes** As part of an overall plan to treat anxiety, patients should be counseled to avoid caffeine, evaluated for hypoglycemia, and encouraged to eat foods that contain tryptophan.

Generalized anxiety symptoms are frequently associated with a common condition known as **reactive hypoglycemia**,

in which blood glucose drops to abnormal low levels following a glucose challenge. Individuals who experience anxiety episodes related to this condition benefit from dietary changes including low carbohydrate intake, high protein, consumption of foods with different glycemic indices, and avoidance of caffeine (Bell & Forse, 1999). Caffeine use is associated with an increased risk of anxiety. Caffeine consumption increases serum epinephrine, norepinephrine, and cortisol levels, and can result in "nervousness" in healthy adults, or increased feelings of generalized anxiety or panic attacks in individuals who are predisposed to panic (Charney, Heninger, & Jatlow, 1985; Uhde et al., 1984). Chronically anxious patients report that anxiety symptoms diminish when they abstain from caffeine (Bruce & Lader, 1989). A dietary deficiency in the amino acid tryptophan leads to reductions in brain serotonin levels. Individuals who are prone to generalized anxiety or panic attacks report more severe symptoms when treated with an amino acid formula that excludes tryptophan (Klaassen et al., 1998).

Medicinal Herbs

◆ **Certain Ayurvedic herbs are probably beneficial for generalized anxiety** Ayurvedic herbal preparations including *Bacopa monniera* and *Centella asiatica* have been used for millennia to treat symptom patterns that resemble generalized anxiety. Double-blind controlled trials suggest that both herbs effectively reduce general anxiety symptoms (Bradwejn, Zhou, Koszycki, & Shlik, 2000; Stough et al., 2001). Emerging evidence suggests that an Ayurvedic compound herbal formula called Geriforte (Himalaya Proselect, Houston, Texas) may also alleviate symptoms of generalized anxiety (Shah, Nayak & Sethi, 1993). Serious adverse effects have not been reported when the above Ayurvedic herbals are used at recommended doses. Ayurveda is an advanced highly integrated system of medicine that employs diverse herbal, mind–body, energetic treatment modalities. Patients who use Ayurvedic herbal preparations should be under the medical supervision of a trained Ayurvedic physician.

Amino Acids and Amino Acid Precursors

◆ **5-HTP may be as effective as conventional medications for generalized anxiety** L-tryptophan and 5-HTP are widely used nonconventional treatments of generalized anxiety; however, to date few double-blind conducted studies have examined their efficacy. Both amino acids are essential precursors for serotonin synthesis, a neurotransmitter that plays a central role in the regulation of mood and anxiety. There is a more extensive research literature on 5-HTP for anxiety than L-tryptophan. In a double-blind study, 58% of generally anxious patients (*N* = 79) randomized to L-tryptophan 3 g/day reported significantly greater reductions in baseline anxiety compared with placebo (Zang, 1991). Animal studies and human clinical trials show that 5-HTP has consistent antianxiety effects (Kahn et al., 1987; Soderpalm & Engel, 1990). Additionally, 5-HTP may inhibit panic attacks induced by carbon dioxide (Schruers, Pols, Overbeek, van Beek, & Griez, 2000). Patients randomized to receive a combination of 5-HTP and carbidopa (a drug that inhibits the enzyme that breaks down 5-HTP in the peripheral blood supply, thus increasing the amount of 5-HTP that crosses the blood–brain barrier) reported significant reductions in anxiety that were comparable to clomipramine, a conventional antianxiety medication. Patients taking a placebo did not improve (Kahn et al., 1987). 5-HTP may be safely combined with conventional antianxiety drugs with monitoring for adverse effects related to excessive brain serotonin, including insomnia, agitation and nervousness. The risk of adverse effects is minimized when 5-HTP is started at doses of 25 mg/day and gradually increased over several weeks to a daily regimen that is well tolerated and produces therapeutic antianxiety effects. In my clinical experience, 5-HTP at 50 to 100 mg 3 times a day is well tolerated without excessive daytime sedation, and is an effective approach for many chronically anxious patients when used alone or in combination with SSRIs or other conventional antianxiety drugs. Gradually increasing a bedtime dose of 5-HTP to 200 to 400 mg often reduces daytime anxiety and improves the quality of sleep in chronically anxious patients who complain of insomnia. Greater research evidence supporting the use of 5-HTP for anxiety, together with smaller effective doses and increased CNS availability, generally make 5-HTP the preferred choice over L-tryptophan.

◆ **Inositol probably reduces the severity and frequency of panic attacks** Inositol has been the focus of renewed research interest because of its role as a precursor of an important second messenger in the brain, phosphatidylinositol, which is an integral part of serotonin, norepinephrine, and other neurotransmitter receptors. Findings of several double-blind studies suggest that high doses of inositol improve many anxiety symptoms that respond to SSRIs, including panic attacks, agoraphobia, obsessions, and compulsions (Belmaker, Levine, & Kofman, 1998). Available conventional drugs are effective in only two thirds of patients who experience panic attacks (Palatnik, Frolov, Fux, & Benjamin, 2001). Inositol in doses up to 20 g/day reduces the severity and frequency of panic attacks (Benjamin, Nemetz, Fux, Bleichman, & Agam, 1997) by interfering with one of the physiological causes of panic (m-CPP). A 4-week double-blind crossover study concluded that inositol (12 g/day) and imipramine, a conventional medication, are equally effective in reducing the frequency and severity of panic attacks and agoraphobia (Benjamin et al., 1995). A 1-month double-blind, placebo-controlled study enrolling 20 patients concluded that inositol (up to 18 g/day) and fluvoxamine (up to 150 mg/day) had similar efficacy in reducing the frequency of panic attacks (Palatnik et al., 2001). The average number of weekly panic attacks in the group taking inositol decreased by 4, compared with an average decrease by 2 in the group treated with fluvoxamine. Serious adverse effects have not been reported by patients taking therapeutic doses of inositol.

Somatic and Mind–Body Approaches

◆ **Regular exercise reduces symptoms of generalized anxiety and may reduce the frequency and severity of panic attacks** Anxious patients frequently engage in strenuous physical activity in efforts to alleviate anxiety symptoms. Open studies suggest that regular aerobic exercise or strength training improves anxiety (Paluska & Schwenk, 2000). An exercise program consisting of at least 20 to 30 minutes of daily exercise can significantly reduce symptoms of generalized anxiety (Osei-Tutu & Campagna, 1998). Findings of a prospective 10-week study of

exercise in individuals prone to panic attacks suggest that regular walking or jogging (4 miles 3 times a week) reduces the severity and frequency of panic attacks (Stevinson, 1999). In my own clinical practice, I have observed that anxious patients who follow a regular exercise program pay more attention to health in general, and tend to respond more rapidly to both conventional and integrative treatments compared with patients who are not physically active. Individuals with heart disease, chronic pain, or other serious medical problems should consult their physician before starting an exercise program.

◆ **Regular massage reduces the severity of chronic moderate anxiety** Massage is widely used to evoke feelings of deep relaxation and reduced anxiety. The anxiety-reducing effects of massage are probably mediated by decreased cortisol and increased parasympathetic tone (Acolet et al., 1993; Serepca, 1996). Few controlled trials on massage have been done; however, a critical review of published studies concluded that there is no strong medical evidence supporting the majority of its therapeutic claims (Ernst & Fialka, 1994). In spite of these criticisms, regular massage as a treatment of chronic stress and anxiety is worthy of serious attention. The subjective physical and psychological benefits of massage are difficult to quantify in controlled trials. Few massage therapists are trained in biomedical research methods or work in institutional settings where sham-controlled trials can be conducted. Consistent anecdotal evidence, a long-standing history of widespread use for stress reduction, and the findings of many open trials support the view that regular massage therapy reduces the severity of chronic moderate anxiety in general, specifically when anxiety is related to test taking or problem solving, work stress, or the anticipation of invasive medical procedures (Field et al., 1996; Kim et al., 2002; McKechnie et al., 1983; Okvat et al., 2002; Shulman & Jones, 1996). In my own clinical experience, regular massage therapy effectively reduces anxiety, improves emotional resilience, and enhances feelings of general well-being in anxious patients.

Treatments Based on Forms of Energy or Information That Are Validated by Western Science

◆ **Listening to soothing music and binaural sound reduce symptoms of generalized anxiety** Music and sound are used in many cultures and healing traditions for their anxiety-reducing benefits. In a randomized study, 40 anxious adult patients were assigned to conventional cognitive therapy versus music-assisted reframing. Patients in the music group experienced greater reductions in overall anxiety on the basis of standardized scales (Kerr, Walsh, & Marshall, 2001). A unique auditory experience occurs when headphones are used to route slightly different frequencies of sound binaurally to the right and left hemispheres. The brainstem "constructs" binaural beats on the basis of the frequency difference between sounds processed in each hemisphere. Functional brain imaging studies suggest that interhemispheric synchronization of information is enhanced by this experience. Certain binaural beats consistently induce a calm, relaxed state, whereas others facilitate increased attention or arousal (Atwater, 1999). In this way, the therapeutic use of certain sound frequency patterns to achieve different therapeutic goals is analogous to the use of different EEG-biofeedback protocols. I encourage anxious patients to listen to soothing music as often as possible without distractions, especially at the start of their day. I have observed that generally anxious patients frequently experience both reduced anxiety and improved mental clarity after listening to binaural sounds of appropriate frequencies. Patients often report significantly reduced anxiety, increased feelings of peace, and a more hopeful outlook after becoming absorbed in a relaxing musical experience.

◆ **Biofeedback training using HRV is beneficial in chronically anxious individuals** In contrast to the documented efficacy of GSR, EMG, and EEG biofeedback, few research studies have examined the efficacy of heart rate variability biofeedback as a treatment of anxiety. Findings from case reports and controlled trials suggest that biofeedback training based on HRV significantly reduces stress and improves general feelings of emotional well-being in individuals who are subjected to acute job-related stress (McCraty, Atkinson, & Tomasino, 2001). Beneficial changes in baseline anxiety following HRV biofeedback are associated with decreased serum cortisol levels and increased serum DHEA levels. Police officers are often subjected to unexpected severe stress. In a 4-month controlled trial, the majority of 29 police officers trained in biofeedback techniques based on HRV (The Institute of HeartMath, Boulder Creek, California) reported significant improvements in baseline anxiety, whereas 36 officers assigned to a wait-list group did not report significant improvements (McCraty, Tomasino, Atkinson, & Sundram, 1999). Chronically anxious patients who undergo HRV biofeedback training report improvements in general emotional well-being and reduced baseline anxiety (McCraty et al., 1998).

Treatments Based on Forms of Energy or Information That Are Not Validated by Western Science

◆ **Acupuncture and electroacupuncture probably reduce symptoms of generalized anxiety** Acupuncture and acupressure are widely used to treat anxiety. Extensive case reports from the Chinese medical literature suggest that different acupuncture protocols are beneficial in the management of anxiety symptom patterns that resemble generalized anxiety and panic attacks (Flaws, 2001). However, at present only a few small prospective controlled studies support the use of these traditional energy therapies, and most studies on the anxiety-reducing effects of acupuncture examine the general benefits of acupuncture on diverse cognitive, affective, and behavioral symptoms, including anxiety.

A narrative review of controlled studies, outcomes studies, and published case reports on acupuncture as a treatment of anxiety and depressed mood was published by the British Acupuncture Council (2002). Sham-controlled studies yielded consistent improvements in anxiety using both regular acupuncture and electroacupuncture. The reviewers noted that significant differences exist between protocols used in both regular and electroacupuncture, pointing to the unresolved issue of a general beneficial effect or possibly a placebo effect. Positive findings of most controlled studies were suggestive of a general anxiety-reducing effect of acupuncture, but were regarded by the reviewers as inconclusive because of study design problems, including the absence of standardized symptom rating scales in most studies, limited follow-up, and poorly defined differences between protocols used in different studies.

In one double-blind study, 36 mildly depressed or anxious patients were randomized to an acupuncture protocol believed to reduce anxiety versus a sham acupuncture protocol. Patients received three sessions. HRV and mean heart rate were measured at 5 and 15 minutes after treatment. Resting heart rate was significantly lower in the treatment group but not the sham group, and changes in HRV indices suggested that acupuncture had modulated autonomic activity in a way that reduced overall anxiety. The significance of these findings is limited by the absence of comments on baseline anxiety before and after treatment (Agelink et al., 2003). In another double-blind study, 55 adults (who had not been diagnosed with an anxiety disorder) were randomized to a bilateral auricular acupuncture protocol called the "shenmen" point—a protocol believed to be effective against anxiety (the so-called relaxation point)—versus a sham acupuncture point. Acupuncture needles remained in place for 48 hours. The "relaxation" group was significantly less anxious at 30 minutes and 24 and 48 hours compared with the other two groups; however, there were no significant intergroup differences in blood pressure, heart rate, or electrodermal activity (Wang & Kain, 2001). A small double-blind sham-controlled trial involving anxious patients with mixed symptoms of moderate depressed mood obtained a response rate of 85% following 10 acupuncture treatment sessions using specific acupuncture points (Du.20, Ex.6, He.7, PC.6, Bl.62) (Eich, Agelink, Lehmann, Lemmer, & Klieser, 2000). Uncommon transient adverse effects associated with acupuncture include bruising, fatigue, and nausea. Very rare cases of pneumothorax have been reported.

◆ **Regular Reiki treatments may reduce symptoms of anxiety associated with chronic pain or depressed mood** The findings of two studies suggest that regular Reiki treatments reduce the severity of anxiety symptoms in individuals who are chronically stressed (Kramer, 1990). Patients with mixed anxious depressed mood experienced significant relief following weekly treatments with contact or noncontact Reiki (Shore, 2004). Reiki treatments may improve state anxiety in chronic pain patients. In one study 120 chronically ill patients were randomized to receive Reiki, sham Reiki, progressive muscle relaxation, and no treatment (Dressen & Singg, 1998). Improvements in state anxiety (and pain) in patients receiving Reiki were significantly greater than the other three groups. Findings of this study are limited because possible differences in the use of anxiety-reducing medications between the active treatment groups and the control groups were not taken into account in the study design.

Possibly Effective Nonconventional Treatments of Anxiety

Table 10–4 outlines the possibly effective nonconventional treatments of anxiety.

Medicinal Herbs

◆ **Passionflower extract may reduce symptoms of generalized anxiety** Passionflower (*P. incarnata*) contains a bioactive ingredient called chrysin that has been demonstrated to bind to CNS benzodiazepine receptors. Although passionflower extract is commonly used to treat anxiety, few double-blind, placebo-controlled studies have been done. In one small study,

Table 10–4 Possibly Effective Nonconventional Treatments of Anxiety

Category	Treatment Approach	Evidence for Claimed Treatment Effect	Comments
Biological	Passionflower (*Passiflora incarnata*)	Passionflower extract may have anxiety-reducing effects comparable to benzodiazepines	Passionflower extract avoids the risk of tolerance or dependence
	Ashwagondha (*Withania somnifera*)	Ashwagondha is an Ayurvedic herbal used to treat anxiety and chronic stress	*Note:* Although serious adverse effects have not been reported with Ashwagondha, individuals who use Ayurvedic herbs should do so only under the supervision of a skilled Ayurvedic physician
	Lavender and rosemary essential oils	When used as aromatherapy or applied to the skin during massage, lavender and rosemary essential oils may reduce generalized anxiety	Lavender aromatherapy may produce relaxed, drowsy feelings; rosemary promotes a relaxed alert state
	D-cycloserine	D-cycloserine 500 mg facilitates the effectiveness of VRGET in acrophobia	A beneficial effect of D-cycloserine was maintained 3 months after VRGET treatment
	Bach flower remedies	Certain Bach flower remedies may reduce test anxiety	Adverse effects have not been reported with Bach flower remedies
	DHEA	DHEA 100 mg/day may reduce anxiety symptoms in psychotic patients	Combining DHEA with conventional medications may reduce the severity of anxiety associated with depressed mood or psychosis
	Vitamins (including thiamine, niacinamide, and vitamins B_6, B_{12}, C, and E)	Two forms of niacin—nicotinamide and niacinamide—may have calming effects. Niacinamide 1–3 g/day may reduce anxiety caused by hypoglycemia	B vitamins are cofactors for the biosynthesis of neurotransmitters implicated in chronic anxiety (and depression) and should be used with conventional anxiety reducing drugs
	Minerals (phosphorus, magnesium, and selenium)	Phosphorus may reduce the frequency of panic attacks. Magnesium 100–200 mg may reduce symptoms of generalized anxiety	Serious adverse effects are not associated with these mineral supplements at doses that are possibly beneficial in anxiety
Somatic and mind–body approaches	Animal-facilitated psychotherapy	Animal-facilitated psychotherapy may improve general emotional well-being and reduce symptoms of generalized anxiety	Socially isolated elderly and medically disabled individuals who are lonely or chronically anxious will probably benefit from frequent contact with domesticated animals
	Lucid dreaming	Training in lucid dreaming induction may reduce the severity of PTSD symptoms	Training in lucid dreaming is a reasonable alternative for patients diagnosed with PTSD who have not responded to other treatments
Energy-information approaches validated by Western science	Paraspinal electrical stimulation	Microcurrent stimulation of the paraspinal regions may reduce the severity of PTSD symptoms	Paraspinal electrical stimulation may be a viable alternative for PTSD patients who have not responded to other treatments
Energy-information approaches not validated by Western science	Healing Touch (HT) and Therapeutic Touch (TT)	HT and TT may reduce symptoms of generalized anxiety and anxiety related to pain or trauma	Sham-controlled studies suggest a nonspecific beneficial effect versus placebo effect
	Qigong and Tai Chi	The regular practice of qigong and Tai Chi may reduce symptoms of generalized anxiety. Tai Chi may be more effective than progressive muscle relaxation in PTSD combat veterans	*Caution:* Psychotic individuals or patients diagnosed with severe personality disorders should practice qigong only under the supervision of a skilled instructor
	Homeopathic remedies	Case reports suggest improvements in social phobia, PTSD, panic attacks, and OCD, but two double-blind studies showed no beneficial effects	*Note:* Inherent experimental design problems limit biomedical studies of homeopathy
	Thought field therapy (TFT) and Emotional Freedom Techniques (EFT)	TFT and EFT claim to reduce anxiety by rebalancing energy in the meridians. Both approaches are widely used to treat different anxiety syndromes	*Note:* Sham-controlled studies suggest that observed benefits of EFT are achieved by desensitization and distraction
	Somatoemotional release and craniosacral therapy	Case reports and one study suggest beneficial effects in trauma survivors	*Note:* The only study on somatoemotional release and craniosacral therapy in PTSD is small and methodologically flawed
	Religious attitudes and affiliation	Individuals who have strong religious beliefs or religious affiliations may be more resilient when facing stressful circumstances	Beneficial effects of religious beliefs on anxiety and stress are probably greater in cultures that provide frameworks for religious or spiritual experiences
	Intercessory prayer	Praying at a distance may be associated with a reduction in symptoms of pain and anxiety	*Note:* Beneficial effects of intercessory prayer on anxiety and emotional well-being may be due to group suggestion

DHEA, dehydroepiandrosterone; OCD, obsessive-compulsive disorder; PTSD, post-traumatic stress disorder; VRGET, virtual reality graded exposure therapy passionflower extract at 45 drops/day and oxazepam (a benzodiazepine) were equally effective in reducing generalized anxiety (Akhondzadeh, Naghavi, Vazirian, Shayeganpour, Rashidi, & Khani, 2001). Significantly, patients taking oxazepam reported significant impairments in job performance at doses that lowered anxiety. In contrast, there were no reports of performance impairment among patients taking effective doses of passionflower extract. Important benefits of passionflower extract (and other herbal treatments) include the absence of excessive daytime sedation and avoidance of the risk of developing tolerance or dependence with prolonged use in chronically anxious patients.

◆ **Ashwagondha may reduce anxiety related to chronic stress** Ashwagondha (*W. somnifera*) is a widely used restorative in Ayurvedic medicine, and is traditionally used to promote feelings of enhanced well-being and to treat cancer, diseases of inflammation, and many psychological symptoms, including chronic stress and anxiety. The anxiety-reducing effects of Ashwagondha are probably related to inhibition of stress-induced dopamine receptors (Sakena, Singh, Dixit, Singh, Seth, & Gupta, 1988). Animal studies suggest that beneficial effects of this herbal remedy are mediated by increased corticosteroid production in the adrenals (Archana & Namasivayam, 1999).

Other Biological Treatments

◆ **The essential oils of lavender and rosemary reduce symptoms of generalized anxiety** Essential oils derived from several species of lavender and other fragrant herbs are widely used to treat anxiety symptoms in the form of aromatherapy or massage. Preliminary evidence suggests that certain essential oils, especially lavender, have moderate antianxiety effects. A randomized controlled trial evaluated changes in EEG and subjective emotional states in 40 adults exposed to lavender or rosemary aromatherapy (Diego et al., 1998). Individuals receiving lavender aromatherapy showed increased β activity and reported decreased state anxiety. Patients receiving rosemary aromatherapy showed decreased frontal α and β power and reported diminished anxiety and increased alertness. These findings suggest that lavender aromatherapy promotes a relaxed drowsy state, and rosemary aromatherapy promotes a relaxed alert state. Although other essential oil preparations are sometimes used to treat anxiety, at present there is not enough evidence to support their use.

◆ **D-Cycloserine may reduce the intensity of phobic anxiety symptoms when combined with exposure therapy** D-cycloserine may function as a cognitive enhancer by stimulating NMDA receptors, and may facilitate extinction of conditioned fear in phobic patients. Animal studies suggest that extinction of a learned fear response is enhanced by D-cycloserine (Walker, Ressler, Lu, & Davis, 2002). In one study 28 individuals with a *DSM-IV* diagnosis of acrophobia were randomized to receive D-cycloserine at 500 mg versus placebo in combination with two sessions of VRGET in a virtual glass elevator environment. Patients receiving D-cycloserine experienced significantly greater improvement in phobic symptoms compared with matched patients undergoing virtual reality exposure therapy alone. This difference was noticeable 1 week following treatment, and was maintained at 3-month follow-up (Ressler et al., 2004).

◆ **Certain Bach flower remedies may reduce test anxiety** Bach flower remedies are widely used as self-administered treatments in North America and Europe for a range of medical and psychological problems, including anxiety. Research findings suggest that certain Bach flower remedies reduce anxiety in some cases. In one double-blind, placebo crossover study, individuals reported significant nonspecific reductions in test anxiety after taking certain Bach flower remedies (Walach, Rilling, & Engelke, 2001).

◆ **DHEA combined with conventional antipsychotic medications may reduce anxiety in schizophrenics** There is substantial evidence that DHEA is an effective treatment of depressed mood; however, few studies have examined possible anxiety-reducing benefits of DHEA. A small double-blind study found that DHEA at 100 mg/day combined with conventional antipsychotic medications significantly improved anxiety, depressed mood, and negative psychotic symptoms in 30 inpatients diagnosed with schizophrenia (Strous et al., 2003).

Vitamins and Minerals

◆ **Niacinamide may reduce generalized anxiety due to hypoglycemia; supplementation with vitamins B$_6$, B$_{12}$, C, and E may reduce the severity of generalized anxiety** Feelings of generalized anxiety are often reported by individuals who are chronically deficient in thiamine and vitamins B$_6$, B$_{12}$, E, and C (Heseker et al., 1992). Several mechanisms of action are probably involved, including diminished conversion of pyruvate to lactate and reduced synthesis of serotonin from dietary L-tryptophan. Two forms of niacin, nicotinamide and niacinamide, reportedly have general calming and quieting effects mediated by GABA, the brain's major inhibitory neurotransmitter (Fomenko, Parkhomets, Stepanenko, & Donchenko, 1994). Anecdotal reports suggest a beneficial calming effect of niacinamide at 1 to 3 g in divided doses in patients whose anxiety is caused by hypoglycemia (Gaby, 1995). Human clinical trials, however, have failed to substantiate a consistent anxiety-reducing effect of niacinamide. Reported calming effects of pyridoxine (vitamin B$_6$) may be related to the fact that this vitamin is an essential cofactor in the synthesis of dopamine, serotonin, and GABA.

◆ **Magnesium may reduce generalized anxiety; phosphorus supplementation may reduce the frequency of panic attacks** Supplementation with magnesium, phosphorus, or selenium is commonly used to treat anxiety and fatigue in naturopathic medicine, although few controlled trials substantiate the use of these minerals for this purpose. Supplemental phosphorus may reduce the frequency of panic attacks in predisposed individuals (Bolon, Yeragani, & Pohl, 1988). Selenium at 100 μg/day (Benton & Cook, 1991) or magnesium at 200 mg/day may improve mood and anxiety in individuals who are deficient in these minerals. The calming effects of magnesium may be enhanced when taken together with calcium (400 mg/day).

Somatic and Mind–Body Approaches

◆ **Animal-facilitated psychotherapy may reduce generalized anxiety** Residing with a pet, having regular contact with a cat, dog, or other domesticated animal, or the regular presence of a domesticated animal during psychotherapy may have general positive effects on emotional well-being and facilitate beneficial physical or psychological responses in anxious individuals (Odendaal, 2002).

◆ **Lucid dreaming may be an effective treatment of traumatized patients who have recurring nightmares** *Lucid dreaming* is a special state of consciousness in which the dreamer is self-aware while dreaming, and able to change or control dream content (LaBerge & Rheingold, 1990). Lucid dreaming takes place during normal rapid eye movement (REM) sleep, which is associated with heightened cortical activation (Brylowski, Levitan, & LaBerge, 1989). Many patients have learned how to "signal" the onset of lucidity to researchers during REM sleep. The recurring vivid nightmares of trauma survivors can be described as a kind of dream-anxiety syndrome. Anecdotal reports and small studies suggest that individuals who have recurring nightmares related to memories of trauma are able to reduce the frequency or intensity of nightmares and experience clinical improvements using lucid dream induction techniques (Brylowski, 1990). Case reports suggest that training in lucid dreaming is probably an effective adjunct to long-term psychotherapy of trauma victims who report intense daytime anxiety and recurring nightmares. Therapeutic training in lucid dreaming methods requires a commitment of 4 to 6 weeks, including daily journaling of dreams and nightmares and weekly sessions for training in lucid dream induction techniques and integration of dream insights with dynamic issues related to themes of a recurrent nightmare.

Different induction techniques have been developed in research settings (Price & Cohen, 1988). A frequently used approach that helps patients to increase their capacity to become lucid is called mnemonic induction of lucid dreaming (MILD). In this approach, before going to sleep the patient repeats to himself or herself, "The next time I am dreaming, I want to remember to realize that I am dreaming."

Case reports suggest that trauma victims experience insights during lucid dreams that translate into measurable clinical improvements in anxiety and mood symptoms when these insights are integrated into long-term psychodynamic therapy (Brylowski et al., 1989). Vietnam War veterans diagnosed with PTSD who had a history of recurring combat-related nightmares were successfully able to change dream content and diminish distressing dream experiences using lucid dreaming methods (Brylowski &McKay, 1991). Veterans who became lucid while dreaming reported being able to remember they were safe at home in bed while dreaming, and to explore and master frightening dream experiences without awakening. However, in most cases agitation or screaming during sleep, hitting spouses while asleep, sleepwalking, and other symptoms did not improve even after patients had learned how to become lucid.

Lucid dreaming methods, including "dialoguing" with or "physically embracing" dream characters, reduce feelings of helplessness and terror as the patient learns that he or she is able to control frightening images or experiences associated with past trauma. Patients who develop skill at lucid dreaming frequently report improved self-confidence in situations that remind them of past trauma.

◆ **Paraspinal electrical stimulation may be effective in some cases of post-traumatic stress disorder** Findings of a case report suggest that the application of pulsed microcurrent along the paraspinal muscles from the base of the skull to the sacrum alleviates symptoms of post-traumatic stress disorder (Gottlieb, 2004). The patient was a 34-year-old torture survivor who had failed to respond to conventional pharmacological and psychotherapy treatments of abdominal pain, nightmares, insomnia, hypervigilance, panic attacks, intrusive thoughts, and irritability. His symptoms had worsened over a 5-year period following his torture, and he had become severely depressed and suicidal. The patient experienced almost complete pain relief following the initial 15-minute treatment, and described "massive euphoria" and difficulty sleeping several hours afterwards. Adverse effects included transient tingling and loss of sensation in small areas of the feet that did not interfere with balance or walking. Subsequent treatments were administered 2 days and 2 weeks later. Symptoms of PTSD initially worsened, but all symptoms had completely disappeared following the third treatment, and the patient's mood remained consistently elevated. He reported being more productive at work and slept less. His marital and social life markedly improved. The patient received 7 more treatments in the following months and had remained asymptomatic for 10 months at the time the case report was written. The researchers attributed the successful outcome to massive release of β endorphins, and suggested that paraspinal electrical stimulation may be a viable alternative to electroconvulsive therapy (ECT) in the treatment of PTSD patients while avoiding the potentially serious adverse effects of ECT including the risk of seizures, post-treatment amnesia, and memory loss.

On the basis of only one case report, this approach must be considered a promising but possibly effective treatment of the severe psychiatric symptoms characteristic of post-traumatic stress disorder. Patients who have been diagnosed with bipolar disorder should be cautioned because of reports of manic symptoms associated with paraspinal stimulation.

Treatments Based on Forms of Energy or Information That Are Not Validated by Western Science

◆ **Healing Touch and Therapeutic Touch may reduce symptoms of stress and generalized anxiety** Most studies done on Healing Touch are pilot studies or small open trials with patients who report anxiety or other cognitive or emotional symptoms in the context of chronic pain, cancer, or other medical conditions. Therapeutic Touch may have beneficial effects in chronically anxious patients (Gagne & Toye, 1994), and in nondemented elderly nursing home patients (Simington & Lang, 1993), but there is limited evidence for anxiety-reducing effects of TT in healthy adults (Collins, 1983). The findings of two studies using sham healers in the control group suggest that both contact and noncontact healing reduces state anxiety in patients hospitalized for heart problems (Heidt, 1979; Quinn, 1982). Unfortunately, neither study adequately controlled for anxiety-reducing effects of medications. Two small open studies suggest that patients who receive HealingTouch therapy experience significant reductions in emotional and physical symptoms associated with trauma (Guevara, Menidas, & Silva, 2002; Wardell, 2000) A small double-blind, sham-controlled trial did not find significant differences in self-reported levels of stress in students treated by Healing Touch practitioners compared with students treated by sham practitioners (Hale, 1986). In one 4-week study, third-year nursing students assigned to one weekly session of Healing Touch plus music versus music only reported significant reductions in transient and chronic stress and improved sleep. Interestingly, among first-year students significant differences between stress levels in the Healing Touch and control group were not reported (Taylor & Lo, 2001).

Negative findings from controlled studies raise the question of a general beneficial effect, a threshold anxiety level above which Healing Touch is ineffective, or a placebo effect related to the quality or frequency of contact between the Healing Touch practitioner and the patient. It has been suggested that different outcomes reflect different skill levels of healers who participate in different studies (Ferguson, 1986).

In spite of the absence of strong empirical evidence, patient satisfaction surveys show that most patients who receive Healing Touch treatments perceive significant benefits to pain and anxiety symptoms (DuBrey, 2004). In one small open study on the perceived effectiveness of Healing Touch, 40% of patients reported that calming effects lasted more than 2 weeks following the end of treatment, and 60% experienced feelings of "spiritual well-being" lasting at least 2 weeks after treatment ended (DuBrey, 2003). The significance of these findings is difficult to interpret because established rating scales were not used to grade symptom severity before and after the trial.

Findings of the above studies should be viewed as preliminary, and suggest that Healing Touch has general beneficial effects on stress and anxiety associated with pain and some medical disorders as well as trauma. However, small sample sizes, inadequate controls, and potential biases preclude generalizations about the clinical benefits of Healing Touch and Therapeutic Touch for anxiety.

◆ **The regular practice of qigong or Tai Chi may reduce symptoms of generalized anxiety and promote overall emotional well-being** Qigong is sometimes practiced in efforts to reduce anxiety, but research findings are limited and inconsistent. Design flaws and small numbers of enrolled patients limit the clinical value of most studies done to date. A review of qigong in mental health care identified five studies on qigong in the treatment of anxiety (Lake, 2001). However, only one open prospective study found consistent anxiety-reducing effects of qigong (Li et al., 1989). In the study 35 adults were randomized to receive qigong versus biofeedback. Qigong was more effective in males (but not females) receiving qigong compared with biofeedback. Other small open studies suggest that regular qigong practice results in decreased subjective feelings of anxiety, possibly mediated by changes in autonomic activity following sustained practice (Kato et al., 1992; Shan et al., 1989).

Tai Chi is an ancient mind–body practice that is similar to qigong. Tai Chi probably has beneficial stress-reducing effects that are comparable to meditation or brisk walking (Jin 1992). A pilot study compared Tai Chi to progressive muscle relaxation in combat veterans diagnosed with PTSD (Hutton et al., 1996). Subjects in the Tai Chi group reported significantly greater decreases in subjective distress compared with the group performing progressive muscle relaxation.

Rare cases of agitation, hysteria, and psychosis have been reported following intensive or "unskillful" qigong practice (Lake, 2001). Psychotic individuals and patients who have been diagnosed with a severe personality disorder should practice qigong only under the guidance of a skillful instructor.

◆ **Case reports and limited research findings suggest that homeopathic preparations may be effective in some cases of generalized anxiety** Homeopathic preparations are widely used to self-treat generalized anxiety and other anxiety symptoms. However, to date research findings on homeopathic remedies for anxiety are inconsistent and based largely on case reports. According to homeopathic theory, anxiety symptoms are associated with different constitutional or personality types corresponding to different homeopathic remedies (Spence, 1990). Case reports of symptomatic improvement following the administration of specific homeopathic remedies have been published for post-traumatic stress disorder (Chapman,, 1993; Morrison, 1993), social phobia, panic disorder (Davidson & Gaylord, 1995; Davidson, Morrison, Shore, Davidson, & Beday, 1997), and obsessive-compulsive disorder (Chand, 1991). The findings of two placebo-controlled studies were negative. Sixty-two students with test anxiety were randomized to a specific homeopathic preparation believed to reduce anxiety (*Argentum nitricum* 12X) versus placebo twice daily for 4 days (Baker, Myers, Hosden, & Brooks, 2003). No significant differences in test anxiety were found between the treatment and placebo groups.

At the time of writing, only one randomized double-blind study has been done on homeopathic remedies for generalized anxiety. In the 10-week prospective study, 44 patients diagnosed with generalized anxiety disorder using *DSM-IV* criteria were randomized to receive an appropriate homeopathic treatment versus placebo. All patients were required to be medication-free at least 1 month before the start of the study. Following enrollment, all patients were individually diagnosed by a classically trained homeopathic physician and treated with a homeopathic remedy addressing identified energetic imbalances. Standardized rating scales were used to assess anxiety symptoms at the start of the study, at midpoint (week 5), and at the end of the study (week 10). Remedies for 5 patients were changed at midpoint following the second assessment. Significant but equivalent improvements in baseline anxiety were found in the placebo and treatment groups at week 5 and at the end of the study. On the basis of these findings, the authors concluded that homeopathic treatments of generalized anxiety are ineffective (Bonne, Shemer, Gorali, Katz, & Shalev, 2003). Biomedical research studies of homeopathy are difficult to perform and probably do not take into account important aspects of treatment selection that are difficult to measure using conventional empirical methods.

◆ **Emotional Freedom Techniques may reduce anxiety symptoms through desensitization and distraction** Emotional Freedom Techniques (EFT) have been investigated as a treatment of specific phobias that are often poorly responsive to conventional exposure desensitization techniques. The use of EFT avoids the risk of retraumatization through in vivo exposure to a small animal, insect, or other phobic stimulus. EFT treatments can be self-administered following an initial training session. No technical expertise is required, and unlike acupuncture, there is no risk of injury or infection. Some case reports suggest that a single EFT treatment can result in rapid improvement in acute anxiety symptoms and that improvement is sustained for months afterwards (Callahan, 2001; Craig, 1999). However, few controlled studies have been done, most studies are methodologically flawed, and findings are highly inconsistent (Herbert & Gaudiano, 2001). In a small pilot study, two 1-hour EFT sessions significantly reduced PTSD symptoms in auto accident victims, and improvements were reportedly sustained for 3 months after treatment ended (Swingle, Pulos, & Swingle, 2001).

In a double blind prospective trial, 35 patients who met *DSM-IV* criteria for a specific phobia were randomized to receive one EFT treatment versus one session of diaphragmatic breathing (DB) while exposed to a feared small animal (Wells, Poglase, Andrews, Carrington, & Baker, 2003). EFT-treated patients reported greater improvement compared with DB-treated patients in four out of five measures of anxiety, and improvements were sustained at 3 months in the absence of further EFT or DB treatments. Possible explanations for observed reductions in anxiety included the effects of conventional desensitization methods. The researchers were careful to avoid concluding that results of this single study demonstrate that EFT rebalances meridian energy or that presumed changes in meridian energy associated with EFT treatment result in reduced anxiety in phobic patients. These findings were subsequently replicated in another study (Baker & Siegel, 2001).

Pooled results from many small pilot studies totaling 29,000 individuals from 11 EFT treatment centers in South America suggest that EFT is more effective in patients diagnosed with any anxiety disorder than combined treatment with cognitive-behavioral therapy and conventional medications (Andrade & Feinstein, 2004). Another study examined EFT and sham-EFT in a nonclinical population, and found no differences in anxiety reduction between sham EFT, a defined EFT protocol, and a sham protocol that consisted of tapping on a doll (Waite & Holder, 2003). The findings of this study do not support the view that EFT stimulates acupuncture meridians and suggests that therapeutic benefits of EFT are attributable to the anxiety-reducing effects of conventional approaches, including desensitization and distraction.

Preliminary evidence suggests that EFT may be an effective alternative to acupuncture or conventional exposure therapies as a treatment of phobias or other anxiety symptoms. Large prospective studies are needed to clarify differences in the effectiveness of EFT, other energy psychology techniques, and conventional desensitization methods.

◆ **Somatoemotional release and craniosacral therapy may be beneficial in some cases of post-traumatic stress**   As in other energy healing methods, a putative mechanism of somatoemotional release and craniosacral therapy has not been empirically demonstrated. Although both techniques are widely used to treat symptoms of psychological or physical trauma, at present there is only limited supporting evidence for their efficacy. A total of 22 Vietnam veterans with a prior diagnosis of post-traumatic stress disorder completed a 2-week intensive program in which they were treated with both craniosacral therapy and somatoemotional release. Pre- and post-treatment assessments showed significant reductions in pain and other symptoms of physical distress, as well as general improvements in depression,

anxiety, suspiciousness, guardedness, and behavioral isolation (Zonderman, 2000). The significance of these findings is limited by the small study size, the absence of a sham treatment arm, lack of follow-up, and the use of nonstandardized symptom rating scales. To date sham-controlled studies have not been conducted, and limited evidence from published case reports does not support the use of these energy methods as treatments of PTSD or other anxiety syndromes. Until there is more convincing evidence, there is no basis for recommending somatoemotional release or craniosacral therapy to trauma survivors or others complaining of anxiety, depression, pain, or other symptoms of physical distress.

◆ **Positive religious attitudes may reduce stress in some cases** Religious attitudes may provide an effective buffer against stress in some individuals, diminishing anxious responses to difficult circumstances. The relationship between religiosity and effective coping strategies is complex and is strongly influenced by the specific religious institutional affiliation and socioeconomic level of the patient, as well as other factors that are difficult to quantify (Kim, Nesselroade, & Featherman, 1996; Koenig, George, Blaze, Pritchett, & Meador, 1993). Cultures that provide a religious framework promoting acceptance of death and other inevitable anxiety-provoking circumstances probably facilitate emotional resilience and lower anxiety during times of personal stress (Thorson, 1998).

◆ **Prayer and distant healing intention may have beneficial effects on anxiety**   Findings of controlled studies suggest that prayer at a distance has beneficial effects on anxiety; however, the effects of group suggestion cannot be ruled out. Patients who were randomly assigned to be prayed for at a distance following pituitary surgery, and who were not aware of being prayed for, reported less postoperative anxiety and required lower doses of pain medications compared with matched patients who were not prayed for (Green, 1993). In another study observed improvements in anxiety and general emotional well-being in 90 volunteers following intercessory prayer were attributed to suggestion (O'Laoire, 1997).

◆ **The Integrative Management Algorithm for Anxiety**

Figure 10–1 is the integrative management algorithm for anxiety. Note that specific assessment and treatment approaches are representative examples of reasonable choices. Moderate symptoms often respond to exercise, dietary modification, mind–body practices, and energy-information therapies. When managing severe symptoms, emphasize biological therapies. Encourage exercise and other lifestyle changes in motivated patients. Consider conventional, nonconventional, and integrative approaches that have not been tried.

See evidence tables and text for complete reviews of evidence-based options.

Before implementing any treatment plan, always check evidence tables and Web site updates at www.thieme.com/mentalhealth for specific assessment and treatment protocols, and obtain patient informed consent.

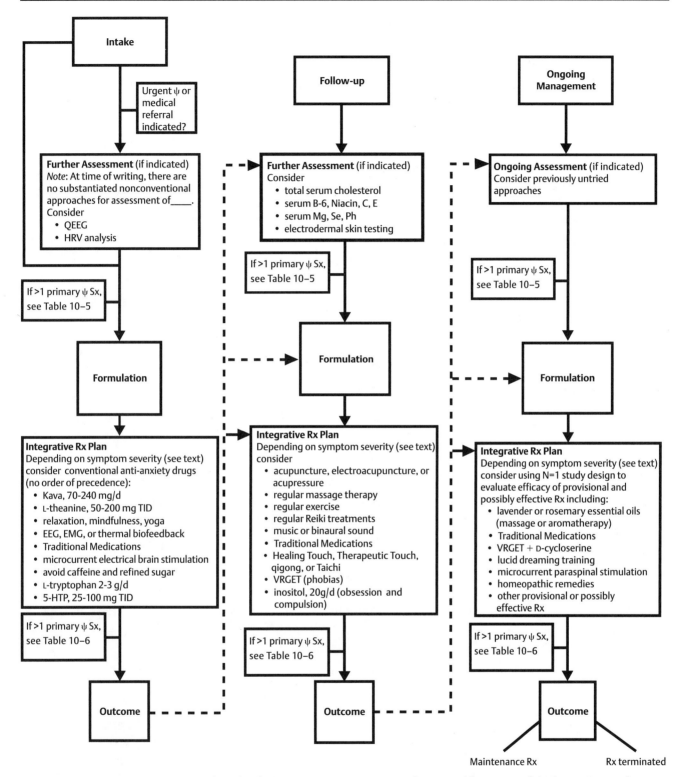

Figure 10–1 Integrative management algorithm for anxiety. Note that specific assessment and treatment approaches are representative examples of reasonable choices. Moderate symptoms often respond to exercise, dietary modification, mind–body practices, and energy-information therapies. Rx, treatment; Sx, symptoms

◆ **Integrated Approaches to Consider When Two or More Core Symptoms Are Present**

Table 10–5 shows the assessment approaches to consider using when anxiety is the focus of clinical attention and one or more other symptoms are being assessed concurrently.

Table 10–6 outlines the treatment approaches to consider using when anxiety is the focus of clinical attention and one or more other symptoms are being treated concurrently.

Table 10–5 Assessment Approaches to Anxiety When Other Symptoms Are Being Assessed Concurrently

Other Symptoms Being Assessed Concurrently	Assessment Approach	Comments
Depressed mood	Serologic studies	Deficiencies of niacin and vitamins B_6, C, and E are sometimes associated with generalized anxiety.
		Limited evidence suggests that total serum cholesterol is elevated in chronically anxious patients.
		Low total serum triglycerides and cholesterol levels correlate with more severe depressed mood and higher risk of suicide.
		Low levels of vitamins B_{12} and E are frequently found in depressed patients
	qEEG brain mapping	Limited evidence suggests that specific qEEG changes correspond to disparate anxiety syndromes.
		In patients diagnosed with OCD, increased α power predicts response to SSRIs, and increased θ power predicts nonresponse to SSRIs.
		Specific qEEG findings may predict differential response of depressed patients to both conventional and nonconventional treatments
Mania and cyclic mood changes	Serologic studies	Low trace lithium levels (i.e., from low nutritional intake) are common in acutely manic patients.
		Limited evidence suggests that pretreatment serum GABA levels predict improved response of mania and cyclic mood changes to divalproex (Depakote) but not other mood stabilizers
	qEEG brain mapping	Limited evidence suggests that pretreatment qEEG findings in acutely manic or cycling patients (showing left-sided abnormalities) predict improved response to conventional treatments
Psychosis	Serologic studies	Limited evidence suggests that abnormally low serum and RBC folate levels correlate with increased risk of schizophrenia and other psychotic syndromes.
		Limited evidence suggests that high pretreatment serum HVA levels predict improved response to lower doses of conventional antipsychotics in acutely manic patients with psychotic symptoms
	qEEG brain mapping	Limited evidence suggests that specific qEEG findings correlate with differential response rates of psychosis to conventional or nonconventional treatments
Cognitive impairment	Serologic studies	Limited evidence suggests that abnormally low serum DHA levels correlate with increased risk of developing Alzheimer's disease
	qEEG brain mapping	qEEG mapping, VEP, and AER studies facilitate early diagnosis and more aggressive treatment of early Alzheimer's and mild cognitive impairment.
		qEEG mapping provides useful information when planning EEG-biofeedback protocols addressing cognitive impairment in general.
		qEEG mapping can be used to evaluate response to conventional and nonconventional cognitive enhancing treatments
Substance abuse or dependence	Serologic studies	In alcohol abuse the magnitude of serum deficiencies of vitamins A and C and some B vitamins, as well as zinc, magnesium, and essential fatty acids, is an indicator of the severity of malnutrition
	qEEG brain mapping	Limited evidence suggests that qEEG brain mapping provides useful information when planning specific EEG-biofeedback protocols for relapsing alcoholics or narcotics abusers
	AER	Conventional treatments of heroin detoxification normalize AER findings
Disturbance of sleep or wakefulness	Serologic studies	Deficiencies in folic acid and vitamins C, E, and B_{12} are correlated with increased daytime sleepiness and insomnia.
		Abnormally low serum levels of magnesium and zinc are often associated with increased daytime sleepiness

AER, auditory evoked response; DHA, docosahexaenoic acid; EEG, electroencephalography; GABA, γ-aminobutyric acid; HVA, homovanillic acid; OCD, obsessive-compulsive disorder; qEEG, quantitative electroencephalography; RBC, red blood cell (count); SSRI, selective serotonin reuptake inhibitor; VEP, visual evoked potential

Table 10–6 Treatment Approaches to Anxiety When Other Symptoms Are Being Treated Concurrently

Other Symptoms Being Treated Concurrently	Treatment Approach	Comments
Depressed mood	Dietary modifications	Limited evidence suggests that avoiding refined sugar and caffeine and increasing protein and foods containing tryptophan reduce symptoms of generalized anxiety and panic.
		Limited evidence suggests that restricting caffeine and refined sugar and increasing consumption of fatty fish and whole foods rich in B vitamins improve depressed mood and reduce the risk of becoming depressed
	L-tryptophan and 5-HTP	L-tryptophan 2–3 g/day or 5-HTP 25–100 mg up to 3 times a day is probably an effective treatment of generalized anxiety.
		Limited evidence suggests that 5-HTP prevents panic attacks.
		5-HTP 300 mg/day is probably as effective as conventional antidepressants for moderate depressed mood
	Exercise	Regular aerobic or strengthening exercise reduces generalized anxiety symptoms, and there is limited evidence that it may reduce may frequency and severity of panic attacks.
		Regular exercise at least 30 minutes 3 times a week is as effective as conventional antidepressants, St. John's wort, and cognitive therapy for moderate depressed mood.
		Exercising under bright light is more effective against depressed than exercise or bright light alone
	Acupuncture	Some acupuncture and electroacupuncture protocols probably reduce symptoms of generalized anxiety.
		Conventional acupuncture may be effective against severe depressed mood
	Combining HRV and EEG-biofeedback	Electroacupuncture alone may be as effective as electroacupuncture combined with amitriptyline or other conventional antidepressants, and there is emerging evidence that computer-controlled electroacupuncture using high-frequency currents is more effective than conventional or standard electroacupuncture.
		EEG, EMG, GSR, and thermal biofeedback are effective treatments of generalized anxiety, and there is limited evidence that regular biofeedback permits dose reductions of conventional drugs.
		Combining GSR biofeedback and relaxation is more effective against anxiety than either approach alone.
		Biofeedback training using HRV probably reduces symptoms of generalized anxiety.
		There is limited evidence that combined EEG-HRV biofeedback (energy cardiology) training improves depressed mood
	Music and binaural sound	Regular listening to soothing music or certain binaural sounds can significantly reduce generalized anxiety.
		Attentive listening to music probably improves moderately depressed mood.
		Combining music with guided imagery is more beneficial than either approach alone.
		Limited evidence suggests that listening to binaural sounds in the beta frequency range (16–24 Hz) improves depressed mood
	Meditation and mindfulness training	Limited evidence suggests that certain meditation practices promote calmness and are beneficial in mania or hypomania.
		Mindfulness training is probably as effective as cognitive therapy in moderate depressed mood
Mania and cyclic mood changes	L-tryptophan and 5-HTP	Limited evidence suggests that L-tryptophan reduces the frequency of depressive mood swings and reduces the severity of mania in bipolar patients.
		L-tryptophan 3 g tid added to lithium may improve symptoms of mania more than lithium alone
Psychosis	DHEA	Combining DHEA 100 mg with a conventional antipsychotic may reduce the severity of negative symptoms and improve symptoms of anxiety and depressed mood
Cognitive impairment	Dietary changes	Moderate wine consumption, reduced saturated fats, and reduced total caloric intake are correlated with reduced risk of developing Alzheimer's disease.
		Limited evidence suggests that diets high in fish or other sources of omega-3 fatty acids and low in omega-6 fatty acids are associated with a reduced risk of developing dementia

(Continued)

Table 10–6 Treatment Approaches to Anxiety When Other Symptoms Are Being Treated Concurrently *(Continued)*

Other Symptoms Being Treated Concurrently	Treatment Approach	Comments
	Ashwagondha (*Withania somnifera*)	Ashwagondha is an Ayurvedic herbal remedy widely used to treat anxiety and chronic stress.
		Note: Individuals who use Ayurvedic herbs should do so only under the supervision of an Ayurvedic physician.
		Ashwagondha 50 mg/kg may improve short- and long-term memory and executive functioning in cognitively impaired individuals.
		Note: Few human trials on Ashwagondha have been published
	DHEA	DHEA 25–50 mg/day may improve mental performance in healthy adults, and 200 mg/day may improve cognitive functioning in vascular dementia
	Music	Regular music therapy probably enhances global functioning in demented individuals, reduces agitation and wandering, enhances social interaction, increases cooperative behavior, and increases baseline cognitive functioning.
		Binaural sounds in the beta frequency range may enhance cognitive functioning in healthy adults
	Microcurrent electrical stimulation	Microcurrent electrical stimulation, including CES, has comparable efficacy to conventional drug treatments of generalized anxiety and phobias, and may permit dose reductions of conventional drugs.
		Limited evidence suggests that microcurrent stimulation improves word recall, face recognition, and motivation in demented individuals
Substance abuse or dependence	Dietary changes	Alcoholics who improve their diets, including reduced intake of refined sugar and caffeine and increased intake of omega-3 fatty acids and protein, probably have an increased chance for maintaining sobriety
	Microcurrent electrical stimulation	Regular CES or TES treatments reduce symptoms of alcohol or opiate withdrawal but not nicotine withdrawal; both approaches reduce anxiety and improve cognitive functioning in alcoholics or drug addicts.
		Note: Optimum therapeutic effects are achieved when specific treatment protocols are employed
	Meditation and mindfulness training	Regular meditation or mindfulness training reduces symptoms of generalized anxiety.
		Mindfulness training reduces the severity of physical symptoms associated with chronic anxiety, including irritable bowel syndrome.
		Abstinent alcoholics and addicts who engage in a regular mindfulness practice or meditation probably have a reduced risk of relapse
Disturbance of sleep or wakefulness	Yoga and other mind–body approaches	Regular yoga practice is beneficial for many anxiety symptoms and may permit reductions in conventional medications.
		Many somatic and mind–body practices. including progressive muscle relaxation, massage, meditation, and guided imagery, are as effective as conventional sedative-hypnotics for mild to moderate insomnia
	Microcurrent electrical stimulation	Limited evidence suggests that microcurrent electrical stimulation is beneficial in some cases of chronic insomnia
	L-tryptophan and 5-HTP	Combining L-tryptophan 2 g with a conventional antidepressant probably enhances antidepressant response and improves sleep quality.
		5-HTP and L-tryptophan probably reduce symptoms of mild or situational insomnia.
		5-HTP increases sleep duration in obstructive sleep apnea and narcolepsy

CES, cranioelectrotherapy stimulation; DHEA, dehydroepiandrosterone; EEG, electroencephalography; EMG, electromyography; 5-HTP, 5-hydroxytryptophan; GSR, galvanic skin response; HRV, heart rate variability; TES, trans-cranial electrical stimulation

Case Vignette

History and Initial Presentation

Steve is a 21-year-old engineering student referred by an emergency room doctor for evaluation and management of chronic anxiety, recent onset panic attacks, and intrusive irrational thoughts. Steve has felt generally anxious since childhood. His first panic attack occurred after studying all night during finals week in his junior year of college. He remembers having sharp chest pains, hyperventilating, and perspiring. He was convinced he was having a heart attack. In the ER Steve's medical workup was unremarkable, including a normal electrocardiogram and chest x-ray, normal cardiac enzymes, and a negative urine toxicology screen. He was given lorazepam 1 mg in the ER and discharged with a prescription for lorazepam 0.5 mg to be taken as needed for recurring panic attacks. He was referred to a psychiatrist in the community.

Steve did not keep his appointment with the psychiatrist and eventually decided to see a cardiologist because he believed the emergency physician had missed a problem having to do with his heart. After reviewing Steve's benign laboratory findings from the ER, including a normal EKG and normal laboratory findings, the cardiologist recommended no further tests and encouraged Steve to see a psychiatrist to address symptoms of generalized anxiety and new onset panic attacks.

Steve felt progressively more anxious during the ensuing months and began to avoid friends. He avoided theaters and shopping malls out of fear that he would have more panic attacks. His second panic attack occurred without warning one afternoon while sitting in front of the campus book store. He was again taken to the ER by paramedics after calling 911, stating that he believed he was having a heart attack. Normal cardiac enzymes and a normal EKG confirmed that Steve's heart was healthy. On reviewing Steve's chart from the initial ER visit 4 months earlier, the on-call physician ordered a psychiatric consultation. After interviewing Steve, the crisis counselor reassured him that his anxiety problem was very real and gave him the names of two local psychiatrists. Steve was discharged from the ER with instructions to take lorazepam 0.5 mg twice daily for 1 week and then as needed for recurring panic episodes, and was referred to a psychiatrist. This time he made an appointment with Dr. Falk, who had a reputation for practicing integrative psychiatry.

Assessment, Formulation and Integrative Treatment Plan

Dr. Falk confirmed that there was no significant medical history, including a history of head injury or seizure disorder, and also confirmed that Steve's panic attacks were spontaneous events. She noted that Steve was sleep deprived and had abused stimulants at the time of his first panic episode. Steve described symptoms of chronic anxiety starting in childhood and more recent symptoms of depressed mood. He denied a history of childhood abuse or recent traumatic experiences, and there was no significant family psychiatric or medical history. Steve felt estranged from people in general, had a very limited social life, and had not exercised for several months, starting around the time of the first panic attack. He had never been in psychotherapy and was a very pragmatic individual who did not appear to be psychologically minded. He reported intrusive thoughts starting at about the time of his initial panic attack, and told Dr. Falk that he had been convinced that he was having a heart attack. Steve disclosed that until 1 week ago (i.e., when he started taking the lorazepam) he had been convinced that he could die at any moment from another heart attack. He denied severe depressed mood and suicidal thoughts, but he reported interrupted sleep and frequent anxious dreams. On mental status examination, his thought process was coherent, and there were no delusions, auditory hallucinations, or paranoid thoughts. Steve disclosed counting to 7 while breathing deeply whenever he found himself worrying about his heart, and denied having these "mental habits" before the time of the first panic attack 4 months ago. He had been using the prescribed lorazepam but was taking twice the recommended dose. He did not take other medications or supplements. Steve described chronic poor nutrition. He often missed breakfast and had a Diet Coke for lunch. He denied symptoms that suggested hypoglycemic episodes during periods of prolonged fasting, and there was no apparent relationship between the timing of panic attacks and his eating habits.

Nevertheless, Dr. Falk decided to order a random serum glucose level. She also ordered a thyroid panel, which had not been part of Steve's initial ER workup.

Dr. Falk's provisional assessment was of a young man with a benign medical history and noncontributory family history who was chronically anxious with a socially avoidant personality and moderately depressed mood and who now reported new onset panic attacks that were not triggered, associated intrusive thoughts, and possibly compulsions. Steve met *DSM-IV* criteria for generalized anxiety disorder but not panic disorder, obsessive-compulsive disorder, major depressive disorder, or a personality disorder. Pending normal results of the thyroid panel and a random glucose level, there were no findings consistent with a medical cause of Steve's symptoms. Dr. Falk recommended improved nutrition, including meals spaced at regular intervals, reduced caffeine consumption, a daily stress management routine, improved sleep hygiene, and exercise. She suggested that Steve consider nonaddictive alternatives to lorazepam, including kava kava, L-theanine, and propranolol. Steve did not wish to try kava because of safety warnings he had read about. He agreed to a trial on L-theanine starting at 200 mg twice daily. Dr. Falk outlined a plan to gradually taper and discontinue routine daily use of the lorazepam after gradually increasing the L-theanine for 1 week, assuming that Steve's baseline anxiety symptoms were adequately controlled. She instructed Steve to use lorazepam no more than once daily only if needed to break a panic attack, and emphasized the importance of good nutrition, physical activity, and an effective daily stress management routine, including possibly meditation, mindfulness training, or yoga. Steve had enjoyed yoga at one time and expressed interest in resuming his former practice. Addressing Steve's moderate insomnia symptoms, Dr. Falk suggested hot baths, relaxing music, and reading during the hours before sleeping. Valerian extract (600 mg) at bedtime was recommended for recurring sleep problems.

At the end of the session, Dr. Falk introduced a few basic ideas from cognitive-behavioral therapy addressing Steve's catastrophic thinking around panic symptoms, and again stressed the importance of regular exercise, good nutrition, and stress management for the management of anxiety.

Two-Week Follow-Up

Steve appeared to be relaxed and rested. He had kept up a daily Yoga practice, had started to walk for 1 hour in the early evening, and had significantly reduced his consumption of caffeine. His serum glucose level had returned in the borderline-low range, and his thyroid studies were normal. Sleep had improved significantly with relaxing music and hot showers before bedtime. He used valerian only occasionally and had taken lorazepam only 3 times for sporadic anxiety symptoms with good effect. There had been no further panic attacks. L-theanine 400 mg twice daily had produced a consistent calming effect, and there were no adverse effects. Steve's mood was somewhat brighter. He had successfully used a Yogic breathing technique and self-talk to reduce anxiety symptoms associated with intrusive thoughts about his heart. Dr. Falk encouraged Steve to continue a daily routine of exercise, good nutrition, and stress reduction while taking his current dose of L-theanine and using valerian extract as needed for sleep and lorazepam only for severe anxiety symptoms. They agreed on a routine 1-month follow-up appointment.

References

Abbey, S. (2004, May). *Mindfulness-based stress reduction groups* [Abstract No. 72C]. Paper presented at the annual meeting of the American Psychiatric Association, New York.

Achterberg, J. (1985). *Imagery in healing: Shamanism and modern medicine.* Boston: New Science Library.

Achterberg, J., Dossey, B., & Kolkmeier, L. (1994). *Rituals of healing: Using imagery for health and wellness.* New York: Bantam Books.

Acolet, D., Modi, N., Giannakoulopoulos, X., Bond, C., Weg, W., Clow, A., & Glover, V. (1993). Changes in plasma and catecholamine concentrations in response to massage in preterm infants. *Archives of Disease in Childhood, 68,* 29–31.

Agelink, M. W., Sanner, D., Eich, H., Pach, J., Bertling, R., Lemmer, W., Klieser, E., & Lehmann, E. (2003). Does acupuncture influence the cardiac autonomic nervous system in patients with minor depression or anxiety disorders? [German]. *Fortschritte der Neurologie-Psychiatrie, 71*(3), 141–149.

Akhondzadeh, S., Naghavi, H. R., Vazirian, M., Shayeganpour, A., Rashidi, H., & Khani, M. (2001). Passionflower in the treatment of generalized anxiety: A pilot double-blind randomized controlled trial with oxazepam. *Journal of Clinical Pharmacy and Therapeutics, 26*(5), 363–367.

Almeida, J. C., & Grimsley, W. (1996). Coma from the health food store: Interaction between kava kava and alprazolam. *Annals of Internal Medicine, 125,* 940–941.

Andrade, J., & Feinstein, D. (2004). Preliminary report of the first large-scale study of energy psychology. In *Energy psychology interactive: An integrated book and CD program for learning the fundamentals of energy psychology.* Ashland, OR: Innersource.

Angst, J. (1994). The epidemiology of obsessive compulsive disorder. In E. Hollander, J. Zohar, D. Marazziti. & B. Olivier (Eds.), *Current insights in obsessive compulsive disorder.* Chichester, UK: Wiley.

Archana, R., & Namasivayam, A. (1999). Antistressor effect of *Withania somnifera. Journal of Ethnopharmacology, 64*(1), 91–93.

Atwater, F. (1999). *The hemi-sync process.* Faber, VA: Monroe Institute.

Baker, A. H., & Siegel, L. (2001). *Effect of emotional freedom techniques upon reduction of fear of rats, spiders and water bugs: A preliminary report of findings.* Paper presented at the annual meeting of the Association for Comprehensive Energy Psychology, Las Vegas, NV.

Baker, D. G., Myers, S. P., Howden, I., & Brooks, L. (2003). The effects of homeopathic argentum nitricum on test anxiety. *Complementary Therapies in Medicine, 2,* 65–71.

Barlow, D. (1988). *Anxiety and its disorders: The nature and treatment of anxiety and panic.* New York: Guilford Press.

Bell, S. J., & Forse, R. A. (1999) Nutritional management of hypoglycemia. *Diabetes Education, 25*(1), 41–47.

Belmaker, R. H., Levine, J. A., & Kofman, O. (1998, June). *Inositol: A novel augmentation for mood disorders* [Abstract No. 84E]. Paper presented at the annual meeting of the American Psychiatric Association, Toronto.

Benjamin, J., Levine, J., Fux, M., et al. (1995). Double-blind placebo-controlled crossover trial of inositol treatment for panic disorder. *American Journal of Psychiatry, 152*(7), 1084–1086.

Benjamin, J., Nemetz, H., Fux, M., Bleichman, I., & Agam, G. (1997). Acute inositol does not attenuate m-CPP-induced anxiety, mydriasis and endocrine effects in panic disorder. *Journal of Psychiatric Research, 31*(4), 489–495.

Benton, D., & Cook, R. (1991). The impact of selenium supplementation on mood. *Biological Psychiatry, 29*(11), 1092–1098.

Bernal, I., Cercos, A., Fuste, I., & Valiverdu, R. (1995). Relaxation therapy in patients with anxiety and somatoform disorders in primary care [Spanish]. *Atencion Primaria, 15*(8), 499–504.

Boerner, R. J., Sommer, H., Berger, W., Kuhn, U., Schmidt, U., & Mannel, M. (2003). Kava-kava extract LI 150 is as effective as opipramol and buspirone in generalised anxiety disorder: An 8-week randomized, double-blind multi-centre clinical trial in 129 out-patients. *Phytomedicine, 10*(Suppl. 4), 38–49.

Bolon, R., Yeragani, V. K., & Pohl, R. (1988). Relative hypophosphatemia in patients with panic disorder. *Archives of General Psychiatry, 45,* 294–295.

Bone ,K. (1993/1994). Kava: A safe herbal treatment for anxiety. *British Journal of Phytotherapy, 3,* 147–153.

Bonne, O., Shemer, Y., Gorali, Y., Katz, M., & Shalev, A. Y. (2003). A randomized, double-blind, placebo-controlled study of classical homeopathy in generalized anxiety disorder. *Journal of Clinical Psychiatry, 64*(3), 282–287.

Botella, C., Banos, R., Guillen, V., et al. (2000). Telepsychology: Public speaking fear treatment on the Internet. *Cyberpsychology and Behavior, 3*(6), 959–968.

Bouchard, S., Paquin, B., Payeur, R., Allard, M., Rivard, V., Fournier, T., Renaud, P., & Lapierre, J. (2004). Delivering cognitive-behavior therapy for panic disorder with agoraphobia in videoconference. *Telemedicine Journal and e-Health, 10*(1), 13–25.

Bouchard, S., Payeur, R., Rivard, V., Allard, M., Paquin, B., Renaud, P., & Goyer, L. (2000). Cognitive behavior therapy or panic disorder with agoraphobia in videoconerence: Preliminary results. *Cyberpsychology and Behavior, 3,* 999–1008.

Bradwejn, J., Zhou, Y., Koszycki, D., & Shlik, J. (2000). A double-blind, placebo-controlled study on the effects of gotu kola (*Centella asiatica*) on acoustic startle response in healthy subjects. *Journal of Clinical Psychopharmacology, 20*(6), 680–684.

British Acupuncture Council. (2002, February). *Depression, anxiety and acupuncture: The evidence for effectiveness* (Briefing Paper No. 9). London: Author.

Bruce, M. S., & Lader, M. (1989). Caffeine abstention in the management of anxiety disorders. *Psychological Medicine, 19,* 211–214.

Brylowski, A. (1990). Nightmares in crisis: Clinical applications of lucid dreaming techniques. *Psychiatric Journal of the University of Ottawa, 15*(2), 79–84.

Brylowski, A., Levitan, L., & LaBerge, S. (1989). H-reflex suppression and autonomic activation during lucid REM sleep: A case study. *Sleep, 12*(4), 374–378.

Brylowski, A., McKay. (1991, April). *Lucid dreaming as a treatment for nightmares in posttraumatic stress of Vietnam combat veterans.* Paper presented at the meeting of the Southern Association for Research in Psychiatry, Tampa, FL.

Burke, J., Regier, A. (1988). Epidemiological catchment area study In J. Talbott, R. Hales, & S. Yudofsky (Eds.), *Textbook of psychiatry.* Washington, DC: American Psychiatric Press.

Bussi, R., Perna, G., Allevi, L., Caldirola, D., & Bellodi, L. (1997, September). *The 35% CO_2 challenge test in patients with generalized anxiety disorder: Preliminary results.* Paper presented at the 10th European College of Neuropsychopharmacology Congress, Vienna.

Callahan, R. J. (2001). Raising and lowering heart rate variability: Some clinical findings of thought field therapy. *Journal of Clinical Psychology, 57*(10), 1175–1186.

Chand, D. (1991, May). *Homeopathy in the treatment of mental disorders: Clinical case, obsessive compulsive disorder.* Paper presented at the 46th Congress of the Liga Medicorum Homeopathica Internationalis, Koln, Germany.

Chapman, E. (1993). The many faces of post-traumatic stress syndrome. *Journal of the American Institute of Homeopathy, 86*(2), 67–71.

Charney, D. S., Heninger, G. R., & Jatlow, P. I. (1985). Increased anxiogenic effects of caffeine in panic disorders. *Archives of General Psychiatry, 42,* 233–243.

Chaudhary, A. K., Bhatnagar, H. N., Bhatnagar, L. K., et al. (1988). Comparative study of the effect of drugs and relaxation exercise (yoga shavasan) in hypertension. *Journal of the Association of Physicians in India, 36*(12), 721–723.

Collins, J. (1983). *The effect of non-contact Therapeutic Touch on the relaxation response.* Master's thesis, Vanderbilt University, Nashville, TN.

Craig, G. (1999). *Emotional Freedom Techniques: The manual.* Coulterville, CA: The Sea Ranch.

Davidson, J., & Gaylord, S. (1995). Meeting of Minds in psychiatry and homeopathy: An example in social phobia. *Alternative Therapies in Health and Medicine, 1*(3), 36–43.

Davidson, J. R., Morrison, R. M., Shore, J., Davidson, R. T., & Bedayn, G. (1997). Homeopathic treatment of depression and anxiety. *Alternative Therapies in Health and Medicine, 3*(1), 46–49.

Davis, M., Eshelman, E., & McKay, M. (1982). *The relaxation and stress reduction workbook* (2nd ed.). Oakland, CA: New Harbinger Press.

Day, S., & Schneider, P. (2002). Psychotherapy using distance technology: Story and science. *Journal of Counseling Psychology, 49,* 499–503.

DeBartolo, P., Hofmann, S., & Barlow, D. (1995). Psychosocial approaches to panic disorder and agoraphobia: assessment and treatment issues for the primary care physician. *Mind/Body Medicine, 1*(3), 133–143.

DeFelice, E. (1997). Cranial electrotherapy stimulation (CES) in the treatment of anxiety and other stress-related disorders: A review of controlled clinical trials. *Stress Medicine, 13,* 31–42.

De Leo, V., La Marca, A., Lanzetta, D., et al. (2000). Assessment of the association of kava-kava extract and hormone replacement therapy in the treatment of postmenopausal anxiety. *Minerva Ginecologica, 52*(6), 263–267.

Delmonte, M. M. (1985). Meditation and anxiety reduction: A literature review. *Clinical Psychology Review, 5,* 91–102.

Diego, M. A., Jones, N. A., & Field, T., Hernandez-Reif, M., Schanberg, S., Kuhn, C., McAdam, V.,Galamaga, R., & Galamaga, M. (1998). Aromatherapy positively affects mood, EEG patterns of alertness and math computations. *International Journal of Neuroscience, 96*(3–4), 217–224.

Difede, J., & Hoffman, H. G. (2002). Virtual reality exposure therapy for World Trade Center post-traumatic stress disorder: A case report. *Cyberpsychology and Behavior, 5*(6), 529–535.

Dragull, K., Yoshida, W. Y., & Tang, C. S. (2003). Piperidine alkaloids from *Piper methysticum*. *Phytochemistry, 63*(2), 193–198.

Dressen, L., & Singg, S. (1998). Effects of Reiki on pain and selected affective and personality variables of chronically ill patients. *Subtle Energies, 9*(1), 51–82.

DuBrey, R. J. (2003). A quality assurance project on the effectiveness of Healing Touch treatments as perceived by patients at the Wellness Institute. In *Healing Touch research summary*. Amsterdam, NY: St. Mary's Hospital.

DuBrey, R. J. (2004). A quality assurance project on the effectiveness of Healing Touch treatments as perceived by patients at the Wellness Institute of St. Mary's Hospital, Amsterdam, NY. In *Healing Touch International, research survey* (4th ed.). Lakewood, CO: Healing Touch International.

Durlach, J., Durlach, V., Bac, P. et al. (1994). Magnesium and therapeutics. *Magnesium Research, 7*(3–4), 313–328.

Eaton, W., Kessler, R., Wittchen, H., & Magee, W. (1994). Panic and panic disorder in the United States. *American Journal of Psychiatry, 151*(3), 413–420.

Eich, H., Agelink, M. W., Lehmann, E., Lemmer, W., & Klieser, E. (2000). Acupuncture in patients with minor depression or generalized anxiety disorders: Results of a randomized study [German]. *Fortschritte der Neurologie Psychiatrie, 68*(3), 137–144.

Emmelkamp, P., Bruynzeel, M., Drost, L., & Van der Mast, C. (2001). Virtual reality treatment in acrophobia: A comparison with exposure in vivo. *Cyberpsychology Behaviour, 4*(3), 335–339.

Epstein, R. M. (1999). Mindful practice. *Journal of the American Medical Association, 282*(9), 833–839.

Ernst, E., & Fialka, V. (1994). The clinical effectiveness of massage therapy—a critical review. *Forsch Komplementarmedizin, 1*, 226–232.

Escher, M., Desmeules, J., Giostra, E., et al. (2001). Hepatitis associated with kava, a herbal remedy for anxiety. *British Medical Journal, 322*, 139.

Fehring, R. J. (1983). Effects of biofeedback-aided relaxation on the psychological stress symptoms of college students. *Nursing Research, 32*(6), 362–366.

Ferguson, C. (1986). *Subjective Experience of Therapeutic Touch Survey (SETTS): Psychometric examination of an instrument*. Doctoral dissertation, University of Texas, Austin.

Field, T., Ironson, G., Scafidi, F., et al. (1996). Massage therapy reduces anxiety and enhances EEG pattern of alertness and math computations. *International Journal of Neuroscience, 86*(3–4), 197–205.

Flaws, B., & Lake, J. (2001). *Chinese medical psychiatry: A textbook and clinical manual*. Boulder, CO: Blue Poppy Press, Book 1, ch. 5; Book 2, ch. 4 and ch. 6; Book 3, ch. 7 and ch. 8.

Fomenko, A., Parkhomets, P., Stepanenko, S., & Donchenko, G. (1994). Participation of benzodiazepine receptors in the mechanism of action of nicotinamide in nerve cells. *Ukraïns'ky Biokhimichny Zhurnal, 66*, 75–80.

Forbes, M. A., Rust, R., & Becker, G. J. (2004). Surface electromyography (EMG) apparatus as a measurement device for biofield research: Results from a single case. *Journal of Alternative and Complementary Medicine, 10*(4), 617–626.

Gaby, A. (1995, December). Vitamin B₃. 2: Powerful tool in nutritional medicine. *Nutrition and Healing*.

Gagne, D., & Toye, R. (1994). The effects of therapeutic touch and relaxation therapy in reducing anxiety. *Archives of Psychiatric Nursing, 8*(3), 184–189.

Gangadhar, B. N., Janakiramaiah, N., Sudarshan, B., et al. (2000, May). *Stress-related biochemical effects of Sudarshan Kriya yoga in depressed patients* (Study No. 6). Paper presented at the Conference on Biological Psychiatry, UN NGO Mental Health Committee, New York.

Glantz, K., Durlach, N., Barnett, R., & Aviles, W. (1996). Virtual reality for psychotherapy: From the physical to the social environment. *Psychotherapy, 33*, 464–473.

Gottlieb, P. D. (2004). Successful treatment of post-traumatic stress disorder and chronic pain with paraspinal square wave stimulation. *Alternative Therapies in Health and Medicine, 10*(1), 92–96.

Green, W. (1993). *The therapeutic effects of distant intercessory prayer and patients' enhanced positive expectations on recovery rates and anxiety levels of hospitalized neurosurgical pituitary patients: A double-blind study*. Doctoral dissertation, California Institute of Integral Studies, San Francisco.

Guevara, E., Menidas, N., & Silva, C. (2002). *Developing a protocol for decreasing post-traumatic stress symptoms in abused women*. Paper presented at the Eighth Nursing Research Pan American Colloquium, Mexico City.

Hale, E. (1986). *A study of the relationship between Therapeutic Touch (TT) and the anxiety levels of hospitalized adults*. Doctoral dissertation, College of Nursing, Texas Woman's University, Denton.

Hale. (2003). The effects of healing touch on stress in college students. In Healing Touch research summary.

Hansel, R. (1996, Winter). Kava-kava in modern drug research: Portrait of a medicinal plant. *Quarterly Review of Natural Medicine*, 259–274.

Heffernan, M. (1995). The effect of a single cranial electrotherapy stimulation on multiple stress measures. *Townsend Letter for Doctors and Patients, 147*, 60–64.

Heidt, P. (1979). *Effect of therapeutic touch on anxiety level of hospitalized patients*. Doctoral dissertation, New York University, New York.

Helzer, J., Robins, L., & McEvoy, E. (1987). Post-traumatic stress disorder in the general population: Findings of the epidemiologic catchment area survey. *New England Journal of Medicine, 317*, 1630–1634.

Herbert, J. D., & Gaudiano, B. (2001). The search for the Holy Grail: Heart rate variability and Thought Field Therapy. *Journal of Clinical Psychology, 57*(10), 1207–1214.

Heseker, H., Kubler, W., Pudel, V., & Westenhoffer, J. (1992). Psychological disorders as early symptoms of a mild-moderate vitamin deficiency. *Annals of the New York Academy of Sciences, 669*, 352–357.

Hughes, J., & Roy, E. (1999). Conventional and quantitative electroencephalography in psychiatry. *Journal of Neuropsychiatry and Clinical Neuroscience, 11*, 190–208.

Hurley, J. D., & Meminger, S. R. (1992). A relapse-prevention program: Effects of electromyographic training on high and low levels of state and trait anxiety. *Perceptual and Motor Skills, 74*(3, Pt. 1), 699–705.

Hutton, D., et al. (1996). *Alternative relaxation training for combat PTSD veterans*. Paper presented at the Third World Conference Acad Exch Med. Qigong.

Ito, K., Nagato, Y., Aoi, N., Juneja, L., Kim, K., Yamamoto, T., & Siugimoto, S. (1998). Effects of L-theanine on the release of alpha-brain waves in human volunteers. *Nippon Nogeika-gaku Kaishi, 72*, 153.

Izzo, A. A., & Ernst, E. (2001). Interactions between herbal medicines and prescribed drugs: A systematic review. *Drugs, 61*(15), 2163–2175.

Jin, P. (1992). Efficacy of Tai Chi, brisk walking, meditation, and reading in reducing mental and emotional stress. *Journal of Psychosomatic Research, 36*(4), 361–370.

Juneja, L. R., Chu, D.-C., Okubo, T., et al. (1999). L-theanine, a unique amino acid of green tea, and its relaxation effect in humans. *Trends in Food Science Technology, 10*, 199–204.

Kabat-Zinn, J. (1990). *Full Catastrophe Living: Using the wisdom of your body and mind to face stress, pain and illness*. New York: Delacorte.

Kabat-Zinn, J., Massion, A. O., Kristeller, J., et al. (1992). Effectiveness of a meditation-based stress reduction program in the treatment of anxiety disorders. *American Journal of Psychiatry,149*(7), 936–943.

Kahn, R. S., Westenberg, H. G., Verhoeven, W. M., et al. (1987). Effect of a serotonin precursor and uptake inhibitor in anxiety disorders: A double-blind comparison of 5-hydroxytryptophan, clomipramine, and placebo. *International Clinical Psychopharmacology, 2*(1), 33–45.

Kakuda, T., Nozawa, A., Unno, T., et al. (2000). Inhibiting effects of theanine on caffeine stimulation evaluated by EEG in the rat. *Bioscience Biotechnology Biochemistry, 64*, 287–293.

Kato, T., Numata, T., & Shirayama, M. (1992). Physiological and psychological study of qigong. *Japanese Mind-Body Science, 1*, 29–38.

Keefer, L., & Blanchard, E. (2001). The effects of relaxation response meditation on the symptoms of irritable bowel syndrome: Results of a controlled treatment study. *Behavior Research and Therapy, 39*(7), 801–811.

Kerr, T., Walsh, J., & Marshall, A. (2001). Emotional change processes in music-assisted reframing. *Journal of Music Therapy, 38*(3), 193–211.

Kessler, R. C., Demler, O., Frank, R. G., Olfson, M., Pincus, H., et al. (2005). Prevalence and treatment of mental disorders. *New England Journal of Medicine, 352*(24), 2515–2523.

Kessler, R. C., McGonagle, K. A., Zhao, S., Nelson, C., Hughes, M., Eshleman, S., Wittehen, H., & Kendler, K. (1994). Lifetime and 12-month prevalence of DSM-III-R psychiatric disorders in the United States: Results from the national comorbidity survey. *Archives of General Psychiatry, 51*, 8–19.

Kim, J., Nesselroade, J., & Featherman, D. (1996). The state component in self-reported world-views and religious beliefs of older adults: The MacArthur Successful Aging Studies. *Psychology and Aging, 11*, 396–407.

Kim, M. S, Cho, K. S., Woo, H., et al. (2002). Effects of hand massage on anxiety in cataract surgery using local anesthesia. *Journal of Cataract Refractory Surgery, 27*(6), 884–890.

Klaassen, T., Klumperbeek, J., Deutz, N. E., van Praag, H. M., & Griez, E. (1998). Effects of tryptophan depletion on anxiety and on panic provoked by carbon dioxide challenge. *Psychiatry Research, 77*(3), 167–174.

Klawansky, S., Yeung, A., Berkey, C., Shah, N., Phan, H., & Chalmers, T. C. (1995). Meta-analysis of randomized controlled trials of cranial electrostimulation: Efficacy in treating selected psychological and physiological conditions. *Journal of Nervous and Mental Disease, 183*(7), 478–484.

Knott, V. J., Bakish, D., Lusk, S., & Barkely, J. (1997). Relaxation-induced EEG alterations in panic disorder patients. *Journal of Anxiety Disorders, 11*(4), 365–376.

Koenig, H., George, L., Blazer, D., Pritchett, J., & Meador, K. (1993). The relationship between religion and anxiety in a sample of community-dwelling older adults. *Journal of Geriatric Psychiatry, 26*, 65–93.

Kraft, M., Spahn, T. W., Menzel, J., et al. (2002). Fulminant liver failure after administration of the herbal antidepressant kava-kava [German]. *Deutsche Medizinische Wochenschrift, 126*, 970–972.

Kramer, N. A. (1990). Comparison of therapeutic touch and casual touch in stress reduction of hospitalized children. *Pediatric Nursing, 16*(5), 483–485.

Kulka, R., Schlenger, W., Fairbank, J., Hough, R., Jordan, B., Marmar, C., & Weiss, D. (1990). *Trauma and the Vietnam War generation: Report of findings from the National Vietnam Veterans Readjustment Study.* New York: Brunner Mazel.

LaBerge, S., & Rheingold, H. (1990). *Exploring the world of lucid dreaming: A workbook of dream exploration and discovery that will help you put the ideas in lucid dreaming into practice.* New York: Ballantine Books.

Lake, J. (2001). Qigong. In *Alternative and complementary therapies in mental health: Innovation and integration* (ch. 9). New York: Academic Press.

Li, L, Qin, C., Yang, S., Wei, B., Jiang, S., Du, C., et al. (1989). *A comparative study of qigong and biofeedback therapy.* Paper presented at the Second International Conference on Qigong.

Malathi, A., & Damodaran, A. (1999). Stress due to exams in medical students: Role of yoga. *Indian Journal of Physiology and Pharmacology, 43*(2), 218–224.

Malsch, U., & Kieser, M. (2001). Efficacy of kava-kava in the treatment of non-psychotic anxiety, following pretreatment with benzodiazepines. *Psychopharmacology, 157*(3), 277–283.

Maltby, N., Kirsch, I., Mayers, M., & Allen, G. J. (2002). Virtual reality exposure therapy for the treatment of fear of flying: a controlled investigation. *Journal of Consulting and Clinical Psychology, 70*(5), 1112–1118.

Manchanda, M., & McLaren, P. (1998). Cognitive behavior therapy via interactive video. *Journal of Telemedicine and Telecare, 4*(Suppl. 1), 53–55.

Mason, R. (2001). 200 mg of Zen: L-theanine boosts alpha waves, promotes alert relaxation. *Alternative and Complementary Therapies, 7,* 91–95.

Mathews, J. D., Riley, M. D., Fejo, L., et al. (1988). Effects of the heavy usage of kava on physical health: Summary of a pilot survey in an aboriginal community. *Medical Journal of Australia, 148,* 548–555.

McCleane, G., & Watters, C. (1990). Pre-operative anxiety and serum potassium. *Anaesthesia, 45*(7), 583–585.

McCraty, R., Atkinson, M., & Tomasino, D. (2001). *Science of the heart: Exploring the role of the heart in human performance-an overview of research conducted by the Institute of HeartMath* (Pub. No. 01–001). Boulder Creek, CA: HeartMath Research Center.

McCraty, R., Barrios-Choplin, B., Rozman, D., Atkinson, M., & Watkins, A. (1998). The impact of a new emotional self-management program on stress, emotions, heart rate variability, DHEA and cortisol. *Integrative Physiological and Behavioral Science, 33*(2), 151–170.

McCraty, R., Tomasino, B., Atkinson, M., & Sundram, J. (1999). Impact of HeartMath self-management skills program on physiological and psychological stress in police officers (Pub. No. 99–075). Boulder Creek, CA: HeartMath Research Center.

McKechnie, A. A., Wilson, F., Watson, N., et al. (1983). Anxiety states: A preliminary report on the value of connective tissue massage. *Journal of Psychosomatic Research, 27*(2), 125–129.

Miller, J. J., Fletcher, K., & Kabat-Zinn, J. (1995). Three-year follow-up and clinical implications of a mindfulness meditation-based stress reduction intervention in the treatment of anxiety disorders. *General Hospital Psychiatry,17*(3), 192–200.

Moran, M. (2004, August 20). Structured interview helps make correct diagnosis. *Psychiatric News,* pp. 27, 33.

Morrison, R. (1993). Materia medica of post-traumatic stress disorder. *Journal of the American Institute of Homeopathy, 86*(2), 110–118.

O'Laoire, S. (1997). An experimental study of the effects of distant, intercessory prayer on self-esteem, anxiety, and depression. *Alternative Therapies in Health and Medicine, 3*(6), 38–53.

Odendaal, J. (2002). *Pets and our mental health: The why, the what and the how.* New York: Vantage Press.

Okvat, H. A., Oz, M. C., Ting, W., et al. (2002). Massage therapy for patients undergoing cardiac catheterization. *Alternative Therapies in Health and Medicine, 8*(3), 68–75.

Osei-Tutu, K. E., & Campagna, P. D. (1998). Psychological benefits of continuous vs. intermittent moderate intensity exercise [Abstract]. *Medicine Science Sports Exercise, 30* (Suppl. 5), 117.

Ossebaard, H. C. (2000). Stress reduction by technology? An experimental study into the effects of brainmachines on burnout and state anxiety. *Applied Psychophysiology and Biofeedback, 2,* 93–101.

Ost, L. G., & Breitholtz, E. (2000). Applied relaxation vs. cognitive therapy in the treatment of generalized anxiety disorder. *Behaviour Research and Therapy, 38*(8), 777–790.

Overcash, S. (1999). A retrospective study to determine the effect of cranial electrotherapy stimulation (CES) on patients suffering from anxiety disorders. *American Journal of Electromedicine, 16*(1), 49–51.

Palatnik, A., Frolov, K., Fux, M., & Benjamin, J. (2001). Double-blind, controlled, crossover trial of inositol versus fluvoxamine for the treatment of panic disorder. *Journal of Clinical Psychopharmacology, 21*(3), 335–339.

Paluska, S. A., & Schwenk, T. L. (2000). Physical activity and mental health. *Sports Medicine, 29*(3), 167–180.

Panjwani, U., Gupta, H. L., Singh, S. H., et al. (1995). Effect of sahaja yoga practice on stress management in patients of epilepsy. *Indian Journal of Physiology and Pharmacology, 39*(2), 111–116.

Pertaub, D., Slater, M., & Barker, C. (2001). An experiment on fear of public speaking in virtual reality. In J. Westwood, H. Hoffman, G. Mogel, & D. Stredney (Eds.), *Medicine meets virtual reality.* Amsterdam: IOS Press.

Peter, H., Tabrizian, S., & Hand, I. (1997, May). *Serum cholesterol in patients with OCD during treatment with behavior therapy and fluvoxamine versus placebo* [Abstract]. Paper presented at the annual meeting of the American Psychiatric Association, San Diego, CA.

Peter, H., Tabrizian, S., & Hand, I. (2000). Serum cholesterol in patents with obsessive compulsive disorder during treatment with behavior therapy and ssri or placebo. *International Journal of Psychiatry in Medicine, 30*(1), 27–39.

Pittler, M. H., & Ernst, E. (2000). Efficacy of kava extract for treating anxiety: Systematic review and meta-analysis. *Journal of Clinical Psychopharmacology, 20*(1), 84–89.

Price, R., & Cohen, D. (1988). Lucid dream induction: An empirical evaluation. In J. Gackenbach & S. LaBerge (Eds.), *Conscious mind, sleeping brain: Perspectives on lucid dreaming* (ch. 6). New York: Plenum Press.

Princhep, L., Mas, F., Hollander, E., et al. (1993). Quantitative electroencephalographic (QEEG) subtyping of obsessive-compulsive disorder. *Psychiatry Research, 50,* 25–32.

Quinn, J. (1982). *An investigation of the effect of therapeutic touch without physical contact on state anxiety of hospitalized cardiovascular patients.* Doctoral dissertation, New York University, New York.

Rees, B. L. (1995). Effect of relaxation with guided imagery on anxiety, depression, and self-esteem in primiparas. *Journal of Holistic Nursing, 13*(3), 255–267.

Ressler, K., Rothbaum, B., Tannenbaum, L., Anderson, P., Graap, K., Zimand, E., Hodges, L., & Davis, M. (2004). Cognitive enhancers as adjuncts to psychotherapy: Use of D-cycloserine in phobic individuals to facilitate extinction of fear. *Archives of General Psychiatry, 61,* 1136–1144.

Rice, K. M., Blanchard, E. B., & Purcell, M. (1993). Biofeedback treatments of generalized anxiety disorder: Preliminary results. *Biofeedback and Self-Regulation, 18*(2), 93–105.

Riva, G., Alcaniz, A., Anolli, L., Bacchetta, M., Banos, R., Beltrame, F., et al. (2001). The VESPY updated project: Virtual environments in clinical psychology. *Cyberpsychology and Behaviour, 4*(4), 449–455.

Robins, L., Helzer, J., Weissman, M., et al. (1984). Lifetime prevalence of psychiatric disorders at three sites. *Archives of General Psychiatry, 41,* 949–959.

Roome, J. R., & Romney, D. M. (1985). Reducing anxiety in gifted children by inducing relaxation. *Roeper Review, 7*(3), 177–179.

Rothbaum, B. O., & Hodges, L. F. (1999). The use of virtual reality exposure in the treatment of anxiety disorders. *Behavior Modification, 23*(4), 507–525.

Rothbaum, B., Hodges, L., & Smith, S. (1999). Virtual reality exposure therapy abbreviated treatment manual: Fear of flying application. *Cognite and Behavioral Practice, 6*(3), 234–244.

Rothbaum, B., Smith, S., Hodges, L., & Lee, J. (2000). A controlled study of virtual reality exposure therapy for the fear of flying. *Journal of Consulting and Clinical Psychology, 68*(6), 1020–1026.

Russell, P., Bakker, D., & Singh, N. (1987). The effects of kava on alerting and speed of access of information from long-term memory. *Bulletin of the Psychonomic Society, 25,* 236–237.

Sakena, A., Singh, S., Dixit, K., Singh, N., Seth, P., & Gupta, G. (1988). Effect of *Withania somnifera* and *Panax ginseng* on dopaminergic receptors in rat brain during stress. In *Proceedings of the 36th Annual Congress on Medicinal Plant Research* (p. 28). Stuttgart and New York: Thieme.

Sarkar, P., Rathee, S. P., & Neera, N. (1999). Comparative efficacy of pharmacotherapy and bio-feedback among cases of generalised anxiety disorder. *Journal of Projective Psychology and Mental Health, 6*(1), 69–77.

Scandrett, S. L, Bean, J. L., Breeden, S., & Powell, S. (1986). A comparative study of biofeedback and progressive relaxation in anxious patients. *Issues in Mental Health Nursing, 8*(3), 255–271.

Schmitt, R., Capo, T., & Boyd, E. (1986). Cranial electrotherapy stimulation as a treatment for anxiety in chemically dependent persons. *Alcoholism, Clinical and Experimental Research, 10*(2), 158–160.

Schroeder, M. J., & Barr, R. E. (2001). Quantitative analysis of the electroencephalogram during cranial electrotherapy stimulation. *Clinical Neurophysiology, 112*(11), 2075–2083.

Schruers, K., Pols, H., Overbeek, T., van Beek, N., & Griez, E. (2000). 5-hydroxytryptophan inhibits 35% CO_2 induced panic. *International Journal of Neuropsychopharmacology 3*(Suppl. 1), S272.

Schulz, V., Hansel, R., & Tyler, V. (2001). *Rational phytotherapy: A physician's guide to herbal medicine* (4th ed.). Berlin: Springer.

Serepca, B. (1996, September). Interview with Dr. Tiffany Field, PhD, director of the Touch Research Institute. *Massage, 63.*

Shah, L. P., Nayak, P. R., & Sethi, A. (1993). A comparative study of Geriforte in anxiety neurosis and mixed anxiety-depressive disorders. *Probe, 32*(3), 195.

Shan, H., et al. (1989). *A preliminary evaluation on Chinese qigong treatment of anxiety.* Paper presented at the Second International Conference on Qigong.

Shannahoff-Khalsa, D. S., Ray, L. E., Levine, S., et al. (1999). Randomized controlled trial of yogic meditation techniques for patients with obsessive-compulsive disorder. *CNS Spectrums, 4*(12), 34–47.

Shore, A. G. (2004). Long-term effects of energetic healing on symptoms of psychological depression and self-perceived stress. *Alternative Therapies in Health Medicine, 10*(3), 42–48.

Shulman, K. R., & Jones, G. E. (1996). The effectiveness of massage therapy intervention on reducing anxiety in the workplace. *Journal of Applied Behavioral Science, 32*(2), 160–173.

Sierles, F., Chen, J., McFarland, R., & Taylor, M. (1983). Post-traumatic stress disorder and concurrent psychiatric illness: A preliminary report. *American Journal of Psychiatry, 140,* 1177–1179.

Simington, J., & Laing, G. (1993). Effects of Therapeutic Touch on anxiety in the institutionalized elderly. *Clinical Nursing Research, 2(4),* 438–450.

Singh, Y. N., & Blumenthal, M. (1996). Kava: An overview. *Herbalgram Special Review, 39,* 33–55.

Smith, R., & Shiromoto, F. (1992). The use of cranial electrotherapy stimulation to block fear perception in phobic patients. *Journal of Current Therapeutic Research, 51*(2), 249–253.

Soderpalm, B., & Engel, J. A. (1990). Serotonergic involvement in conflict behavior. *European Neuropsychopharmacology, 1*(1), 7–13.

Spence, D. (1990). Day to day management of anxiety and depression. *British Homeopathic Journal, 79,* 39–44.

Spiegel, H., & Spiegel, D. (1978). *Trance and treatment.* New York: Basic Books, pp. 22–23.

Stevinson, C. (1999). Exercise may help treat panic disorder. *Focus on Alternative and Complementary Therapies, 4*(2), 84–85.

Stouffer, D., Kaiser, D., Pitman, G., Rolf, W. (2003) Electrodermal testing to measure the effect of a Healing Touch treatment. Healing Touch Research Summary. *Journal of Holistic Nursing.*

Stough, C., Lloyd, J., Clarke, J., Downey, L. A., Hutchison, C. W., Rodgers, T., & Nathan, P. J. (2001). The chronic effects of an extract of *Bacopa monniera* (Brahmi) on cognitive function in healthy human subjects. *Psychopharmacology (Berlin), 156*(4), 481–484.

Strous, R. D., Maayan, R., Lapidus, R., Stryjer, R., Lustig, M., Kotler, M., & Weizman, A. (2003). Dehydroepiandrosterone augmentation in the management of negative, depressive, and anxiety symptoms in schizophrenia. *Archives of General Psychiatry, 60*(2), 133–141.

Swingle, P., Pulos, L., & Swingle, M. (2001, May). *Effects of a meridian-based therapy, EFT, on symptoms of PTSD in auto accident victims.* Paper presented at the annual meeting of the Association for Comprehensive Energy Psychology, Las Vegas, NV.

Taylor, B. (2001, February). The effects of healing touch on the coping ability, self-esteem and general health of undergraduate nursing students. *Complementary Therapies in Nursing and Midwifery,* pp. 34–42.

Thorson, J. (1998). Religion and anxiety: Which anxiety? Which religion? In H. Koenig (Ed.), *Handbook of religion and mental health* (pp. 147–160). San Diego, CA: Academic Press.

Titlebaum, H. M. (1988). Relaxation. *Holistic Nursing Practice, 2*(3), 17–25.

Uhde, T., et al. (1984). Caffeine and behavior: Relation to psychopathology and underlying mechanisms. *Psychopharmacology Bulletin, 20*(3), 426–430.

Vanathy, S., Sharma, P. S. V. N, & Kumar, K. B. (1998). The efficacy of alpha and theta neurofeedback training in treatment of generalized anxiety disorder. *Indian Journal of Clinical Psychology, 25*(2), 136–143.

Vincelli, F., Anolli, L., Bouchard, S., Wiederhold, B., Zurloni. V., & Riva, G. (2003). Experiential cognitive therapy in the treatment of panic disorders with agoraphobia: A controlled study. *Cyberpsychology and Behavior, 6*(3), 321–328.

Vincelli, M., Choi, Y., Molinari, E., Wiederhold, B., & Riva, G. (2000). Experiential cognitive therapy for the treatment of panic disorder with agoraphobia: Definition of a protocol. *Cyberpsychology and Behavior, 3*(3), 375–385.

Waite, W., & Holder, M. (2003, Spring/Summer). Assessment of the emotional freedom technique: An alternative treatment for fear. *Science Review of Mental Health Practice, 2*(1), 20–26.

Walach, H., Rilling, C., & Engelke, U. (2001). Efficacy of Bach-flower remedies in test anxiety: A double-blind, placebo-controlled, randomized trial with partial crossover. *Journal of Anxiety Disorders, 15*(4), 359–366.

Walker, D., Ressler, K., Lu, K., & Davis, M. (2002). Facilitation of conditioned fear extinction by systemic administration or intra-amygdala infusions of D-cycloserine as assessed with fear-potentiated startle in rats. *Journal of Neuroscience, 22,* 2343–2352.

Waller, D. (2002). *DABT's review of adverse events reportedly associated with kava.* Silver Spring, MD: American Herbal Products Association.

Wang, S. M., & Kain, Z. N. (2001). Auricular acupuncture: A potential treatment for anxiety. *Anesthesia and Analgesia, 92*(2), 548–553.

Wardell, W. (2000). The trauma release technique: How it is taught and experienced in Healing Touch. *Alternative and Complementary Therapies, 6*(1), 20–27.

Watkins, L. L., Connor, K. M., & Davidson, J. R. (2001). Effect of kava extract on vagal cardiac control in generalized anxiety disorder: Preliminary findings. *Journal of Psychopharmacology, 15*(4), 283–286.

Webb, W., & Gehi, M. (1981). Electrolyte and fluid imbalance: Neuropsychiatric manifestations. *Psychosomatics, 22*(3), 199–203.

Weissman, M., Klerman, G., Markowitz, J., et al. (1990). Suicidal ideation and suicide attempts in panic disorder and panic attacks. *New England Journal of Medicine, 321*(18),1209–1214.

Weissman, M., & Merikangas, K. (1986). The epidemiology of anxiety and panic disorders: An update. *Journal of Clinical Psychopharmacology, 46*(Suppl. 6), 11–17.

Wells, S., Polglase, K., Andrews, H. B., Carrington, P., & Baker, A. H. (2003). Evaluation of a meridian-based intervention, Emotional Freedom Techniques (EFT), for reducing specific phobias of small animals. *Journal of Clinical Psychology, 59*(9), 943–966.

Wenck, L. S., Leu, P. W., & D'Amato, R. C. (1996). Evaluating the efficacy of a biofeedback intervention to reduce children's anxiety. *Journal of Clinical Psychology, 52*(4), 469–473.

Westen, D., & Morrison, K. (2001). A multidimensional meta-analysis of treatments for depression, panic and generalized anxiety disorder: An empirical examination of the status of empirically supported therapies. *Journal of Consulting and Clinical Psychology, 69*(6), 875–899.

Wiederhold, B., Jang, D., Gevirtz, R., Kim, S., Kim, Y., & Wiederhold, M. (2002). The treatment of fear of flying: A controlled study of imaginal and virtual reality graded exposure therapy. *IEEE Transactions on Information Technology in Biomedicine, 6*(3), 218–223.

Wiederhold, B., & Wiederhold, M. (2005). Side effects and contraindications. In *Virtual reality therapy for anxiety disorders: Advances in evaluation and treatment* (ch. 5). Washington, DC: American Psychological Association.

Zahourek, R. (1998). Imagery. *Alternative Health Practitioner, 4*(3), 203–231.

Zang, D. X. (1991). A self body double blind clinical study of L-tryptophan and placebo in treated neurosis. *Zhonghua Shen Jing Jing Shen Ke Za Zhi, 24*(2), 77–80, 123–124. Chinese.

Zonderman, R. (2000). *The Upledger Foundation Vietnam veteran intensive program.* Palm Beach, FL: The Upledger Institute.

11

Integrative Management of Psychosis

The judicious use of nonconventional therapies in conjunction with established conventional treatments of schizophrenia and other psychotic syndromes holds promise for enhancing outcomes while potentially reducing risks of serious adverse effects associated with conventional antipsychotics and improving the patient's overall level of functioning and quality of life.

◆ Background

Causes of Schizophrenia and Other Psychotic Syndromes Are Poorly Understood

Approximately 1% of the world adult population fulfills criteria established by the fourth edition of the *Diagnostic and Statistical Manual of Mental Disorders* (*DSM-IV*) for schizophrenia or another syndrome characterized by chronic psychosis. Many

theories have been advanced in efforts to explain the pathogenesis of schizophrenia. Close relatives of schizophrenics have a 10 times greater risk of developing schizophrenia compared with the population at large (Gottesman, 1991). However, the findings of twin studies show that a significant part of the risk of developing schizophrenia cannot be attributed to genetic factors (Kringlen, 1995). Genetic theories of schizophrenia have been further weakened by the failure of genetic linkage studies to identify specific genes or mutations that are consistently associated with schizophrenia. Adoption studies suggest that genetically determined vulnerability plays a significant role, and the risk of developing schizophrenia in the adopted offspring of a schizophrenic parent is a function of both genetic predisposition and exposure to psychopathology in the adoptive parents. Offspring of schizophrenics who are adopted by high-functioning parents are at significantly lower risk of developing schizophrenia compared with those adopted by parents who have psychotic syndromes or other chronic severe mental illnesses (Wahlberg et al., 1997). Exposure of the fetal brain to the influenza virus during the second trimester of pregnancy is correlated with a significantly increased risk of adult-onset schizophrenia (Munk-Jørgensen & Ewald, 2001). Correlations have also been found between obstetric complications at the time of birth and an increased risk of schizophrenia (Dassa et al., 1996). Abnormal development of certain brain circuits during critical fetal growth periods has been proposed as a general neurodevelopmental model of schizophrenia (Tsuang, Stone, & Faraone, 2001).

It is likely that complex interactions between disparate environmental, genetic, and nongenetic biological factors contribute to the risk of developing schizophrenia (McGuffin et al., 1994). One controversial hypothesis for which there is limited direct evidence ascribes the complex findings of schizophrenia to the end product of a transmethylation reaction involving norepinephrine, resulting in the formation of hallucinogenic compounds in the brain (Smythies, 1997). According to this theory, imbalances or deficiencies of several vitamins, minerals, and other nutritional factors, including tryptophan, vitamins B_3, B_6, and B_{12}, ascorbic acid, essential fatty acids, and zinc, potentially affect normal biosynthetic pathways, resulting in dyregulation of neurotransmitters and, subsequently, psychotic symptoms (Smythies, Gottfries, & Regland, 1997).

Western Diagnostic Criteria for Psychotic Disorders Continue to Evolve

Western diagnostic criteria used to define schizophrenia and other psychotic syndromes have undergone considerable evolution in recent decades, reflecting emerging findings about the course, causes, and duration of schizophrenia and other symptom patterns characterized by psychosis. Successive editions of the *DSM* have defined schizophrenia and other psychotic disorders on the basis of different core criteria of symptom type, duration, and presumed etiology. The three major psychotic symptom patterns defined in the current version of the *DSM* are distortions in the perception of reality; impairment in the capacity to reason, speak, or behave rationally; and impairment in the capacity to respond socially with appropriate affect and motivation (Fauman, 1994). *DSM-IV* criteria have placed renewed emphasis on the importance of so-called negative symptoms, including flat affect, paucity of thought, and paucity of speech. Negative symptoms are contrasted to so-called positive symptoms of auditory hallucinations, delusions, paranoia, disorganized speech, catatonic behavior, and ideas of reference that have historically been regarded by Western psychiatry as the most important symptoms of schizophrenia and other psychotic disorders. Positive and negative psychotic symptoms compose the core criteria (referred to as criteria A symptoms) required for a diagnosis of schizophrenia and other psychotic disorders. The *DSM-IV* stipulates that two or more criteria A symptoms must persist for at least 1 month (the "active" phase of illness) before a diagnosis of **schizophrenia** can be made. Severe impairment in social and occupational functioning, a minimum duration of symptoms (including a so-called prodromal phase that sometimes takes place prior to the active phase), and residual symptoms following the initial active phase are required before a diagnosis of schizophrenia can be made. The total duration of all phases of the illness must be at least 6 months. Five subtypes of schizophrenia have been put

forward with respect to the dominant symptom pattern of psychosis: paranoid type, disorganized type, catatonic type, undifferentiated type, and residual type.

Other *DSM-IV* psychotic disorders are characterized by symptoms of shorter duration. A psychotic symptom pattern that resolves within 1 month is called a brief psychotic disorder. A psychotic syndrome of intermediate duration (longer than 1 month but shorter than 6 months) is called schizophreniform disorder. Delusional disorder is diagnosed when a "nonbizarre" (i.e., within the cultural context of the patient) delusion persists at least 1 month in the absence of other prominent psychotic or mood symptoms. Schizoaffective disorder is another *DSM-IV* psychotic disorder in which depressed, manic, or mixed mood symptoms take place for a "substantial" period during the active phase (i.e., the period of time when criteria A are fulfilled), in which delusions or hallucinations occur for at least 2 weeks in the absence of prominent mood symptoms.

Schizophrenia, schizophreniform disorder, delusional disorder, brief psychotic disorder, and schizoaffective disorder can be diagnosed only when other psychiatric disorders with overlapping symptoms have been excluded, and medical causes and substance abuse have been ruled out as causes. However, the *DSM-IV* also includes psychotic disorders in which a medical condition or substance abuse is the identified cause of psychosis.

Psychotic Symptom Patterns Do Not Clearly Segregate According to *DSM-IV* Disorders

Many individuals experience transient or chronic psychosis in the context of a mental or medical illness. However, relatively few patients fulfill the complex criteria of psychotic symptoms, severity, and duration required to formally diagnose the subtypes of schizophrenia or the other *DSM-IV* psychotic disorders.

In clinical practice disparate psychotic symptom patterns seldom segregate into different populations according to *DSM-IV* criteria. Psychotic patients who have prominent delusions often have prominent negative symptoms that are missed because the focus of attention is on the treatment of delusions or other so-called positive symptoms. The interpretation of a delusional belief as "bizarre" is clearly related to the cultural lens of the mental health professional making that judgment. What is bizarre in the context of one culture is frequently regarded as within the range of normal thought or behavior in a different culture. The prodromal phase of schizophrenia or another psychotic symptom pattern can only be established retrospectively, and in the absence of close monitoring, the residual phase is often difficult to distinguish from the patient's baseline social or psychological functioning. Individuals who experience predominantly negative symptoms are sometimes misdiagnosed as withdrawn and chronically depressed. Patients who have a history of psychosis in the context of repeated episodes of mania or persisting cyclic mood changes are frequently diagnosed with bipolar disorder (and not schizoaffective disorder) because it is difficult to determine from self-reported history whether an isolated psychotic episode occurred in the absence of mood symptoms. Many Western psychiatrists view schizoaffective disorder as a "garbage" diagnosis, and there is ongoing debate over whether this disorder has construct validity as a diagnostic entity. Patients who fulfill strict *DSM-IV* criteria for schizoaffective disorder are often subsequently diagnosed with either schizophrenia or bipolar disorder. For these reasons it is likely that future versions of the *DSM* will either omit schizoaffective disorder as a discrete entity or substantially modify criteria used to diagnose it.

The accurate Western psychiatric diagnosis of any psychotic disorder becomes even more problematic when differences in professional training, practical difficulties in obtaining reliable patient history, and the cognitive- and affective-blunting effects of conventional antipsychotics on baseline functioning are taken into account. In Western countries the majority of chronically psychotic patients have been taking conventional antipsychotic medications for many years. Significant impairments in cognitive functioning and other adverse neurological effects are frequently associated with prolonged use of conventional antipsychotic medications, giving the appearance of negative symptoms, including cognitive blunting, social withdrawal, and diminished spontaneous behavior. Although some positive psychotic symptoms respond to conventional treatments, negative symptoms are poorly responsive to most conventional antipsychotic medications. Furthermore, chronically psychotic patients are frequently unable to describe changes in positive or negative symptoms over time.

◆ The Integrative Assessment of Psychosis

Overview of Conventional Approaches Used to Assess Psychosis

At present, there are no specific biological markers for schizophrenia or other symptom patterns of chronic psychosis. Brain-imaging studies have identified nonspecific changes that occur at relatively higher rates in schizophrenic patients, including enlargement of the ventricles and structural abnormalities in the temporal lobes. Conventionally trained mental health professionals rely on the history and mental status examination when assessing a psychotic patient. Collateral information from a reliable third party, including a family member or friend, is helpful when confirming the history and course of illness. In unusual cases, brain tumors, hyperthyroidism (or other endocrinological disease), seizure disorders, systemic lupus erythematosus (SLE), or other medical illnesses may result in symptoms that resemble schizophrenia. Chronic substance abuse, especially of stimulants or hallucinogens, can result in a chronic psychotic state. In Western medicine it is first necessary to rule out a primary medical cause before a psychiatric disorder can be diagnosed or appropriately treated. After conventional treatment has been initiated, effectiveness is assessed on the basis of beneficial changes in positive and negative symptoms using standardized instruments (e.g., the Positive and Negative Symptom Scale, or PANSS). Less tangible outcome measures are also important indicators of successful treatment. These include improved quality of life, enhanced social skills, and improved capacity for successful vocational rehabilitation.

Overview of Nonconventional Approaches Used to Assess Psychosis

At the time of writing, nonconventional approaches used to assess psychosis are not substantiated by consistent or reliable research findings. However, many promising biological assays are on the horizon. Four biological assessment approaches are supported by provisional evidence at this time:

◆ Red blood cell (RBC) fatty acid levels
◆ Serum and RBC folate levels
◆ Serum dehydroepiandrosterone (DHEA) levels
◆ Serum estradiol levels (in women)

Preliminary evidence suggests that abnormal findings of these assays reflect dysregulation at the level of neurotransmitter systems or hormones implicated in the pathogenesis of schizophrenia or other psychotic symptom patterns. Quantitative electroencephalography (qEEG) analysis of electrical brain activity is another significant emerging method used to assess psychosis. This approach will be increasingly used to identify treatments that have a high probability of ameliorating psychotic symptom patterns that correspond to different qEEG findings. Limited evidence suggests that two biological assays may provide useful information pertaining to putative causes of psychosis: serum phospholipase A_2 levels and serum homovanillic acid (HVA) levels. Research is ongoing to determine the clinical significance of abnormally high levels of brain glutamate (by magnetic resonance spectroscopy) in first-degree relatives of schizophrenics.

Table 11–1 outlines the assessment approaches that are substantiated or that probably yield specific diagnostic information about the cause(s) of psychosis.

Substantiated Approaches Used to Assess Psychosis

There are no substantiated assessment approaches at the time of writing.

Provisional Approaches Used to Assess Psychosis

Biological Assessment Approaches

◆ **Low RBC fatty acid levels may correlate with increased risk of schizophrenia and dissociative symptoms**   Consistently reduced red blood cell membrane levels of two fatty acids, arachidonic acid and decosahexanoic acid (DHA—an omega-3 essential fatty acid), have been reported in nonmedicated schizophrenics compared with medicated schizophrenics and normal controls (Arvindakshan, Sitasawad, et al., 2003; Assies, Lieverse, Vreken, Wanders, Dingemans, & Linszen, 2001; Horrobin, 1998). Low peripheral fatty acid and cholesterol levels are a marker of abnormally low brain levels because these molecules move freely across the blood–brain barrier and are principal components of nerve cell membranes. It has been suggested that low brain levels of fatty acids and cholesterol indirectly affect the number and activity of neurotransmitter receptors by modifying their three-dimensional structure in the lipid bilayer of nerve cell membranes (Engelberg, 1992). An open study compared serum lipid levels in 16 patients diagnosed with dissociative disorder according to *DSM-IV* criteria with 16 normal controls. Patients diagnosed with dissociative disorder had consistently lower total serum cholesterol, triglycerides, low-density lipoprotein (LDL) and very low-density lipoprotein (VLDL) levels compared with matched controls. The relationship between RBC levels of omega-3 fatty acids is confounded by the high rate of smoking in schizophrenics and patients with other chronic psychotic

Table 11–1   Assessment Approaches That May Yield Specific Diagnostic Information about the Cause of Psychosis

	Assessment Approach	Evidence for Specific Diagnostic Information	Positive Finding Suggests Efficacy of This Treatment
Substantiated	None at time of writing		
Provisional			
Biological	RBC fatty acid levels	Consistently low RBC levels of two fatty acids (arachidonic acid and DHA) suggest low brain levels in schizophrenia	Fatty acid supplementation may partially correct brain deficits and ameliorate symptoms
	Serum DHEA levels	Abnormally low serum DHEA may correlate with increased risk of schizophrenia	Supplementation may reduce severity of negative psychotic symptoms in patients who are DHEA deficient
	Niacin challenge test	Schizophrenics exhibit a reduced flushing response to niacin	The niacin challenge test may provide a semiquantitative way to distinguish between schizophrenia and other severe symptom patterns
	Serum estradiol levels (in women)	Abnormally low serum estradiol levels in women may correspond to increased risk of developing psychosis	Estradiol supplementation may ameliorate psychotic symptoms in women who are deficient
	Serum and RBC folate levels	Abnormally low serum and RBC folate levels may correlate with increased risk of schizophrenia and other psychotic syndromes	Folate supplementation may ameliorate psychotic symptoms (i.e., by indirectly affecting brain glutamate levels)
Somatic	None at time of writing		
Energy-information assessment approaches validated by Western science	qEEG	Specific qEEG findings may correlate with disparate symptom patterns	Specific qEEG findings may correlate with differential response rates to conventional or nonconventional treatments
Energy-information assessment approaches not (yet) validated by Western science	None at time of writing		

DHA, docosahexaenoic acid; DHEA, dehydroepiandrosterone; qEEG, quantitative electroencephalography; RBC, red blood cell (count)

syndromes. Smoking is correlated with reduced consumption of foods rich in omega-3s and also with abnormally low RBC omega-3 essential fatty acid levels (Hibbeln, Makino, Martin, Dickerson, Boronow, & Fenton, 2003; Leng et al., 1994).

◆ **Abnormally low serum DHEA and estradiol levels found in schizophrenia** Abnormally low serum levels may provide markers for vulnerability to depression, anxiety, and schizophrenia. Serum dehydroepiandrosterone (but not cortisol) levels increased significantly in chronically psychotic patients who improved when treated with DHEA. Lower serum DHEA may correlate with increased severity of psychotic symptoms on standardized scales (Harris, Wolkowitz, & Reus, 2001). Increases in serum DHEA correlated with reductions in negative psychotic symptoms (Strous et al., 2003). In a prospective study of 26 active duty military personnel, higher serum DHEA levels correlated with fewer symptoms of dissociation and overall improved performance during periods of extreme stress (Morgan et al., 2004). Women diagnosed with schizophrenia or other chronic psychotic syndromes frequently have abnormally low serum estradiol levels, and it has been suggested that women may be more susceptible to developing a psychotic syndrome when estrogen levels are low, including the premenstrual and postpartum periods, and following discontinuation of oral contraceptives (Huber et al., 2001).

◆ **The niacin challenge test may help distinguish schizophrenia from other severe syndromes** Emerging evidence suggests that the flushing response to niacin (and associated elevation

in skin temperature) is attenuated in schizophrenia and other chronic psychotic syndromes. The mechanism of action probably involves dysregulation of phospholipid-dependent signal transduction and increased phospholipase A_2 activity (Messamore, Hoffman, & Janowsky, 2003; Tavares, Yacubian, Talib, Barbosa, & Gattaz, 2003). Approximately 80% of schizophrenics do not flush when challenged with niacin compared with healthy controls. In one series, 43% of schizophrenics experienced abnormally low vasodilation in response to a 200 mg challenge dose of niacin, compared with only 6% of individuals diagnosed with bipolar disorder. Response to niacin is significantly affected by the dose used, age, and gender (Smesny et al., 2004). For example, at low doses healthy men are more likely to be nonresponders compared with women, suggesting that these factors should be considered when determining normative responses to a niacin challenge in male versus female schizophrenics. Continued refinement of the niacin challenge test may eventually provide a specific and sensitive clinical method for differentiating schizophrenia from other severe psychiatric syndromes (Hudson, Lin, Cogan, Cashman, & Warsh, 1997; Puri, Hirsch, Easton, & Richardson, 2002).

◆ **RBC and serum folate levels are consistently low** Low folate is probably related to abnormally low brain glutamate activity and increased negative psychotic symptoms (see discussion below). Findings from case reports and open trials suggest that serum folate levels are consistently low in schizophrenics and patients with other chronic psychotic syndromes (Goff & Coyle, 2001).

Somatic Assessment Approaches

There are no substantiated assessment approaches in this category at the time of writing.

Assessment Approaches Based on Forms of Energy or Information that are Validated by Western Science

◆ **qEEG may prove a useful adjunct to conventional assessment methods** Quantitative electroencephalography uses mathematical methods to analyze brain electrical activity that is unavailable from conventional EEG studies. It may prove a useful adjunct to conventional assessment methods when the underlying causes of psychotic symptoms are not clearly established or when a psychotic patient fails to respond to conventional treatment. Decreased α power in the frontal lobes is a typical finding in chronically psychotic schizophrenic patients who exhibit positive symptoms (Merrin & Floyd, 1992), and conventional antipsychotic medications are known to increase α power (Galderisi et al., 1994). Conversely, negative psychotic symptoms are more often associated with changes in slow wave (delta, δ) activity in the temporal lobes (Gattaz et al., 1992). However, other research findings are inconsistent with these reports, suggesting that there are no simple correlations between EEG changes and psychosis (Lifshitz & Gradijan, 1974). The range of findings suggests wide variation in the neurophysiological correlates of disparate psychotic symptom patterns (John et al., 1994). This view is consistent with differential response rates to conventional antipsychotic drugs in psychotic patients exhibiting different qEEG findings (Czobor & Volavka, 1991, 1993). Differences in interhemispheric EEG coherence may prove useful in differentiating depressed or bipolar patients who are psychotic from patients who are schizophrenic (Pockberger et al., 1989). The ability to reliably make this distinction will help psychiatrists develop treatment strategies employing potentially beneficial conventional and nonconventional approaches. It is reasonable to consider

obtaining a qEEG map when a psychotic patient has failed to respond to conventional or nonconventional treatments.

Assessment Approaches Based on Forms of Energy or Information That Are Not Validated by Western Science

At the time of writing, there are no assessment approaches in this category.

Assessment Approaches That May Yield Specific Diagnostic Information about the Causes of Psychosis

Table 11–2 outlines the current assessment approaches that possibly yield specific information about the causes of psychosis.

Biological Assessment Approaches

◆ **High serum phospholipase A$_2$ levels may be correlated with increased risk of developing schizophrenia or other severe psychiatric syndromes** Preliminary evidence suggests that serum levels of phospholipase A$_2$ are abnormally high in patients diagnosed with schizophrenia. In normal individuals this enzyme is involved in the turnover of phospholipids in nerve cell membranes. According to Horrobin's phospholipid membrane hypothesis (Horrobin, 1996, 1998), schizophrenia and other severe psychiatric syndromes may be caused by abnormally high levels of this enzyme in the brain, resulting in a general deficiency of phospholipids in nerve cell membranes and associated abnormalities in neurotransmission.

◆ **Abnormally high serum HVA levels may be correlated with lower effective doses of first-generation antipsychotics** Pretreatment serum homovanillic acid levels may predict response to certain conventional antipsychotic medications in the treatment of acutely manic or psychotic inpatients. Abnormal

Table 11–2 Assessment Approaches That May Yield Specific Information about the Causes of Psychosis

Category	Assessment Approach	Evidence for Specific Diagnostic Information	Comments
Biological	Serum phospholipase A$_2$	Abnormally high serum phospholipase A$_2$ levels may be correlated with increased risk of schizophrenia or other severe psychiatric syndromes	Supplementation with omega-3 fatty acids may compensate for the acquired trait of abnormally high phospholipase A$_2$ levels
	Serum HVA levels	Abnormally high pretreatment serum HVA levels may correlate with higher turnover of brain dopamine	Abnormally high serum HVA levels may predict lower effective doses of first-generation antipsychotics
	Brain glutamate levels	Pilot study data suggest abnormally high brain glutamate activity in relatives of schizophrenics	Dietary modifications addressing abnormal brain glutamate activity may ameliorate psychotic symptoms
Somatic	None at time of writing		
Energy-information assessment approaches validated by Western science	None at time of writing		
Energy-information assessment approaches not validated by Western science	VAS	The VAS reflex may provide clinically useful information for identifying treatments and doses that will be effective in previously nonresponsive patients	The VAS reflex is easy and inexpensive to measure, and there are no safety issues

HVA, homovanillic acid; VAS, vascular autonomic system

high serum HVA levels may reflect an increased turnover rate of brain dopamine and correspond to lower effective doses of dopamine-blocking antipsychotics in the management of psychotic symptoms. Higher serum HVA levels predicted an improved response rate to lower doses of first-generation antipsychotics including haloperidol (e.g., 5 mg/day). In contrast, lower pretreatment HVA levels correlated with a need for higher dosing strategies of typical antipsychotics (e.g., up to 25 mg/day; Chou et al., 2000). It is unclear whether these findings generalize to treatment strategies using atypical antipsychotics or other conventional medications.

◆ **Abnormally high brain glutamate levels may be correlated with risk of developing schizophrenia** The excitatory neurotransmitter glutamate has long been implicated in the pathogenesis of schizophrenia. Findings of a pilot study suggest that adolescent offspring of schizophrenic parents have abnormally high levels of glutamate in the medial prefrontal cortex (Tibbo, Hanstock, Valiakalayil, & Allen, 2004). A functional brain-imaging technique known as 3-T proton magnetic resonance spectroscopy (MRS) was used to obtain data on glutamate brain levels. MRS is a highly specialized research tool, and the possible future clinical relevance of this finding awaits the development of a more practical screening method.

Approaches Based on Forms of Energy or Information That Are Not Validated by Western Science

◆ **Analysis of the VAS** A case report suggests that information obtained from measuring the vascular autonomic signal (VAS) reflex may provide useful information when evaluating the potential effectiveness of conventional antipsychotic medications (Morton & Dlouhy, 1989). The VAS reflex was used in consultation with a 25-year-old schizophrenic who had not responded to conventional antipsychotics. After screening several medications, a specific dose of lithium carbonate was identified as the treatment choice that would most likely result in desirable energetic changes. Subsequently lithium carbonate at 600 mg/day was initiated, and the patient reportedly experienced a significant reduction in anxiety and was soon able to function at a higher level in social contexts.

◆ The Integrative Treatment of Psychosis

Conventional Western Treatments of Schizophrenia and Other Psychotic Symptoms Are Limited in Effectiveness and Have Significant Unresolved Safety Problems

Different classes of antipsychotics are based on disparate mechanisms of action and are associated with different kinds of adverse effects. A significant advantage of more recently introduced "atypical" antipsychotics over first-generation antipsychotics (e.g., haloperidol and chlorpromazine) is the relatively reduced risk of serious permanent neurological syndromes, including tardive dyskinesia and tardive dystonia. At the time of writing, six atypical antipsychotics are widely prescribed in North America and Western Europe: clozapine, risperidone, olanzapine, quetiapine, ziprasidone, and aripiprazole. In spite of the early promise of the atypical agents, a meta-analysis concluded that they have only a slight advantage over

first-generation antipsychotics in both efficacy and frequency of adverse neurological effects (Geddes, Freemantle, Harrison, & Bebbington, 2000). Atypical and first-generation antipsychotic medications have equal efficacy in the short-term management of schizophrenia and other psychotic syndromes. A meta-analysis comparing outcomes of all randomized controlled trials of conventional antipsychotics conducted between 1953 and 2002 concluded that only one atypical agent, clozapine, yielded outcomes that were significantly better than first-generation antipsychotics (Davis, Chen, & Glick, 2003). The same meta-analysis concluded that the antipsychotic efficacy of haloperidol, an important first-generation antipsychotic, was superior to all atypical agents. Unfortunately, a 1% risk of a potentially fatal blood disorder (agranulocytosis) with clozapine generally restricts the use of this medication to patients who are refractory to other antipsychotics (Alvir, Lieberman, Safferman, Schwimmer, & Schaaf, 1993). The efficacy of conventional antipsychotic medications is difficult to evaluate for many reasons (Preskhorn, 2004):

◆ Published studies tend to be biased in favor of those reporting favorable outcomes.

◆ Many patients become sedated on doses of antipsychotic medications that are regarded as "effective." Although such patients may appear to have improved, their symptoms may not have diminished.

◆ Western-trained physicians often increase antipsychotic doses before allowing a reasonable amount of time for the initial dosing strategy to become effective. This approach results in significant risk of adverse effects and obscures efforts to determine efficacy.

◆ There is an increasing trend toward polypharmacy, in which patients are treated with many antipsychotics in spite of significantly more adverse effects with multiple drug regimens and no clear research evidence supporting this approach (Centorrino, Goren, Hennen, Salvatore, Kelleher, & Baldessarini, 2004).

◆ Schizophrenic patients often fail to disclose noncompliance to their psychiatrists, who assume that prescribed antipsychotics are working (when in fact there may be noncompliance or partial compliance), making it difficult to determine the efficacy or adverse effects associated with conventional antipsychotics.

Few studies have been done to evaluate the long-term effectiveness of conventional antipsychotic medications in the management of schizophrenia and other chronic psychotic syndromes. At the same time, there are increasing safety concerns over the long-term use of antipsychotics. Many atypical agents cause a metabolic syndrome, including weight gain, with a significant associated risk of acquiring non-insulin-dependent diabetes. Other serious medical consequences associated with atypical antipsychotics are hypotension, cardiac arrhythmias, and a potentially fatal condition called Stevens-Johnson syndrome. The U.S. Food and Drug Administration now requires drug companies to issue warnings to physicians and patients about the risk of developing hyperglycemia and diabetes associated with prolonged use of most atypical agents, potentially progressing to diabetic coma and death.

The conventional pharmacological management of schizophrenia and other psychotic symptom patterns is complicated by the fact that many psychotic patients also experience depressed mood, agitation, and anxiety. Although severe cognitive impairment is frequently associated with psychotic syndromes, it can also be an adverse effect of antipsychotic medications. Conventional treatment regimens often combine two or more antipsychotics, or an antipsychotic with antidepressants, mood stabilizers, and antianxiety agents, in an effort to address complex symptom patterns. However, meta-analyses reveal limited evidence of efficacy and underscore unresolved safety issues when two or more conventional treatments are combined in the management of schizophrenia (Atre-Vaidya & Taylor, 1989; Freudenreich & Goff, 2002; Plasky, 1991; Wolkowitz & Pickar, 1991). The inherent limitations of conventional pharmacological treatments of the complex symptom patterns associated with psychosis invites open-minded consideration of the promising nonconventional strategies reviewed in this chapter.

Lack of Effectiveness, Noncompliance, and Adverse Effects Limit Conventional Pharmacologic Treatments of Psychosis

It is estimated that, while taking conventional antipsychotic medications, as many as 3.5% of schizophrenics relapse every month (Csernansky & Schuchart, 2002). Eighty-two percent of patients who discontinue an antipsychotic medication following an initially successful response relapse within 5 years, and this group of patients is much more likely to have subsequent relapses compared with patients who continue on long-term maintenance antipsychotic therapy (Robinson et al., 1999). Nonadherence with conventional antipsychotics is correlated with a significantly increased risk of repeat hospitalization, high outpatient service utilization, and chronic losses in productivity (Knapp, King, Pugner, & Lapuerta, 2004). Many patients who have chronic psychotic syndromes use conventional medications on an as-needed basis, significantly increasing the risk of relapse (Kane, 1996).

Noncompliance with conventional antipsychotic medications places schizophrenics and patients who suffer from other chronic psychotic syndromes at considerable risk. The findings of one survey study suggest that only one third of chronically psychotic patients are fully compliant with prescribed antipsychotic medications, one third are partially compliant, and the remaining one third do not take any conventional antipsychotic medications (Wright, 1993). A systematic review and meta-analysis of 86 studies on treatment adherence in schizophrenics concluded that 25% of all schizophrenics who use conventional pharmacologic treatments do not adhere to their prescribed medications (Barbui et al., 2003). Another systematic review of 103 studies assessing medication compliance among outpatients and inpatients being treated for psychotic symptoms concluded that ~30% of chronically psychotic patients stop taking medications after a short time, and thus obtain little benefit from their use. Twenty-five percent of patients who take conventional antipsychotics do not keep regular appointments with their psychiatrist (Nose, Barbui, & Tansella, 2003).

A review of eight meta-analyses of studies published since 1990 on the effectiveness of interventions aimed at increasing compliance with antipsychotics concluded that neither psychoeducation nor cognitive-behavioral approaches significantly improve compliance (Puschner, Born, Giessler, Helm, Becker, & Angermeyer, 2005). Many factors are related to noncompliance, including negative attitudes toward medications,

infrequent visits with a mental health professional, severe psychopathology impairing a patient's capacity to take medications, the high cost of many drugs, and concerns over adverse effects (Rettenbacher et al., 2004). Schizophrenics frequently refuse conventional antipsychotic medications because of concerns over severe potential neurological or other medical complications, including akathisia and tardive dyskinesia, and more recently (with the atypical agents) non-insulin-dependent diabetes and cardiac arrhythmias.

The benefits of antipsychotic therapy must be weighed against the cumulative risks of adverse effects that become more likely with continued treatment, including debilitating neurological effects and adult-onset diabetes. Many chronically psychotic patients who fail to respond to conventional antipsychotic medications or discontinue them due to adverse effects or because they cannot afford them are seeking viable alternatives. For these reasons it is important for mental health professionals to become familiar with the evidence for nonconventional treatments of schizophrenia and other psychotic symptom patterns.

Overview of Nonconventional and Integrative Treatments of Psychosis

At the time of writing, nonconventional treatments of psychotic symptoms have not been substantiated by compelling research evidence. Provisional findings support the use of four biological treatments for the management of psychotic symptoms. Omega-3 fatty acids, especially ecosapentanoic acid (EPA), may improve outcomes when combined with conventional antipsychotics, and may have robust beneficial effects in the early stages of psychosis in nonmedicated individuals. Taking folate in the form of methylfolate together with a conventional antipsychotic may improve outcomes. Large doses of glycine may ameliorate some symptoms of psychosis. Adding estrogen to conventional antipsychotics may improve outcomes in postpartum psychosis or other psychotic symptom patterns in women. An innovative form of spiritually focused group therapy combined with Yogic breathing practices probably improves global functioning in chronically psychotic patients. Recent interest has focused on an intriguing new treatment from Chinese medicine in which laser acupuncture is used to stimulate a specific acupoint associated with psychosis.

Possibly effective dietary approaches to psychosis include increased intake of unsaturated fats, including foods rich in omega-3 fatty acids, reduced intake of saturated fats and gluten, and improved dietary regulation of glucose. Limited evidence suggests that combining *Ginkgo biloba* with antipsychotic medications may improve outcomes while reducing adverse effects of conventional medications. Supplementing conventional antipsychotics with DHEA may also improve outcomes. Manganese, selenium, and zinc may be beneficial in some cases of psychosis, but limited evidence supports their use at this time. Although religious involvement is probably beneficial for individuals who are stable or who have residual symptoms, intense religious or spiritual interests or activities should be actively discouraged in patients who are acutely psychotic or chronically symptomatic. Stable chronically psychotic patients may benefit from yoga, qigong, or other energetic or mind–body approaches, but they should be instructed to practice these techniques only under the

Table 11–3 Nonconventional Treatments of Psychosis That Are Probably Effective

	Treatment Approach	Evidence for Modality or Integrative Approaches	Comments (Including Safety Issues or Contraindications)
Substantiated	None at time of writing		
Provisional			
Biological	Brahmyadiyoga and Mentat	Brahmyadiyoga 8–12 g may be as effective as conventional antipsychotics; Mentat may reduce severity of negative psychotic symptoms	Brahmyadiyoga is a widely used compound herbal formula in Ayurvedic medicine. *Note:* Reports of elevated liver enzymes
	Korean compound herbal formulas	Many Korean traditional herbal formulas may be beneficial in psychosis	Few human trials have been done on Korean herbal formulas, and safety issues have not been clearly defined
	EPA, an omega-3 fatty acid	EPA (1–4 g) alone or in combination with conventional antipsychotics (especially clozapine) may improve outcomes. This effect may be more robust in the early acute phase of the illness	*Note:* High doses of omega-3 fatty acids may cause GI distress
	DHEA	Combining DHEA 100 mg with a conventional antipsychotic may reduce the severity of negative symptoms and improve depressed mood and anxiety	*Caution:* DHEA can be activating and should be taken in the morning. Patients with a history of BPH or prostate cancer should consult their physician before taking DHEA
	Estrogen supplementation	Estrogen replacement therapy may be an effective treatment for postpartum psychosis. Adding estrogen to conventional antipsychotics may improve outcomes	*Caution:* Estrogen supplementation may increase risk of breast cancer or heart disease in susceptible women
	Niacin, folate, and thiamine	Combining niacin 3–8 g (in the form of nicotinamide), folate 15 mg (in the form of methylfolate), or thiamine 500 mg tid with conventional antipsychotics may improve outcomes	*Note:* Flushing and discomfort are associated with large doses of niacin and are reportedly diminished with niacinamide
	Glycine	Combining glycine 60 g with a conventional antipsychotic may improve both positive and negative symptoms. Glycine supplementation may improve mood and overall cognitive functioning in chronic psychotics	*Caution:* Case reports suggest that therapeutic doses of glycine may precipitate acute psychosis
Somatic or mind–body approaches	Spiritually oriented group therapy	Combining spiritually oriented group therapy with Yogic breathing practice and conventional medications improves global functioning in stable chronically psychotic patients	*Note:* Support groups for psychotic individuals should be led only by qualified therapists *Caution:* Patients who are delusional or have other acute psychotic symptoms should be discouraged from participating in spiritual or religious practices
Validated energy-information approaches	None at time of writing		
Nonvalidated energy-information approaches	Religious or spiritual involvement	Patients who have well-controlled psychotic symptoms may benefit from social support in organized religious activity	*Caution:* Patients who are actively psychotic should be advised to avoid intense religious or spiritual activity
	Qigong	Patients who have well-controlled psychotic symptoms may benefit from the regular practice of certain qigong exercises	*Caution:* Patients who have a history of psychosis should practice qigong only under the supervision of a qualified instructor

BPH, benign prostatic hypertrophy; DHEA, dehydroepiandrosterone; EPA, ecosapentanoic acid; GI, gastrointestinal

skillful supervision of an instructor who is aware of the risks associated with certain Yogic or qigong practices.

Table 11–3 outlines nonconventional treatments of psychosis that are considered effective or that are probably effective.

Substantiated Treatments of Psychosis

There are no substantiated nonconventional treatment approaches at the time of writing.

Provisional Treatments of Psychosis

Biological Treatments

◆ **Brahmyadiyoga, an Ayurvedic compound herbal medicine, holds significant promise for the management of psychosis**
Brahmyadiyoga is a compound herbal formula used in Ayurvedic medicine for the treatment of symptom patterns that resemble the Western psychiatric diagnosis of schizophrenia. The

formula contains six herbs including *Rauwolfia serpentina*, from which reserpine was isolated in the early 20th century and shown to have significant antipsychotic efficacy. Reserpine is seldom used to treat schizophrenia in Western countries today because of concerns over reports of severe depressed mood. In a 2-month double-blind, placebo controlled study, 108 chronically psychotic patients were randomized to Brahmyadiyoga (8–12 g in four divided doses), valerian (8–12 g in four divided doses), chlorpromazine (200–300 mg/day), and placebo (Mahal, Ramu, Chaturvedi, Thomas, Senapati, & Murthy, 1976). Patients treated with Brahmyadiyoga (but not valerian) and chlorpromazine reported significant and comparable improvements in symptom severity. No significant adverse effects were reported in the group taking Brahmyadiyoga. A subsequent study confirmed the antipsychotic efficacy of Brahmyadiyoga (Ramu, Venkataram, Mukundan, Shankara, Leelavathy, & Janakiramaiah, 1992). Preliminary research findings suggest that another compound herbal formula, Mentat, may reduce negative psychotic symptoms (Das & De Sousa, 1989). Ayurvedic herbal medicines should be used only under the supervision of a qualified Ayurvedic physician.

◆ **Some Korean traditional medicinal herbs reportedly reduce the severity of psychotic symptoms** Korean traditional medicine includes over 200 medicinal plants administered as compound herbal formulas to treat psychotic symptom patterns (Chung, Kim, & Kim, 1992). Formal Western-style research studies of these natural substances have not been conducted in populations diagnosed with schizophrenia or other *DSM-IV* psychotic disorders. However, consistent anecdotal reports and findings of in vitro studies suggest that many Korean herbal formulas are promising candidates for future antipsychotic treatments in Western countries. Receptor-binding studies show that some biologically active ingredients of Korean herbal formulas used to treat psychosis have strong binding affinities to receptors (including serotonin and dopamine) that would be expected to be activated when antipsychotic effects are present (Chung et al., 1995). Safety issues associated with the use of Korean traditional medicinal herbs have not been well described.

◆ **Supplementation with omega-3 fatty acids may improve both positive and negative psychotic symptoms** Findings from case reports (Puri et al., 2000; Su, Shen, & Huang, 2001) suggest that omega-3 fatty acids improve psychotic symptoms. In a small open study (Arvindakshan, Ghate, Ranjekar, Evans, & Mahadik, 2003), chronically psychotic patients experienced significant clinical improvements when treated with omega-3s (EPA and DHA, at 300 mg), and antioxidant vitamins twice daily over a 4-month period. Sustained improvements in psychotic symptoms were reported throughout the trial. A small double-blind study (Peet, Laugharne, Mellor, & Ramchand, 1996) demonstrated sustained improvement in both positive and negative psychotic symptoms in chronically psychotic patients treated with omega-3 fatty acids, with or without conventional antipsychotic medications. In a more recent and larger study (Peet & Horrobin, 2002), 115 treatment-refractory schizophrenics were randomized to receive 1, 2, or 4 g/day of EPA versus placebo together with their conventional antipsychotic medications. Only patients taking clozapine (but not other antipsychotics) experienced improvements greater than those reported by the group taking EPA. Clinical

improvements were observed in all EPA-treated groups taking clozapine, but the group receiving 2 g/day benefited most. However, another double-blind, placebo-controlled study revealed no differences in response between EPA (3 g/day) and placebo over a 4-month period in a group of 87 chronically psychotic patients taking conventional antipsychotics concurrently (Fenton, Dickerson, Boronow, Hibbeln, & Knable, 2001). In contrast to earlier studies, patients in the Fenton study were treated for residual psychotic symptoms but did not receive omega-3 fatty acids while in the early acute phase of illness. Interestingly, the results of a similar study (Emsley, Myburgh, Oosthuizen, & van Rensburg, 2002) using ethyl-EPA instead of EPA concluded that EPA was an effective augmentation treatment.

On the basis of research findings to date, specific treatment recommendations for the use of omega-3 fatty acids in psychotic patients cannot be made at this time. However, the above provisional findings suggest that patients in the early phase of a psychotic illness, or chronically psychotic patients taking clozapine, benefit more from augmentation with EPA compared with other groups. One can infer that synergistic antipsychotic effects take place when EPA is combined with clozapine (and perhaps other atypical antipsychotics). In view of the general health benefits of omega-3 fatty acid supplementation, and the absence of significant risks or adverse effects, patients who report psychotic symptoms should be encouraged to add a quality brand EPA supplement (2 g/day) to their conventional medication regimen. Transient gastrointestinal distress is sometimes reported by patients who take omega-3 fatty acids.

◆ **DHEA may be an effective adjunctive treatment, especially for negative psychotic symptoms** The sulfated form of DHEA—DHEA-S—is the most abundant steroid in the body. DHEA is an important neuroactive steroid because it acts as an antagonist to the γ-aminobutyric acid (GABA) receptor complex, thus modulating neuronal excitability (Howard, 1992). Possible mechanisms of action include increased dopamine release in the frontal cortex and enhanced activity of *N*-methyl-D-asparate (NMDA) and sigma receptors (Majewska, 1987; Maurice, Urani, Phan, & Romieu, 2001). In a 6-week randomized placebo-controlled study, 30 schizophrenic inpatients treated with DHEA at 100 mg/day in addition to their regular antipsychotic medications experienced significant improvements in negative psychotic symptoms, including reduced apathy and social withdrawal. Patients taking DHEA also reported marked improvement in depressed mood and anxiety (Strous et al., 2003). There were no significant changes in positive psychotic symptoms, including auditory hallucinations and delusions. Findings of another small double-blind study ($N = 30$) suggest that DHEA augmentation (100 mg/day for 6 weeks) of conventional antipsychotic medications is well tolerated, significantly reduces negative symptoms, and may be especially effective in women (Strous, 2005). Combining DHEA with conventional medications is a reasonable and conservative integrative treatment strategy for chronically psychotic patients, especially in view of frequent complex symptom patterns in this population, including anxiety and depressed mood. DHEA is generally well tolerated at therapeutic doses, but acne, hirsutism, voice deepening, and rare cases of mania have been reported with chronic high doses (Wolkowitz et al., 1997). Patients who have a history of benign prostatic hypertrophy or prostate cancer should consult their primary care physician before starting DHEA.

◆ **Estrogen replacement may diminish psychotic symptoms in predisposed women** Estrogen may be a "protective" factor in schizophrenic women (Bergemann et al., 2002). The serum estrogen level is related to brain dopamine activity, and estrogen withdrawal has been proposed as a model for psychosis (Deuchar & Brockington, 1998). A case report suggests that acute psychosis associated with chronically low estrogen levels completely remits with appropriate hormonal replacement therapy using estrogen and progesterone (Rettenbacher, Mechtcheriakov, Bergant, Brugger, & Fleischhacker, 2004). The findings of a pilot study suggest that estrogen replacement is an effective treatment of postpartum psychosis (Ahokas, Aito, & Rimon, 2000). Adding estrogen to conventional antipsychotics may improve response (Kulkarni et al., 2001). Women who use estrogen replacement therapy are at increased risk for heart disease and breast cancer.

◆ **Combining folic acid and thiamine with conventional antipsychotics may reduce symptom severity, but there is inconsistent evidence for niacin and vitamin B$_6$** Findings of double-blind, placebo-controlled trials suggest that niacin and folic acid have beneficial effects in some cases of chronic schizophrenia; however, results have been inconsistent. Numerous case reports and three small double-blind, placebo-controlled studies suggest that niacin in the form of nicotinamide (3–8 g/day), taken together with a conventional antipsychotic medication, results in greater improvement in psychotic symptoms compared with conventional antipsychotics alone (Ananth, Vacaflor, Kekhwa, Sterlin, & Ban, 1972; Denson, 1962; Osmond & Hoffer, 1962). The negative findings of an early double-blind study suggest that a particular subgroup of schizophrenics differentially benefits from niacin supplementation (Wittenborn, 1974). However, a review of 53 trials on niacin and other vitamins in the treatment of schizophrenia and other chronic mental illnesses identified shortcomings in research design methods and concluded that reported findings had only marginal statistical significance (Kleijnen & Knipschild, 1991). There is ongoing debate over the effectiveness of high doses of vitamins in the management of psychosis; however, numerous case reports suggest that some chronically psychotic patients experience significant and sustained benefits from this therapy (personal communications, A. Hoffer, M.D., June–December 2004). Practitioners who treat medical and psychiatric illnesses with high doses of niacin and other micronutrients have formed the Society of Orthomolecular Medicine, which publishes a peer-reviewed research journal. To date, controlled studies using the orthomolecular approach have enrolled chronic schizophrenics or patients diagnosed with Bipolar disorder or schizoaffective disorder. However, it has recently been suggested that the orthomolecular approach may be more effective in the initial phases of schizophrenia and other psychotic syndromes, and that patients who are chronically psychotic may experience less overall improvement when taking large doses of niacin and other vitamins. A double-blind, placebo-controlled trial of a high-dose regimen of niacin, other B-vitamins and vitamin C as an adjunctive treatment of patients hospitalized with first-episode acute psychosis in their first year of illness is currently in the open pilot phase at the Ben Gurion University of the Negev and the Beersehva Mental Health Center, Beersheva University, Israel (personal communication May 4 and 5, 2006, Professor R.H. Belmaker). On admission, all patients will be treated with risperidone (an atypical antipsychotic) 2-8mg/day and randomized to a vitamin regimen versus placebo. The dose will be lowered as soon as the patient is stable according to standardized rating scales including the BPRS (Brief Psychiatric Rating Scale). In the pilot phase patients will receive risperidone and a vitamin regimen but there will not be a placebo arm. In the 6-month controlled trial patients randomized to the orthomolecular treatment group will receive ascorbic acid (vitamin C) 1.5g twice daily, a B-complex (twice daily) containing 150 mg vitamin B6 per day and approximately 1 mg of folic acid and 100–200 μg of vitamin B$_{12}$ per day, and niacin or niacinamide starting at 1.5 gm twice daily and gradually increased. Both groups will receive a multivitamin (Centrum Forte) with breakfast. During the 6-month follow-up all patients will receive supportive psychotherapy. A registered dietician will meet with each patient weekly and discourage refined sugar or excess fat and encourage regular fruit and vegetable consumption. A high protein breakfast will be emphasized. Outcome measures will include BPRS, Clinical Global Assessment at the end of the study period, and recording of the dose of risperidone required to maintain sustained improvement in global functioning. In view of a large number of positive case reports and the growing level of professional interest in the use of high doses of niacin and other vitamins to treat psychotic syndromes, the theory and clinical methods of orthomolecular medicine warrant serious consideration.

Chronically psychotic patients who take daily folic acid in the form of methylfolate (15 mg) together with their conventional antipsychotic medication have fewer positive and negative psychotic symptoms and improve more rapidly compared with patients taking conventional drugs alone (Carney, 1979; Godfrey et al., 1990; Procter, 1991). Folate deficiency in schizophrenics is probably the result of both chronic malnutrition and the indirect effects of conventional antipsychotic medications on absorption (Ramchand, Ramchand, & Hemmings, 1992). Low brain levels of folate may also result from a heritable deficiency in the enzyme glutamate carboxypeptidase II (GCPII), required for folate absorption through the gut. When taken together with a conventional antipsychotic medication, thiamine supplementation at 500 mg 3 times daily may lessen the severity of psychotic symptoms in chronic schizophrenics (Sacks, Cowen, Green, Esser, Talarico, & Cankosyan, 1989; Sacks, Esser, Feitel, & Abbott, 1988). Vitamin B$_6$ deficiency due to a metabolic disorder may be an indirect cause of chronic psychosis (Cruz & Vogel, 1978), but in industrialized countries it is generally not a significant contributory factor. Furthermore, most schizophrenics do not improve with B$_6$ supplementation (Kleijnen & Knipschild, 1991). Emerging research findings suggest that some cases of chronic psychosis may be related to diffuse oxidative injury in the brain. Abnormalities in the body's antioxidant defense system may contribute to the pathogenesis of schizophrenia. Supplementation with antioxidant vitamins, including vitamins C and E and beta-carotene, may be beneficial in such cases (Mahadik & Scheffer, 1996).

◆ **Adding glycine to conventional antipsychotics may improve negative symptoms** Some cases of chronic psychosis may be related to abnormally low activity of the excitatory neurotransmitter glutamate or dysregulation of NMDA receptors to which glutamate binds. NMDA receptors function best when both glutamate and glycine bind to them, increasing their excitatory activity (Ishimaru et al., 1997). Provisional evidence is consistent with the hypothesis that atypical antipsychotics increase brain glutamate. In one small open series, 11 patients switched from a first-generation antipsychotic to a newer atypical agent were found to have significantly higher brain glutamate concentrations (Goff & Coyle, 2001). Increased glutamate correlated with significant improvements in negative psychotic symptoms, including reduced social withdrawal and apathy. A small open trial resulted in beneficial effects of glycine at doses up to 60 g/day (Leiderman, Zylberman, Zukin, Cooper, & Javitt, 1996). In a 6-week double-blind crossover study, 22 treatment-resistant schizophrenics were randomized to glycine (0.8 g/kg) versus placebo in addition to their conventional antipsychotic medication (Heresco-Levy et al., 1999). Negative symptoms and global functioning improved by 20 to 30% with glycine augmentation (up to 60 g/day) compared with conventional treatment alone, and glycine was well tolerated at doses that were therapeutic. Case reports suggest that glycine supplementation may improve mood and overall cognitive functioning in some chronic schizophrenics (Heresco-Levy et al., 1996; Javitt, Zylberman, Zukin, Heresco-Levy, & Lindenmayer, 1994). Glycine has few adverse effects; however, there are case reports of acute psychosis in some chronically psychotic patients treated with large doses. The clinical use of glycine is complicated by the fact that it is impractical for many chronically psychotic patients to take large doses of glycine (or quality brands of other nutritional supplements) that can potentially ameliorate their symptoms. Provisional research findings suggest that an indirect relationship exists between low levels of folate, reduced brain glutamate, and negative psychotic symptoms. The same enzyme that regulates glutamate activity at NMDA receptors is necessary for absorption of folate through the gut. This enzyme, GCPII, is consistently low in schizophrenic patients (Goff & Coyle, 2001).

Somatic and Mind–Body Approaches

◆ **Yogic breathing combined with spiritually oriented group psychotherapy improves overall functioning in chronic schizophrenics** Complex relationships exist between religious or spiritual beliefs and practices and psychotic symptoms. Individuals who have a history of schizophrenia or another chronic psychotic illness and are stable or have well-controlled residual symptoms often benefit from social support that comes with involvement in organized religion. A spiritual orientation can provide encouragement, social support, and valuable insights to people who struggle daily with schizophrenia (Sullivan, 1993). Innovative efforts to build support groups for chronic schizophrenics around spiritual themes and mind–body practices have identified important benefits of this approach (Sageman, 2004). Individuals who participated in a spiritually oriented support group reported significant improvements in general self-esteem and increased hopefulness, together with a deeper sense of connection with their peers and communities. Group prayer, reading passages from various spiritual traditions, and Yogic breathing practices are valuable components of the group process. A style of yoga called Sudarshan kriya is especially effective in reducing anxiety and improving mental clarity (Brown & Gerbarg, 2002). The researchers felt that schizophrenic patients who attended spiritually oriented support groups improved more than patients in more conventional support groups. Significant clinical benefits of regular spiritually oriented groups included improved range of affect, enhanced feelings of subjective well-being, improved cognitive functioning during groups, deeper experiences of interpersonal

bonding with other group members, and enhanced capacity for empathy. Patients benefited by discussing dynamic personal and interpersonal themes from a spiritual perspective, including loss and separation, feelings of empowerment achieved through a spiritual practice, and spirituality as a satisfying substitute for interpersonal intimacy. There were no reports of worsening or new-onset psychotic symptoms during or following group meetings.

◆ **Caveats when exploring spiritual issues with patients who are acutely psychotic** Mental health practitioners should use good clinical judgment when considering whether it is appropriate to invite any patient with a history of psychosis to explore spiritual issues. Although particular religious beliefs or spiritual practices do not place an individual at risk of developing schizophrenia or other psychotic symptom patterns, chronically psychotic patients sometimes experience religious delusions, including identification with the devil or a deity. Intense religious or spiritual interest when delusions or other psychotic symptoms are poorly controlled can amplify delusional content, cause acute anxiety, and have profound destabilizing effects. The delusional patient is at risk of acting on his or her beliefs, potentially harming himself or herself or others. For these reasons, individuals who are experiencing religious delusions or other severe psychotic symptoms should be actively discouraged from pursuing religious or spiritual practices, including spiritually oriented group therapy.

Treatments Based on Forms of Energy or Information Validated by Western Science

At the time of writing, there are no treatment approaches in this category.

Treatments Based on Forms of Energy or Information Not Validated by Western Science

◆ **Qigong should be practiced under supervision only** Patients who have a history of psychosis but are currently stable may benefit from the regular practice of qigong under the supervision of a skilled qigong instructor who is aware of particular exercises that may place the patient at risk of symptomatic worsening. Schizophrenics or patients diagnosed with other psychotic disorders, including dissociative disorder and schizoaffective disorder, as well as severe personality disorders, including borderline personality, risk an acute exacerbation of symptoms when practicing qigong and should do so only under the supervision of a skilled instructor, preferably a qigong master (Flaws & Lake, 2001; Lake, 2002).

Possibly Effective Treatments of Psychosis

Table 11–4 outlines treatment approaches to psychosis that may be effective.

◆ **Certain dietary modifications may ameliorate psychotic symptoms** Findings from epidemiological studies suggest that schizophrenic patients who consume a diet high in saturated fats have more severe symptoms compared with patients who follow diets with moderate fat intake (Christensen & Christensen, 1988). However, chronically psychotic patients who consume

Table 11–4 Treatment Approaches to Psychosis That Are Possibly Effective

Category	Treatment Approach	Evidence for Claimed Treatment Effect	Comments
Biological	Dietary changes, including decreased intake of saturated fats and increased intake of omega-3 fatty acids, reduced gluten, and improved glucose regulation	Chronically psychotic patients with higher intake of unsaturated fats, reduced gluten, and improved glucose regulation may experience milder symptoms	*Caution:* Patients should consult a nutritionist or other qualified specialist before undertaking dietary changes of any kind
	Ginkgo biloba	Combining *G. biloba* (360 mg/day) with a conventional antipsychotic may be more effective for both positive and negative symptoms compared with conventional treatments alone	*Note:* Combining *G. biloba* with a conventional antipsychotic may reduce adverse neurological effects
	Mineral supplements	Manganese, selenium, or zinc supplementation may improve psychotic symptoms in some cases	*Note:* The evidence for beneficial effects of mineral supplementation in schizophrenia is limited and inconsistent
	Evening primrose (*Oenothera biennis*) oil	Putative mechanism of action involves restoring deficient prostaglandins with essential fatty acids. May improve psychotic symptoms in some cases	*Note:* Few double-blind studies; inconsistent findings
Somatic and mind–body	Yoga	The regular practice of certain Yogic breathing routines and postures may reduce the severity of psychotic symptoms in some cases	*Caution:* Certain Yogic breathing practices can cause agitation and transient worsening of psychotic symptoms. Chronically psychotic patients should practice yoga only under the guidance of a skilled instructor
	The Wilbarger intervention	The Wilbarger method is a sensory stimulation technique involving frequent passive stretching and touching of the body. Preliminary findings suggest improved sensory integration in schizophrenics	*Note:* Beneficial effects of this technique may be related to frequent human contact
Energy-information approaches validated by Western science	None at time of writing		
Energy-information approaches not validated by Western science	Laser acupuncture	Daily 15-minute laser acupuncture treatments of the yamen point may reduce psychotic symptoms in schizophrenics	*Note:* Safety issues have not been described when laser acupuncture is used in clinical settings

large amounts of unsaturated fats, including omega-3 fatty acids, generally have milder symptoms (Emsley, Oosthuizen, & van Rensburg, 2003). A specialized high-carbohydrate, low-protein diet that is also low in the amino acids glycine and serine may be beneficial in some patients who have intermittent psychotic symptoms due to a rare metabolic derangement called porphyria (Bruinvels, Pepplinkhuizen, & Fekkes, 1988). However, case reports suggest that glycine supplementation may diminish negative symptoms (see discussion above).

There is preliminary evidence that some schizophrenic patients become more symptomatic when they eat foods containing gluten, a major constituent of wheat protein. It has been hypothesized that a breakdown product of normal gluten metabolism can precipitate psychotic symptoms in genetically predisposed individuals (Reichelt et al., 1990). Research findings suggest that eliminating gluten from the diet may be beneficial in some cases of schizophrenia; however, most reports are anecdotal, and at least three controlled studies have failed to show any beneficial effects on symptom severity after gluten is eliminated (Potkin et al., 1981; Storms, Clopton, & Wright, 1982; Vlissides, Venulet, & Jenner, 1986).

Future studies may reveal causal relationships between disparate psychotic syndromes and specific dietary deficiencies associated with dysregulations of specific neurotransmitter systems. It may eventually be possible to develop dietary modifications addressing specific symptom patterns and putative underlying neurotransmitter "imbalances." In a double-blind, randomized, placebo-controlled trial, schizophrenics, stable bipolar patients, and healthy controls were randomized to receive a large bolus of dextrose (which is rapidly converted to glucose) versus saccharin (Newcomer et al., 1999). Significant improvements in verbal memory and overall cognitive functioning were correlated with blood glucose levels in schizophrenic patients, but not bipolars or healthy controls. These findings suggest that dietary modifications or future treatments directed at increasing brain glucose levels may result in significant cognitive improvements in schizophrenic patients.

◆ ***Ginkgo biloba* may enhance the efficacy of conventional antipsychotics** Findings from a double-blind study (Zhang et al., 2001) suggest that combining *Ginkgo biloba* extract 360 mg/day with a conventional antipsychotic drug (haloperidol) versus haloperidol alone resulted in a greater reduction in both negative and positive psychotic symptoms in patients diagnosed with schizophrenia. Significantly, fewer neurological side effects were reported by patients taking the combined regimen.

◆ **Mineral supplements may be beneficial in some cases of chronic psychosis** Supplementation with manganese, selenium, or zinc may improve psychotic symptoms in some schizophrenic patients; however, findings of studies conducted to date are inconsistent. Oral manganese increases urinary excretion of copper, which may be associated with some cases of chronic psychosis due to metabolic disease (Pfeiffer & Iliev, 1972). Selenium may be required for normal functioning of a transport protein whose deficiency results in a subtype of schizophrenia that includes paranoia and negative symptoms (Berry, 1994). Observational studies and case reports suggest a possible relationship between low selenium or zinc intake and the incidence of schizophrenia (Brown, 1994), but controlled trials on these supplements in schizophrenic patients have not been conducted, and anecdotal evidence is weak and inconsistent.

◆ **Inconsistent efficacy findings of evening primrose oil in psychosis** Evening primrose (*Oenothera biennis*) oil has been investigated as a potential treatment of psychotic symptoms, in the belief that abnormal prostaglandin levels in psychotic patients are corrected through oral supplementation with the essential fatty acids contained in this natural oil, including linoleic acid and γ-linolenic acid (Vaddadi, 1981). However, the prostaglandin deficiency hypothesis has not been validated, there are limited anecdotal reports, and findings from few controlled double-blind studies conducted to date on the efficacy of this fatty acid supplementation in psychosis are inconsistent and ambiguous (Holman & Bell, 1983; Manku, Morse-Fischer, & Horrobin, 1988).

Somatic and Mind–Body Approaches

◆ **Regular yoga practice may reduce agitation and anxiety in chronically psychotic patients** Anecdotal reports and observations from spiritually focused support groups that combine yoga with conventional group activities (see discussion above) suggest that yoga has general beneficial effects on psychotic symptoms. To date few studies have examined the effectiveness of yoga alone in chronically psychotic patients. Two open studies suggest that the regular practice of relaxing Yogic breathing and postures reduces agitation and anxiety in psychotic patients (Higashi, 1964; Jordan, 1989). Certain Yogic breathing exercises are potentially "activating." Chronically psychotic patients should be cautioned to practice only "calming" forms of yoga and to do so under the guidance of a qualified instructor.

◆ **The Wilbarger intervention may improve sensory integration deficits in psychotic patients** The Wilbarger intervention is a sensory stimulation approach that includes passive stretching of the wrists, elbows, shoulders, knees, and ankles, together with gentle brushing of the arms, back, and legs. The method has been successfully used to treat children with sensory integration deficits, which commonly occur in schizophrenia. In a 4-week pilot study, 30 schizophrenic patients were treated 5 times daily without days off. The majority of patients completed the study and showed significant improvements on measures of sensory integration, including

reduced left-right confusion (Withersly, Stout, Mogge, Nesland, & Allen, 2005). The significance of these preliminary findings is confounded by the likely beneficial effects of frequent human contact and touch.

Treatments Based on Forms of Energy or Information Not Validated by Western Science

◆ **Daily laser acupuncture treatments may improve global functioning in schizophrenics** The use of laser light to stimulate specific acupuncture points reportedly results in significant clinical improvements in patients diagnosed with schizophrenia based on standardized symptom rating scales. Researchers at the Institute of Mental Health, Beijing College of Medicine, have developed a protocol that uses laser light of different wavelengths to stimulate the yamen acupoint in schizophrenics (Lio, Wang, Zhang, Chen, & Liu, 1986). The protocol is based on daily 10-minute sessions, excluding Sundays, and reportedly reduces the severity of auditory hallucinations and other positive psychotic symptoms. In a single-blind study, 15 schizophrenic patients with a 5-year or shorter history of active symptoms were randomly assigned to receive laser acupoint therapy with a 25 versus 5.9 mW laser for a total number of 30 consecutive daily treatments (Jia, Luo, Zhan, Jia, & Yan, 1987). Patients did not know the specifications of the laser used. Conventional antipsychotic drugs were not taken throughout the 30-day trial. Protocols using both lasers reportedly resulted in significant and equivalent clinical improvement by blind physician raters on the Brief Psychiatric Rating Scale (BPRS), the Clinical Global Impression (CGI), and other standardized symptom rating instruments. No significant between-group differences were observed. Changes in blood chemistries or adverse physical or psychological effects of laser acupoint treatment in this population have not been reported. A subsequent controlled study of 33 individuals diagnosed with schizophrenia concluded that laser acupuncture following the above protocol and daily chlorpromazine were equally effective as measured by standardized rating scales of positive and negative psychotic symptoms (Zhang, 1991). Larger studies, including a sham laser treatment arm, a sham acupuncture protocol, and double-blinding, are needed to confirm the significance of these findings.

◆ The Integrative Management Algorithm for Psychosis

Figure 11–1 is the integrative management algorithm for psychosis. Note that specific assessment and treatment approaches are representative examples of reasonable choices. Moderate symptoms often respond to exercise, dietary modification, mind–body practices, and energy-information therapies. When managing severe symptoms, emphasize biological therapies. Encourage exercise and other lifestyle changes in motivated patients. Consider conventional, nonconventional, and integrative approaches that have not been tried.

See evidence tables and text for complete reviews of evidence-based options.

Before implementing any treatment plan, always check evidence tables and Web site updates at www.thieme.com/mentalhealth for specific assessment and treatment protocols, and obtain patient informed consent.

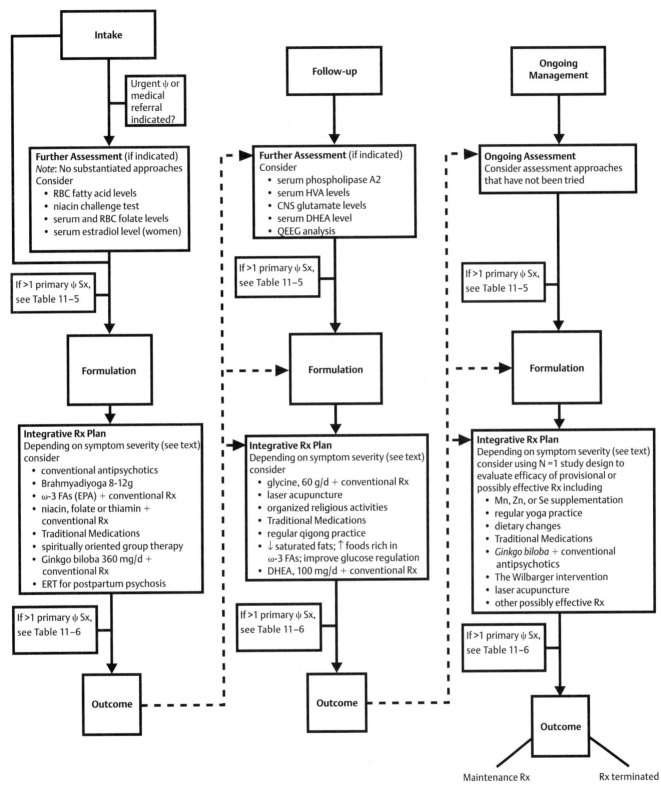

Figure 11–1 Integrative management algorithm for psychosis. Note that specific assessment and treatment approaches are representative examples of reasonable choices. Moderate symptoms often respond to exercise, dietary modification, mind–body practices, and energy-information therapies. Rx, treatment; Sx, symptoms.

◆ Integrated Approaches to Consider When Two or More Core Symptoms Are Present

Table 11–5 shows the assessment approaches to consider using when psychosis is the focus of clinical attention and one or more other symptoms are being assessed concurrently.

Table 11–6 outlines the treatment approaches to consider using when psychosis is the focus of clinical attention and one or more other symptoms are being treated concurrently.

Table 11–5   Assessment Approaches to Psychosis When Other Symptoms Are Being Assessed Concurrently

Other Symptoms Being Assessed Concurrently	Assessment Approach	Comments
Depressed mood	Serologic studies	Limited evidence suggests that consistently low RBC levels of two fatty acids (arachidonic acid and DHA) correspond to low brain levels of these fatty acids in chronic psychosis.
		Limited evidence suggests that abnormally low serum and RBC folate levels correlate with increased risk of schizophrenia and other chronic psychotic syndromes.
		Low serum folate levels predict nonresponse to conventional and nonconventional treatments of depressed mood.
		Low RBC omega-3 fatty acids are correlated with more severe depressed mood
	qEEG brain mapping	Limited evidence suggests that specific qEEG findings correlate with differential response rates of psychotic symptoms to both conventional and nonconventional treatments.
		Specific qEEG findings predict differential response of depressed mood to both conventional and nonconventional treatments
Mania and cyclic mood changes	Serologic studies	Low trace lithium levels (i.e., from low nutritional intake) are common in acutely manic patients.
		Limited evidence suggests that pretreatment serum GABA levels predict improved response of mania and cyclic mood changes to divalproex (Depakote) but not other mood stabilizers
	qEEG brain mapping	Limited evidence suggests that pretreatment qEEG in acutely manic or cycling patients (showing left-sided abnormalities) predicts improved response to conventional treatments
Anxiety	Serologic studies	Deficiencies of niacin and vitamins B_6, C, and E are sometimes associated with generalized anxiety.
		Limited evidence suggests that total serum cholesterol is elevated in chronically anxious patients
	qEEG brain mapping	Limited evidence suggests that specific qEEG changes correspond to disparate anxiety syndromes
Cognitive impairment	Serologic studies	Limited evidence suggests that abnormally low levels of zinc and magnesium correlate with the risk of developing Alzheimer's disease.
		Limited evidence suggests that abnormally low serum DHA levels correlate with increased risk of developing Alzheimer's disease
	qEEG brain mapping	qEEG mapping and VEP and AER studies facilitate early diagnosis and more aggressive treatment of early Alzheimer's and mild cognitive impairment.
		qEEG mapping provides useful information when planning EEG-biofeedback protocols addressing cognitive impairment in general.
		qEEG mapping can be used to evaluate response to conventional and nonconventional cognitive-enhancing treatments
Substance abuse or dependence	Serologic studies	In alcohol abuse the magnitude of serum deficiencies of vitamins A and C, some B vitamins, and zinc, magnesium, and essential fatty acids is an indicator of the severity of malnutrition.
		Elevated serum homocysteine is an indicator of chronic alcohol abuse and returns to normal levels soon after cessation of alcohol abuse
	qEEG brain mapping	Limited evidence suggests that qEEG brain mapping provides useful information when planning specific EEG-biofeedback protocols for relapsing alcoholics or narcotics abusers
	AER	Conventional treatments of heroin detoxification normalize AER findings
Disturbance of sleep or wakefulness	Serologic studies	Deficiencies in vitamins B_{12}, C, and E and folic acid are correlated with increased daytime sleepiness and insomnia.
		Abnormally low serum levels of magnesium and zinc are often associated with increased daytime sleepiness.
		Limited evidence suggests that abnormally high nighttime serum norepinephrine levels and abnormally low nighttime serum IL-6 and TNF levels are associated with increased rates of chronic insomnia.

AER, auditory evoked response; DHA, docosahexaenoic acid; EEG, electroencephalography; GABA, γ-aminobutyric acid; IL, interleukin; qEEG, quantitative electroencephalography; RBC, red blood cell (count); TNF, tumor necrosis factor; VEP, visual evoked potential

Table 11–6 Treatment Approaches to Psychosis When Other Symptoms Are Being Treated Concurrently

Other Symptoms Being Treated Concurrently	Treatment Approach	Comments
Depressed mood	Dietary modifications	Limited evidence suggests that chronically psychotic patients with higher intake of unsaturated fats, reduced gluten, and improved glucose regulation may experience milder symptoms.
		Limited evidence suggests that restricting caffeine and refined sugar and increasing consumption of fatty fish and whole foods rich in B vitamins improve depressed mood and reduce the risk of becoming depressed
	Vitamins	Combining niacin (in the form of nicotinamide 3–8 g), folate (in the form of methylfolate 15 mg), or thiamine (500 mg tid) with conventional antipsychotics may improve outcomes.
		Note: Flushing and discomfort are associated with large doses of niacin and reportedly diminish when niacin is taken in the form of niacinamide.
		Folate 0.5–1 mg/day augments the effects of conventional antidepressants and SAMe
	Omega-3 essential fatty acids	Limited evidence suggests that EPA (1–4 g) alone or in combination with conventional antipsychotics (especially clozapine) improves outcomes. Beneficial effects of omega-3 essential fatty acids may be more robust in the early acute phase of the illness.
		Combining omega-3 fatty acids (especially EPA) 1–2 g/day with conventional antidepressants improves response and may accelerate response rate.
		Limited evidence suggests that EPA alone is an effective treatment of severe depressed mood
	DHEA and estrogen	Limited evidence suggests that combining DHEA 100 mg with a conventional antipsychotic may reduce the severity of negative symptoms and improve depressed mood and anxiety.
		Caution: DHEA can be activating and should be taken in the morning. Patients with a history of BPH or prostate cancer should consult their physician before taking DHEA.
		DHEA 90–450 mg/day is beneficial for mild to moderate depressed mood.
		DHEA has synergistic effects when combined with conventional antidepressants and may be an effective monotherapy for moderate depressed mood.
		Estrogen replacement therapy may be an effective treatment for postpartum psychosis. Adding estrogen to conventional antipsychotics may improve outcomes.
		Caution: Estrogen supplementation may increase risk of breast cancer or heart disease in susceptible women
	Ayurvedic herbs	Limited evidence suggests that Brahmyadiyoga 8–12 g is as effective as conventional antipsychotics, and Mentat reduces the severity of negative psychotic symptoms.
		Several Ayurvedic herbs and compound herbal formulas are probably beneficial for depression.
		Note: Patients taking Ayurvedic herbs should be supervised by an Ayurvedic physician
	Ginkgo biloba	Limited evidence suggests that combining *G. biloba* (360 mg/day) with a conventional antipsychotic is more effective for both positive and negative symptoms compared with conventional treatments alone.
		Note: There is limited evidence that combining *G. biloba* with a conventional antipsychotic reduces adverse neurological effects.
		G. biloba may provide a safe alternative to conventional augmentation strategies.
		Caution: *G. biloba* should not be taken with warfarin or other drugs that affect bleeding time
	Somatic approaches	Limited evidence suggests that a sensory stimulation technique known as the Wilbarger method improves sensory integration in schizophrenics.
		Regular exercise at least 30 minutes 3 times a week is probably as effective as conventional antidepressants, St. John's wort, and cognitive therapy for moderate depressed mood.
		Exercising under bright light is more effective against depressed mood than exercise or bright light alone
	Acupuncture	Limited evidence suggests that daily 15-minute laser acupuncture treatments of the yamen point reduces psychotic symptoms in schizophrenics.
		Limited evidence suggests that conventional acupuncture is effective against severe depressed mood.
		Limited evidence suggests that electroacupuncture alone is as effective as electroacupuncture combined with amitriptyline or other conventional antidepressants, and there is also limited evidence that computer-controlled electroacupuncture using high-frequency currents is more effective than conventional or standard electroacupuncture

(Continued)

Table 11–6 Treatment Approaches to Psychosis When Other Symptoms Are Being Treated Concurrently *(Continued)*

Other Symptoms Being Treated Concurrently	Treatment Approach	Comments
	Spiritually oriented group therapy and mindfulness training	Combining spiritually oriented group therapy with Yogic breathing practice and conventional medications improves global functioning in stable chronically psychotic patients.
		Caution: Patients who are delusional or have other acute psychotic symptoms should be discouraged from participating in spiritual or religious practices.
		Limited evidence suggests that patients who have well-controlled psychotic symptoms benefit from social support in organized religious activity.
		Caution: Patients who are actively psychotic should be advised to avoid intense religious or spiritual activity.
		Mindfulness training is probably as effective as cognitive therapy in moderate depressed mood
Mania and cyclic mood changes	Vitamins and minerals	Limited evidence suggests that folic acid 200 μg/day augments the effects of lithium in mania and that monthly vitamin B$_{12}$ injections reduce the risk of recurring manic episodes.
		Limited evidence suggests that magnesium supplementation 40 mEq/day is an effective treatment of rapid cycling episodes, and that potassium 20 mEq bid reduces lithium-induced tremor and improves compliance
	Omega-3 fatty acids	Limited evidence suggests that EPA 1–2 g/day in combination with conventional mood stabilizers reduces the severity and frequency of manic episodes.
		Note: At the time of writing, there is one case report of EPA-induced hypomania
	Mind–body approaches	Limited evidence suggests that certain yogic breathing practices and postures reduce the severity of mania or hypomania
	Mindfulness training	Limited evidence suggests that certain meditation practices promote calmness and are beneficial in mania or hypomania
Anxiety	Dietary modifications	Limited evidence suggests that avoiding refined sugar and caffeine and increasing protein and foods containing tryptophan reduce symptoms of generalized anxiety and panic
	DHEA	Combining DHEA 100 mg with a conventional antipsychotic may reduce the severity of negative symptoms and improve symptoms of anxiety and depressed mood
	Somatic approaches	Regular aerobic or strengthening exercise reduces generalized anxiety symptoms, and there is limited evidence that exercise may also reduce the frequency and severity of panic attacks
	Acupuncture	Some acupuncture and electroacupuncture protocols probably reduce symptoms of generalized anxiety
Cognitive impairment	Dietary changes	Moderate wine consumption, reduced saturated fats, and reduced total caloric intake are correlated with reduced risk of developing Alzheimer's disease
	Vitamins	Limited evidence suggests that diets high in fish or other sources of omega-3 fatty acids and low in omega-6 fatty acids are associated with a reduced risk of developing dementia.
		Limited evidence suggests that high niacin intake from food or supplements significantly reduces the risk of developing dementia and decreases the rate of cognitive decline in healthy elderly individuals
	Ashwagondha (*Withania somnifera*)	Limited evidence suggests that Ashwagondha 50 mg/kg improves short- and long-term memory and executive functioning in cognitively impaired individuals.
		Note: Individuals who use Ayurvedic herbs should do so only under the supervision of an Ayurvedic physician
	DHEA and estrogen	Limited evidence suggests that DHEA 25–50 mg/day improves mental performance in healthy adults, and 200 mg/day improves cognitive functioning in vascular dementia
		Note: Meta-analyses fail to show that hormonal replacement with estrogen/progesterone slows progression of dementia in postmenopausal women diagnosed with Alzheimer's disease or prevents cognitive decline in healthy postmenopausal women.
		Caution: Estrogen replacement therapy is associated with increased risk of breast cancer, heart disease, and stroke
Substance abuse or dependence	Dietary changes	Alcoholics who improve their diets, including reduced intake of refined sugar and caffeine and increased intake of omega-3 fatty acids and protein, probably have an increased chance for maintaining sobriety
	Vitamins and minerals	Limited evidence suggests that thiamine reduces alcohol craving, nicotinic acid reduces the risk of alcohol dependence in chronic drinkers, and taking antioxidant vitamins soon before drinking reduces the severity of hangover symptoms.
		Limited evidence suggests that supplementation of chronic alcoholics with magnesium and zinc improves global neuropsychological functioning and protects the brain against free radical damage

Table 11–6 Treatment Approaches to Psychosis When Other Symptoms Are Being Treated Concurrently *(Continued)*

Other Symptoms Being Treated Concurrently	Treatment Approach	Comments
	Somatic approaches	Limited evidence suggests that regular aerobic exercise or strength training in abstinent alcoholics improves general emotional well-being.
		Caution: All patients should consult with their primary care physician before starting a rigorous exercise program
	Mindfulness training	Abstinent alcoholics and addicts who engage in a regular mindfulness practice or meditation probably have a reduced risk of relapse
	Acupuncture	Some acupuncture points and protocols are probably more effective than others in reducing symptoms of alcohol or cocaine withdrawal
Disturbance of sleep or wakefulness	Somatic and mind–body approaches	Many somatic and mind–body practices, including progressive muscle relaxation, massage, meditation, and guided imagery, are as effective as conventional sedative-hypnotics for mild to moderate insomnia
	Acupuncture	Some acupuncture and auriculotherapy protocols probably reduce the severity of sleep disturbances, including insomnia related to a mental or emotional problem

BPH, benign prostatic hypertrophy; DHEA, dehydroepiandrosterone; EPA, ecosapentanoic acid; SAMe, *S*-adenosylmethionine

Case Vignette

History and Initial Presentation

William is a 28-year-old single, unemployed male on long-term disability because of a diagnosis of schizophrenia. His medical and psychiatric history was unremarkable throughout childhood. Although William briefly experimented with hallucinogenic mushrooms, he did not abuse other drugs or drink heavily. William experienced his first psychotic episode at the age of 19 toward the end of his freshman year of college. His symptoms included auditory hallucinations, confusion, paranoia, and agitation. During a 3-day psychiatric hospitalization, he was started on haloperidol but experienced an acute dystonic reaction with jaw clenching, which resolved when the medication was discontinued. He was then treated with perphenazine with good response and no significant adverse effects. William was discharged with a routine follow-up appointment in 1 month and was able to resume his college coursework. After 6 months he discontinued the perphenazine against the advice of his psychiatrist and began to experience psychotic symptoms a few days later, including paranoid thoughts and auditory hallucinations. He was hospitalized again and started on the atypical antipsychotic olanzapine (Zyprexa), 10 mg at bedtime. He experienced no adverse effects, and his symptoms soon resolved. Soon after discharge William went on psychiatric disability and chose to take time away from school. He began to see a vocational rehabilitation counselor and decided to enter a training program for sheet metal workers. He continued to take olanzapine 5 g twice daily with good control of psychotic symptoms, saw a psychiatrist every 3 months for medication management, and found employment as a sheet metal worker. William continued to feel disorganized and was becoming more and more isolated, though he was not depressed or anxious. He became progressively less physically active and was chronically fatigued. He paid little attention to nutrition and steadily gained weight. Eventually he scheduled a consultation with Dr. Richards, a local naturopathic physician, to discuss nutrition and his general health.

Assessment, Formulation, and Treatment Plan

Dr. Richards confirmed that William had not experienced psychotic symptoms for more than 6 years while taking olanzapine. He told William that his weight problem and fatigue were probably related to both medication side effects and chronic poor nutrition. William reported moderately depressed mood. Dr. Richards ordered RBC folate levels and serum fatty acid levels and recommended that William start taking omega-3 fatty acids, B vitamins, and DHEA (100 mg/day) while continuing on olanzapine and working to improve his general nutrition, including more grains and fish. He encouraged William to begin a regular exercise program to address symptoms of fatigue and his weight problem.

Follow-Up

One month later William appeared to have more energy and had lost a noticeable amount of weight. There had been no psychotic symptoms since the initial appointment, and William's mood had improved. He was noticeably less fatigued since beginning to take a B-vitamin complex and omega-3 fatty acids, and had started to jog several times a week. His serum lipid levels were elevated, and his folate and fatty acid levels were in the low-normal range. William asked Dr. Richards if it would be "safe" to discontinue the olanzapine in view of his progress since beginning the recommended supplements, starting an exercise plan, and improving his diet. Dr. Richards told William that he was not qualified to make recommendations about medication changes and referred William to Dr. Jenkins, a local psychiatrist familiar with evidence-based uses of nonconventional treatments. Dr. Richards obtained William's written consent to send his records to Dr. Jenkins.

Ongoing Follow-Up Appointments

William arrived on time at Dr. Jenkins's office and was neatly groomed. He maintained good eye contact throughout the hour-long consultation with Dr. Jenkins, who had reviewed Dr. Richards's notes earlier that day. William confirmed that he been taking omega-3 fatty acids, B vitamins, and DHEA while continuing his daily olanzapine regimen. He described his commitment to a healthy diet and regular exercise. He had increased his dose of omega-3s to 2 g/day with no adverse effects. William disclosed that he had decreased the olanzapine from 5 mg twice daily to 7.5 mg at bedtime 1 month earlier, realizing this decision was against Dr. Richards's medical advice. There had been no recurring psychotic symptoms on the reduced dose, and his mood remained stable. Dr. Jenkins remarked that William's current dose of olanzapine was apparently effective and cautioned William not to further reduce the dose at this time.

On routine follow-up 2 months later, William remained stable, and there had been no recurring symptoms of psychosis or depressed mood. He had lost another 5 pounds and was now on a regular morning exercise program. He continued to take the recommended supplements. After carefully reviewing the pros and cons of continuing his present dose of olanzapine versus further reducing it, Dr. Jenkins cautiously agreed with William's wish to reduce the dose to 5 mg. William agreed to contact Dr. Jenkins immediately in the event of recurring psychotic symptoms or changes in mood, and agreed to a return appointment in 2 weeks. Following 2 weeks on olanzapine at 5 mg, William reported some difficulty staying asleep at night, but there were no changes in his previous baseline. Dr. Jenkins prescribed a mild nonaddictive sedative called zolpidem to be used as needed for insomnia.

During the ensuing 3 months, William remained stable on olanzapine at 5 mg. Dr. Jenkins agreed with William's request to discontinue the antipsychotic while continuing the supplements and carefully monitoring for recurring psychotic symptoms or mood changes. One month after reducing his dose to 2.5 mg, there were no recurring symptoms, and William disclosed that he felt "safe" off medications. Dr. Jenkins advised William of the risk that discontinuing olanzapine might precipitate another psychotic episode and documented this conversation in William's chart.

References

Ahokas, A., Aito, M., & Rimon, R. (2000). Positive treatment effect of estradiol in postpartum psychosis: A pilot study. *Journal of Clinical Psychiatry, 61,* 166–169.

Alvir, J., Lieberman, J., Safferman, A., Schwimmer, J., & Schaaf, J. (1993). Clozapine-induced agranulocytosis: Incidence and risk factors in the United States. *New England Journal of Medicine, 329*(3), 162–167.

Ananth, J. V., Vacaflor, L., Kekhwa, G., Sterlin, C., & Ban, T. A. (1972). Nicotinic acid in the treatment of newly admitted schizophrenic patients: A placebo controlled study. *Internationale Zeitschrift für Klinische Pharmakologie, Therapie und Toxikologie, 5,* 406–410.

Arvindakshan, M., Ghate, M., Ranjekar, P. K., Evans, D. R., & Mahadik, S. P. (2003). Supplementation with a combination of omega-3 fatty acids and antioxidants (vitamins E and C) improves the outcome of schizophrenia. *Schizophrenia Research, 62*(3), 195–204.

Arvindakshan, M., Sitasawad, S., Debsikday, V., Ghate, M., Evans, D., Horrobin, D. F., Bennett, C., Ramjekar, P. K., & Mahadik, S. P. (2003). Essential polyunsaturated fatty acid and lipid peroxide levels in never-medicated and medicated schizophrenic patients. *Biological Psychiatry, 53,* 56–64.

Assies, J., Lieverse, R., Vreken, P., Wanders, R. J., Dingemans, P. M., & Linszen, D. H. (2001). Significantly reduced docosahexenoic acid concentrations in erythrocyte membranes from schizophrenic patients compared with a carefully matched control group. *Biological Psychiatry, 49,* 510–522.

Atre-Vaidya, N., & Taylor, M. (1989). Effectiveness of lithium in schizophrenia: Do we really have an answer? *Journal of Clinical Psychiatry, 50,* 170–173.

Nose, M., Barbui, N., Gray, R., et al. (2003). Clinical interventions for treatment non-adherence in psychosis: Meta-analysis. *British Journal of Psychiatry, 183,* 197–206.

Bergemann, N., Parzer, P., Nagl, I., et al. (2002). Acute psychiatric admission and menstrual cycle phase in women with schizophrenia. *Archives of Women's Mental Health, 5,* 119–126.

Berry, T. (1994). A selenium transport protein model of a sub-type of schizophrenia. *Medical Hypotheses, 43*(6), 409–414.

Brown, J. (1994). Role of selenium and other trace elements in the geography of schizophrenia. *Schizophrenia Bulletin, 20*(2), 387–398.

Brown, R. P., & Gerbarg, P. L. (2002). *Yogic breathing and meditation: When the thalamus quiets the cortex and rouses the limbic system.* Paper presented at the "Science of Breath" International Symposium on Sudarshan Kriya, Pranayam, and Conciousness, New Delhi, India.

Bruinvels, J., Pepplinkhuizen, L., & Fekkes, D. (1988). Derangement of one-carbon metabolism in episodic schizoaffective psychoses. *Pharmacopsychiatry, 21*(1), 28–32.

Carney, M. (1979). Psychiatric aspects of folate deficiency. In M. I. Botez & E. H. Reynolds (Eds.), *Folic acid in neurology, psychiatry and internal medicine.* New York: Raven Press.

Centorrino, F., Goren, J. L., Hennen, J., Salvatore, P., Kelleher, J. P., & Baldessarini, R. J. (2004). Multiple versus single antipsychotic agents for hospitalized psychiatric patients: Case-control study of risks versus benefits. *American Journal of Psychiatry, 161,* 700–706.

Chou, J. C., Czobor, P., Tuma, I., Charles, O., Bebe, R., Cooper, T. B., Chang, W. H., Lane, H. Y., & Stone, D. L. (2000). Pretreatment plasma HVA and haloperidol response in acute mania. *Journal of Affective Disorders, 59*(1), 55–59.

Christensen, O., & Christensen, E. (1988). Fat consumption and schizophrenia. *Acta Psychiatrica Scandinavica, 78,* 587–591.

Chung, I., Kim, Y., Ahn, J., Lee, H., Chen, G., Manji, H., Potter, W., & Pickar, D. (1995). Pharmacologic profile of natural products used to treat psychotic illnesses. *Psychopharmacology Bulletin, 31,* 139–145

Chung, I., Kim, Y., Ahn, J., et al. (1995). Pharmacologic profile of natural products used to treat psychotic illnesses. *Psychopharmacology Bulletin, 31*(1), 139–145.

Cruz, R., & Vogel, W. (1978). Pyroluria: A poor marker in chronic schizophrenia. *American Journal of Psychiatry, 135*(10), 1239–1240.

Csernansky, J., & Schuchart, E. (2002). Relapse and rehospitalisation rates in patients with schizophrenia: Effects of second generation antipsychotics. *CNS Drugs, 16*(7), 473–484.

Czobor, P., & Volavka, J. (1991). Pretreatment EEG predicts short-term response to haloperidol treatment. *Biological Psychiatry, 30,* 927–942.

Czobor P, Volavka, J. (1993). Quantitative EEG electroencephalogram effect of risperidone in schizophrenic patients. *Journal of Clinical Psychopharmacology, 13,* 332–342.

Das, S., & De Sousa, A. (1989). Mentat (BR-16A) in schizophrenia. *Journal of Community Psychiatry, 12*(2–4), 15.

Dassa, D., Sham, P. C., van Os, J., et al. (1996). Relationship of birth season to clinical features, family history, and obstetric complications in schizophrenia. *Psychiatry Research, 64,* 11–17.

Davis, J., Chen, N., & Glick, I. (2003). A mata-analysis of the efficacy of second-generation antipsychotics. *Archives of General Psychiatry, 60*(6), 553–564.

Denson, S. (1962). The value of nicotinamide in the treatment of schizophrenia. *Diseases of the Nervous System, 23,* 167–172.

Deuchar, N., & Brockington, I. (1998). Puerperal and menstrual psychoses: The proposal of a unitary etiological hypothesis. *Journal of Psychosomatic Obstetrics and Gynaecology, 19*(2), 104–110.

Emsley, R., Myburgh, C., Oosthuizen, P., & van Rensburg, S. J. (2002). Randomized, placebo-controlled study of ethyl-eicosapentaenoic acid as supplemental treatment in schizophrenia. *American Journal of Psychiatry, 159,* 1596–1598.

Emsley, R., Oosthuizen, P., & van Rensburg, S. J. (2003). Clinical potential of omega-3 fatty acids in the treatment of schizophrenia. *CNS Drugs, 17*(15), 1081–1091.

Engelberg, H. (1992). Low serum cholesterol and suicide. *Lancet, 339,* 727–729.

Fauman, M. (1994). *Study guide to DSM-IV.* Washington, DC: American Psychiatric Press.

Fenton, W. S., Dickerson, F., Boronow, J., Hibbeln, J. R., & Knable, M. (2001). A placebo-controlled trial of omega-3 fatty acid (ethyl eicosapentaenoic acid) supplementation for residual symptoms and cognitive impairment in schizophrenia. *American Journal of Psychiatry, 158*(12), 2071–2073.

Flaws, B., & Lake, J. (2001). Psychological disturbances due to erroneous qigong. In *Chinese Medical Psychiatry: A textbook and clinical manual* (Book 3, pp. 433–442). Boulder, CO: Blue Poppy Press.

Freudenreich, O., & Goff, D. (2002). Antipsychotic combination therapy in schizophrenia: A review of efficacy and risks of current combinations. *Acta Psychiatrica Scandinavia, 106,* 323–330.

Galderisi, S., Maj, M., Mucci, A., et al. (1994). QEEG alpha 1 changes after a single dose of high-potency neuroleptics as a predictor of short-term response to treatment in schizophrenic patients. *Biological Psychiatry, 35,* 367–374.

Gattaz, W., Mayer, S., Ziegler, P., et al. (1992). Hypofrontality on topographic EEG in schizophrenia: Correlations with neuropsychological and psychopathological parameters. *European Archives of Psychiatry and Clinical Neuroscience, 241,* 328–332.

Geddes, J., Freemantle, N., Harrison, P., & Bebbington, P. (2000). Atypical antipsychotics in the treatment of schizophrenia: Systematic overview and meta-regression analysis. *British Medical Journal, 321*(7273), 1371–1376.

Godfrey, P., Toone, B., Carney, M., et al. (1990). Enhancement of recovery from psychiatric illness by methylfolate. *Lancet, 336,* 392–395.

Goff, D., & Coyle, J. (2001). The emerging role of glutamate in the pathophysiology and treatment of schizophrenia. *American Journal of Psychiatry, 158,* 1367–1377.

Gottesman, I. I. (1991). *Schizophrenia genesis: The origin of madness.* New York: Freeman.

Harris, D., Wolkowitz, O., & Reus, V. (2001). Movement disorder, psychiatric symptoms and serum DHEA levels in schizophrenic and schizoaffective patients. *World Journal of Biologial Psychiatry, 2,* 99–102.

Heresco-Levy, U., Javitt, D., Ermilov, M., et al. (1996). Double-blind, placebo-controlled crossover trial of glycine adjuvant therapy for treatment-resistant schizophrenia. *British Journal of Psychiatry, 169,* 610–617.

Heresco-Levy, U., Javitt, D., Ermilov, M., et al. (1999). Efficacy of high-dose glycine in the treatment of enduring negative symptoms of schizophrenia. *Archives of General Psychiatry, 56,* 29–36.

Hibbeln, J. R., Makino, K. K., Martin, C. E., Dickerson, F., Boronow, J., & Fenton, W. S. (2003). Smoking, gender, and dietary influences on erythrocyte essential fatty acid composition among patients with schizophrenia or schizoaffective disorder. *Biological Psychiatry, 53*(5), 431–441.

Higashi, M. (1964). Pranayama as a psychiatric regimen [Letter]. *Lancet, 14,* 1177–1178.

Holman, C., & Bell, A. (1983). A trial of evening primrose oil in the treatment of chronic schizophrenia. *Journal of Orthomolecular Psychiatry, 12,* 302–304.

Horrobin, D. F. (1996). Schizophrenia as a membrane lipid disorder which is expressed throughout the body. *Prostaglandins, Leukotreines, and Essential Fatty Acids, 55*(1–2), 3–7.

Horrobin, D. F. (1998). The membrane phospholipid hypothesis as a biochemical basis for the neurodevelopmental concept of schizophrenia. *Schizophrenia Research, 30,* 193–208.

Howard, J. (1992). Severe psychosis and the adrenal androgens. *Integrative Physiological and Behavioral Science, 27,* 209–215.

Huber, T., Rollnik, J., Wilhelms, J., et al. (2001). Estradiol levels in psychotic disorders. *Psychoneuroendocrinology, 26,* 27–35.

Hudson, C. J., Lin, A., Cogan, S., Cashman, F., & Warsh, J. J. (1997). The niacin challenge test: Clinical manifestation of altered transmembrane signal transduction in schizophrenia? *Biological Psychiatry, 41*(5), 507–513.

Goff, D. C., Coyle, J. T. (2001). The emerging rold of glutamate in the pathophysiology and treatment of schizophrenia. *American Journal of Psychiatry, 7*(1), 47–67.

Javitt, D. C., Zylberman, I., Zukin, S. R., Heresco-Levy, U., & Lindenmayer, J. P. (1994). Amelioration of negative symptoms in schizophrenia by glycine. *American Journal of Psychiatry, 151 (9),* 1367–1377.

Jia, Y. K., Luo, H. C., Zhan, L., Jia, T. Z., & Yan, M. (1987). A study on the treatment of schizophrenia with He-Ne laser irradiation of acupoint. *Journal of Traditional Chinese Medicine, 7*(4), 269–272.

John, E., Princhep, L., Alper, K., et al. (1994). Quantitative electrophysiological characteristics and subtyping of schizophrenia. *Biological Psychiatry, 36,* 801–826.

Jordan, N. (1989). Psychotherapy with expressive technics in psychotic patients. *Acta Psiquiátrica y Psicológica de America Latina, 35*(1–2), 55–60.

Kane J. (1996). Schizophrenia. *New England Journal of Medicine, 334*(1), 34–42.

Kleijnen, J., & Knipschild, P. (1991). Niacin and vitamin B$_6$ in mental functioning: A review of controlled trials in humans. *Biological Psychiatry, 29*(9), 931–941.

Knapp, M., King, D., Pugner, K., & Lapuerta, P. (2004). Non-adherence to antipsychotic medication regimens: Associations with resource use and costs. *British Journal of Psychiatry, 184,* 509–516.

Kringlen, E. (1995). Twin studies in mental disorder. *Baillière's Clinical Psychiatry, 1,* 47–62.

Kulkarni, J., Riedel, A., de Castella, A., et al. (2001). Estrogen: A potential treatment for schizophrenia. *Schizophrenia Research, 48,* 137–144.

Lake, J. (2002). Qigong. In S. Shannon (Ed.), *Handbook of complementary and alternative therapies in mental health education* (ch. 9, pp. 183–208). New York: Academic Press.

Leiderman, E., Zylberman, I., Zukin, S., Cooper, T., & Javitt, D. (1996). Preliminary investigation of high-dose oral glycine on serum levels and negative symptoms in schizophrenia: An open-label trial. *Biological Psychiatry, 39,* 213–215.

Leng, G. C., Smith, F. B., Fowkes, F. G., et al. (1994). Relationship between plasma essential fatty acids and smoking, serum lipids, blood pressure and haemostatic and rheological factors. *Prostaglandins, Leukotrienes, and Essential Fatty Acids, 51,* 101–108.

Lifshitz, K., & Gradijan, J. (1974). Spectral evaluation of the electroencephalogram: Power and variability in chronic schizophrenics and control subjects. *Psychophysiology, 11,* 479–490.

Lio, Z. Z., Wang, Y., Zhang, S., He, A., Chen, Y., & Liu, X. (1986). Therapeutic effect of He-Ne laser irradiation of point erman in schizophrenic auditory hallucination—a clinical assessment. *Journal of Traditional Chinese Medicine, 6*(4), 253–256.

Mahadik, S., & Scheffer, R. (1996). Oxidative injury and potential use of antioxidants in schizophrenia. *Prostaglandins, Leukotriences, and Essential Fatty Acids, 55*(1–2), 45–54.

Mahal, A., Ramu, N., Chaturvedi, D., Thomas, K., Senapati, H., & Murthy, N. (1976). Double-blind controlled study of brahmyadiyoga and tagara in the management of various types of unmade (schizophrenia). *Indian Journal of Psychiatry, 18,* 283–292.

Majewska, M. (1987). Steroids and brain activity: Essential dialogue between body and mind. *Biochemical Pharmacology, 36,* 3781–3788.

Manku M, Morse-Fischer N, & Horrobin D. (1988). Changes in human plasma essential fatty acid levels as a result of administration of linoleic acid and gamma-linolenic acid. *European Journal of Clinical Nutrition, 42,* 55–60.

Maurice, T., Urani, A., Phan, V. L., & Romieu, P. (2001). The interaction between neuroactive steroids and the signal receptor 1 function: Behavioral consequences and therapeutic opportunities. *Brain Research Reviews, 37,* 116–132.

McGuffin, P., Asherson, P., Owen, M, et al. (1994). The strength of the genetic effect: Is there room for an environmental influence in the aetiology of schizophrenia? *British Journal of Psychiatry, 164,* 593–599.

Merrin, E., & Floyd, T. (1992). Negative symptoms and EEG alpha activity in schizophrenic patients. *Schizophrenia Research, 8,* 11–20.

Messamore, E., Hoffman, W. F., & Janowsky, A. (2003). The niacin skin flush abnormality in schizophrenia: A quantitative dose-response study. *Schizophrenia Research, 62*(3), 251–258.

Morgan, C., Southwick, S., Hazlett, G., et al. (2004). Relationships among plasma dehydroepiandrosterone sulfate and cortisol levels, symptoms of dissociation, and objective performance in humans exposed to acute stress. *Archives of General Psychiatry, 61,* 819–825.

Morton, M., Dlouhy, C. (1989). *Energy fields in medicine: A study of device technology based on acupuncture meridians and chi energy.* Kalamazoo, Michigan: Fetzer Foundation, 124–189.

Munk-Jørgensen, P., & Ewald, H. (2001). Epidemiology in neurobiological research: Exemplified by the influenza-schizophrenia theory. *British Journal of Psychiatry, 40*(Suppl.), S30–S32.

Newcomer, J. W., Craft, S., Fucetola, R., Moldin, S. O., Selke, G., Paras, L., & Miller, R. (1999). Glucose-induced increase in memory performance in patients with schizophrenia. *Schizophrenia Bulletin, 25*(2), 321–335.

Nose, M., Barbui, C., & Tansella, M. (2003). How often do patients with psychosis fail to adhere to treatment programmes? A systematic review. *Psychological Medicine, 33,* 1149–1160.

Osmond, H., & Hoffer, A. (1962). Massive niacin treatment in schizophrenia: Review of a nine-year study. *Lancet, 1,* 316–320.

Peet, M., & Horrobin, D. F. (2002). E-E Multicentre Study Group: A dose-ranging exploratory study of the effects of ethyl-eicosapentaenoate in patients with persistent schizophrenic symptoms. *Journal of Psychiatric Research, 36*(1), 7–18.

Peet, M., Laugharne, J. D., Mellor, J., & Ramchand, C. N. (1996). Essential fatty acid deficiency in erythrocyte membranes from chronic schizophrenic patients, and the clinical effects of dietary supplementation. *Prostaglandins, Leukotrienes, and Essential Fatty Acids, 55*(1–2), 71–75.

Pfeiffer, C., & Iliev, V. (1972). A study of zinc deficiency and copper excess in the schizophrenias. *International Review of Neurobiology, 72,* 141

Plasky, P. (1991). Antidepressant usage in schizophrenia. *Schizophrenia Bulletin, 17*(4), 649–657.

Pockberger, H., Thau, K., Lovrek, A., et al. (1989). Coherence mapping reveals differences in the EEG between psychiatric patients and healthy persons. In M. K. Berlin (Ed.), *Topographic brain mapping of EEG and evoked potentials* (pp. 451–457). Heidelberg, Germany: Springer-Verlag.

Potkin, S. G., Weinberger, D., Kleinman, J., et al. (1981). Wheat gluten challenge in schizophrenic patients. *American Journal of Psychiatry, 138*(9), 1208–1211.

Preskorn, S. H. (2004). The recommended dosage range: How is it established and why would it ever be exceeded? *Journal of Psychiatric Practice,10*(4), 249–254.

(1989). Energy fields in medicine: A study of device technology based on acupuncture meridians and chi energy. Proceedings from the conference sponsored by the John E. Fetzer Foundation, 124–189.

Procter, A. (1991). Enhancement of recovery from psychiatric illness by methylfolate. *British Journal of Psychiatry, 159*, 271–272.

Puri, B. K., Counsell, S. J., Richardson, A. J., & Horrobin, D. F. (2002). Eicosapentaenoic acid in treatment-resistant depression. *Archives of General Psychiatry, 59*(1), 91–92.

Puri, B. K., Hirsch, S. R., Easton, T., & Richardson, A. J. (2002). A volumetric biochemical niacin flush-based index that noninvasively detects fatty acid deficiency in schizophrenia. *Progress in Neuro-psychopharmacology and Biological Psychiatry, 26*(1), 49–52.

Puri, B. K., Richardson, A. J., Horrobin, D. F., et al. (2000). Eicosapentaenoic acid treatment in schizophrenia associated with symptom remission, normalisation of blood fatty acids, reduced neuronal membrane phospholipid turnover and structural brain changes. *International Journal of Clinical Practice, 54*(1), 57–63.

Puschner, B., Born, A., Giessler, A., Helm, H., Becker, T., & Angermeyer, M. (2005). Effects of interventions to improve compliance with antipsychotic medication in people suffering from schizophrenia: Results of recent reviews [German]. *Psychiatrische Praxis, 32*(2), 62–67.

Ramchand C, Ramchand R, & Hemmings G. (1992). RBC and serum folate concentrations in neuroleptic-treated and neuroleptic-free schizophrenic patients. *Journal of Nutrition and Medicine, 3*, 303–309.

Ramu, M., Venkataram, B., Mukundan, H., Shankara, M., Leelavathy, S., & Janakiramaiah, N. (1992). A controlled study of Ayurvedic treatment in the acutely ill patients with schizophrenia (Unmada)—rationale and results. *NIMHANS Journal, 10*(1), 1–16.

Reichelt, K., Sagedal, E., landmark, J., et al. (1990). The effect of gluten-free diet on urinary peptide excretion and clinical state in schizophrenia. *Journal of Orthomolecular Medicine, 5*(4), 223–239.

Rettenbacher, M., Hofer, A., Eder, U., Hummer, M., Kemmler, G., Weiss, E., & Fleischhacker, W. (2004). Compliance in schizophrenia: Psychopathology, side effects, and patients' attitudes toward the illness and medication. *Journal of Clinical Psychiatry, 65*, 1211–1218.

Rettenbacher, M., Mechtcheriakov, S., Bergant, A., Brugger, A., & Fleischhacker, W. W. (2004). Improvement of psychosis during treatment with estrogen and progesterone in a patient with hypoestrogenemia [Letter to the Editor]. *Journal of Clinical Psychiatry, 65*(2), 275–277.

Robinson, D., Woerner, M. G., Alvir, J. M., Bilder, R., Goldman, R., Geisler, S., Koreen, A., Sheitman, et al. (1999). Predictors of relapse following response from a first episode of schizophrenia or schizoaffective disorder. *Archives of General Psychiatry, 56*, 241–247.

Sacks, W., Cowen, M. A., Green, M. R., Esser, A. H., Talarico, P., & Cankosyan, G. (1988). Acetazolamide and thiamine (A + T): A preliminary report of an ancillary therapy for chronic mental illness. *Journal of Clinical Psychopharmacology, 8*, 70.

Sacks, W., Esser, A. H., Feitel, B., & Abbott, K. (1989). Acetazolamide and thiamine: An ancillary therapy for chronic mental illness. *Psychiatry Research, 28*, 279–288.

Sageman, S. (2004). Breaking through the despair: Spiritually oriented group therapy as a means of healing women with severe mental illness. *Journal of the American Academy of Psychoanalysis and Dynamic Psychiatry, 32*(1), 125–141.

Smesny, S., Rosburg, T., Klemm, S., et al. (2004). The influence of age and gender on niacin skin test results: Implications for the use as a biochemical marker in schizophrenia. *Journal of Psychiatry Research, 38*(5), 537–543.

Smythies, J. R. (1997). Oxidative reactions and schizophrenia: A review-discussion. *Schizophrenia Research, 24*, 357–364.

Smythies, J. R., Gottfries, C. G., & Regland, B. (1997). Disturbances of one-carbon metabolism in neuropsychiatric disorders: A review. *Biological Psychiatry, 41*, 230–233.

Storms, L. H., Clopton, J. M., & Wright, C. (1982). Effects of gluten on schizophrenics. *Archives of General Psychiatry, 39*, 323–327.

Strous, R. D. (2005). Dehydroepiandrosterone (DHEA) augmentation in the management of schizophrenia symptomatology. *Essential Psychopharmacology, 6*(3), 141–147.

Strous, R. D., Maayan, R., Lapidus, R., Stryjer, R., Lustig, M., Kotler, M., & Weizman, A. (2003). Dehydroepiandrosterone augmentation in the management of negative, depressive, and anxiety symptoms in schizophrenia. *Archives of General Psychiatry, 60*(2), 133–141.

Su, K. P., Shen, W. W., & Huang, S. Y. (2001). Omega-3 fatty acids as a psychotherapeutic agent for a pregnant schizophrenic patient. *European Neuropsychopharmacology, 11*(4), 295–299.

Sullivan, W. P. (1993). "It helps me to be a whole person": The role of spirituality among the mentally challenged. *Psychosocial–Rehabilitation Journal, 16*(3), 125–134.

Tavares, H., Yacubian, J., Talib, L. L., Barbosa, N. R., & Gattaz, W. F. (2003). Increased phospholipase A2 activity in schizophrenia with absent response to niacin. *Schizophrenia Research, 61*(1), 1–6.

Tibbo, P., Hanstock, C., Valiakalayil, A., & Allen, P. (2004). 3-T proton MRS investigation of glutamate and glutamine in adolescents at high genetic risk for schizophrenia. *American Journal of Psychiatry, 161*, 1116–1118.

Tsuang, M. T., Stone, W. S., & Faraone, S. V. (2001). Genes, environment and schizophrenia. *British Journal of Psychiatry, 40*(Suppl.), S18–S24.

Vaddadi, K. (1981). The use of gamma-linoleic acid and linoleic acid to differentiate between temporal lobe epilepsy and schizophrenia. *Prostaglandins and Medicine, 27*, 313–323.

Vlissides, D. N., Venulet, A., & Jenner, F. A. (1986). A double-blind gluten-free/gluten-load controlled trial in a secure ward population. *British Journal of Psychiatry, 148*, 447–452.

Wahlberg, K. E., Wynne, L. C., Oja, H., et al. (1997). Gene-environment interaction in vulnerability to schizophrenia: findings from the Finnish Adoptive Family Study of Schizophrenia. *American Journal of Psychiatry, 154*, 355–362.

Withersly, D., Stout, J., Mogge, N., Nesland, A., & Allen, G. (2005). Evaluating the use of the Wilbarger intervention with schizophrenic patients: A pilot study. *Psychiatry, 47–49.*

Wittenborn, J. (1974). A search for responders to niacin supplementation. *Archives of General Psychiatry, 31*, 547–552.

Wolkowitz, O. M., & Pickar, D. (1991). Benzodiazepines in the treatment of schizophrenia: A review and reappraisal. *American Journal of Psychiatry, 148*(6), 714–726.

Wolkowitz, O. M., Reus, V. I., Roberts, E., et al. (1997). Dehydroepiandrosterone (DHEA) treatment of depression. *Biological Psychiatry, 41*, 311–318.

Wright, E. (1993). Non-compliance or how many aunts has Mathilda? *Lancet, 342*, 909–913.

Zhang, B. (1991). A controlled study of clinical therapeutic effects of laser acupuncture for schizophrenia [Chinese]. *Zhonghua Shen Jing Jing Shen Ke Za Zhi, 24*(2), 81–3, 124.

Zhang, X. Y., Zhou, D. F., Zhang, P. Y., et al. (2001). A double-blind, placebo-controlled trial of extract of *Ginkgo biloba* added to haloperidol in treatment-resistant patients with schizophrenia. *Journal of Clinical Psychiatry, 62*, 878–883.

12

Dementia and Mild Cognitive Impairment

This chapter focuses on the conventional and nonconventional approaches to dementia and mild cognitive impairment, including Alzheimer's disease and other neurodegenerative disorders and impairment resulting from traumatic brain injuries. It begins with a discussion of the presumed causes of the main categories of cognitive impairment, then moves to a review of assessment methods, in particular quantitative electroencephalographic brain mapping. It then describes the different cost-effective treatment approaches to cognitive impairment that are available to health care professionals today. The approaches presented in this chapter are discussed with respect to their usefulness in the assessment or treatment of moderate or severe cognitive impairment in general. Emerging assessment and treatment approaches have broad potential relevance to the clinical management of both moderate and severe cognitive impairment associated with a wide range of causes.

◆ Background Issues

The Health Care and Economic Burden of Dementia and Other Syndromes of Severe Cognitive Impairment Will Continue to Increase

Criteria for a diagnosis of dementia include severe persisting impairment of short-term and long-term memory in addition to severe deficits in at least one other area of cognitive functioning, including language, the capacity to perform tasks, the capacity to recognize familiar objects or people, and impaired reasoning. The vast majority of underlying medical causes of dementia are irreversible. Dementia can be caused by Alzheimer's disease, vascular disease of the brain, Parkinson's disease, other neurodegenerative disorders, traumatic brain injury, severe cerebrovascular accidents (stroke), and toxic effects of chronic alcohol and substance abuse.

Traumatic brain injury is the most common cause of severe cognitive impairment. Almost 2 million new cases of traumatic brain injury resulting from automobile accidents, sports injuries, falls, and other accidents are reported each year in the United States alone at an annual cost of $48 billion (National Center for Injury Prevention and Control, 1999). Alzheimer's disease is the most common form of dementia. This progressive neurodegenerative disease accounts for 60 to 70% of all cases of dementia and afflicts between 5 and 10% of the population over age 65 (Evans et al., 1989). After 65 the incidence of Alzheimer's doubles approximately every 5 years, and it is estimated that 50% of individuals over 85 have Alzheimer's disease (National Institute on Aging, 1998). Seventy-five percent of Americans confined to nursing homes suffer from Alzheimer's disease or other forms of dementia (Chandler & Chandler, 1988). It is estimated that 12 million people worldwide and 4.5 million elderly adults in the United States have Alzheimer's disease. In the United States, annual health care costs associated with Alzheimer's disease exceed $100 billion. If current population trends continue, and effective treatments are not found, the number of patients with Alzheimer's disease in the United States is projected to increase to over 13 million by the year 2050 (Hebert, Scherr, Bienias, Bennett, & Evans, 2003). Developing cost-effective assessment and treatment approaches for Alzheimer's disease is clearly an urgent priority. Approximately 500,000 individuals suffer from stroke annually in the United States, and over half of stroke survivors have varying degrees of cognitive impairment as a result. The annual health care cost of stroke in the United States was estimated at $43 billion in 1997 (National Stroke Association, 1997).

Alzheimer's Disease and Milder Forms of Cognitive Impairment Are Caused by Multiple Genetic, Biological, and Environmental Factors

Alzheimer's Disease

Chronic nutrient deficiencies, toxic injury to the brain, coronary artery disease, chronic stress, and prolonged restricted intellectual activity probably contribute to the risk of developing Alzheimer's disease and other syndromes of severe cognitive impairment (Kidd, 1999). Dementia of the Alzheimer's type is influenced by genetic risk factors but probably has several other biological causes that have cumulative destructive effects on specialized acetylcholine-producing neurons. Neurofibrillary tangles and amyloid-β plaques are two specific pathological findings in Alzheimer's disease. Abnormal deposits of a protein called amyloid-β are believed to trigger an inflammatory response resulting in the widespread destruction of neurons. Chronic inflammation in turn leads to the accumulation of free radicals, which further damage the brain (Ames, Shigenaga, & Hagen, 1993). Degenerative changes in the brain that lead to Alzheimer's disease are probably also a consequence of age-related changes in calcium homeostasis that affect neuroplasticity of the hippocampus, as well as elevated cortisol secondary to chronic stress or psychological trauma (McEwen, 1998). Inconsistent findings of twin cohort studies show a wide range of concordance rates between identical twins, suggesting that nongenetic factors significantly affect the risk of developing

Alzheimer's disease (Bergem, Engedal, & Kirnglen, 1997; Gatz et al.,1997). However, a small subset of Alzheimer's patients share common mutations affecting the presenilin genes on chromosomes 1, 14, and 21, resulting in excessive production of amyloid precursor protein (Lendon, Ashall, & Goate, 1997). Individuals who are homozygous for the apolipoprotein E gene on chromosome 19 also have a significantly greater risk of developing Alzheimer's disease compared with the nonaffected population (Nalbantoglu et al., 1994). Together these genetic factors account for a very small percentage of the total prevalence rate of Alzheimer's disease, especially among the very elderly. There is even less evidence for genetic factors influencing dementias caused by vascular injury to the brain. Nongenetic risk factors that predispose an individual to develop Alzheimer's disease include early brain trauma and late maternal age at birth (Van Duijn et al., 1994). Approximately one third of individuals who survive early brain trauma are affected by abnormal levels of amyloid β-protein deposits similar to the pathological changes of Alzheimer's disease (Roberts et al., 1994). Recent studies have focused on the putative role of chronic stress and elevated cortisol in the pathogenesis of Alzheimer's disease. There is emerging evidence that the severity of cognitive impairment in Alzheimer's patients is correlated with neurotoxic effects of cortisol on the hippocampus, a region of the brain in which memories are formed (Pomara, Greenberg, Brandord, & Doraiswamy, 2003).

Milder Forms of Cognitive Impairment

The other diagnostic category given in the *Diagnostic and Statistical Manual of Mental Disorders* (4th ed., *DSM-IV*) describing severe persisting cognitive impairment is called **amnestic syndrome**. Amnestic syndrome is characterized by either the inability to recall previously learned information or the inability to learn new information. It does not involve the severe global deficits in cognitive functioning that are typically seen in Alzheimer's disease and other forms of dementia. *DSM-IV* criteria stipulate that this symptom pattern must be caused by a medical condition or substance abuse. Milder forms of cognitive impairment are associated with normal aging, chronic nutritional deficiencies, less severe cerebrovascular accidents, thyroid disease, and other medical disorders, as well as chronic alcohol and narcotic abuse. Research evidence supports the use of specific pharmacological treatments to manage cognitive impairment associated with a particular neurobiological or medical cause.

◆ The Integrative Assessment of Cognitive Impairment

Overview of Conventional Approaches Used to Assess Cognitive Impairment

Any discussion of cognitive impairment assumes a range of normal cognitive functioning outside of which the existence of deficits can be reasonably inferred. The conventional practitioner's task is to distinguish between mild, moderate, and severe degrees of cognitive impairment; establish the causes of symptoms; accurately diagnose the symptom pattern as a delirium, an amnestic syndrome, or dementia; and initiate appropriate treatment. Normal aging is associated with gradual declines in the speed of information processing and reduced efficiency of memory formation and recall. ***Mild cognitive impairment*** (MCI) describes less severe deficits in cognitive functioning that are common with aging but do not fulfill criteria for a *DSM-IV* disorder. Mild cognitive impairment may foreshadow progressive cognitive decline, and it is estimated that individuals with MCI become demented at a rate of 10 to 15% per year, in contrast to healthy unimpaired elderly individuals who have a 2% annual risk of becoming demented (Petersen et al., 2001).

When evaluating a cognitively impaired individual, conventionally trained mental health professionals begin with a comprehensive medical, social, and psychiatric history. A careful history clarifies the course, severity, and type of cognitive impairment. However, impaired patients are frequently unable to provide a reliable history, and collateral information must be obtained from a friend or family member. If history suggests a medical cause of persisting cognitive impairment, the appropriate laboratory studies are ordered, possibly including thyroid studies, complete blood count, liver panel, electrolytes, serum glucose, blood urea nitrogen, and serum vitamin levels. Functional neuroimaging may be indicated if there is evidence of injury, infection, stroke, or brain tumor. Cognitive impairment is frequently seen in delirium caused by a medical problem or substance abuse. Medically complicated cases, acute substance intoxication or withdrawal, or unexplained rapidly evolving symptoms of cognitive impairment warrant urgent medical referral. When acute medical causes have been ruled out by history and normal laboratory findings, the evaluation continues largely on the basis of the clinical interview. Conventionally trained mental health professionals obtain detailed information about the course, severity, and rate of progression of cognitive symptoms, including problems with short- or long-term memory, reasoning, and language. The Mini-Mental State Examination (MMSE) is a brief 11-question screening instrument that is sensitive to dementia and other severe forms of cognitive impairment, but is of little clinical value in the evaluation of mild or moderate symptoms. A formal neuropsychological evaluation using specialized tests of memory, problem solving, and abstraction sometimes helps to clarify the specific characteristics and severity of cognitive impairment. On the basis of history, the clinical interview, laboratory studies, and the MMSE, inferences are made about the primary causes of cognitive impairment. Disparate symptom patterns, including depressed mood, mania, anxiety, psychosis, and chronic substance abuse, are frequently associated with varying degrees and kinds of cognitive impairment. For example, moderately impaired short-term memory is often associated with depressed mood and generalized anxiety. Reasoning and expressive language are often profoundly compromised in psychosis and mania, and also during acute intoxication or withdrawal from alcohol or illicit substances. Psychiatric symptoms that are associated with cognitive impairment are managed with conventional drugs and psychotherapy. When other major psychiatric disorders have been ruled out, a primary disorder of cognitive impairment is assumed to be present.

Although rigorous biomedical standards have been established for the assessment of severe cognitive impairment, in the routine day-to-day practice of medicine it is frequently impractical to identify a medical cause. A consequence of this fact is the increasing rate of newly diagnosed cases of Alzheimer's disease even when multiple medical etiologies have not been formally excluded and possible contributing factors from psychiatric history have not been thoroughly evaluated. Available historical information is often incomplete and inaccurate, insurance coverage is limited, and the cognitively impaired individual (and his or her family) is seldom able to advocate for an appropriate and thorough evaluation. These issues are amplified by the growing scarcity of outpatient mental health resources in the context of the rapidly growing elderly population and the increasing prevalence rate of dementia in developed Western countries. Failure to adequately characterize complex medical or psychiatric causes of severe cognitive impairment leads to shortcomings in treatment planning, and patients who might otherwise benefit from appropriate treatment remain impaired. Emerging assessment approaches will permit mental health professionals to more accurately and reliably identify the various causes of cognitive impairment, and to create integrative treatment strategies that effectively address those causes.

Overview of Nonconventional Approaches Used to Assess Cognitive Impairment

At the time of writing, quantitative electroencephalographic (qEEG) brain mapping is the only nonconventional approach used to assess cognitive impairment that is strongly substantiated by consistent research findings. Quantitative EEG mapping will probably emerge as a standard tool for evaluating cognitive impairment in dementia, traumatic brain injury, and post-stroke patients and will facilitate effective treatment planning. Other applications of qEEG mapping rest on provisional evidence at this time, including measurements of visual- or auditory-evoked potentials in both dementia and mild cognitive impairment. Virtual reality (VR) testing environments will probably become an important adjunct to contemporary neuropsychological tests used to assess the range of symptoms in both mild and severe forms of cognitive impairment. There is provisional evidence that abnormally low serum levels of zinc or magnesium may correlate with an increased risk of developing Alzheimer's disease. Measuring serum vitamin levels and serum docosahexaenoic acid (DHA) levels are two emerging approaches used to assess cognitive impairment that are based on limited evidence at this time. **Table 12–1** summarizes substantiated and provisional nonconventional approaches used to assess cognitive impairment. It gives the evidence for assessment approaches that possibly yield specific findings pertaining to cognitive impairment.

Substantiated Approaches Used to Assess Cognitive Impairment

Biological Approaches

At the time of writing, there are no assessment approaches in this category.

Somatic and Mind–Body Approaches

At the time of writing, there are no assessment approaches in this category.

Table 12–1 Assessment Approaches That Are Substantiated or Probably Yield Specific Accurate Information about the Causes of Cognitive Impairment

	Assessment Approach	Evidence for Specific Diagnostic Information	Positive Finding Suggests Efficacy of This Treatment
Substantiated			
Biological	None at time of writing		
Somatic	None at time of writing		
Energy-information assessment approaches validated by Western science	qEEG and neurometric brain mapping	qEEG qapping shows correlations between cognitive impairment related to dementia or stroke (CVA) and diminished activity in the α and β ranges.	qEEG mapping provides information that is useful when planning EEG-biofeedback protocols addressing cognitive impairment.
		Neurometric brain mapping compares qEEG findings with normative age-matched brain activity	qEEG mapping can be used to evaluate response to cognitive-enhancing treatments
Energy-information assessment approaches not (yet) validated by Western science	None at time of writing		
Provisional			
Biological	Serum zinc and magnesium levels	Abnormally low levels of zinc and magnesium may be correlated with the risk of developing Alzheimer's disease; however, findings are inconsistent	*Note:* Supplementation may correct a chronic deficiency in zinc but not magnesium due to a metabolic error that interferes with magnesium transport into neurons
Somatic	None at time of writing		
Energy-information assessment approaches validated by Western science	qEEG and visual or auditory evoked potentials	Specific qEEG findings correlate with Alzheimer's, whereas specific VEP or AEP findings correlate with milder cognitive impairment	qEEG mapping and VEP/AEP studies may permit early diagnosis and more aggressive treatment of early Alzheimer's and mild cognitive impairment
	Virtual reality (VR) testing	VR testing environments will permit earlier and more accurate assessment of moderate and severe cognitive impairment	Neuropsychological assessment using VR environments will permit more individualized and more effective rehabilitation strategies in traumatic brain injury, dementia, and post-stroke patients
Energy-information assessment approaches not validated by Western science	None at time of writing		

AEP, auditory evoked potential; CVA, cerebrovascular accident; EEG, electroencephalography; qEEG, quantitative electroencephalography; VEP, visual evoked potential

Approaches Based on Forms of Energy or Information Validated by Western Science

◆ **Quantitative electroencephalography and neurometric brain mapping will become standard tools for predicting long-term clinical outcomes** Quantitative EEG has been the subject of intensive research for many years. In spite of compelling research evidence supporting the use of qEEG to predict the long-term course and response of Alzheimer's disease to conventional treatments, this method is still primarily a research tool. Quantitative EEG measures include power, left-right interhemispheric symmetry, and phase coherence of electrical brain activity in homologous regions in both hemispheres (Senf, 1988). Measures of absolute power, relative power, coherence, and symmetry are used to characterize abnormal brain electrical activity associated with cognitive decline. Quantitative EEG changes that take place at different stages of Alzheimer's disease and other syndromes of severe cognitive

impairment reflect decreased regional brain energy metabolism or cerebral blood flow that is frequently not apparent in conventional computed tomography (CT) or magnetic resonance imaging (MRI) studies (Passero et al., 1992; Soininen et al., 1989). The rate of deterioration in normal θ (theta) activity (3.5–7.5 Hz) in the early stages of dementia is highly predictive of long-term clinical outcomes (Richards et al., 1993; Rodriguez et al., 1996). Abnormal decreases in slow-wave δ (delta) activity (1.5–3.5 Hz) take place after normal θ activity has deteriorated, and correspond to severe dementia. Quantitative EEG is a reasonable assessment approach in cases where conventional treatments for severe cognitive impairment have failed, or the psychiatric or neurological diagnosis remains unclear.

Neurometric brain mapping is a specialized qEEG approach that compares EEG characteristics of the individual being evaluated with normative databases for the same age. Neurometric mapping helps to clarify functional brain correlates of cognitive impairment, and yields information that is useful for planning EEG-biofeedback protocols addressing specific kinds of dysfunction. Neurometric brain mapping is an evolving diagnostic tool that is increasingly used in clinical settings to differentiate cognitive impairments that are due to head injuries, medical disorders, progressive dementia, alcohol or substance abuse, depressed mood, learning disorders, or other underlying biological causes.

Assessment Approaches Based on Forms of Energy or Information Not Validated by Western Science

At the time of writing, there are no assessment approaches in this category.

Provisional Approaches Used to Assess Cognitive Impairment

Biological Assessment Approaches

◆ **Abnormally low serum zinc and magnesium levels may correlate with the risk of developing Alzheimer's disease** The risk of developing Alzheimer's disease may be associated with chronic low blood levels of zinc and magnesium, but research findings are inconsistent. The relationship between zinc and Alzheimer's disease is poorly understood. High levels of zinc are neurotoxic and are believed to promote formation of amyloid plaques, whereas histopathology studies of the brains of Alzheimer's patients reveal deficient zinc in the brain (Cuajungco & Lees, 1997). Low plasma levels of zinc bound to thymulin in Alzheimer's patients suggests that impaired zinc metabolism contributes to the pathogenesis of this neurodegenerative disease (Cuajungco & Lees, 1997; Licastro, 1996;). It has been suggested that amyloid plaques indirectly cause a zinc deficiency, which leads to formation of neurofibrillary tangles (Constantinidis, 1990). Low serum zinc levels result in impaired zinc transport to the brain and have been cited as a possible factor in the formation of amyloid plaques. Dysregulation of magnesium transport into neurons may be a metabolic abnormality of Alzheimer's disease in spite of adequate magnesium intake in the diet (Glick, 1990). In this case, checking serum magnesium levels does not provide useful information, and magnesium supplementation is not an effective intervention.

Somatic and Mind–Body Approaches

At the time of writing, there are no assessment approaches in this category.

Approaches Based on Forms of Energy or Information Validated by Western Science

◆ **qEEG, visual evoked potentials, and auditory evoked potentials may help to distinguish early Alzheimer's from vascular dementia and mild cognitive impairment** Emerging research findings suggest that qEEG and EEG evoked potentials are useful assessment tools for the evaluation of mild cognitive impairment, early stages of Alzheimer's disease, and symptoms of inattention and cognitive slowing following stroke or traumatic brain injury. Pilot studies have used visual evoked potentials (VEPs) to reliably differentiate patients with mild cognitive impairment or frank Alzheimer's disease from cognitively intact subjects on the basis of qEEG findings alone (Benvenuto, Jin, Casale, Lynch, & Granger, 2002). The pilot data suggest that specific abnormal EEG signals are correlated with Alzheimer's disease, and abnormal auditory evoked potentials (AEPs) provide specific markers of milder forms of cognitive impairment. Slowing of global α activity below 8 Hz, increased θ activity, and a decrease in the α to θ ratio are typical findings in Alzheimer's disease. In contrast, vascular dementia is associated with normal EEG activity interspersed with regions of focal slowing. Researchers have confirmed a pattern of prefrontal cortical disinhibition using qEEG mapping, a typical finding in Alzheimer's disease and other forms of dementia. A significant percentage of mildly cognitively impaired adults eventually progress to frank dementia. Therefore, early qEEG evaluation of at-risk individuals may facilitate early aggressive treatment.

◆ **Virtual reality tools will permit earlier and more accurate assessment of cognitive impairment** Virtual reality (VR) tools may enhance the diagnostic accuracy of existing conventional neuropsychological assessment methods used to evaluate cognitive impairment in degenerative neurological disorders, stroke, developmental disorders, and traumatic brain injury (Rizzo & Wiederhold, 2000). Virtual performance testing environments will lead to the development of novel methods for earlier and more accurate assessment of cognitive impairment. Prototype VR environments have already yielded promising results for assessment of memory, attention, executive functioning, sensorimotor integration, and many activities of daily living. Future neuropsychological assessment approaches will combine VR technology with functional MRI (fMRI) and other functional brain-imaging technologies, dramatically advancing our understanding of the dynamic causes of moderate and severe forms of cognitive impairment. The use of VR environments to assess neuropsychological functioning will lead to individualized rehabilitation strategies that more effectively address performance deficits on a case by case basis.

Assessment Approaches Based on Forms of Energy or Information Not Validated by Western Science

At the time of writing, there are no assessment approaches in this category.

Table 12–2 lists assessment approaches that may yield specific information about the causes of cognitive impairment.

◆ **Abnormally low serum levels of certain vitamins and trace elements may correlate with the risk of developing Alzheimer's disease** Malnutrition due to malabsorption of essential dietary factors may play a significant causative role in dementia. Chronic brain deficiencies of vitamins and certain trace elements may contribute to the formation of neurofibrillary tangles and other pathological changes in the brain that eventually manifest as Alzheimer's disease or other degenerative disorders (Evans, 1987). However, clear correlations have not been established between the risk of developing Alzheimer's disease and abnormally low serum levels of vitamins or trace elements (Scileppi, Blass, & Baker, 1984).

Table 12–2 Assessment Approaches That Possibly Yield Specific Information about Causes of Cognitive Impairment

Category	Assessment Approach	Evidence for Specific Diagnostic Information	Comments
Biological	Serum levels of vitamins and trace elements	Chronic malnutrition caused by malabsorption of essential dietary factors may increase the risk of developing Alzheimer's disease or mild cognitive impairment	Relationships between serum levels of vitamins and trace elements and risk of dementia are inconsistent
	Serum DHA levels	Abnormally low serum DHA levels may be correlated with increased risk of developing Alzheimer's disease	*Note:* Findings of correlations between serum DHA levels and cognitive impairment risk are inconsistent
Somatic	None at time of writing		
Energy-information assessment approaches validated by Western science	None at time of writing		
Energy-information assessment approaches not validated by Western science	None at time of writing		

DHA, docosahexaenoic acid

◆ **Low serum DHA levels may correspond to relatively greater cognitive impairment** Case studies suggest that abnormally low levels of serum DHA (an omega-3 fatty acid) may be correlated with the severity of cognitive impairment in demented patients (Kyle, Schaefer, & Patton, 1998; Tully et al., 2003). However, the results of other studies contradict this finding (Laurin, Verreault, Lindsay, Dewailly, & Holub, 2003). Testing serum DHA levels in demented patients should not be regarded as a useful clinical approach pending future research findings that demonstrate consistent correlations between serum omega-3 fatty acid levels and the relative risk of developing severe cognitive impairment.

◆ The Integrative Treatment of Cognitive Impairment

Existing Conventional Treatments Are Sometimes Beneficial in Early Stages of Mild to Moderate Dementia

The research emphasis on conventional biomedical treatments of dementia has shifted from vasodilators and nootropic agents to drugs that increase brain levels of acetylcholine. Current biomedical treatments of Alzheimer's disease work by inhibiting the enzyme that breaks down acetylcholine, thus increasing available levels of the neurotransmitter that is critical for learning and memory. Commercially available cholinesterase inhibitors have significant adverse effects and are only effective against mild or early symptoms of Alzheimer's disease, not other forms of dementia. Early promising results of studies on tacrine, the first commercially marketed acetylcholinesterase inhibitor, were offset by findings of significant hepatotoxicity. Second-generation acetylcholinesterase inhibitors (donepezil, rivastigmine, and galantamine) are no more effective than tacrine but require less frequent dosing and have fewer associated safety issues. Other drug classes that have been investigated for possible cognitive-enhancing benefits in dementia include the monoamine oxidase inhibitors (MAOIs), estrogen replacement therapy (i.e., in cognitively impaired postmenopausal women), naloxone, and various neuropeptides, including vasopressin and somatostatin (Zandi et al., 2005). Most studies on conventional agents have yielded equivocal or negative results. Promising novel biomedical treatments of Alzheimer's disease currently being investigated in clinical trials include a vaccine that may immunize individuals against formation of amyloid-β, secretase inhibitors, anti-inflammatory agents, and statins.

Severely cognitively impaired individuals frequently experience depressed mood, anxiety, and psychotic symptoms (Burns, Jacoby, & Levy, 1990; Wragg & Jeste, 1989). Western medical management of mixed symptom patterns uses combinations of conventional drugs. Behavioral disturbances, including agitation and aggressive behavior toward caregivers, are commonly encountered in demented individuals. Even though acetylcholinesterase inhibitors offer only transient improvements in the early stages of dementia, these drugs have become the standard biomedical approach to Alzheimer's disease and other forms of dementia in Western countries because of consistent findings of reduced agitation. In addition to pharmacological management, behavioral interventions, environmental enrichment, and social support mitigate some of the cognitive and behavioral symptoms of dementia.

An Overview of Nonconventional Treatments of Cognitive Impairment

Many nonconventional modalities have been substantiated as effective treatments of cognitive impairment related to Alzheimer's disease, stroke, traumatic brain injury, or normal aging. Dietary changes that are correlated with a reduced risk of developing Alzheimer's disease include restricted intake of saturated fats and moderate wine consumption. Regular aerobic exercise also reduces the risk of developing any kind of dementia. *Ginkgo biloba* is an effective treatment of cognitive impairment in early or moderate cases of Alzheimer's disease and vascular dementia. Phosphatidylserine and huperzine A will probably play increasingly important roles as adjunctive agents and stand-alone treatments in the management of early or moderate Alzheimer's disease, mild cognitive impairment, and age-related cognitive decline. Cytidine diphosphate (CDP)-choline holds promise as a treatment of cognitive impairment following stroke or traumatic brain injury.

At the time of writing, provisional nonconventional biological treatments of dementia related to various underlying causes include paracetam, Choto-san, golden root (*Rhodiola rosea*), Kami-untan-to (KUT), centrophenoxine (CPH), idebenone, acetyl-L-carnitine, dehydroepiandrosterone (DHEA), certain B vitamins, and a combined regimen of vitamins E and C. The essential oils of lemon balm (*Melissa officinalis*) and common sage (*Salvia officinalis*) probably reduce agitation and "sundowning" in demented individuals when applied to the arms and face. Snoezelen is an emerging sensory stimulation therapy that probably improves global functioning. Cranioelectrotherapy stimulation of the brain is based on microcurrent pulses of electricity and purportedly results in transient improvements in word recall, face recognition, and motivation. Regular music therapy reportedly results in transient improvements in agitated behavior and cognitive functioning in Alzheimer's pa-

tients. Research findings suggest that regular Healing Touch and Therapeutic Touch have beneficial calming effects and improve global functioning in Alzheimer's disease.

Possibly effective nonconventional biological treatments of cognitive impairment include medicinal herbs or herbal formulas from several systems of medicine, including Ashwagondha, lemon balm, common sage, ginseng, Qian Jin Yi Fang, Trasina, and Mentat. Nonherbal biologicals that may prove to be effective treatments of dementia, cognitive impairments following stroke or traumatic brain injury, or age-related cognitive decline include dronabinol, dehydroevodiamine (DHED), niacin, piracetam, CPH, picamilon, α-lipoic acid, pyritinol, and melatonin. Regular massage therapy and bright light exposure are two emerging approaches used to manage agitation or inappropriate behavior in demented individuals. Preliminary findings suggest that certain EEG-biofeedback protocols improve cognitive functioning following stroke or traumatic brain injury. Finally, intriguing case reports suggest that regular qigong treatments or the practice of certain qigong exercises can slow or potentially reverse the underlying neurobiological causes of dementia. **Table 12–3** summarizes the evidence for substantiated and provisional nonconventional treatments of dementia and less severe forms of cognitive impairment.

Table 12–3 Nonconventional Treatments of Dementia and Less Severe Forms of Cognitive Impairment That Are or Probably Are Effective

	Substantiated Treatment Approach	Evidence for Modality or Integrative Approaches	Comments (Including Safety Issues or Contraindications)
Biological treatments	Dietary modification	Moderate wine consumption, reduced saturated fats, and reduced total caloric intake are correlated with reduced risk of developing Alzheimer's disease	***Caution:*** Elderly people should be cautioned about excessive alcohol consumption. Consuming more than 2 to 4 glasses of wine per day increases the risk of dementia
	Ginkgo biloba	Standardized extracts of *G. biloba* 120 to 600 mg/day improve memory and cognitive performance in mild to moderate Alzheimer's disease, vascular dementia, and post-stroke patients and may slow cognitive decline in severe dementia. Combining *G. biloba* with ginseng enhances cognitive performance in nonimpaired healthy adults. Combining *G. biloba* with piracetam or CDP-choline may improve outcomes	***Caution:*** *G. biloba* is contraindicated in patients taking anticoagulants. Cases of serotonin syndrome have been reported when combined with SSRIs
	Huperzine A (*Huperzia serrata*)	Huperzine A 200 to 400 μg/day may have beneficial effects in age-related memory loss and Alzheimer's disease that are comparable to conventional cholinesterase inhibitors	***Note:*** Transient adverse effects of huperzine A include dizziness, nausea, and diarrhea
	CDP-choline	CDP-choline enhances the rate of cognitive recovery following stroke and may be beneficial in traumatic brain–injured patients	***Note:*** CDP-choline may not improve attention, but it does improve global functioning and memory
	Phosphatidylserine (PS)	PS 300 mg/day is beneficial for age-related cognitive decline and Alzheimer's disease	***Caution:*** Bovine brain–derived PS is probably more effective than the soy-derived product, but there is growing concern over acquiring a slow virus from infected brain tissue
	Idebenone	Idebenone 360 mg/day may be more effective than conventional cholinesterase inhibitors in the treatment of mild to moderate Alzheimer's disease. Post-stroke recovery may be enhanced by combining idebenone with vinpocetine	***Note:*** Use of idebenone in post-stroke patients is based on animal studies and must be confirmed by human clinical trials before being recommended

(Continued)

Table 12–3 Nonconventional Treatments of Dementia and Less Severe Forms of Cognitive Impairment That Are or Probably Are Effective *(Continued)*

	Substantiated Treatment Approach	Evidence for Modality or Integrative Approaches	Comments (Including Safety Issues or Contraindications)
Somatic or mind–body	Exercise	Regular physical exercise in healthy elderly individuals significantly reduces the risk of all categories of dementia	*Note:* Exercise is probably not an effective intervention after the onset of dementia *Caution:* Individuals who have been sedentary or who have a chronic pain syndrome or a major medical illness should be evaluated by a physician before starting a rigorous exercise program
Energy-information approaches validated by Western science	None at time of writing		
Energy-information approaches not validated by Western science	None at time of writing		
Provisional			
Biological treatments	Dietary modifications	Diets high in fish or other sources of omega-3 fatty acids and low in omega-6 fatty acids may be associated with reduced risk of dementia	*Note:* Epidemiologic data on relationships between specific foods and the risk of developing dementia are inconsistent
	Ginkgo biloba	*G. biloba* extract (1.9 mL/day) may improve the efficiency and speed of information processing in healthy elderly individuals. *G. biloba* may slow progression of mild cognitive impairment	*Caution:* *G. biloba* should be avoided in patients taking aspirin or anticoagulant drugs
	Kami-untan-to (KUT)	KUT, a compound herbal formula, stimulates production of nerve growth factor and the synthetic enzyme for acetylcholine and may slow the rate of progression of Alzheimer's disease	*Note:* One open study used KUT combined with vitamin E and a nonsteroidal anti-inflammatory drug, making it difficult to attribute cognitive-enhancing effects to KUT alone
	Golden root (*Rhodiola rosea*)	*R. rosea* 500 mg/day improves memory and performance in healthy adults and may accelerate recovery of normal cognitive functioning following head injury. Neuroprotective effects may be enhanced by piracetam, *Ginkgo biloba,* or ginseng	*Caution:* *R. rosea* may induce mania in bipolar patients and should be avoided in this population
	Choto-san	Choto-san, a compound herbal formula, affects dopamine and serotonin receptors and has strong antioxidant properties. Choto-san improves global functioning and cognition in vascular dementia	*Note:* There is evidence that Choto-san reduces symptoms of psychosis in demented individuals
	Acetyl-L-carnitine (ALC)	ALC 1500 to 3000 mg/day may be beneficial for mild cognitive decline and Alzheimer's disease. ALC may improve cognitive performance in healthy adults, and in depressed individuals and abstinent alcoholics. Neuroprotective effects of ALC may be enhanced when combined with CoQ10, α–lipoic acid, or omega-3 fatty acids	*Note:* Initial beneficial cognitive effects in dementia may not be sustained beyond 1 year with continuous treatment
	B vitamins (folate, B_{12}, and thiamine)	Daily folate, B_{12}, or thiamine supplementation may be beneficial in some cases of age-related cognitive decline and Alzheimer's disease. Folate 50 mg/day may improve mood and cognition in depressed demented individuals	*Note:* The evidence for vitamin B_{12} is limited and largely anecdotal. A systematic review did not find strong evidence for folate or B_{12} in dementia or other forms of severe cognitive impairment

Table 12–3 Nonconventional Treatments of Dementia and Less Severe Forms of Cognitive Impairment That Are or Probably Are Effective *(Continued)*

	Substantiated Treatment Approach	Evidence for Modality or Integrative Approaches	Comments (Including Safety Issues or Contraindications)
	Vitamins C and E	Daily combined use of vitamin C (at least 500 mg) and vitamin E (at least 400 IU) may significantly reduce the risk of developing Alzheimer's disease	*Note:* There is probably little protective benefit from taking either vitamin C or vitamin E alone. A systematic review did not find strong evidence for a beneficial effect of vitamin E in dementia. *Caution:* High doses of vitamin E may increase the risk of stroke in at-risk patients
	DHEA and testosterone	DHEA 25 to 50 mg/day may improve mental performance in healthy adults, and 200 mg/day may improve cognitive functioning in vascular dementia. Testosterone 75 mg/day may slow the rate of progression of Alzheimer's disease	*Note:* There is no evidence for a cognitive-enhancing effect of DHEA in Alzheimer's disease. *Caution:* DHEA can cause insomnia or agitation and should be taken in the morning; testosterone replacement can increase the risk of prostate cancer
	Essential oils	Essential oils of lavender and lemon balm applied to the face and arms (but not as aromatherapy) have beneficial calming effects on agitation in demented patients	*Caution:* Essential oils can cause skin allergies and phototoxic reactions. Lavender oil increases the sedating effects of conventional sedatives. Pregnant women should not apply essential oils to the skin because of systemic absorption and potential toxic effects on the fetus
Somatic and mind–body approaches	Snoezelen, a multimodal sensory stimulation therapy	Four to 8 weekly Snoezelen sessions may reduce apathy and psychomotor agitation while enhancing language in demented individuals	*Note:* The significance of systematic review findings is limited by inclusion of only two studies. Four studies are in progress at the time of writing
Energy-information approaches validated by Western science	TENS and CES	TENS and CES treatments resulted in improvements in word recall, face recognition, and motivation in demented individuals	*Note:* The beneficial effects of weak electrical stimulation are not sustained several weeks after treatment ends
	Music therapy and binaural sound	Regular music therapy probably enhances global functioning in demented individuals, reduces agitation and wandering, enhances social interaction, improves depressed mood, increases cooperative behavior, and increases baseline cognitive functioning. Binaural sounds in the beta frequency range may enhance cognitive functioning in healthy adults	*Note:* Most studies on music in dementia are small, and findings are limited by the absence of quantitative outcome measures, randomization, and blinding
Energy-information approaches not validated by Western science	Healing Touch (HT) and Therapeutic Touch (TT)	Regular HT or TT treatments may reduce agitation, improve global functioning, improve sleep schedule, and enhance compliance with nursing home routines. Patients who receive regular HT treatments may require lower doses of medications for agitated behavior	*Note:* Findings of HT and TT as treatments of agitation in dementia are limited by study design flaws, including lack of blinding, small size, and the absence of control groups receiving sham treatments in most studies

CDP, cytidine diphosphate; CES, cranioelectrotherapy stimulation; CoQ10, coenzyme Q10; DHEA, dehydroepiandrosterone; HT, Healing Touch; IU, international unit; SSRI, selective serotonin reuptake inhibitor; TENS, transcranial electrical nerve stimulation; TT, Therapeutic Touch

Substantiated Treatments of Cognitive Impairment

Dietary Modifications

◆ **Moderate wine consumption and diets low in saturated fat and total calories reduce the risk of Alzheimer's disease** Individuals who consume a high-fat, high-calorie diet are at significantly greater risk of developing Alzheimer's dementia compared with individuals who have moderate fat intake and restrict total calories. It has been suggested that excess caloric intake and high fat intake promote formation of damaging free radicals that cause many neuropathological changes in the brain. A meta-analysis of findings from 18 community-wide studies concluded that the risk of Alzheimer's disease increased linearly at a rate of 0.3% with every 100-calorie increase in daily intake (Grant, 1997). Average daily fat consumption was highly correlated with increased risk of developing dementia. The same meta-analysis showed that fish consumption was the only specific dietary factor associated with a measurable reduction in the risk of developing Alzheimer's disease. Fish are an important source of omega-3 fatty acids, for which there is emerging evidence of beneficial and possibly preventive effects in dementia and less severe forms of cognitive impairment (see discussion below). Moderate but not heavy consumption of wine (2–4 glasses/day) is also associated with reduced risk of Alzheimer's disease (Orgogozo et al., 1997). In a large 5-year cohort study, 19,000 women ages 70 to 80 years who drank 14 g alcohol daily (the equivalent of $1^1/_2$ glasses of wine or one 12 oz. beer) were 20% less likely to experience significant cognitive impairment compared with nondrinkers. Greater average consumption of alcohol was associated with increased risk of cognitive impairment during the study period (Weuve, Kang, Manson, Breteler, Ware, & Grodstein, 2004).

Medicinal Herbs

◆ **Standardized extracts of *Ginkgo biloba* are effective treatments of mild to moderate symptoms of Alzheimer's disease and vascular dementia**   Standardized preparations of this herb are widely used in Europe to treat dementia and other neurodegenerative diseases, and in recent years its use has become widespread in North America. Most commercially available ginkgo preparations are standardized to two bioactive constituents: 24% flavone glycosides and 6% terpenoids. The flavonoid constituent functions as a strong antioxidant and is believed to have a general neuroprotective effect (Seif-El-Nasr & El-Fattah, 1995). Animal studies have confirmed that the terpenoid fraction antagonizes platelet activating factor (PAF), facilitating post-stroke recovery through vascular reperfusion by decreasing thrombosis and nerve cell death associated with cerebral ischemia (Smith, Maclennan, & Darlington, 1996). Constituents of ginkgo may inhibit neurotoxicity and nerve cell death caused by nitric oxide (Zhao & Li, 2002). Other putative therapeutic actions include vasodilation of small blood vessels in the brain and anti-inflammatory effects (Blumenthal, Goldberg, & Brinckmann, 2000). EEG changes associated with increased alertness have been found in healthy adults taking ginkgo preparations (Pidoux, 1986). Therapeutic doses range from 40 mg 3 times daily up to 600 mg/day in divided doses, and sustained improvement in cognitive functioning is usually observed following 3 months of treatment. Systematic reviews and meta-analyses of double-blind studies have concluded that standardized preparations of *G. biloba* in doses between 120 and 600 mg/day taken over durations of several weeks to 1 year result in consistent modest improvements in memory, general cognitive functioning, and activities of daily living in mild to moderate cases of both Alzheimer's dementia and multi-infarct dementia that are equivalent to improvements seen with donepezil, a conventional cholinesterase inhibitor (Ernst, 1999; Itil et al., 1998; Kanowski, Herrmann, Stephan, Wierich, & Horr, 1997; Le Bars, Katz, Berman, Turan, Freedman, & Schatzberg, 1997; Oken , Storzbach, & Kaye, 1998; Wong, Smith, & Boon, 1998). However, a more recent meta-analysis pointed out inconsistent findings of three trials based on more rigorous methodologies and commented on research design problems in both recent and early trials, including the absence of standardized ginkgo preparations and the use of different dementia rating scales across studies (Birks & Grimley, 2004). Although most controlled studies fail to support the claim that ginkgo

significantly improves memory in severely demented patients, the findings of one double-blind study suggest that the rate of overall cognitive decline is moderately slowed in this population (Le Bars, Velasco, Ferguson, Dessain, Kieser, & Hoerr, 2002).

Standardized preparations of ginkgo are also used to treat cognitive impairments due to vascular insufficiency and traumatic brain injury (Gaby, 1996). A systematic review of 40 studies (Kleijnen & Knipschild, 1992) concluded that ginkgo improves many cognitive symptoms associated with cerebral vascular insufficiency, including impaired concentration and memory loss. In contrast to Alzheimer's patients, greater improvement was reported with ginkgo in individuals diagnosed with vascular dementia who had severe memory impairment compared with individuals with mild memory impairment.

◆ **Combining *Ginkgo biloba* with ginseng (*panax ginseng*) enhances memory performance in nonimpaired individuals more than either herbal alone**   Randomized, placebo-controlled studies have concluded that a compound herbal product containing both *Ginkgo biloba* (160 or 320 mg) and *Panax ginseng* (400 mg) significantly improves recall performance in healthy middle-aged adults (Kennedy, Scholey, & Wesnes, 2001; Wesnes et al., 1997, 2000). Enhanced cognitive functioning appears to reach its peak ~6 hours after the herbal preparation is taken. Combining ginkgo with another traditional Chinese herbal, Dangshen (*Codonopsis pilosula*), may also have more beneficial effects on learning and memory in healthy adults compared with either herbal alone (Singh et al., 2004).

Side effects associated with ginkgo are infrequent and typically mild, including rash and headache. Ginkgo taken alone does not increase the risk of bleeding; however, the use of ginkgo preparations is contraindicated in patients taking anticoagulants. An ongoing study funded by the National Center for Complementary and Alternative Medicine (NCCAM) is evaluating the safety of *G. biloba* extract in diabetic patients because of evidence that ginkgo results in progressive insulin resistance by accelerating pancreatic β-cell dysfunction. The reader is invited to check the companion Web site (www.thieme.com/mentalhealth) for preliminary findings.

Safety problems associated with G. biloba   All practitioners should become familiar with important safety issues before recommending *G. biloba* to patients. Informed consent should be documented in the patient's chart at the time of the consultation when *G. biloba* is discussed. Because of its strong antiPAF profile, *G. biloba* extract increases the risk of bleeding, and concurrent use should be avoided in patients taking aspirin, warfarin, heparin, or other medications that interfere with platelet activity and increase bleeding time. Because of the risk of increased bleeding, *G. biloba* preparations should be discontinued at least 2 weeks prior to surgery. *G. biloba* preparations have been reported to result in the elevation of hepatic enzymes, and there are case reports of possible serotonin syndrome when ginkgo is taken with selective serotonin reuptake inhibitors (SSRIs). Mild transient adverse effects include upset stomach, dizziness, and headaches.

◆ **Huperzine A may be more effective than conventional cholinesterase inhibitors for age-related memory loss and dementia**   Huperzine A is an alkaloid derivative of the herb *Huperzia serrata*, and is an important ingredient of many compound herbal formulas used in Chinese medicine to treat cognitive impairment related to normal aging. Huperzine A reversibly inhibits acetylcholinesterase and may also slow production of nitric oxide in the brain, reducing age-related neurotoxicity (Zhao & Li, 2002). Findings from animal studies suggest that huperzine A may be a more potent and more specific inhibitor of acetylcholinesterase than available conventional cholinesterase inhibitors. Controlled trials show consistent beneficial effects in both age-related memory loss (i.e., benign senescent forgetfulness) and Alzheimer's disease at doses between 200 and 400 μg/day (Wang, Ren, Shen, 1994; Zucker, 1999). Huperzine A is more effective than piracetam for age-related memory loss (Wang et al., 1994). Infrequent adverse effects include transient dizziness, nausea, and diarrhea.

◆ **Phosphatidylserine is beneficial for age-related cognitive decline and Alzheimer's disease** Phosphatidylserine is one of the most important phospholipids in the brain and is an essential component of nerve cell membranes. Commercial phosphatidylserine products are derived from soy or bovine brains and are usually dosed at 300 mg/day. The mechanism of action is believed to be enhanced fluidity of nerve cell membranes, indirectly increasing brain levels of many important neurotransmitters (Pepeu, Pepeu, & Amaducci, 1996). Brain-derived phosphatidylserine is probably more effective than the soy-derived product (Hibbeln & Salem, 1995), possibly due to the higher content in DHA, an omega-3 fatty acid (see discussion on DHA and ecosapentanoic acid below), but recent concerns have been raised over the risk of slow viruses in infected bovine tissue. The findings of many large double-blind, placebo-controlled studies confirm improved global functioning and memory in Alzheimer's disease and age-related cognitive decline at typical doses of 300 mg/day (Amaducci, 1988; Cenacchi et al., 1993; Crook et al., 1991; Palmieri et al., 1987; Villardita et al., 1987).

◆ **CDP-choline has beneficial effects on memory and behavior in post-stroke patients and possibly also in traumatic brain injury and Alzheimer's disease** Like acetyl-L-carnitine, CDP-choline increases mitochondrial energy production and in many parts of the world is used to treat cognitive impairments resulting from neurodegenerative diseases. The findings of one study suggest that CDP-choline at 500 mg to 1000 mg/day improves overall energy metabolism in the brain, increases brain levels of dopamine and norepinephrine (Secades & Frontera, 1995), and enhances short-term memory in Alzheimer's patients (Alvarez et al., 1997). Two Cochrane systematic reviews concluded that CDP-choline has consistent positive effects on the rate of recovery in post-stroke patients, as well as in elderly individuals who are cognitively impaired due to cerebrovascular disease (Fioravanti & Yanagi, 2004; Mitka, 2002). An interesting finding was the absence of beneficial effects on attention in spite of significant improvements in global functioning and memory. There is preliminary but promising evidence of a beneficial effect following traumatic brain injury (Spiers & Hochanadel, 1999). The findings of one small study suggest a possible effect of CDP-choline 1000 mg/day in the early stages of Alzheimer's disease (Alvarez et al., 1999).

◆ **Idebenone may be more effective than conventional treatments of Alzheimer's disease** Idebenone is a naturally occurring substance that is related to ubiquinone (coenzyme Q10, or CoQ10), and like that compound also increases intracellular energy production in mitochondria. Animal and human studies have shown that idebenone 360 mg/day may be more effective than tacrine (Gutzmann, 2002) and possibly other conventional treatments (i.e., cholinesterase inhibitors) of cognitive impairment in mild to moderate cases of Alzheimer's dementia (Gutzmann, 1998). Preliminary evidence from animal studies suggests that combining idebenone with vinpocetine accelerates recovery following stroke (Ishihara, 1989).

Somatic and Mind–Body Approaches

◆ **Regular exercise reduces the risk of developing dementia but does not reduce symptoms of cognitive impairment in demented individuals** Physical exercise increases levels of brain-derived neurotrophic factor, probably enhancing neural plasticity and new synapse formation (Cotman, 2002). Regular exercise is associated with increases in the relative size of the frontotemporal and parietal lobes, which are important centers for learning, memory, and executive functioning (Haier, 1993). Long-term regular physical activity, including walking, is associated with reduced risk of all categories of dementia in elderly men and women. In one study, over 2000 physically nonimpaired men ages 71 to 93 years were followed with routine neurological assessments at 2-year intervals starting in 1991 (Abbott, White, Ross, Masaki, Curb, & Petrovitch, 2004). At the end of the study period, men who walked less than 0.25 mile daily had an almost twofold greater probability of being diagnosed with any category of dementia (including Alzheimer's disease and vascular dementia) compared with men who walked at least 2 miles each day. Factors other than the level of physical activity were accounted for, including the possibility that limited activity could be a result of early but undiagnosed dementia. Findings of the Nurses' Health Study based on biannual mailed surveys over 10 years showed that elderly women ages 70 to 81 years who engaged in regular vigorous physical activity were significantly less likely to have been diagnosed with dementia compared with women with more sedentary lifestyles (Weuve et al., 2004). Although regular exercise is an important preventive strategy, it is probably not an effective intervention once dementia has started. A randomized controlled trial showed that regular daily exercise in moderately demented individuals receiving in-home care reduces depressed mood, but it does not improve cognitive functioning (Teri et al., 2003).

Treatments Based on Forms of Energy or Information Validated by Western Science

At the time of writing, there are no treatment approaches in this category.

Treatments Based on Forms of Energy or Information Not Validated by Western Science

At the time of writing, there are no treatment approaches in this category.

Provisional Treatments of Cognitive Impairment

Dietary Modifications

◆ **Diets rich in omega-3 fatty acids may reduce the risk of Alzheimer's disease** Evidence from epidemiologic studies suggests that regular intake of foods rich in omega-3 fatty acids may be inversely related to cognitive impairment or the rate of overall cognitive decline in nondemented elderly individuals. However, findings to date are inconclusive. Regular consumption of foods rich in omega-3, especially fish, may reduce oxidative stress and associated atherosclerotic changes in the brain, indirectly lowering the risk of cognitive decline due to cerebrovascular disease. In contrast, high dietary intake of omega-6 polyunsaturated fatty acids, including linoleic acid, may contribute to increased oxidative stress in the brain, indirectly promoting atherosclerosis and thrombosis, which eventually manifest as declines in overall cognitive functioning. A large epidemiologic study concluded that fish consumption 2 to 3 times weekly significantly reduces the risk of cognitive decline in elderly populations (Kalmijn, Feskens, Launer, & Kromhout, 1997). Cognitive impairment scores were analyzed for two groups of elderly men (ages 69–89) with different dietary preferences. High fish consumption (containing large amounts of omega-3 fatty acids) was inversely correlated with cognitive impairment. In contrast, a preference for foods rich in linoleic acid (an omega-6 fatty acid) was associated with significantly higher rates of cognitive decline. Findings from a prospective cohort study (Morris et al., 2003) suggest that individuals who consume fish at least weekly have a 60% lower risk of developing Alzheimer's disease compared with individuals who seldom eat fish. However, a similar study failed to show a correlation between fish consumption and the risk of developing Alzheimer's disease (Engelhart et al., 2002b). Another cohort study concluded that enhanced cognitive performance in nonimpaired middle-aged individuals is correlated with high intake of fatty fish and other foods rich in omega-3 fatty acids (Kalmijn, van Boxtel, Ocke, Vershuren, Kromhout, & Launer, 2004). The findings of one study (Barberger-Gateau, Letenneur, Deschamps, Peres, Dartigues, & Renaud, 2002) suggest that lifestyle factors and educational level are associated with healthy dietary preferences, including increased fish consumption, and that a lower risk of developing Alzheimer's disease cannot be ascribed to fish consumption alone. A systematic review of six case control studies and three cohort studies examining dietary preferences in dementia concluded that there is no compelling evidence for causal relationships between specific dietary factors and the risk of becoming demented (Ernst, 1999). The findings of the case control studies examining the relationship between dietary protein, vitamins, and minerals and the risk of dementia were highly inconsistent. One of the cohort studies reviewed by Ernst (1999) concluded that the risk of dementia was slightly reduced with moderate consumption of wine or fish, and slightly increased in patients who followed diets high in animal fat and cholesterol, but this finding was not corroborated by the results of other cohort studies examined in the meta-analysis.

Medicinal Herbs

◆ *Ginkgo biloba* **may prevent or slow the rate of progression of some cases of mild cognitive impairment** In addition to compelling evidence supporting its use as a treatment of early or moderate dementia, other research findings suggest that *Ginkgo biloba* is beneficial in mildly impaired elderly individuals who are experiencing age-related cognitive decline. It is not clear whether mildly impaired individuals who benefit from *G. biloba* are exhibiting early signs of Alzheimer's disease or vascular dementia. A meta-analysis of 11 clinical trials of *G. biloba* extract in elderly individuals who reported cognitive difficulties

but did not meet full criteria for dementia confirmed consistent cognitive-enhancing effects (Hopfenmuller, 1994). A 24-week multicenter trial randomized 241 patients (ages 55–86) complaining of mild cognitive impairments to a low-dose ginkgo extract (0.9 mL), a high-dose of ginkgo extract (1.9 mL), versus placebo 3 times daily. The high-dose ginkgo group experienced significantly greater improvement in cognitive performance compared with the low-dose and placebo groups, suggesting a dose–response effect in this population (Brautigam et al., 1998). Other large studies on ginkgo in mild cognitive impairment have yielded negative findings (Van Dongen et al., 2003). Long-term use of *G. biloba* extract in nonimpaired elderly individuals may improve the efficiency and speed of information processing and delay onset of mild cognitive impairment (Allain et al., 1993; Semlitsch et al., 1995). However, a more recent large study failed to confirm a preventive effect (Cheuvront & Carter, 2003). High doses of *G. biloba* extract may be beneficial in some individuals who are mildly cognitively impaired. In contrast to strong evidence supporting its use as a treatment of early or moderate dementia, available research findings suggest that ginkgo should be regarded as a provisional approach for the prevention or treatment of mild cognitive impairment.

◆ **Kami-untan-to is probably an effective treatment of age-related cognitive decline and early or mild Alzheimer's disease** Kami-untan-to is a compound herbal formula consisting of 13 different herbs that is used in Japanese traditional healing (Kampo) to treat cognitive impairment and frank dementia, as well as other psychiatric symptoms. Animal studies suggest that KUT increases brain levels of both nerve growth factor (NGF) and choline acetyltransferase, the enzyme that makes acetylcholine (Yabe, Toriizuka, & Yamada, 1996; Yabe & Yamada, 1996/1997). The putative mechanism of action of KUT is thus the converse of conventional cholinesterase inhibitors, which inhibit the enzyme that degrades acetylcholine in the synaptic cleft. KUT also protects against cognitive impairment due to thiamine deficiency in mice, suggesting possible beneficial effects in delirium tremens and other syndromes of cognitive impairment related to thiamine deficiency (Nakagawasai et al., 2004). In a 12-month open trial, 20 moderately demented Alzheimer's patients treated with KUT alone and 7 treated with a combined regimen of vitamin E, estrogen, and a nonsteroidal anti-inflammatory drug deteriorated at a significantly slower rate compared with 32 moderately demented control patients who received no treatment. The beneficial effects of KUT were most notable 3 months into the study (Arai, Suzuki, Sasaki, Hanawa, Toriizuka, & Yamada, 2000).

◆ **Golden root may enhance memory in healthy adults and speed up recovery following traumatic brain injury** Golden root was the object of intense research interest in the former Soviet Union because of its use as an adaptogen and performance enhancer in athletes, soldiers, and cosmonauts. In traditional Russian society, this herb is prepared as a tea. It is widely consumed and is believed to contribute to improved general health and longevity. Information on the diverse medical benefits of golden root has only recently been available in Western countries, but the herbal is already in widespread use in western Europe. A comprehensive review of the research evidence for golden root is available in Brown and Gerbarg (2004). Psychiatric benefits are probably related to increased dopamine, serotonin, and norepinephrine (Petkov eet al., 1990), and include improved memory, increased mental stamina, and a general calming effect. Results from open studies suggest that golden root at 500 mg improves overall mental performance and stamina in normal individuals (Spasov et al., 2000), and may accelerate return to normal cognitive functioning following traumatic brain injury. Brown and Gerberg (2004) speculated that golden root may be more effective when combined with piracetam, ginseng, or ginkgo. There are no reports of toxicities or serious drug–drug interactions; however, practitioners should advise patients diagnosed with bipolar disorder to avoid use of this herb because of reports of possible induction of mania (Saratikov & Krasnov, 1987).

◆ **Choto-san, a Kampo herbal formula, may be beneficial for vascular dementia** Choto-san is a Kampo herbal formula in current use in Japan to treat symptoms associated with cerebrovascular disease. Putative mechanisms of action include activating effects at serotonin and dopamine receptors, and strong antioxidant effects. Two controlled, double-blind studies have demonstrated consistent beneficial effects in the treatment of vascular dementia, including improved global functioning, improved sleep, reduced psychotic symptoms, and improved cognitive functioning (Shimada et al., 1994; Terasawa et al., 1997).

Amino Acids and Their Precursors

◆ **Acetyl-l-carnitine may be beneficial in early Alzheimer's disease and mild cognitive impairment** Acetyl-L-carnitine (ALC) occurs naturally in the brain and liver. Research findings suggest that ALC may stabilize nerve cell membranes, stimulate synthesis of acetylcholine, and increase the efficiency of mitochondrial energy production. Although commonly used to treat cognitive impairments related to dementia or other neurodegenerative diseases, findings of human clinical trials are inconsistent (Pettegrew, Levine, & McClure, 2000). Double-blind, placebo-controlled studies show that ALC at 1500 to 3000 mg/day improves overall performance on tests of reaction time, memory, and cognitive performance in demented patients and may slow the overall rate of progression of cognitive impairment (Arrigo, Casale, Buonocore, & Ciano, 1990; Calvani et al., 1992; Thal et al., 1996). The findings of these studies suggest that younger demented individuals (i.e., individuals with presenile dementia) benefit more than older individuals and that 62 years may be the optimal age beyond which ALC loses much of its efficacy (Pettegrew et al., 2000). A Cochrane systematic review of 11 double-blind, placebo-controlled studies of ALC in dementia confirmed significant positive effects at weeks 12 and 24 that were not sustained (as measured by the Clinical Global Impression scale) at 1 year with continued treatment (Hudson & Tabet, 2004). Findings from placebo-controlled studies suggest that ALC 1.5 to 3.0 g/day improves age-related symptoms of cognitive impairment in healthy non-demented elderly individuals and depressed elderly patients (Bella, Biondi, Raffaele, & Bennisi, 1990; Cipolli & Chiari, 1990). At high doses (2 g/day) ALC improves memory, word recall, and visuospatial deficits in cognitively impaired abstinent alcoholics (Tempesta et al., 1990). Preliminary evidence from animal studies suggests that the neuroprotective effect of ALC may be enhanced when combined with other natural products, including α-lipoic acid, CoQ10, or omega-3 fatty acids (Lolic, Fiskum, & Rosenthal, 1997). ALC is well tolerated, and there are few reports of adverse effects.

Vitamins

◆ **Folic acid, vitamin B$_{12}$, and thiamine improve cognitive functioning in some cases of dementia** Many B vitamins are essential enzyme cofactors in the synthesis of neurotransmitters. Low serum levels of folic acid, niacin, and thiamine are associated with cognitive impairment in general (Hassing et al., 1999). A diet low in folic acid and vitamin B$_{12}$ leads to elevated blood levels of homocysteine and decreased synthesis of S-adenosylmethionine (SAMe), resulting in reduced synthesis of several neurotransmitters critical for normal cognitive functioning. Dietary deficiencies of folate and B$_{12}$ ultimately manifest as moderate to severe degrees of cognitive impairment. Clinical trial results suggest that healthy adults who take a B complex experience improvements in overall cognitive functioning (Benton, 1997). A daily B vitamin supplement may slow deterioration of cognitive functioning in mild to moderate dementia (Pelka & Leuchtgens, 1995). Findings from case studies and controlled trials suggest that a large daily dose of folic acid reduces the severity of dementia in some cases. In one double-blind, placebo-controlled study, depressed demented patients treated with 5-methyl-tetrahydrofolate (5-MTHF), a form of folate, at 50 mg/day experienced significant improvements in both mood and memory after 4 weeks of therapy (Passeri et al., 1993). However, the relationship between cognitive functioning and folate remains unclear. For example, demented individuals often have normal red blood cell folate levels and fail to improve with supplementation (Levitt & Karlinsky, 1992). Furthermore, a Cochrane systematic review of four studies concluded that there is insufficient evidence to support the use of folic acid with or without B$_{12}$ as a treatment of dementia or other forms of severe cognitive impairment (Malouf, Areosa, & Sastre, 2004). It is important to note that many positive studies and case reports of beneficial effects of folic acid or B$_{12}$ in dementia were omitted from the Cochrane review. Supplementation with large doses of thiamine 3 to 8 g/day may result in mild improvement in cognitive impairment in Alzheimer's patients (Mimori, Katsuoka, & Nakamuri, 1996). Vitamin B$_{12}$ is often recommended for elderly patients who complain of impaired cognition; however, this effect is largely anecdotal, research findings are inconsistent, and no large controlled trials have been conducted.

A few small open studies have evaluated the efficacy of B$_{12}$ as a cognitive-enhancing agent in moderately impaired, non-demented elderly patients. In one study, 18 elderly patients with abnormally low serum B$_{12}$ levels were treated with injections of B$_{12}$ following a strict protocol: daily 1 mg injections for the first week, followed by weekly 1 mg injections for 1 month, then monthly 1 mg injections for 6 months. All patients in the study improved, and those who had been cognitively impaired less than 1 year experienced the most significant gains (Martin, Francis, Protetch, & Huff, 1992).

◆ **Taking vitamins C and E together may reduce the prevalence and incidence of Alzheimer's disease** Vitamins C and E are important antioxidants and function as free-radical scavengers throughout the body and brain, possibly slowing progression of Alzheimer's disease and other neurodegenerative diseases. The findings of a large epidemiologic study show a correlation between intake of vitamins C and E in the form of supplements and reduced risk of Alzheimer's disease (Englehart et al., 2002a). This effect was greatest for vitamin E. Anecdotal reports suggest that supplementation with vitamins C and E improves cognitive functioning in Alzheimer's patients;

however, few controlled studies have been done, and the findings of several observational studies are inconclusive or negative (Jama et al., 1996; Kalmijn et al., 1997). A Cochrane review identified only one study of vitamin E in dementia that met rigorous inclusion criteria, and that study failed to provide clear evidence of improved global or cognitive functioning or reduced behavioral disturbances in moderately demented individuals (Tabet, Birks, Grimley, Orrel, & Spector, 2004).

Combining vitamin E and vitamin C may reduce the prevalence and incidence of Alzheimer's disease. A prospective 5-year study followed 4740 adults ages 65 and older (Zandi et al., 2004). At the end of the study there were 104 new cases of Alzheimer's disease. A strong inverse correlation was found between the incidence and prevalence of Alzheimer's disease and combined use of vitamin C (at least 500 mg/day) and vitamin E (at least 400 IU/day). However, there was no association between the use of vitamin C alone, vitamin E alone, or a multivitamin alone and the incidence or prevalence of Alzheimer's disease. The significance of these findings is limited by the fact that almost 1500 individuals in the study were lost to 5-year follow-up, suggesting that the incidence of new cases of Alzheimer's disease could have been higher than reported.

Large doses of vitamin E are associated with an increased risk of bleeding. Individuals who are at increased risk of stroke should consult their physician before starting a high-dose vitamin E regimen.

Other Natural Products

DHEA may improve memory and general cognitive functioning in healthy older people, testosterone may slow the rate of decline in early or mild Alzheimer's disease Dehydroepiandrosterone is a precursor of testosterone and other hormones. It is widely used in Europe and North America to self-treat decline in cognitive functioning associated with normal aging. DHEA binds to both γ-aminobutyric acid (GABA) receptors and N-methyl-D-asparate (NMDA) receptors, but it is not clear whether these receptor affinities are related to its putative cognitive-enhancing role (Friess et al., 1995). There is preliminary evidence from anecdotal reports and pilot studies that DHEA at 25 to 50 mg/day improves memory and enhances general cognitive functioning in healthy adults (Wolkowitz, 199). However, research findings are inconsistent, and negative findings have been reported at doses lower than 90 mg/day (Wolf et al., 1997). It is likely that DHEA improves memory in elderly patients who have low DHEA serum levels more than in healthy adults. A Cochrane systematic review and meta-analysis found no support for the use of DHEA as a cognitive enhancer in healthy older individuals (Huppert & Van Niekerk, 2004). However, the Cochrane findings are limited by several factors: only four studies met inclusion criteria, all studies reviewed were 3 months in duration or shorter, and doses tested ranged between 25 and 50 mg only. There is evidence that DHEA at 200 mg/day may improve symptoms of cognitive impairment in multi-infarct dementia (Azuma et al., 1999). To date, no controlled trials have been done on DHEA in Alzheimer's disease.

Limited evidence suggests that testosterone replacement therapy may improve global functioning in mild Alzheimer's disease. In a 6-month randomized, double-blind, placebo-controlled study, 47 men ages 50 and older were randomized to receive testosterone 75 mg (in the form of a dermal gel) versus placebo together with their usual medications. The study included healthy controls and individuals diagnosed with mild dementia. Global quality of life improved in both the mildly demented group and healthy controls. Mildly demented patients who received testosterone experienced less decline in overall functioning and visuospatial abilities. Men who have benign prostatic hypertrophy or prostate cancer should avoid use of testosterone.

Mild insomnia is an infrequent side effect of DHEA, which should be dosed in the morning. There is no evidence that DHEA replacement doses of 25 to 50 mg/day increase the risk of prostate cancer in middle aged men.

◆ **Applying certain essential oils to the skin has beneficial calming effects in agitated demented patients** Essential oils can be used as aromatherapy or applied directly to the skin during massage. Recent findings suggest that certain essential oils have beneficial calming effects on agitation in demented patients. A Cochrane systematic review was able to identify only one study that met inclusion criteria, and although the outcome of that study was positive, the reviewers concluded that methodological problems limited the significance of findings (Thorgrimsen, Spector, Wiles, & Orrell, 2004). The essential oils of lemon balm and lavender reduced agitated behavior in demented individuals when topically applied directly to the face and arms (Ballard et al., 2002; Holmes et al., 2002). It is likely that essential oil therapies in agitated demented patients do not act primarily through the sense of smell, as olfaction is frequently impaired in severely demented individuals. In fact, a recent controlled study determined that aromatherapy alone in the absence of massage using essential oils was no more effective than placebo (unscented grapeseed oil) in agitated demented patients (Snow, Hovanec, & Brandt, 2004). This finding supports the hypothesis that essential oils are effective in agitated demented patients through systemic absorption or the combined effects of massage and olfaction, but not through olfaction alone.

Possible adverse effects of essential oil therapies include skin allergies, phototoxic reactions, and potentiation of sedative-hypnotics when used with lavender or other oils known to have sedating effects. Pregnant women should exercise caution when considering aromatherapy because of possible effects on the fetus and uterus caused by systemic absorption of certain essential oils.

Somatic and Mind–body Approaches

◆ **Snoezelen, a multimodal sensory therapy, may reduce symptoms of apathy, agitation, and impaired communication in dementia** *Snoezelen* is an integrative treatment of dementia and other forms of severe cognitive impairment in which music, light patterns, tactile surfaces, essential oils, and other forms of sensory stimulation are employed to stimulate sight, hearing, touch, taste, and smell. This multimodal therapy is based on the belief that stimulation of multiple senses improves global cognitive functioning. Snoezelen sessions are usually administered 2 or 3 times weekly to demented patients in skilled nursing homes. A systematic review of controlled double-blind studies suggests that apathy, speech skills, and psychomotor agitation improve in demented patients after four to eight sessions of Snoezelen therapy (Chung, Lai, Chung, & French, 2004). The significance of these findings is limited by the fact that only two studies met strict criteria required by the reviewers, and those studies were difficult to compare because of differences in methodology and nonstandardized control conditions.

Treatments Based on Forms of Energy or Information Validated by Western Science

◆ **Weak electrical stimulation of the brain using transcranial electrical nerve stimulation or cranioelectrotherapy stimulation may result in transient improvement in some symptoms of dementia** The application of weak electrical current to the head or neck may improve memory, behavior, and activities of daily living in demented patients (Scherder, Bouma & Steen, 1995; Van Someren, Scherder, & Swaab, 1998). It has been suggested that the daily application of weak electrical current to the neck or head stimulates global brain activity and causes beneficial changes in neurotransmitters implicated in dementia. A Cochrane meta-analysis of three studies on transcranial electrical nerve stimulation (TENS) or cranio-electrotherapy stimulation (CES) devices used to treat demented patients found evidence of significant but transient improvements in word recall, face recognition, and motivation immediately following treatment (Cameron, Lonergan, & Lee, 2004). Beneficial effects of TENS and CES on other cognitive or behavioral symptoms of dementia were not observed. Significantly, most research findings show that improvements are not sustained 6 weeks or more after treatment is terminated.

◆ **Music therapy and binaural sound patterns probably improve global functioning in dementia** Music is used in many healing traditions to calm the mind and reduce agitated behavior. Findings of a meta-analysis evaluating studies of music therapy in demented individuals show that various approaches—singing, dance, listening to music, and musical games—are associated with improvements in cognitive and behavioral functioning in severely demented individuals, including reduced agitation, reduced wandering, enhanced social interaction, improved mood, reduced irritability and anxiety, increased cooperative behavior, and increased performance on standardized scales such as the Mini-Mental State Examination (Koger, Chapin, & Brotons, 1999). The significance of these findings is limited by the absence of quantitative outcomes measures, failure to specify end points before trials began, small study sizes, and the absence of randomization or blinding in most studies.

Calming background music significantly reduced irritable behavior, anxiety, and depressed mood in demented nursing home patients (Ragneskog, Brane, Karlsson, & Kihlgren, 1996). Regular music therapy reduces irritability and improves expressive language in demented individuals (Suzuki et al., 2004). Improvements in global behavior and sleep following music therapy may be mediated by increased melatonin levels (Kumar et al., 1999). Listening to binaural sounds in the β-frequency range (16-24 Hz) using headphones may enhance performance on tests of attention and short-term and immediate recall in healthy volunteers (Kennerly, 1996). In non-impaired individuals, EEG biofeedback using a beta-training protocol may result in substantial improvements in average intelligence as measured by standardized tests. In demented individuals, regular exposure to binaural beats at particular frequencies may have beneficial effects on dynamic brain organization that are analogous to those induced by EEG-biofeedback training.

Treatments Based on Forms of Energy or Information Not Validated by Western Science

◆ **Regular Healing Touch and Therapeutic Touch may reduce agitation and improve global functioning in patients with Alzheimer's disease** Open studies, case reports, and one double-blind trial suggest that Healing Touch (HT) and Therapeutic Touch (TT) have beneficial effects on agitation in demented patients. In one small open study, measures of agitation were significantly improved in 14 demented residential patients who received 3 HT treatments weekly over a 4-week period (Wang, & Hermann, 1999). Diminished need for (presumably sedating) psychotropic medications was observed in three patients during the active treatment phase, and two residents required dose increases in the first 2 weeks after HT treatments were stopped. In another small sham-controlled study (Ostuni & Pietro, 2000, 2001) two weekly 10- to 20-minute HT treatments were administered to Alzheimer's patients over a 5-week period. Patients who received regular healing touch treatments were found to have consistent reductions in disruptive behaviors, and globally improved emotional and cognitive functioning including enhanced socialization, a more regular sleep schedule, improved compliance with nursing home routines, greater emotional stability, and improved communication with staff. Of note, agitation as measured by the frequency and intensity of outbursts was significantly reduced in the healing touch group but did not change in the control group. Demented patients who received Healing Touch treatments complained of physical distress or discomfort significantly less often compared with patients in the control group. In a double-blind study ($N = 57$) that included mock TT in the control arm, agitated demented patients who received two brief TT treatments daily for 3 days exhibited significantly fewer behavioral symptoms of dementia, including reduced restlessness and fewer disruptive vocalizations, compared with patients who received mock TT (Woods, Craven, & Whitney, 2005). Because this short study lasted only 3 days, findings cannot be generalized to possible long-term benefits of TT in agitated demented patients. Promising early research findings on TT and HT in dementia are limited by study design flaws including lack of blinding, the likely beneficial confounding influence of frequent human contact, small numbers of enrolled patients, the lack of standardized methods, and the absence of control groups receiving sham HT or TT treatments in most studies.

Nonconventional Approaches That Are Possibly Effective for the Treatment of Cognitive Impairment

Table 12–4 lists the possibly effective nonconventional treatments of cognitive impairment.

Medicinal Herbs

◆ **Vinpocetine may enhance cognitive functioning in Alzheimer's disease and vascular dementia** Vinpocetine is a semisynthetic derivative of the periwinkle plant. Animal studies suggest a cerebral vasodilation effect and possibly a cerebral metabolic stimulant effect. Vinpocetine 30 to 60 mg/day may

Table 12–4 Possibly Effective Nonconventional Treatments of Cognitive Impairment

Category	Treatment Approach	Evidence for Claimed Treatment Effect	Comments
Biological	Vinpocetine	Vinpocetine 30 to 60 mg/day may be beneficial in both Alzheimer's disease and vascular dementia	**Note:** Only a few small human trials on vinpocetine in dementia have been done, and findings are inconsistent
	Ashwagondha (*Withania somnifera*)	Ashwagondha 50 mg/kg may improve short- and long-term memory and executive functioning in cognitively impaired individuals	**Note:** Few human trials on Ashwagondha have been published
	Ginseng (*Panax ginseng*)	Ginseng may enhance memory and overall cognitive performance in healthy adults	**Note:** Some negative trials with ginseng, and at least one reported case of mania induction
	Lemon balm (*Melissa officinalis*) and common sage (*Salvia officinalis*)	Extracts of lemon balm and common sage (60 drops/day) may slow the rate of decline in Alzheimer's disease	Teas made of both herbs are traditionally are used to enhance general cognitive functioning and to treat dementia
	Dronabinol	Dronabinol may reduce agitated behavior, improve global functioning, and enhance mental status in Alzheimer's disease	There are no reports of significant adverse effects with dronabinol
	Dehydroevodiamine (DHED), Qian Jin Yi Fang, Trasina, Mentat, and lobeline	Dehydroevodiamine (DHED) may be more effective than cholinesterase inhibitors in Alzheimer's disease. A Chinese compound herbal formula called Qian Jin Yi Fang reportedly reduces symptoms of dementia. Two proprietary Ayurvedic compound herbal formulas, Trasina and Mentat, may be beneficial in Alzheimer's disease and age-related cognitive impairment. Lobeline is a promising memory-enhancing agent	**Note:** Human clinical trials data for these herbals are extremely limited or entirely absent
	Niacin	Findings of a single study suggest that high niacin intake from food or supplements may significantly reduce the risk of developing dementia and decrease the rate of cognitive decline in healthy elderly individuals	**Note:** Only epidemiologic studies have been done on niacin and dementia. Confirmation of a protective effect of niacin will require a large controlled trial
	Centrophenoxine (CPH), phosphatidylcholine, and lecithin	CPH may improve global functioning and cognitive performance in Alzheimer's disease. Benefits of CPH are possibly enhanced when combined with vitamins. Phosphatidylcholine and lecithin are probably ineffective	**Note:** Beneficial findings for CPH in dementia are still preliminary
	Piracetam	Piracetam alone may be ineffective, but piracetam (up to 4800 mg/day) in combination with vinpocetine or CDP-choline may improve cognitive performance in mild to moderate dementia. Piracetam in combination with *Ginkgo biloba* may improve overall cognitive performance in dyslexic individuals	**Note:** Few human trials, and findings of a Cochrane review on piracetam in dementia were equivocal
	Nicergoline	Nicergoline may be beneficial in cognitive decline caused by various underlying pathologies, including vascular dementia and Alzheimer's disease	**Note:** A systematic review of 14 double-blind studies found only some evidence of efficacy
	α-lipoic acid (ALA)	Animal studies suggest that ALA may enhance recovery following stroke. Human case reports suggest that ALA may accelerate return of cognitive function after traumatic brain injury	**Note:** Findings on ALA in dementia are largely from case studies, and a Cochrane review identified no controlled trials
	Estrogen and progesterone replacement in women	Case reports suggest efficacy; however, meta-analyses fail to show that hormonal replacement with estrogen/progesterone slows progression of dementia in postmenopausal women diagnosed with Alzheimer's disease or prevents cognitive decline in healthy postmenopausal women	**Caution:** Estrogen replacement therapy is associated with increased risk of breast cancer, heart disease, and stroke
	SAMe	SAMe (up to 3200 mg/day) may improve post-stroke survival and enhance return to baseline cognitive functioning. SAMe (150 mg/day) may accelerate return of normal cognitive functioning following traumatic brain injury	**Note:** Findings of small studies on SAMe in Alzheimer's disease are inconsistent. **Caution:** SAMe at high doses may cause agitation, and there are rare reports of hypomania in bipolar patients

Table 12–4 Possibly Effective Nonconventional Treatments of Cognitive Impairment *(Continued)*

Category	Treatment Approach	Evidence for Claimed Treatment Effect	Comments
	Picamilon	Picamilon (50 mg 3 times/day) may reduce cognitive impairments related to cerebrovascular disease and accelerate recovery following traumatic brain injury	*Note:* Few human trials have been done on picamilon in dementia or traumatic brain injury
	Pyritinol	Pyritinol (600 mg/day) may have general beneficial effects on cognitive functioning following traumatic brain injury	*Note:* Few studies on pyritinol and inconsistent findings
	Melatonin	Melatonin 3 mg at bedtime may improve alertness and wakefulness while reducing agitation in Alzheimer's patients	Melatonin has no significant adverse effects at therapeutic doses
Somatic and mind–body approaches	Massage	Regular massage therapy may reduce agitated behavior in demented nursing home patients	*Note:* Anecdotal reports and open studies provide the only evidence for calming effects of massage in dementia
	Wander garden	Wander gardens permit demented or post-stroke patients to enjoy nature-related activities and reportedly improve baseline functioning in the early stages of dementia	*Note:* Although there may be no measurable benefits, time spent in a beautiful natural setting is almost always a source of pleasure
Approaches based on forms of energy-information validated by Western science	Bright light exposure	Regular bright light (10,000 lux) exposure may improve sleep, reduce "sundowning," reduce agitation and other inappropriate behaviors, and delay the time of peak agitation in Alzheimer's patients	*Note:* Combining melatonin and bright light exposure does not result in differential improvements in behavior compared with bright light alone
	EEG and HRV biofeedback	EEG- and HRV-biofeedback training may enhance cognitive performance in healthy adults. EEG biofeedback may accelerate recovery following stroke or traumatic brain injury	*Caution:* Certain EEG-biofeedback protocols can cause seizures and should be avoided in patients who have epilepsy
Approaches based on forms of energy-information not validated by Western science	Qigong	Regular qigong practice or external qigong treatments may normalize EEG slowing and reverse cerebral atrophy associated with dementia	*Note:* Controlled studies of qigong in dementia have not been done, but there are case reports of dramatic beneficial effects

EEG, electroencephalography; HRV, heart rate variability; SAMe, *S*-adenosylmethionine

reduce symptoms of cognitive impairment and improve global functioning in patients who have mild Alzheimer's disease or mild vascular dementia (Balestreri, Fontana, & Astengo, 1987; Blaha et al., 1989). The cognitive benefits of vinpocetine may be enhanced when combined with idebenone (see discussion above). It is difficult to evaluate the clinical significance of vinpocetine because most studies are small, and findings to date have been inconsistent (Thal et al., 1989).

◆ **Ashwagondha may improve memory and executive functioning in cognitively impaired individuals** Ashwagondha (*Withania somnifera*) is widely used in traditional Ayurvedic medicine as a restorative and is being investigated in Western countries because of strong anecdotal evidence for its reported memory-enhancing, antiseizure, anticancer, and anti-inflammatory benefits. The postulated mechanism of action underlying its beneficial cognitive effects is the stimulation of increased acetylcholine activity in the cerebral cortex and basal forebrain (Ghosal et al., 1989; Schliebs et al., 1997). In vitro studies point to another possible mechanism of action involving stimulation of dendritic and axonal sprouting in human nerve cells (Kubyoyama et al., 2005). Anecdotal reports and human trials suggest that Ashwagondha extract at 50 mg/kg improves short- and long-term memory and executive functioning in cognitively impaired individuals (Bhattacharya, Khumar, & Ghosal, 1995).

◆ **Ginseng may enhance learning capacity and mental performance in healthy adults** Ginseng is a popular herb used to increase stamina and alertness. Findings of a systematic review of controlled studies support the use of standardized ginseng extract at 200 to 400 mg/day to enhance learning and overall mental performance in healthy adults (Sorensen & Sonne, 1996; Vogler, Pittler, & Ernst, 1999). However, some negative findings have been reported (Cardinal & Engels, 2001). In one double-blind study, ginseng had no effects on memory or concentration (Sorensen & Sonne, 1996). Genseng is regarded as very safe; however, there is one case report of a possible manic episode induced by ginseng (Gonzalez-Seijo, Ramos, & Lastra, 1995).

◆ **Lemon balm and common sage may improve global functioning in mild Alzheimer's dementia** Teas made from lemon balm and common sage have been used traditionally for centuries to enhance cognition. Animal studies have confirmed that components of both plant extracts have high binding affinities for brain acetylcholine receptors. In a 4-month randomized, double-blind study, mildly demented individuals received a standardized lemon balm extract (60 drops/day) versus placebo. By the end of the study, the group taking lemon balm extract showed significantly less decline in global cognitive functioning and less agitation compared with the control group (Akhondzadeh et al., 2003). In a separate 4-month study, 30 mildly demented patients were randomized to receive an extract of common sage (60 drops/day) versus placebo. Findings were similar to those seen with lemon balm. No adverse effects were reported in either study. Larger studies are required to replicate these preliminary findings and evaluate the potential therapeutic benefits of both herbal preparations in Alzheimer's disease and other syndromes of cognitive impairment (Akhondzadeh et al., 2003).

◆ **A synthetic derivative of marijuana may reduce symptoms of agitation in dementia** Dronabinol, a synthetic derivative of marijuana, may significantly reduce agitated behavior and improve global functioning in demented individuals. In a retrospective review, patients who had previously been nonresponsive to conventional treatments of agitation received dronabinol 10 mg/day over a 2-week period. At the end of the study period, 65% exhibited no further agitated behavior, 37% had moderately improved MMSE scores, and global functioning had improved in almost 70%. Adverse effects were not reported, including dizziness, worsening of agitated behavior, or a drug-induced "high."

◆ **Several Korean, Chinese, and Ayurvedic herbals may be beneficial in Alzheimer's disease and age-related cognitive decline** Dehydroevodiamine (DHED) is a biologically active constituent of *Evodia rutaecarpa*, a plant used in traditional Korean medicine, and may prove to be more effective in the treatment of age-related cognitive decline and Alzheimer's disease compared with cholinesterase inhibitors (Park et al., 1996). Qian Jin Yi Fang is a compound herbal formula used in Chinese medicine that reportedly reduces symptoms of dementia (Nishiyama, Chu, & Saito, 1996). Trasina and Mentat are compound herbal formulas used in Ayurvedic medicine to treat symptoms that resemble Alzheimer's disease and age-related cognitive impairment (Bhattacharya & Kumar, 1997; Bhattacharya et al., 1995). Animal studies suggest that Trasina has beneficial effects on experimental models of Alzheimer's disease (Bhattacharya & Kumar, 1997). Preparations of the herb lobeline have been studied as a memory-enhancing agent in rats with excellent results (Decker, Majchrzak, & Arneric, 1993).

Other Biological Treatments

◆ **Niacin may reduce the risk of developing Alzheimer's disease** A 6-year prospective study found that elderly individuals who consumed the highest amount of niacin in the form of supplements or food had a 70% reduced risk of developing Alzheimer's disease (i.e., during the study period) compared with individuals who used the least amount of niacin (Morris et al., 2004). Furthermore, nondemented individuals who consumed the highest amount of niacin experienced less than half of the average cognitive decline observed in the group with the lowest niacin intake. There was no difference in protective benefits of niacin obtained through diet or supplements. Large controlled studies are needed to confirm a putative causal relationship between high niacin intake and a reduced risk of developing Alzheimer's disease or age-related cognitive decline.

◆ **Centrophenoxine, but not lecithin, choline, and phosphatidylcholine, may be beneficial in Alzheimer's disease and age-related cognitive decline** These related substances are naturally occurring biological products used in many European countries to treat age-related cognitive decline in healthy elderly individuals, and as adjuncts to conventional drug treatments of Alzheimer's disease, vascular dementia, and other neurodegenerative disorders. Lecithin is a natural product that is frequently used to self-treat symptoms of cognitive decline. Many individuals diagnosed with Alzheimer's disease lack the capacity to convert choline, a principle constituent of lecithin, into acetylcholine. In spite of the widespread use of these natural products, few large studies have been done, and findings are inconsistent. Early small trials of choline in dementia failed to show a clinical benefit (Growon & Corkin, 1980). A Cochrane review of 12 randomized controlled trials concluded that lecithin is not an effective treatment of Alzheimer's disease or other severe forms of cognitive impairment (Higgins & Flicker, 2004). The significance of this conclusion is limited by the fact that all but one of the reviewed studies were excluded from the meta-analysis, and the reviewers commented on dramatic findings of one study (not included in the review) showing a significant differential benefit (i.e., of lecithin over placebo) in individuals with subjective memory complaints who had not been previously diagnosed with Alzheimer's disease. The findings of two small studies on phosphatidylcholine in dementia were negative or inconclusive (Heyman et al., 1987; Little et al., 1985). Centrophenoxine is a natural product required for the synthesis of choline. Its putative neuroprotective mechanism of action involves enhanced transport of dimethylaminoethanol (DMAE) across the blood–brain barrier, where the latter compound is taken up in neuronal membranes to function as a powerful free radical scavenger. Preliminary findings (Pek, Fulop, & Zs-Nagy, 1989) suggest that centrophenoxine improves general cognitive performance and activities of daily living in Alzheimer's patients.

◆ **Piracetam in combination with conventional drugs or other natural products may have beneficial effects in mild to moderate dementia** Piracetam is widely used in Western Europe to treat memory loss and cognitive impairments associated with dementia, stroke, or traumatic brain injury. Piracetam functions in a way that is similar to phosphatidylserine and omega-3 fatty acids by increasing nerve cell membrane fluidity, indirectly enhancing brain levels of important neurotransmitters. Its cognitive-enhancing mechanism of action may also involve enhanced oxygen and glucose utilization in the brain as well as improved cerebral microcirculation. Research findings to date are inconsistent, and improvements in mildly to moderately demented patients who use piracetam alone (up to 4800 mg/day) are equivocal (Itil et al., 1986). A Cochrane systematic review was inconclusive (Flicker & Grimley, 2004). However, animal studies (Gouliaev & Senning, 1994) suggest that beneficial effects on learning and memory can be further enhanced when piracetam is combined with conventional drugs or other natural products (including CDP-choline, vinpocetine, and idebenone). For example, piracetam can be safely combined with ginkgo to enhance cognitive performance in dyslexic patients (Enderby et al., 1994).

◆ **Nicergoline may reduce the severity of cognitive impairment related to cerebrovascular disease** Nicergoline is a semisynthetic derivative of ergot used in many European countries to treat vascular dementia and other cerebrovascular syndromes associated with severe cognitive impairment. Findings of a review of 14 double-blind, randomized controlled studies on nicergoline confirm "some evidence of positive effects" on both cognitive functioning and behavior in dementias of various pathologies including Alzheimer's disease (Fioravanti & Flicker, 2004). Although available research findings do not strongly support the use of nicergoline in Alzheimer's disease, there is evidence for general beneficial effects in dementia regardless of the underlying pathophysiology.

◆ **Alpha-lipoic acid may accelerate cognitive recovery following stroke**   Alpha-lipoic acid (ALA) occurs naturally in the human body and facilitates the synthesis of glutathione, a powerful antioxidant and free radical scavenger. Preliminary findings from animal studies suggest that ALA enhances the rate of cognitive recovery to baseline following stroke (Lonnrot, Porsti, Alho, Wu,, Hervonen, & Tolvanen,1998). There are case reports of accelerated recovery of cognitive functioning following traumatic brain injury when ALA is dosed at 300 mg 3 times a day. However, a Cochrane systematic review identified no published studies on ALA in dementia, and concluded that there is no basis for recommending this treatment for dementia at present (Sauer, et al., 2004).

◆ **Hormonal replacement therapy in women is probably of little benefit in the prevention of age-related cognitive decline or Alzheimer's disease**   The use of hormones to treat mental health problems remains controversial because of associated significant medical risks. There is some evidence that estrogen replacement therapy reduces the rate of progression of Alzheimer's disease in postmenopausal women by interfering with synthesis of a protein called amyloid-precursor protein (APP) (Baker et al., 2003). However, a Cochrane meta-analysis failed to show that hormonal replacement slows the rate of progression of dementia in postmenopausal women diagnosed with Alzheimer's disease (Hogervorst, Yaffe, Richards, & Hupper, 2004b). A separate Cochrane meta-analysis of 9 trials concluded that there is little evidence for beneficial effects of hormone replacement therapy (HRT) with estrogens or combined estrogens and progestagens in the prevention of cognitive decline in general in postmenopausal women (Hogervorst, Yaffe, Richards, & Hupper, 2004a). An independent review (Yaffe , Sawaya, Lieberburg, & Grady, 1998) and findings from the Women's Health Initiative Memory Study (WHIMS) are in agreement with the Cochrane meta-analysis. That review concluded that estrogen replacement in elderly women does not reduce the risk of developing Alzheimer's disease, while significantly increasing the risk of breast cancer, heart disease, and stroke (Shumaker et al., 2004).

◆ **SAMe may enhance cognitive recovery following stroke or traumatic brain injury**   Although SAMe is used mainly to treat depressed mood, preliminary findings of double blind studies suggest that SAMe may enhance recovery of normal cognitive functioning following stroke or traumatic brain injury. Post-stroke survival was greater in patients who took SAMe at doses up to 3200 mg/day (Monaco et al., 1996). Patients who had experienced closed head injury returned to their previous baseline of cognitive functioning more rapidly when taking SAMe 150 mg/day (Bacci Ballerini et al., 1983). Small studies on SAMe in Alzheimer's disease have yielded inconsistent findings (Cohen, Satlin, & Zubenko, 1988; Bottiglieri, et al., 1990).

◆ **Picamilon may enhance cognitive recovery following stroke or head injury**   This natural product consists of GABA (the brain's principal inhibitory neurotransmitter) and niacin. It is in common use in Russia to enhance overall mental performance and alertness. Findings from a large Russian study suggest that picamilon 50 mg taken 3 times daily enhances recovery from cognitive impairments related to head injury or cerebrovascular disease (Kruglikova, 1997).

◆ **Pyritinol may facilitate cognitive recovery following closed head injury**   This molecule is related to vitamin B_6 (pyridoxine), and is believed to improve the efficiency of energy production and utilization in the brain at several levels including increased glucose uptake and increased release of acetylcholine, a principal neurotransmitter in learning and memory. Pyritinol 600 mg/day has been used to treat cognitive impairment following closed head injuries. Findings to date are inconsistent however a few studies suggest a nonspecific cognitive-enhancing effect (Kitamura, 1981).

◆ **Reduced melatonin levels may be associated with progressive cognitive decline**   Progressive cognitive impairment may be related to a decline in the secretion of melatonin in the brain with normal aging. Melatonin is required for maintenance of sleep-wake rhythms, which are typically disturbed in dementia (Ghali, Hopkins, & Rindlisbacher, 1995). Chronically disrupted sleep is associated with global impairment in cognitive functioning, including short-term memory problems. Melatonin has strong antioxidant properties which may help to reduce pathological consequences of oxidative damage in the aging brain, including amyloid formation (Varadarajan, Yatin, Aksenova, & Butterfield, 2000). Findings from one open study suggest that melatonin 3 mg taken at bedtime may reduce agitation while improving wakefulness and alertness in demented individuals (Cohen-Mansfield, Garfinkel, & Lipson, 2000).

Somatic and Mind–Body Approaches

◆ **Massage therapy may reduce agitated behavior in demented individuals**   Skilled nursing homes frequently provide regular massage therapy to demented residents. There is anecdotal evidence of calming effects and reduced agitation following massage. Findings from open trials suggest that massage decreases agitated behavior in demented individuals (Fraser & Kerr, 1993; Snyder, Egan, & Burns, 1995).

◆ **Wander gardens provide stimulation and pleasure for demented individuals and may reduce anxiety in post-stroke patients**   Regularly spending time in nature is beneficial for physical and psychological well-being in healthy individuals and is probably therapeutic in Alzheimer's dementia and individuals recovering from a stroke. A wander garden is a protected outdoor area in which individuals can safely walk, socialize, or explore nature. Wander gardens are increasingly used to provide visual, auditory, and tactile stimulation as well as pleasure and autonomy for institutionalized demented patients. There is emerging evidence that nature-related activities, including strolling in a park or gardening, can improve baseline functioning in the early stages of dementia and provide a source of pleasure and relaxation in the later stages of dementia (Ebel, 1991; Epstein, Hansen, & Hazen, 1991). Findings of a case report suggest that time spent in a wander garden reduces anxiety in post-stroke patients (Detweiler & Warf, 2005).

*Treatments Based on Forms of Energy or
Information Validated by Western Science*

◆ **Regular exposure to bright light may improve sleep and reduce sundowning in demented patients** Bright light exposure alone may improve sleep and reduce sundowning in Alzheimer's patients (Satlin, Volicer, Ross, Herz, & Campbell, 1992). The results of a Cochrane meta-analysis of studies on bright light therapy in the management of sleep, behavior, and mood in demented individuals were inconclusive (Forbes, Morgan, Bangma, Peacock, Pelletier, & Adamson, 2004). However, only three of five studies reviewed were included in the meta-analysis. Furthermore, the reviewers were unable to retrieve all of the required data for analysis, and were thus unable to assess the relative strength of evidence for beneficial claims of bright light exposure. In a controlled study, 92 severely demented institutionalized patients exposed to daily morning bright light experienced a delay of 1.5 hours in the peak time of agitated behavior, but significant reductions in overall agitated behavior were not observed (Ancoli-Israel et al., 2003). In a small 7-day double-blind, placebo-controlled trial, six demented residential patients were randomly given melatonin 2.5 mg versus placebo and exposed to bright light (10,000 lux) every night at 10:00 P.M. for 30 minutes. Each patient served as his or her own control on random nights (Haffmans, Lucius, & Sival, 1998). Patients taking a placebo during bright light exposure displayed significantly reduced motor restlessness, but no improvements in inappropriate behaviors including aggression, confusion or repetitive behavior. No significant changes in behavior or restlessness were observed in patients who took melatonin while exposed to bright light. Research findings to date suggest that, although bright light exposure is beneficial for symptoms of restlessness and delays the peak time of agitated behavior, it probably does not significantly reduce the severity of agitation or other inappropriate behaviors in demented individuals.

◆ **EEG-biofeedback training may enhance recovery following stroke and traumatic brain injury** EEG-biofeedback training, sometimes called neurotherapy, employs light or sound as feedback with the goal of entraining changes in brain electrical activity that result in improved cognitive functioning. Biofeedback training directed at improving coherence in heart rate variability (HRV) may improve performance in concentration tasks in healthy adults (McCraty, 2002). Target symptoms of both EEG and HRV biofeedback include inattention, global decline in cognitive functioning following stroke or head injury, anxiety states, and mood. EEG-biofeedback training is sometimes done following initial assessment of brain electrical activity using a qEEG "map" (see earlier discussion), but it is more often done without the benefit of an initial "Q." The findings of a case study suggest that EEG-biofeedback training improves the speed of cognitive rehabilitation following stroke, including enhanced word finding, attention, speech, and concentration (Rozelle & Budzinski, 1995). Findings from one small open study suggest that EEG-biofeedback training may improve memory following traumatic brain injury (TBI; Thornton, 2000). A small controlled, double-blind study showed that regular EEG-biofeedback sessions improved cognitive functioning and mood in TBI patients (Schoenberger, Shif, Esty, Ochs, & Matheis, 2001).

EEG biofeedback has been successfully used to treat cognitive deficits associated with seizures; however, patients with a history of epilepsy should be cautioned that certain EEG-biofeedback protocols can potentially trigger seizure activity.

*Treatments Based on Forms of Energy or
Information Not Validated by Western Science*

◆ **Regular qigong practice may normalize EEG activity and slow the rate of cognitive decline in Alzheimer's disease** Case reports using advanced functional brain-imaging methods suggest that the consistent practice of qigong may normalize EEG slowing and possibly reverse cerebral cortical atrophy associated with cognitive impairment in the elderly. Three-dimensional positron emission tomography (PET) and EEG were used to examine relationships between brain electrical activity and changes in regional cerebral blood flow in a qigong practitioner (Manabu et al., 1996). Findings included significant increases in high-frequency (α and β) EEG domains and reduced slow-frequency (δ) activity following qigong. Enhanced β activity in the frontal lobes following qigong practice was correlated with increased cerebral blood flow in the same region and relatively decreased regional blood flow in posterior brain regions. In another case report, researchers claimed that regular qigong practice resulted in the reversal of cerebral atrophy (Zhao, Guang, & Wie, 1988) in a 79-year-old male. The patient had gradually lost his capacity to read and work, complained of dizziness and "inert thinking," and was observed to have "stupid facial expressions." A pretreatment CT scan reportedly confirmed the presence of significant generalized cerebral atrophy consistent with dementia. After failing to respond to Western medicines, Chinese acupuncture, and Chinese herbal treatments, the patient was advised to follow a twice-daily routine of a meditative qigong practice called Quan Zhen Gong. The patient also received an unspecified number of qigong treatments from a qigong master, reportedly with observable improvements in cognitive symptoms. After 6 months of daily qigong practice and regular qigong treatments, the patient had returned to his previous baseline of cognitive functioning and was no longer assessed as demented. Following several more months of continued qigong practice but no further qigong treatments, a repeat CT scan confirmed reversal of generalized cerebral atrophy identified in the initial scan. Replication of these findings under controlled conditions in a population of cognitively impaired elderly patients using blind raters to assess pre- and post-treatment mental status and to establish clinical correlation between changes in cognitive functioning and EEG or CT findings would constitute a truly remarkable finding.

◆ The Integrative Management Algorithm for Dementia and Mild Cognitive Impairment

Figure 12–1 is the integrative management algorithm for dementia and mild cognitive impairment. Note that specific assessment and treatment approaches are representative examples of reasonable choices. Moderate symptoms often respond to exercise, dietary modification, mind–body practices, and energy-information therapies. When managing severe symptoms, emphasize biological therapies. Encourage exercise and other lifestyle changes in motivated patients. Consider conventional, nonconventional, and integrative approaches that have not been tried.

See evidence tables and text for complete reviews of evidence-based options.

Before implementing any treatment plan, always check evidence tables and Web site updates at www.thieme.com/mentalhealth for specific assessment and treatment protocols, and obtain patient informed consent.

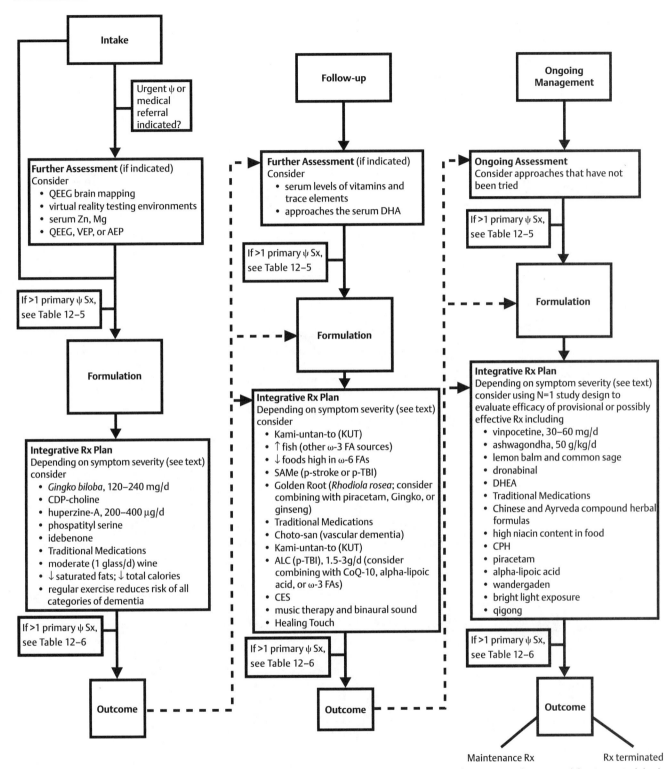

Figure 12–1 Integrative management algorithm for dementia and cognitive impairment. Note that specific assessment and treatment approaches are representative examples of reasonable choices. Moderate symptoms often respond to exercise, dietary modification, mind–body practices, and energy-information therapies. Rx, treatment; Sx, symptoms.

◆ Integrated Approaches to Consider When Two or More Core Symptoms Are Present

Table 12–5 shows the assessment approaches to consider using when cognitive impairment is the focus of clinical attention and one or more other symptoms are being assessed concurrently.

Table 12–6 outlines the treatment approaches to consider using when cognitive impairment is the focus of clinical attention and one or more other symptoms are being treated concurrently.

Table 12–5 Assessment Approaches to Cognitive Impairment When Other Symptoms Are Being Assessed Concurrently

Other Symptom(s) Being Assessed Concurrently	Assessment Approach	Comments
Depressed mood	Serologic studies	Limited evidence suggests that abnormally low serum DHA (an omega-3 essential fatty acid) levels correlate with increased risk of developing Alzheimer's disease.
		Limited evidence suggests that abnormally low levels of zinc and magnesium correlate with the risk of developing Alzheimer's disease.
		Low serum folate levels predict nonresponse to both conventional and nonconventional treatments of depressed mood.
		Low RBC omega-3 essential fatty acids are correlated with more severe depressed mood
	qEEG brain mapping	qEEG mapping provides useful information when planning EEG-biofeedback protocols addressing cognitive impairment in general.
		Specific qEEG findings correlate with Alzheimer's; specific VEP or AER findings correlate with milder cognitive impairment.
		Specific qEEG findings predict differential response rates of depressed mood to both conventional and nonconventional treatments
Mania and cyclic mood changes	Serologic studies	Low trace lithium levels (i.e., from low nutritional intake) are common in acutely manic patients.
		Limited evidence suggests that pretreatment serum GABA levels predict improved response of mania and cyclic mood changes to divalproex (Depakote) but not other mood stabilizers
	qEEG brain mapping	Emerging evidence suggests that pretreatment qEEG in acutely manic or cycling patients (showing left-sided abnormalities) predicts improved response to conventional treatments
Anxiety	Serologic studies	Deficiencies of niacin and vitamins B_6, C, and E are sometimes associated with generalized anxiety.
		Limited evidence suggests that total serum cholesterol is elevated in chronically anxious patients
	qEEG brain mapping	Limited evidence suggests that specific qEEG changes correspond to disparate anxiety syndromes
Psychosis	Serologic studies	Limited evidence suggests that abnormally low serum and RBC folate levels correlate with increased risk of schizophrenia and other psychotic syndromes.
		Limited evidence suggests that high pretreatment serum HVA levels predict improved response to lower doses of conventional antipsychotics in acutely manic patients with psychotic symptoms
	qEEG brain mapping	qEEG mapping, VEP, and AER studies facilitate diagnosis and more aggressive treatment of early Alzheimer's and mild cognitive impairment.
		qEEG mapping can be used to evaluate response to conventional and nonconventional cognitive enhancing treatments.
		Specific qEEG findings may correlate with disparate syndromes of chronic psychosis
Substance abuse or dependence	Serum micronutrient levels	Abnormally low levels of zinc and magnesium may correlate with the risk of developing Alzheimer's disease; however, findings are inconsistent.
		In alcohol abuse the magnitude of serum deficiencies of vitamins A and C, some B vitamins, and zinc, magnesium, and essential fatty acids is an indicator of the severity of malnutrition
	qEEG brain mapping	Limited evidence suggests that qEEG brain mapping provides useful information when planning specific EEG-biofeedback protocols for relapsing alcoholics or narcotics abusers
Disturbance of sleep or wakefulness	Serologic studies	Limited evidence suggests that chronic malnutrition caused by malabsorption of essential dietary factors increases the risk of developing Alzheimer's disease or mild cognitive impairment.
		Deficiencies in vitamins B_{12}, C, and E and folic acid are correlated with increased daytime sleepiness and insomnia.
		Abnormally low serum levels of magnesium and zinc are often associated with increased daytime sleepiness

AER, auditory evoked response; DHA, docosahexaenoic acid; EEG, GABA, γ-aminobutyric acid; HVA, homovanillic acid; qEEG, quantitative electroencephalography; RBC, red blood cell (count); VEP, visual evoked potential

Table 12–6 Treatment Approaches to Cognitive Impairment When One or More Other Symptoms Are Being Treated Concurrently *(Continued)*

Other Symptom(s) Being Treated Concurrently	Treatment Approach	Comments
Depressed mood	Dietary modifications	Moderate wine consumption, reduced saturated fats, and reduced total caloric intake are correlated with reduced risk of developing Alzheimer's disease.
		Limited evidence suggests that restricting caffeine and refined sugar and increasing consumption of fatty fish and whole foods rich in B vitamins improves depressed mood and reduces the risk of becoming depressed
	Omega-3 essential fatty acids	Limited evidence suggests that diets high in fish or other sources of omega-3 fatty acids and low in omega-6 fatty acids are associated with a reduced risk of developing dementia.
		Combining omega-3 fatty acids (especially EPA) 1 to 2 g/day with conventional antidepressants improves response and may accelerate response rate.
		Limited evidence suggests that EPA alone is an effective treatment of severe depressed mood
	Vitamins	Limited evidence suggests that high niacin intake from food or supplements significantly reduces the risk of developing dementia and decreases the rate of cognitive decline in healthy elderly individuals.
		Folate 0.5 to 1 mg/day augments the effects of conventional antidepressants and SAMe
	DHEA and estrogen	Limited evidence suggests that DHEA 25 to 50 mg/day improves mental performance in healthy adults, and 200 mg/day also improves cognitive functioning in vascular dementia.
		DHEA 90 to 450 mg/day is beneficial for mild to moderate depressed mood.
		DHEA has synergistic effects when combined with conventional antidepressants and may be an effective monotherapy for moderate depressed mood.
		Estrogen replacement therapy may be an effective treatment for postpartum psychosis. Adding estrogen to conventional antipsychotics may improve outcomes.
		Note: Meta-analyses fail to show that hormonal replacement with estrogen/progesterone slows progression of dementia in postmenopausal women diagnosed with Alzheimer's disease or prevents cognitive decline in healthy postmenopausal women.
		Caution: Estrogen replacement therapy is associated with increased risk of breast cancer, heart disease, and stroke.
		Estrogen supplementation may increase risk of breast cancer or heart disease in susceptible women
	Ayurvedic herbs	Limited evidence suggests that Ashwagondha 50 mg/kg improves short- and long-term memory and executive functioning in cognitively impaired individuals.
		Several Ayurvedic herbs and compound herbal formulas are probably beneficial for depression.
		Note: Individuals who use Ayurvedic herbs should do so only under the supervision of an Ayurvedic physician
	Ginkgo biloba	Standardized extracts of *G. biloba* 120 to 600 mg/day improve memory and cognitive performance in mild to moderate Alzheimer's disease, vascular dementia, and post-stroke patients and may slow cognitive decline in severe dementia.
		Combining *G. biloba* with ginseng enhances cognitive performance in nonimpaired healthy adults.
		Limited evidence suggests that *G. biloba* slows progression to mild cognitive impairment.
		Possibly enhanced effect when combined with piracetam or CDP-choline.
		Caution: *G. biloba* is contraindicated in patients taking anticoagulants.
		Cases of serotonin syndrome have been reported when combined with SSRIs
	Rhodiola rosea (golden root)	*R. rosea* 500 mg/day improves memory and performance in healthy adults and may accelerate recovery of normal cognitive functioning following head injury.
		Neuroprotective effects may be enhanced by piracetam, *Ginkgo biloba,* or ginseng.
		Caution: *R. rosea* may induce mania in bipolar patients and should be avoided in this population
	Somatic and mind–body approaches	Wander gardens permit demented or post-stroke patients to enjoy nature-related activities and reportedly improve baseline functioning in the early stages of dementia.
		Regular exercise at least 30 minutes 3 times a week is probably as effective as conventional antidepressants, St. John's wort, and cognitive therapy for moderate depressed mood.
		Exercising under bright light is more effective against depression than exercise or bright light alone

(Continued)

Table 12–6 Treatment Approaches to Cognitive Impairment When One or More Other Symptoms Are Being Treated Concurrently *(Continued)*

Other Symptom(s) Being Treated Concurrently	Treatment Approach	Comments
	Music and sound	Regular music therapy probably enhances global functioning in demented individuals, reduces agitation and wandering, enhances social interaction, improves depressed mood, increases cooperative behavior, and increases baseline cognitive functioning. Binaural sounds in the beta frequency range (16–24 Hz) may enhance cognitive functioning in healthy adults.
		Note: Most studies on music in dementia are small, and findings are limited by the absence of quantitative outcomes measures, randomization, and blinding
	Microcurrent electrical stimulation	Two forms of microcurrent electrical stimulation—TENS and CES—resulted in improvements in word recall, face recognition, and motivation in demented individuals
		Note: The beneficial effects of weak electrical stimulation are not sustained several weeks after treatment ends
	Qigong Vitamins and minerals	Limited evidence suggests that regular qigong practice or external qigong treatments normalize EEG slowing and reverse cerebral atrophy associated with dementia
		Regular qigong practice results in generally improved emotional well-being.
		Note: Controlled studies of qigong in dementia have not been done, but case reports suggest dramatic beneficial effects
Mania and cyclic mood changes		Limited evidence suggests that folic acid 200 μg/day augments the effects of lithium in mania and that monthly B$_{12}$ injections reduce the risk of recurring manic episodes.
		Limited evidence suggests that magnesium supplementation 40 mEq/day is an effective treatment of rapid cycling episodes, and that potassium 20 mEq bid reduces lithium-induced tremor and improve compliance
	Omega-3 fatty acids	Limited evidence suggests that EPA 1 to 2 g/day in combination with conventional mood stabilizers reduces the severity and frequency of manic episodes.
		Note: At the time of writing, there is one case report of EPA-induced hypomania
	Mind–body approaches	Limited evidence suggests that certain yogic breathing practices and postures reduce the severity of mania or hypomania
	Mindfulness training	Limited evidence suggests that certain meditation practices promote calmness and are beneficial in mania or hypomania
Anxiety	Dietary modifications	Limited evidence suggests that avoiding refined sugar and caffeine and increasing protein and foods containing tryptophan reduce symptoms of generalized anxiety and panic
	Somatic approaches	Regular aerobic or strengthening exercise reduces generalized anxiety symptoms, and there is limited evidence that exercise may also reduce the frequency and severity of panic attacks
Psychosis	Dietary changes	Limited evidence suggests that chronically psychotic patients with higher intake of unsaturated fats, reduced gluten, and improved glucose regulation may experience milder symptoms
	Vitamins	Combining niacin (in the form of nicotinamide 3–8 g), folate (in the form of methylfolate 15 mg), or thiamine (500 mg tid) with conventional antipsychotics may improve outcomes.
		Note: Flushing and discomfort are associated with large doses of niacin and reportedly diminished when niacin is taken in the form of niacinamide
	Omega-3 fatty acids	Limited evidence suggests that EPA (1–4 g) alone or in combination with conventional antipsychotics (and especially clozapine) improves outcomes. Beneficial effects of omega-3 essential fatty acids may be more robust in the early acute phase of the illness
	Ayurvedic herbs	Limited evidence suggests that Brahmyadiyoga 8 to 12 g is as effective as conventional antipsychotics; Mentat may reduce severity of negative psychotic symptoms
	Ginkgo biloba	Limited evidence suggests that combining *G. biloba* (360 mg/day) with a conventional antipsychotic is more effective for both positive and negative symptoms compared with conventional treatments alone.
		Note: There is limited evidence that combining *G. biloba* with a conventional antipsychotic reduces adverse neurological effects
	DHEA and estrogen	Limited evidence suggests that combining DHEA 100 mg with a conventional antipsychotic may reduce the severity of negative symptoms and improve depressed mood and anxiety.
		Caution: DHEA can be activating and should be taken in the morning. Patients with a history or benign prostatic hypertrophy or prostate cancer should consult their physician before taking DHEA

Table 12–6   Treatment Approaches to Cognitive Impairment When One or More Other Symptoms Are Being Treated Concurrently *(Continued)*

Other Symptom(s) Being Treated Concurrently	Treatment Approach	Comments
	Somatic approaches	Limited evidence suggests that a sensory stimulation technique known as the Wilbarger method improves sensory integration in schizophrenics
	Spiritually oriented group therapy and mindfulness training	Combining spiritually oriented group therapy with yogic breathing practice and conventional medications improves global functioning in stable chronically psychotic patients
		Caution: Patients who are delusional or have other acute psychotic symptoms should be discouraged from participating in spiritual or religious practices
	Religious or spiritual activity	Limited evidence suggests that patients who have well-controlled psychotic symptoms benefit from social support in organized religious activity.
		Caution: Patients who are actively psychotic should be advised to avoid intense religious or spiritual activity
Substance abuse or dependence	Dietary changes	Alcoholics who improve their diets, including reduced intake of refined sugar and caffeine and increased intake of omega-3 fatty acids and protein, probably have an increased chance for maintaining sobriety
	Vitamins and minerals	Limited evidence suggests that thiamine reduces alcohol craving, nicotinic acid reduces the risk of alcohol dependence in chronic drinkers, and taking antioxidant vitamins soon before drinking reduces the severity of hangover symptoms.
		Limited evidence suggests that supplementation of chronic alcoholics with magnesium and zinc improves global neuropsychological functioning and protects the brain against free radical damage
	Somatic approaches	Limited evidence suggests that regular aerobic exercise or strength training in abstinent alcoholics improves general emotional well-being.
		Caution: All patients should consult with their primary care physician before starting a rigorous exercise program
	Mindfulness training	Abstinent alcoholics and addicts who engage in a regular mindfulness practice or meditation probably have a reduced risk of relapse
	Acupuncture	Some acupuncture points and protocols are probably more effective than others in reducing symptoms of alcohol or cocaine withdrawal
Disturbance of sleep or wakefulness	Somatic and mind–body approaches	Many somatic and mind–body practices, including progressive muscle relaxation, massage, meditation, and guided imagery, are as effective as conventional sedative-hypnotics for mild to moderate insomnia
	Acupuncture	Some acupuncture and auriculotherapy protocols probably reduce the severity of sleep disturbances, including insomnia related to a mental or emotional problem

AER, auditory evoked response; CES, cranioelectrotherapy stimulation; DHEA, dehydroepiandrosterone; EEG, electroencephalography; EPA, ecosapentanoic acid; qEEG, quantitative electroencephalography; RBC, red blood cell (count); SAMe, S-adenosylmethionine; TENS, transcranial electrical nerve stimulation; VEP, visual evoked potential

Case Vignette

History and Initial Presentation

Margaret graduated summa cum laude in economics from Yale in 1943 and still recalls her first job during "the war days" as the assistant manager for the logistics and planning division of a munitions factory. Her intelligence and creativity had soon propelled her through the ranks, and by 1950, at the age of 30, she had become the first woman vice president in the history of the company. New successes followed a growing record of achievements, and the years passed without emotional turmoil. Margaret had always been in excellent health and was an avid tennis player. At the age of 70 she decided to retire. Within 2 years she had become a master gardener and spent much of her time at the local garden club. At the age of 74 Margaret first noticed "slowness in finding the right French verb." Six months after returning from a 3-week vacation in France, Margaret became "stuck" when trying to recall a word. On one occasion she became temporarily lost while driving home from the supermarket where she had shopped for the past 20 years. A friend finally encouraged Margaret to make an appointment with her

internist to evaluate her memory problem. Dr. Harris became concerned as Margaret described progressive difficulty finding words, recognizing familiar faces, and becoming disoriented in her neighborhood but denied neurological symptoms, including transient numbness or weakness of the extremities, changes in vision, and headaches. There was no history of head injury, stroke, or seizures, and Margaret confirmed that there had been no recent medication changes. There was no history of major medical problems including cancer, and only moderately elevated blood pressure, for which Margaret took an antihypertensive. Margaret denied feeling depressed or anxious, had no financial or social stresses, and there was no known family history of dementia or other psychiatric or neurological problems. Her pulse was a regular 78, and her temperature and blood pressure were normal. On the MMSE, Margaret scored 23 out of 30. She was unable to recall three words after 5 minutes, and was unable to calculate serial 7s counting backward from 100 below 79. She could not recall what she had eaten for lunch the previous day. Margaret's long-term memory was intact. Dr. Harris ordered routine blood chemistries and a thyroid panel to rule out possible medical causes of Margaret's cognitive symptoms.

Assessment, Formulation, and Treatment Plan

On her return appointment, Margaret appeared tense. All laboratory findings were unremarkable, including normal serum electrolytes, a normal hematocrit, and normal thyroid hormone levels. Dr. Harris explained to Margaret that it wasn't clear whether she was in the early stages of Alzheimer's disease or experiencing the effects of chronic deficiencies of nutrients that were now impairing her memory and general cognitive functioning. Margaret had already started to practice guided imagery on a daily basis, addressing her fear that she might have Alzheimer's disease. Dr. Harris suggested that because Margaret had been a strict vegan for many decades and had never used supplements, it would be prudent to check a serum DHA level as well as serum B_{12} and folate levels. She encouraged Margaret to take vitamin supplements (i.e., following the blood work) including folate, thiamine, and vitamins B_{12}, C, and E, and also suggested dietary modifications to increase her intake of foods rich in omega-3 fatty acids. Dr. Harris also recommended daily 30-minute walks. A follow-up appointment was scheduled in 1 month.

Follow-Up

Dr. Harris noticed that Margaret's eyes appeared brighter as she entered the examination room. She now walked briskly at least an hour every morning, and had been taking daily supplements, including recommended brands of vitamins C, E, B_{12}, folate, and omega-3 fatty acids. Her short-term memory had noticeably improved. Dr. Harris told Margaret that her serum folate and DHA levels had been in the borderline low range and remarked that her rapid improvement suggested that her symptoms were caused by chronic deficiencies in important nutrients. Margaret commented that she felt less anxious after her morning guided imagery session. She had read about the cognitive-enhancing properties of an herb called golden root, and had been taking it at a dose of 500 mg/day for 3 weeks. She told Dr. Harris that she believed the herb had made a difference in both her short-term memory and anxiety. Dr. Harris was unfamiliar with golden root, and Margaret gave her a copy of a peer-reviewed article she had obtained through a Web site summarizing the research evidence for its use as a cognitive enhancer. The monograph confirmed the absence of significant adverse effects and potential interactions with β-blockers. Dr. Harris agreed that it was reasonable for Margaret to continue taking golden root at her current dose. The session ended with the understanding that Margaret would return for a routine follow-up appointment in 6 months. Margaret agreed to contact Dr. Harris in the event of any recurring problems with memory, anxiety, or mood.

References

Abbott, R., White, L., Ross, W., Masaki, K., Curb, D., & Petrovitch, H. (2004). Walking and dementia in physically capable elderly men. *Journal of the American Medical Association, 292*(12), 1447–1453.

Akhondzadeh, S., Noroozian, M., Mohammadi, M., et al. (2003a). *Melissa officinalis* extract in the treatment of patients with mild to moderate Alzheimer's disease: A double-blind, randomized, placebo-controlled trial. *Journal of Neurology, Neurosurgery, and Psychiatry, 74*, 863–866.

Akhondzadeh, S., Noroozian, M., Mohammadi, M., et al. (2003b). *Salvia officinalis* extract in the treatment of patients with mild to moderate Alzheimer's disease: A double-blind, randomized and placebo-controlled trial. *Journal of Clinical Pharmacy and Therapeutics, 28*, 53–59.

Allain, H., Raoul, P., Lieury, A., et al. (1993). Effect of two doses of Ginkgo biloba extract (EGb 761) on the dual-coding test in elderly subjects. *Clinical Therapeutics; 15*(3), 549–558.

Alvarez, X., Laredo, M., Corzo, D., et al. (1997). Citicoline improves memory performance in elderly subjects. *Methods and Findings in Experimental and Clinical Pharmacology, 19*(3), 201–210.

Alvarez, X. A., Mouzo, R., Pichel, V., et al. (1999). Double-blind placebo-controlled study with citicoline in APOE genotyped Alzheimer's disease patients: Effects on cognitive performance, brain bioelectrical activity and cerebral perfusion. *Methods and Findings in Experimental and Clinical Pharmacology, 21*, 633–644.

Amaducci, L. (1988). Phosphatidylserine in the treatment of Alzheimer's disease: Results of a multicenter study. *Psychopharmacology Bulletin, 24*, 130–134.

Ames, B., Shigenaga, M., & Hagen, T. (1993). Oxidants, antioxidants and the degenerative diseases of aging. *Proceedings of the National Academy of Sciences of the United States of America, 90*, 7915–7922.

Ancoli-Israel, S., Martin, J., Gehrman, P., Shochat, T. Corey-Bloom, J., et al. (2003). Effect of light on agitation in institutionalized patients with severe Alzheimer's disease. *American Journal of Geriatric Psychiatry, 11*(2), 194–203.

Arai, H., Suzuki, T., Sasaki, H., Hanawa, T., Toriizuka, K., & Yamada, H. (2000). A new interventional strategy for Alzheimer's disease by Japanese herbal medicine [in Japanese]. *Nippon Ronen Igakkai Zasshi, 37*(3), 212–215.

Arrigo, A., Casale, R., Buonocore, M., & Ciano, C. (1990). Effects of acetyl-L-carnitine on reaction times in patients with cerebrovascular insufficiency. *International Journal of Clinical Pharmacology Research, 10*, 133–137.

Azuma, T., Nagai, Y., Saito, T., et al. (1999). The effect of dehydroepiandrosterone sulfate administration to patients with multi-infarct dementia. *Journal of the Neurological Sciences, 162*(1), 69–73.

Bacci Ballerini, F., Lopez Anguera, A., Alcaraz, P., & Hernandez Reyes, N. (1983). Treatment of postconcussion syndrome with S-adenosylmethionine. *Medica Clínica (Barcelona), 80*, 161–164.

Baker, L., Sambarmurti, K., Craft, S., Cherrier, M., Raskind, M., Stanczyk, F., et al. (2003). Beta-estradiol reduces plasma beta for HRT-naïve postmenopausal women with Alzheimer's disease: A preliminary study. *American Journal of Geriatric Psychiatry, 11*(2), 239–244.

Balestreri, R., Fontana, L., & Astengo, F. (1987). A double-blind placebo controlled evaluation of the safety and efficacy of vinpocetine in the treatment of patients with chronic vascular senile cerebral dysfunction. *Journal of the American Geriatrics Society, 35*, 425–430.

Ballard, C. G., O'Brien, J. T., Reichelt, K., et al. (2002). Aromatherapy as a safe and effective treatment for the management of agitation in severe dementia: The results of a double-blind, placebo-controlled trial with *Melissa*. *Journal of Clinical Psychiatry, 63*(7), 553–558.

Barberger-Gateau, P., Letenneur, L., Deschamps, V., Peres, K., Dartigues, J. F., & Renaud, S. (2002). Fish, meat, and risk of dementia: Cohort study. *British Medical Journal, 325*(7370), 932–933.

Bella, R., Biondi, R., Raffaele, R., & Bennisi, G. (1990). Effect of acetyl-L-carnitine on geriatric patients suffering from dysthymic disorders. *International Journal of Clinical Pharmacology Research, 10*, 355–360.

Benton, D., Griffiths, R., & Haller, J. (1997). Thiamine supplementation mood and cognitive functioning. *Phsychopharmacology, 129*, 66–71.

Benvenuto, J., Jin, Y., Casale, M., Lynch, G., & Granger, R. (2002). Identification of diagnostic evoked response potential segments in Alzheimer's disease. *Experimental Neurology, 176*(2), 269–276.

Bergem, A. L., Engedal, K., & Kringlen, E. (1997). The role of heredity in late-onset Alzheimer disease and vascular dementia: A twin study. *Archives of General Psychiatry, 54*, 264–270.

Bhattacharya, S., & Kumar, A. (1997). Effect of Trasina, an Ayurvedic herbal formulation, on experimental models of Alzheimer's disease and central cholinergic markers in rats. *Journal of Alternative and Complementary Medicine, 3*(4), 327–336.

Bhattacharya, S. K., Kumar, A., & Ghosal, S. (1995). Effects of glycowithanolides from *Withania somnifera* on an animal model of Alzheimer's disease and perturbed central cholinergic markers of cognition in rats. *Phytotherapy Research, 9*(2), 110–113.

Birks, J., & Grimley, E. (2004). Ginkgo biloba for cognitive impairment and dementia (Cochrane Review). In *The Cochrane Library* (Issue 2). Chichester, UK: John Wiley & Sons.

Blaha, L., Erzigkeit, H., Adamczyk, A., et al. (1989). Clinical evidence of the effectiveness of vinpocetine in the treatment of organic psychosyndrome [Abstract]. *Human Psychopharmacology, 4*, 103–111.

Blumenthal, M., Goldberg, A., & Brinckmann, J. (Eds.). (2000). *Herbal medicine: Expanded Commission E monographs*. Newton, MA: Integrative Medicine Communications, pp. 160–169.

Bottiglieri, T., Godfrey, P., Flynn, T., et al. (1990). Cerebrospinal fluid S-adeno-sylmethionine in depression and dementia: effects of treatment with par-enteral and oral S-adenosylmethionine. *Journal of Neurology, Neurosurgery, an Psychiatry, 53*(12), 1096–1098.

Brautigan, M. R., Blommaert, F. A., Verleye, G., et al. (1998). Treatment of age-related memory complaints with *Ginkgo biloba* extract: A randomized dou-ble blind placebo-controlled study. *Phytomedicine, 5*(6), 425–434.

Brown, R., & Gerbarg, P. (2004). *The rhodiola revolution: Transform your health with the herbal breakthrough of the 21st century.* Emmaus, Pennsylvania: Rodale.

Burns, A., Jacoby, R., & Levy, R. (1990). Psychiatric phenomena in Alzheimer's disease: 2. Disorders of perception. *British Journal of Psychiatry, 157,* 86–94.

Calvani, M., Carta, A., Caruso, G., et al. (1992). Action of acetyl-L-carnitine in neurodegeneration and Alzheimer's disease. *Annals of the New York Academy of Sciences, 663,* 483–486.

Cameron, M., Lonergan, E., & Lee, H. (2004). Transcutaneous electrical nerve stimulation (TENS) for dementia (Cochrane Review). In *The Cochrane Library* (Issue 2). Chichester, UK John Wiley & Sons.

Cardinal, B. J., & Engels, H. J. (2001). Ginseng does not enhance psychological well-being in healthy, young adults: Results of a double-blind, placebo-controlled, randomized clinical trial. *Journal of the American Dietetic Asso-ciation, 101*(6), 655–660.

Cenacchi, T., Bertoldin, T., Farina, C., et al. (1993). Cognitive decline in the eld-erly: A double-blind placebo-controlled multicenter study on efficacy of phosphatidylserine administration. *Aging (Milano), 5,* 123–133.

Chandler, J., & Chandler, J. E. (1988). The prevalence of neuropsychiatric dis-orders in a nursing home population. *Journal of Geriatric Psychiatry and Neurology, 1*(2), 71–76.

Cheuvront, S. N., & Carter, R. III. (2003). Ginkgo and memory. *Journal of the American Medical Association, 289*(5):547–548.

Chung, J. C. C., Lai, C. K. Y, Chung, P. M. B, & French, H. P. (2004). Snoezelen for dementia (Cochrane Review). In *The Cochrane Library* (Issue 2). Chichester, UK: John Wiley & Sons.

Cipolli, C., & Chiari, G. (1990). Effects of L-acetylcarnitine on mental deterio-ration in the aged: Initial results. *La Clínica Terapeutica, 132,* 479–510.

Cohen, B., Satlin, A., & Zubenko, G. (1988). S-adenosyl-L-methionine in the treatment of Alzheimer's disease. *Journal of Clinical Psychopharmacology, 8*(1), 43–47.

Cohen-Mansfield, J., Garfinkel, D., & Lipson, S. (2000). Melatonin for treatment of sundowning in elderly persons with dementia—a preliminary study. *Archives of Gerontology and Geriatrics, 31,* 65–76.

Constantinidis, J. (1990). Alzheimer's disease and the zinc theory [in French]. *L'Encéphale, 16*(4), 231–239.

Growdon, J. H., & Corkin, S. (1980). Neurochemical approaches to the treat-ment of senile demntia. *Proceedings annual Meeting of the American Psychopathology Association, 69,* 281–296.

Cotman, C. W., & Berchtold, N. C. (2002). Exercise: A behavioral intervention to enhance brain health and plasticity. *Trends in Neurosciences, 25*(6), 295–301.

Crook, T., Tinklenberg, J., Yesavage, J., et al. (1991). Effects of phosphatidylser-ine in age-associated memory impairment. *Neurology, 41,* 644–649.

Cuajungco, M. P., & Lees, G. J. (1997). Zinc and Alzheimer's disease: Is there a direct link? *Brain Research Reviews, 23,* 219–236.

Decker, M., Majchrzak, M., & Arneric, S. (1993). Effects of lobeline, a nicotinic receptor agonist, on learning and memory. *Pharmacology, Biochemistry, and Behavior, 45,* 571–576.

Detweiler, M. B., & Warf, C. (2005). Dementia wander garden aids post cere-brovascular stroke restorative therapy: A case study. *Alternative Therapies in Health and Medicine, 11*(4), 54–58.

Ebel, S. (1991). Designing state-specific horticultural therapy interventions for patients with Alzheimer's disease. *Journal of Therapeutic Horticulture, 6,* 3–9.

Enderby, P., Broeckx, J., Hospers, W., et al. (1994). Effect of piracetam on recovery and rehabilitation after stroke: A double-blind, placebo-controlled study. *Clinical Neuropharmacology, 17,* 320–331.

Engelhart, M., Geerlings, M., Ruitenberg, A., et al. (2002a). Dietary intake of antioxidants and risk of Alzheimer's disease. *Journal of the American Medical Association, 287,* 3223–3229.

Engelhart, M. J., Geerlings, M. I., Ruitenberg, A., Van Swieten, J. C., Hofman, A., Witteman, J. C., et al. (2002b). Diet and risk of dementia: Does fat matter? The Rotterdam Study. *Neurology, 59*(12), 1915–1921.

Epstein, M., Hansen, V., & Hazen, T. (1991). Therapeutic gardens: Plant cen-tered activities meet sensory, physical and psychosocial needs. *Oregon's Journal on Aging, 9,* 8–14.

Ernst E. (1999). Diet and dementia, is there a link? A systematic review. *Nutritional Neuroscience, 2,* 1–6.

Evans, D., Funkenstein, H., Albert, M., et al. (1989). Prevalence of Alzheimer's disease in a community population of older persons: Higher than previ-ously reported. *Journal of the American Medical Association, 262*(18), 2551–2556.

Evans, J. (1987). Alzheimer's dementia: Some possible mechanisms related to vitamins, trace elements and minerals suggesting a possible treatment. *Journal of Orthomolecular Medicine, 1*(4), 249–254.

Fioravanti, M., & Flicker, L. (2004). Nicergoline for dementia and other age associated forms of cognitive impairment (Cochrane Review). In *The Cochrane Library* (Issue 2). Chicester, UK: John Wiley & Sons.

Fioravanti, M., & Yanagi, M. (2004). Cytidinediphosphocholine (CDP choline) for cognitive and behavioral disturbances associated with chronic cerebral disorders in the elderly (Cochrane Review). In *The Cochrane Library* (Issue 2). Chichester, UK: John Wiley & Sons.

Flicker, L., & Grimley, D. (2004). Piracetam for dementia or cognitive impair-ment (Cochrane Review). In *The Cochrane Library* (Issue 2). Chichester, UK: John Wiley & Sons.

Forbes, D., Morgan, D., Bangma, J., Peacock, S., Pelletier, N., & Adamson, J. (2004). Light therapy for managing sleep, behavior, and mood disturbances in dementia (Cochrane Review). In *The Cochrane Library* (Issue 2). Chich-ester, UK: John Wiley & Sons.

Fraser, J., & Kerr, J. R. (1993). Psychophysiological effects of back massage on eld-erly institutionalized patients. *Journal of Advanced Nursing, 18*(2), 238–245.

Friess, E., Trachsel, L., Guldner, J., et al. (1995). DHEA administration increases rapid eye movement sleep and EEG power in the sigma frequency range. *American Journal of Physiology, 268*(1, Pt. 1), E107–E113.

Gaby, A. R. (1996). Ginkgo biloba extract: A review. *Alternative Medicine Review, 1,* 236–242.

Gatz, M., Pedersen, N. L., Berg, S., et al. (1997). Heritability for Alzheimer's disease: The study of dementia in Swedish twins. *Journals of Gerontology. Series A: Biological and Medical Sciences, 52,* M117–M125.

Ghali, L., Hopkins, R. W., & Rindlisbacher, P. (1995). The fragmentation of the rest/activity cycles in Alzheimer's disease. *International Journal of Geriatric Psychiatry, 10,* 299–304.

Ghosal, S., Lal, J., Srivastava, R., et al. (1989). Immunomodulatory and CNS effects of sitoindosides IX and X, two new glycowithanolides from *Withania somnifera. Phytotherapy Research, 3*(5), 201–206.

Glick J. (1990). Dementias: The role of magnesium deficiency and an hypothesis concerning the pathogenesis of Alzheimer's disease. *Medical Hypotheses, 31*(3), 211–225.

Gonzalez-Seijo, J. C., Ramos, Y. M., & Lastra, I. (1995). Manic episode and ginseng: Report of a possible case. *Journal of Clinical Psychopharmacology, 15*(6), 447–448.

Gouliaev, A. H., & Senning, A. (1994). Piracetam and other structurally related nootropics. *Brain Research Reviews, 19,* 180–222.

Grant W. (1997). Dietary links to Alzheimer's disease. *Alzheimer's Disease Re-view, 2,* 42–55.

Gutzmann, H., Kuhl, K.P., hadler, D., et al. (2002). Safety and efficacy of idebenone versus tacrine in patients with alzheimer's disease: results fo a randomized, double-blind, parallel–group multicenter study. *Pharma-copysychiatry, 35,* 12–18.

Haffmans, P. M. J., Lucius, S. A. P., & Sival, R. C. (1998, October 31-November 4). *Bright light therapy and melatonin in motor restlessness in dementia* (Abstract P.4.006). Paper presented at the 11th European College of Neuropsychopharmacology Congress, Paris.

Haier, R. (1993). Cerebral glucose metabolism and intelligence. In P. A. Vernon (Ed.), *Biological approaches to the study of intelligence* (pp. 318–332). Westport, CT: Ablex Publishing Corp.

Hassing, L., Wahlin, A., Winblad, B., et al. (1999). Further evidence of the effects of vitamin B_{12} and folate levels on episodic memory functioning: A population-based study of healthy very old adults. *Biological Psychiatry, 45,* 1472–1480.

Hebert, L., Scherr, P., Bienias, J., Bennett, D., & Evans, D. (2003). Alzheimer dis-ease in the U.S. population: Prevalence estimates using the 2000 census. *Archives of Neurology, 60,* 1119–1122.

Heyman, A., et al. (1987). In R. J. Wurtman et al. (Eds.), *Proceedings of the Fourth Meeting of the International Study Group on Pharmacology of Memory Disorders Associated with Aging* (pp. 293–304).

Hibbeln, J. R., & Salem, N., Jr. (1995). Dietary polyunsaturated fatty acids and depression: When cholesterol does not satisfy. *American Journal of Clinical Nutrition, 62,* 1–9.

Higgins, J. P. T., & Flicker, L. (2004). Lecithin for dementia and cognitive im-pairment (Cochrane Review). In *The Cochrane Library* (Issue 2). Chichester, UK: John Wiley & Sons.

Hogervorst, E., Yaffe, K., Richards, M., & Huppert F. (2004a). Hormone replace-ment therapy for cognitive function in postmenopausal women (Cochrane Review). In: *The Cochrane Library,* Issue 2. Chichester, U.K.: John Wiley & Sons, Ltd.

Hogervorst, E., Yaffe, K., Richards, M., & Huppert, F. (2004b). Hormone replace-ment therapy to maintain cognitive function in women with dementia (Cochrane Review). In *The Cochrane Library* (Issue 2). Chichester, UK: John Wiley & Sons.

Holmes, C., Hopkins, V., Hensford, C., et al. (2002). Lavender oil as a treatment for agitated behaviour in severe dementia: A placebo controlled study. *International Journal of Geriatric Psychiatry, 17*(4):305–308.

Hopfenmuller, W. (1994). Evidence for a therapeutic effect of *Ginkgo biloba* special extract: Meta-analysis of 11 clinical studies in patients with cerebrovascular insufficiency in old age. *Arzneimittelforschung, 44,* 1005–1013.

Hudson, S., & Tabet, N. (2004). Acetyl-L-carnitine for dementia (Cochrane Review). In *The Cochrane Library* (Issue 2). Chichester, UK: John Wiley & Sons.

Huppert, F., & Van Niekerk, J. (2004). Dehydroepiandrosterone (DHEA) supplementation for cognitive function (Cochrane Review). In *The Cochrane Library* (Issue 2). Chichester, UK: John Wiley & Sons.

Ishihara, K., Katsuki, H., Sugimura, M., et al. (1989). Idebenone and vinpocetine augment long-term potentiation in hippocampal slices in the guinea pig. *Neuropharmacology, 28,* 569–573.

Itil, T. M., Eralp, E., Ahmed, I., et al. (1998). The pharmacological effects of ginkgo biloba, a plant extract, on the brain of dementia patients in comparison with tacrine. *Psychopharmacology Bulletin, 34,* 391–397.

Itil, T. M., Menon, G. N., Songar, A., et al. (1986). CNS pharmacology and clinical therapeutic effects of oxiracetam. *Clinical Neuropharmacology, 9*(Suppl. 3), S70–S72.

Jama, J., Launer, L., Witteman, J., et al. (1996). Dietary antioxidants and cognitive function in a population-based sample of older persons: The Rotterdam study. *American Journal of Epidemiology, 144,* 275–279.

Kalmijn, S., Feskens, E. J., Launer, L. J., & Kromhout, D. (1997). Polyunsaturated fatty acids, antioxidants, and cognitive function in very old men. *American Journal of Epidemiology, 145*(1), 33–41.

Kalmijn, S., van Boxtel, M., Ocke, M., Verschuren, W., Kromhout, D., & Launer, L. (2004). Dietary intake of fatty acids and fish in relation to cognitive performance at middle age. *Neurology, 62*(2), 275–280.

Kanowski, S., Herrmann, W. M., Stephan, K., Wierich, W., & Horr, R. (1996). Proof of efficacy of the *Ginkgo biloba* special extract EGb 761 in outpatients suffering from mild to moderate primary degenerative dementia of the Alzheimer type or multi-infarct dementia. *Pharmacopsychiatry, 29*(2), 47–56.

Kennedy, D. O., Scholey, A. B, & Wesnes, K. (2001). A direct comparison of the cognitive effects of acute doses of ginseng, ginkgo biloboa and their combination in healthy volunteers. *Journal of Psychopharmacology, 15*(Suppl.), A56.

Kennerly, R. (1996). An empirical investigation into the effect of beta frequency binaural beat audio signals on four measures of human memory. *Hemi-Sync Journal, 14*(3), i–iv.

Kidd, P. (1999). A review of nutrients and botanicals in the integrative management of cognitive dysfunction. *Alternative Medicine Review, 4*(3), 144–161.

Kleijnen, J., & Knipschild, P. (1992). Ginkgo biloba. *Lancet, 340,* 1136–1139.

Koger, S., Chapin, K., & Brotons, M. (1999). Is music therapy an effective intervention for dementia? A meta-analytic review of literature. *Journal of Music Therapy, 36*(1), 2–15.

Kruglikova, R. P. (1997, July). How and why picamilon works. *Life Extension,* pp. 34–38.

Kitamuram, K. (1981). Therapeutic effect of pyritinol on sequelae of head injuries. *Journal of International Medical Research, 9,* 215–221.

Kubyoyama, T., Tohda, C., Komatsu, K., et al. (2005). Neuritic regeneration and synaptic reconstruction induced by withanolide A. *British Journal of Pharmacology, 144* (7), 961–971.

Kumar, A. M., Tims, F., Cruess, D. G., Mintzer, M. J., Ironson, G., Loewenstein, D., et al. (1999). Music therapy increases serum melatonin levels in patients with Alzheimer's disease. *Alternative Therapy, 5,* 49–57.

Kyle, D. J., Schaefer, E., & Patton, G. (1998, June 1–5). *Low serum docosahexanoic acid is a significant risk factor for Alzheimer's dementia.* Paper presented at the Third Issfal Congress, Lyons, France.

Laurin, D., Verreault, R., Lindsay, J., Dewailly, E., & Holub BJ. (2003). Omega-3 fatty acids and risk of cognitive impairment and dementia. *Journal of Alzheimer's Disease, 5*(4), 315–322.

Le Bars, P. L., Katz, M. M., Berman, N., Turan, M., Freedman, A. M., & Schatzberg, A. F. (1997). A placebo-controlled, double-blind, randomized trial of on extract of *Ginkgo biloba* for dementia. *Journal of the American Medical Association, 278,* 1327–1332.

Le Bars, P. L., Velasco, F. M., Ferguson, J. M., Dessain, E. C., Kieser, M., & Hoerr, R. (2002). Influence of the severity of cognitive impairment on the effect of the ginkgo biloba extract EGB 761 in Alzheimer's disease. *Neuropsychobiology, 45,* 19–26.

Lendon, C. L., Ashall, F., & Goate, A. M. (1997). Exploring the etiology of Alzheimer's disease using molecular genetics. *Journal of the American Medical Association, 277,* 825–831.

Levitt, A., & Karlinsky, H. (1992). Folate, vitamin B$_{12}$ and cognitive impairment in patients with Alzheimer's disease. *Acta Psychiatrica Scandinavica, 86*(4), 301–305.

Licastro, F. (1996). Impaired peripheral zinc metabolism in patients with senile dementia of probable Alzheimer's type as shown by low plasma concentrations of thymulin. *Biological Trace Element Research, 51,* 55–61.

Little, A., Levy, R., Chuaqui-Kidd, P., et al. (1985). A double-blind, placebo-controlled trial of high-dose lecithin in Alzheimer's disease. *Journal of Neurology, Neurosurgery, and Psychiatry, 48,* 736–742.

Lolic, M. M., Fiskum, G., & Rosenthal, R. E. (1997). Neuroprotective effects of acetyl-L-carnitine after stroke in rats. *Annals of Emergency Medicine, 29,* 758–765.

Lonnrot, K., Porsti, I., Alho, H., Wu, X., Hervonen, A., & Tolvanen, J. P. (1998). Control of arterial tone after long-term coenzyme Q10 supplementation in senescent rats. *British Journal of Pharmacology, 124,* 1500–1506.

Malouf, R., & Areosa Sastre, A. (2004). Vitamin B$_{12}$ for cognition (Cochrane Review). In *The Cochrane Library* (Issue 2). Chichester, UK: John Wiley & Sons.

Manabu, T., et al. (1996). Three-dimensional PET: An approach in psychology. *Journal of the International Society of Life Information Science, 14*(2), 282–284.

Martin, D., Francis, J., Protetch, J., & Huff, F. (1992). Time dependency of cognitive recovery with cobalamin replacement: Report of a pilot study. *Journal of the American Geriatrics Society, 40*(2), 168–172.

McCraty, R. (2002). Influence of cardiac afferent input on heart brain synchronization and cognitive performance. *International Journal of Psychophysiology.* 45(1–2), 72–73

McEwen, B. (1998). Excitotoxity, stress hormones and the aging nervous system [Commentary]. *Integrative Medicine, 1*(3), 135–141.

Mimori, Y., Katsuoka, H., & Nakamuri, S. (1996). Thiamine therapy in Alzheimer's disease. *Metabolic Brain Disease, 11*(1), 89–94.

Mitka, M. (2002). News about neuroprotectants for the treatment of stroke. *Journal of the American Medical Association, 287,* 1253–1254.

Monaco, P., Pastore, L., Rizzo, S., et al. (1996, September 1–5). *Safety and tolerability of adometionine (ADE) SD for inpatients with stroke: A pilot randomized, double-blind, placebo controlled study.* Paper presented at the Third World Stroke Conference and Fifth European Stroke Conference, Munich, Germany.

Morris, M., Evans, D., Bienias, J., Scherr, P., Tangney, C., Hebert, L., et al. (2004). Dietary niacin and the risk of incident Alzheimer's disease and of cognitive decline. *Journal of Neurology, Neurosurgery, and Psychiatry, 75,* 1093–1099.

Morris, M., Evans, D., Bienias, J., Tangney, C., Bennett, D., et al. (2003). Consumption of fish and omega-3 polyunsaturated fatty acid-rich diets and risk of incident Alzheimer's disease. *Archives of Neurology, 60*(7), 940–946.

Nakagawasai, O., Yamadera, F., Iwasaki, K., Arai, H., Taniguchi, R., Tan-No, K., et al. (2004). Effect of kami-untan-to on the impairment of learning and memory induced by thiamine-deficient feeding in mice. *Neuroscience, 125*(1), 233–241.

Nalbantoglu, J., Gilfix, B. M., Bertrand, Y., et al. (1994). Predictive value of apolipoprotein E genotyping in Alzheimer's disease: Results of an autopsy series and several combined studies. *Annals of Neurology, 36,* 889–895.

National Center for Injury Prevention and Control. (1999). *Acute care, rehabilitation and disabilities.* Available at www.www.ced.gov.ncipc/dacrrdp/dacrrdp.htm

National Institute on Aging. (1998). Progress report on Alzheimer's disease (NIH Pub. No 99–3616). Washington, DC: U.S. Government Printing Office. Available at www.alzheimers.org/pr98.html

National Stroke Association. (1997). *The stroke/brain attack reporter's handbook.* Englewood, CO: Author.

Nishiyama, N., Chu, P., & Saito, H. (1996). An herbal prescription, S-113m, consisting of biota, ginseng and schizandra improves learning performance in senescence accelerated mouse. *Biological and Pharmaceutical Bulletin, 19*(3), 388–393.

Oken, B. S., Storzbach, D. M., & Kaye, J. A. (1998). The efficacy of *Ginkgo biloba* on cognitive function in Alzheimer's disease. *Archives of Neurology, 55,* 1409–1415.

Orgogozo, J. M., Dartigues, J. F., Lafont, S., et al. (1997). Wine consumption and dementia in the elderly: A prospective community study in the Bordeaux area. *Revue Neurologique (Paris), 153*(3), 185–192.

Ostuni, E., & Pietro, M. J. (2000, July 18). Paper presented at the World Alzheimer's Congress, Washington, D.C.

Ostuni, E., & Pietro, M. J. (2001, January). *Effects of healing touch on nursing home residents in later stages of Alzheimer Disease.* Paper presented at the Healing Touch International Fifth Annual Conference, Denver, Colorado.

Palmieri, G., Palmieri, R., Inzoli, M., et al. (1987). Double-blind controlled trial of phosphatidylserine in patients with senile mental deterioration. *Clin Trials Journal, 24,* 73–83

Park, C., Kim, S., Choi, W., Lee, Y., Kim, J., Kang, S., et al. (1996). Novel anticholinesterase and antiamnesic activities of dehydroevodiamine, a constituent of *Evodia rutaecarpa. Planta Medica, 62,* 405–409.

Passeri, M., Cucinotta, D., Abate, G., et al. (1993). Oral 5-methyltetrahydrofolic acid in senile organic mental disorders with depression: Results of a double-blind multi-center study. *Aging (Milano), 5*(1):63–71.

Passero, S., Rocchi, R., Vatli, G., et al. (1992). Quantitative EEG mapping, regional cerebral blood flow and neuropsychological function in Alzheimer's disease. *Dementia, 6,* 148–156.

Pek, G., Fulop, T., & Zs-Nagy, I. (1989). Gerontopsychological studies using NAI ('Nurnberger Alters-Inventar') on patients with organic psychosyndrome (DSM III, Category 1) treated with centrophenoxine in a double blind, comparative, randomized clinical trial. *Archives of Gerontology and Geriatrics, 9,* 17–30.

Pelka, R. B., & Leuchtgens, H. (1995). Pre-Alzheimer study: Action of a herbal yeast preparation (Biol-Strath) in a randomised double-blind trial. *Ars Neducu, 85.*

Pepeu, G., Pepeu, I. M., & Amaducci, L. (1996). A review of phosphatidylserine pharmacological and clinical effects: Is phosphatidylserine a drug for the ageing brain? *Pharmacology Research, 33,* 73–80.

Petersen, R., Doody, R., Kurz, A., et al. (2001). Current concepts in mild cognitive impairment. *Archives of Neurology, 58,* 1985–1992.

Petkov, V. D., Stancheva, S. L., Tocuschieva, L., et al. (1990). Changes in brain biogenic monoamines induced by the nootropic drugs adafenoxate and meclofenoxate and by citicholine (experiments on rats). *General Pharmacology, 21,* 71–75.

Pettegrew, J., Levine, J., & McClure, R. (2000). Acetyl-L-carnitine physical-chemical, metabolic and therapeutic properties: Relevance for its mode of action in Alzheimer's disease and geriatric depression. *Molecular Psychiatry, 5,* 616–632.

Pidoux, B. (1986). Effects of *Ginkgo biloba* extract on functional brain activity: An assessment of clinical and experimental studies [in French]. *Presse Médicale, 15*(31), 1588–1591.

Pomara, N., Greenberg, W., Brandord, M., & Doraiswamy, P. (2003). Therapeutic implications of HPA axis abnormalities in Alzheimer's disease: Review and update. *Psychopharmacology Bulletin, 37*(2), 120–134.

Ragneskog, H., Brane, G., Karlsson, I., & Kihlgren, M. (1996). Influence of dinner music on food intake and symptoms common in dementia. *Scandinavian Journal of Caring Sciences, 10*(1), 11–17.

Richards, M., Folstein, M., Albert, M., et al. (1993). Multicenter study of predictors of disease course in Alzheimer disease (the "predictors study"). 2: Neurological, psychiatric and demographic influences on baseline measures of disease severity. *Alzheimer Disease and Associated Disorders, 7,* 22–32.

Rizzo, A., & Wiederhold, B. (2000, November 16–20). *Applications and issues for the use of virtual reality technology for cognitive-behavioral/neuropsychological assessment and intervention.* Workshop at the annual convention of the Association for Advancement of Behavior Therapy, New Orleans.

Roberts, G. W., Gentleman, S. M., Lynch A., et al. (1994). Beta-amyloid protein deposition in the brain after severe head-injury: Implications for the pathogenesis of Alzheimer's disease. *Journal of Neurology, Neurosurgery, and Psychiatry, 57,* 419–425.

Rodriguez, G., Nobili, F., Arrigo, A., et al. (1996). Prognostic significance of quantitative electroencephalography in Alzheimer patients: Preliminary observations. *Electroencephalography and Clinical Neurophysiology, 99,* 123–128.

Rozelle, G. R., & Budzinski, T. H. (1995). Neurotherapy for stroke rehabilitation: A single case study. *Biofeedback Self-Regulation, 20*(3), 211–228.

Saratikov, A. S., & Krasnov, E. A. (1987). Clinical studies of *Rhodiola.* In A. S. Saratikov & E. A. Krasnov (Eds.), *Rhodiola rosea is a valuable medicinal plant (golden root)* (pp. 216–227). Tomsk, Russia: Tomsk State University.

Satlin, A., Volicer, L., Ross, V., Herz, L., & Campbell, S. (1992). Bright light treatment of behavioral and sleep disturbances in patients with Alzheimer's disease. *American Journal of Psychiatry, 149*(8), 1028–1032.

Sauer, J., Tabet, N., & Howard, R. (2004). Alpha lipoic acid for dementia. *Cochrane Database Systematic Reviews,* (1), CD004244.

Scherder, E. J., Bouma, A., & Steen, A. M. (1995). Effects of short-term transcutaneous electrical nerve stimulation on memory and affective behaviour in patients with probable Alzheimer's disease. *Behavioural Brain Research, 67*(2), 211–219.

Schliebs, R., Liebmann, A., Bhattacharya, S. K., et al. (1997). Systemic administration of defined extracts from *Withania somnifera* (Indian ginseng) and shilajit differentially affects cholinergic but not glutamatergic and gabaergic markers in rat brain. *Neurochemistry International, 30*(2), 181–190.

Schoenberger, N. E., Shif, S. C., Esty, M. L., Ochs, L., & Matheis, R. J. (2001). Flexyx Neurotherapy System in the treatment of traumatic brain injury: An initial evaluation. *Journal of Head Trauma Rehabilitation, 16*(3), 260–274.

Scileppi, K., Blass, J., & Baker H. (1984). Circulating vitamins in Alzheimer's dementia as compared to other dementias. *Journal of the American Geriatrics Society, 32*(10), 709–711.

Secades, J. J., & Frontera, G. (1995). CDP-choline: Pharmacological and clinical review. *Methods and Findings in Experimental and Clinical Pharmacology, 17*(Suppl. B), 1–54.

Seif-El-Nasr, M., & El-Fattah, A. A. (1995). Lipid peroxide, phospholipids, glutathione levels and superoxide dismutase activity in the rat brain after ischemia: Effect of *Ginkgo biloba* extract. *Pharmacology Research, 32,* 273–278.

Semlitsch, H. V., Anderer, P., Saletu, B., et al. (1995). Cognitive psychophysiology in nootropic drug research: Effects of *Ginkgo biloba* on event-related potentials (P300) in age-associated memory impairment. *Pharmacopsychiatry, 28*(4), 134–142.

Senf, G. (1988, November–December). Neurometric brian mapping in the diagnosis and rehabilitation of cognitive dysfunction. *Cognitive Rehabilitation,* 20–37.

Shimada, Y., Terasawa, K., Yamamoto, T., Maruyama, I., Saitoh, Y., Kanaki, E., et al. (1994). A well-controlled study of Cho-to-san and placebo in the

treatment of vascular dementia. *Journal of Traditional Medicine, 11,* 246–255.

Shumaker, S., Legault, C., Kuller, L., Rapp, S., Thal, L., Lane, D., et al., for the Women's Health Initiative Memory Study. (2004). Conjugated equine estrogens and incidence of probable dementia and mild cognitive impairment in postmenopausal women. *Journal of the American Medical Association, 291,* 2947–2958.

Singh, B., Song, H., Siao-Dong, L., Hardy, M., Gan-Zhong, L. et al. (2004). Dangshen (*Codonopsis pilosula*) and Bai Guo (*Ginkgo biloba*) enhance learning and memory [Review] *Alternative Therapies, 10*(4), 52–56.

Smith, P. F., Maclennan, K., & Darlington, C. L. (1996). The neuroprotective properties of the *Ginkgo biloba* leaf: A review of the possible relationship to platelet-activating factor (PAF). *Journal of Ethnopharmacology, 50,* 131–139.

Snow, L. A., Hovanec, L., & Brandt, J. (2004). A controlled trial of aromatherapy for agitation in nursing home patients with dementia. *Journal of Alternative and Complementary Medicine, 10*(3), 431–437.

Snyder, M., Egan, E. C., & Burns, K. R. (1995). Efficacy of hand massage in decreasing agitation behaviors associated with care activities in persons with dementia. *Geriatric Nursing, 16*(2), 60–63.

Soininen, H., Partanen, J., Laulumaa, V., et al. (1989). Longitudinal EEG spectral analysis in early stage of Alzheimer's disease. *Electroencephalography and Clinical Neurophysiology, 72,* 290–297.

Sorensen, H., & Sonne, J. (1996). A double-masked study of the effects of ginseng on cognitive function. *Current Therapeutic Research, 57*(12), 959–968.

Spasov, A. A., Wikman, G. K., Mandrikov, V.B., et al. (2000). A double-blind, placebo-controlled pilot study of the stimulating and adaptogenic effect of *Rhodiola rosea* SHR-5 extract on the fatigue of students caused by stress during an examination period with a repeated low-dose regimen. *Phytomedicine, 7,* 85–89.

Spiers, P. A., & Hochanadel, G. (1999). Citicoline for traumatic brain injury: Report of two cases, including my own. *Journal of the International Neuropsychological Society, 5,* 260–264.

Suzuki, M., Kanamori, M., Watanabe, M., et al. (2004). Behavioral and endocrinological evaluation of music therapy for elderly patients with dementia. *Nursing and Health Sciences, 6,* 11–18.

Tabet, N., Birks, J., Grimley, E., Orrel, M., & Spector, A. (2004). Vitamin E for Alzheimer's disease (Cochrane Review). In *The Cochrane Library* (Issue 2). Chichester, U.K.: John Wiley & Sons.

Tempesta, E., Troncon, R., Janiri, L., et al. (1990). Role of acetyl-L-carnitine in the treatment of cognitive deficit in chronic alcoholism. *International Journal of Clinical Pharmacology Research, 10,* 101–107.

Terasawa, K., Shimada, Y., Kita, T., Yamamoto, T., Tosa, H., Tanaka, N., et al. (1997). Choto-san in the treatment of vascular dementia: A double-blind, placebo-controlled study. *Phytomedicine, 4*(1):15–22.

Teri, L., Gibbons, L., McCurry, S., et al. (2003). Exercise plus behavioral management in patients with Alzheimer's disease. *Journal of the American Medical Association, 290,* 2015–2022.

Thal, L., Carta, A., Clarke, W., et al. (1996). A one-year multicenter placebo-controlled study of acetyl-L-carnitine in patients with Alzheimer's disease. *Neurology, 47,* 705–711.

Thal, L. J., Salmon, D. P., Lasker, B., et al. (1989). The safety and lack of efficacy of vinpocetine in Alzheimer's disease. *Journal of the American Geriatrics Society, 37,* 515–520.

Thorgrimsen, L., Spector, A., Wiles, A., & Orrell, M. (2004). Aroma therapy for dementia (Cochrane Review). In *The Cochrane Library* (Issue 2). Chichester, U.K.: John Wiley & Sons.

Thornton, K. (2000). Improvement/rehabilitation of memory functioning with neurotherapy/QEEG biofeedback. *Journal of Head Trauma Rehabilitation, 15*(6), 1285–1296.

Tully, A. M., Roche, H. M., Doyle, R., Fallon, C., Bruce, I., Lawlor, B., et al. (2003). Low serum cholesteryl ester-docosahexaenoic acid levels in Alzheimer's disease: A case-control study. *British Journal of Nutrition, 89*(4), 483–489.

Van Dongen, M., van Rossum, E., Kessels, A., et al. (2003). Ginkgo for elderly people with dementia and age-associated memory impairment: A randomized clinical trial. *Journal of Clinical Epidemiology, 56*(4), 367–376.

Van Duijn, C. M., Clayton, D. G., Chandra, V., et al. (1994). Interaction between genetic and environmental risk factors for Alzheimer's disease: A reanalysis of case-control studies. *Genetic Epidemiology, 11,* 539–551.

Van Someren, E. J., Scherder, E. J., & Swaab, D. F. (1998). Transcutaneous electrical nerve stimulation (TENS) improves circadian rhythm disturbances in Alzheimer disease. *Alzheimer Disease and Associated Disorders, 12*(2), 114–118.

Varadarajan, S., Yatin, S., Aksenova, M., & Butterfield, D. A. (2000). Alzheimer's amyloid beta-peptide-associated free radical oxidative stress and neurotoxicity [Review]. *Journal of Structural Biology, 130*(2–3), 184–208.

Villardita, C., et al. (1987). Multicentre clinical trial of brain phosphatidylserine in elderly patients with intellectual deterioration. *Clinical Trials Journal, 24,* 84–93.

Vogler, B. K., Pittler, M. H., & Ernst E. (1999). The efficacy of ginseng: A systematic review of randomised clinical trials. *European Journal of Clinical Pharmacology, 55*(8), 567–575.

Wang, K., & Hermann, C. (1999). Healing touch on agitation levels to dementia. *Healing Touch Newsletter, 9*(3), 3.

Wang, Z., Ren, Q., & Shen, Y. (1994, May). A double-blind controlled study of Huperzine A and piracetam in patients with age-associated memory impairment and Alzheimer's disease [Abstract S-181-770]. *Neuropsychopharmacology, 10*(3S, Part 1), 763S.

Wesnes, K. A., Faleni, R. A., Hefting, N. R., et al. (1997). The cognitive, subjective, and physical effects of a *Ginkgo biloba/Panax ginseng* combination in healthy volunteers with neurasthenic complaints. *Psychopharmacology Bulletin, 33*(4), 677–683.

Wesnes, K. A., Ward, T., McGinty, A., et al. (2000). The memory enhancing effects of a *Ginkgo biloba/Panax ginseng* combination in healthy middle-aged volunteers. *Psychopharmacology (Berlin), 152*(4), 353–361.

Weuve, J., Kang, J., Manson, J., Breteler, M., Ware, J., & Grodstein, F. (2004). Physical activity, including walking, and cognitive function in older women. *Journal of the American Medical Association, 292*(12), 1454–1461.

Wolf, O. T., Neumann, O., Hellhammer, D. H., et al. (1997). Effects of a two-week physiological dehydroepiandrosterone substitution on cognitive performance and well-being in healthy elderly women and men. *Journal of Clinical Endocrinology and Metabolism, 82*(7), 2363–2367.

Wolkowitz, O.M., Reus, V.I., Roberts, E., et al. (1995). Antidepressant and cognition-enhancing effects of DHEA in major depression. *Annuals of the New York Academy of Science, 774,* 337–339.

Wong, A. H., Smith, M., & Boon, H. S. (1998). Herbal remedies in psychiatric practice. *Archives of General Psychiatry, 55,* 1033–1043.

Woods, D. L., Craven, R. F., & Whitney, J. (2005). The effect of therapeutic touch on behavioral symptoms of persons with dementia. *Alternative Therapies in Health and Medicine, 11,* 66–74.

Wragg, R. E., & Jeste, D. V. (1989). Overview of depression and psychosis in Alzheimer's disease. *American Journal of Psychiatry, 146,* 577–587.

Yabe, T., Toriizuka, K., & Yamada, H. (1996). Kami-untan-to (KUT) improves cholinergic deficits in aged rats. *Phytomedicine, 2*(3), 253–258.

Yabe, T., & Yamada, H. (1996/1997). Kami-untan-to enhances choline acetyltransferase and nerve growth factor mRNA levels in brain cultured cells. *Phytomedicine, 3,* 361–367.

Yaffe, K., Sawaya, G., Lieberburg, I., & Grady, D. (1998). Estrogen therapy in postmenopausal women: Effects on cognitive function and dementia. *Journal of the American Medical Association, 279*(9), 688–695.

Zandi, P. P., Anthony, J. C., Khachaturian, A. S., et al. (2004). Reduced risk of Alzheimer disease in users of antioxidant vitamin supplements. *Archives of Neurology, 61,* 82–88.

Zandi, P., Sparks, L., Khachaturian, A., Tschanz, J., Norton, M., et al. (2005). Do statins reduce risk of incident dementia and Alzheimer disease? *Archives of General Psychiatry, 62,* 217–224.

Zhao, G. I., & Wie, Q. (1988). *A case of cerebral atrophy cured by qigong.* Paper presented at the First World Conference for Academic Exchange of Medical Qigong, Beijing, China.

Zhao, H. W., & Li, X. Y. (2002). Ginkgolide A, B, and huperzine A inhibit nitric oxide-induced neurotoxicity. *International Immunopharmacology, 2*(11), 1551–1556.

Zucker, M. (1999, May). Huperzine-A: The newest brain nutrient. *Let's Live,* 47–48.

13

Integrative Management of Substance Abuse and Dependence

This chapter reviews the evidence for nonconventional approaches used to assess alcohol or drug abuse; treat physical and psychological symptoms associated with substance abuse, intoxication, and withdrawal; and reduce relapse risk in abstinent alcoholics and addicts. The enormous cost of alcohol and drug abuse reflects an epidemic that has not been adequately addressed by available conventional treatments. The annual direct and indirect costs associated with alcohol and drug abuse in the United States alone are estimated to be in the range of $300 billion (Rice, Kelman, & Miller, 1991). In addition to the social and financial costs of alcohol and illicit substance abuse, prescription drug abuse is becoming a major public health issue in the United States and other Western countries. Abuse of benzodiazepines, barbiturates, and other prescription drugs is a matter of particular concern to psychiatrists, who frequently prescribe potentially addictive drugs when treating anxiety, psychosis, insomnia, and other mental health problems. The prolonged use of prescription benzodiazepines frequently results in dependence and withdrawal while causing significant impairments in social and occupational functioning and cross-tolerance with illicit drugs or alcohol (Golombok, Moodley, & Lader, 1988).

◆ Overview

Abuse and Dependence of Alcohol and Drugs Impact Millions of Lives

In the United States during the most recent year for which survey data are available (2004) approximately 19 million used illicit drugs. The National Household Survey on Drug Abuse (NHSDA) was conducted over a three year period starting in 1999, surveyed 200,000 Americans including 75,000 youths between age 12 and 17 (cite "Results from the 2004 National Survey on Drug Use and Health: National Findings," available online from SAMHSA (Substance Abuse and Mental Health Service Administration) under "publications."). The survey found that the prevalence of drug abuse over-all increased substantially between 1992 and 2001 due to disproportionate increase in illicit substance abuse among the youth (10.8 percent in 2001 vs 5.3 percent in 1992), and steady growth in the U.S. population. In spite of these alarming trends the current prevalence of illicit substance abuse is roughly one half of the rate in 1979—the peak year for drug abuse in the U.S. since national surveys have been conducted.

On average, approximately 7% of adults at any time fulfill criteria established by the *Diagnostic and Statistical Manual of Mental Disorders* (4th ed., *DSM-IV*) for substance abuse or dependence (Myers et al., 1984). Alcohol and nicotine are the most widely abused substances in North America and Europe because they can be readily obtained by anyone over a minimum legal age. It is estimated that approximately 10% of the U.S. population—over 30 million people—abuse alcohol, and roughly one third are alcohol dependent. Similar rates probably apply to most Western countries. As a group, adolescents are at greatest risk for alcohol abuse, whereas the elderly are at lowest risk. All ethnic groups in North America are affected by alcohol abuse and dependence, but African Americans and Asian Americans are at significantly lower risk compared with Caucasians, Hispanics, and Native Americans. According to a recent epidemiologic survey an estimated 66.8 million Americans used tobacco products on a regular basis, and over 30% of the population aged 12 and older smokes or uses other tobacco products. Cigarette smoking is the most common form of tobacco abuse followed by cigars, smokeless tobacco and pipes (2004 National Survey on Drug Use and Health, SAMSHA; available at the Web site for SAMHSA. See above.) Approximately 60 million Americans smoke cigarettes, and recent epidemiologic surveys suggest that the use of tobacco products is increasing, especially among young people Smokers are more likely to drink and use illicit drugs compared to non-smokers. According to the most recent national survey of the Substance Abuse and Mental Health Services Administration (SAMSHA), 20% of smokers use an illicit substance concurrently.

Use rates of drugs that are not legally available, including marijuana, cocaine, methamphetamine, and heroin, are difficult to estimate. However, indirect evidence suggests that marijuana (*Cannabis saativa*) continues to be a widely used recreational drug in North America. A large survey study found that the number of adolescents and adults using marijuana remained relatively unchanged between 1991 and 2001 however the prevalence of marijuana abuse and dependence increased significantly especially among young African-Americans and young Hispanic men (Compton, W., Grant, B., Colliver, J., et al., 2004). It is possible that the increased prevalence of marijuana abuse and dependence in the absence of over-all growth in use, reflects the increased potency of recently introduced strains of Cannibis sativa. It should be noted that marijuana is widely regarded as a recreational or medicinal drug in the United States, where it is regularly used by millions of individuals who do not meet *DSM-IV* criteria for either abuse or dependence. Because marijuana use is widely accepted by many segments of the population, the legal debate over its appropriate use has received considerable media attention. Highly politicized positive and negative distortions of both the putative therapeutic benefits and the potential negative health consequences of marijuana use have resulted in public confusion about use patterns that constitute abuse.

Abuse rates of methamphetamine, cocaine and heroin are difficult to estimate, but recent epidemiological survey data suggest increasing abuse of illicit narcotics especially in major metropolitan areas (Epidemiologic Trends in Drug Abuse, NIDA Advance Report, June 2005). Cocaine continues to be the most widely abused narcotic in large cities and 50% to 90% of hospital admissions for treatment of cocaine intoxication are related to crack cocaine. The number of heroin addicts in the United States has been estimated at a half million, the majority of whom live in New York City, Baltimore, Philadelphia, and other large metropolitan areas. Abuse of methamphetamine is also continuing to grow, especially in the south and southwestern U.S., and there is a trend toward increasing abuse among Hispanic populations. Marijuana continues to be the most widely abused non-prescription narcotic and hospitalizations or admissions to rehabilitation programs related to marijuana abuse exceeded those for other illicit drugs in four major U.S. metropolitan areas. In addition to abuse of illicit drugs, the abuse of and dependence on prescription sedative-hypnotics, especially benzodiazepines, has become a significant public health issue in the United States. Approximately 2% of the adult U.S. population uses benzodiazepines on a chronic basis, and an undefined percentage of users are dependent on these prescribed drugs. Individuals who abuse prescription benzodiazepines also frequently abuse alcohol or cocaine (Coach, 1990).

Biological, Psychological, and Social Theories Have Been Proposed to Explain Substance Abuse and Dependence

Many social, psychological, and biological theories have been advanced in efforts to explain alcohol and drug abuse and dependence. Drinking patterns are strongly influenced by cultural and social variables, including religious attitudes toward the use of alcohol, the cost of alcohol, and the legal drinking age (Grant, 1997). The risk of developing alcohol dependence is probably determined by multiple interacting environmental, psychological, and biological factors, family dynamics, cultural influences, and genetic predisposition. An early psychoanalytic theory viewed *alcoholism* as a maladaptive defense mechanism employed to resolve neurotic conflicts between feelings of dependence and anger (Fenichel, 1945). More recently proposed psychological models explain *substance abuse* as the use of pharmacological substances to reduce distress that cannot be effectively addressed by an individual's own psychological resources (Wieder & Kaplan, 1969). Because the magnitude of risk associated with social factors is difficult to quantify, there are still no widely accepted theories explaining the social and cultural dynamics of alcohol abuse and dependence. However, poverty, unemployment, what has been described as the "ghettoization" of American cities, and an increasing divorce rate are strong predictors of the risk of alcohol and drug abuse (Johnson & Muffler, 1997). A large cross-sectional study of 300 adoptees failed to find genetic or environmental factors that were highly predictive of the risk of developing alcohol abuse or dependence (Cutrona et al., 1994). The findings of other studies suggest that genetic factors sometimes influence the risk of developing a pattern of alcohol abuse. First-degree relatives or identical twins of alcoholics are significantly more likely to have abuse or dependence problems compared with the population at large (Merikangas & Swendsen, 1997; Prescott & Kendler, 1999). Abnormal functioning of dopamine or serotonin receptors may be related to genetically determined changes in the enzymes that break down alcohol or its metabolite, aldehyde (Health et al., 2001). A decreased genetic risk of alcohol dependence is associated with flushing when a small amount of alcohol is consumed. However, this genetic factor explains only a small percentage of the total number of individuals who account for the high prevalence rate of alcohol abuse.

Drug-seeking behavior is probably related to activity in limbic brain circuits regulated by dopamine, serotonin, γ-aminobutyric acid (GABA) and endogenous opioid peptides. Dopamine release is associated with intense feelings of reward, pleasure, and reduced stress. The so-called **reward cascade** is a complex series of neurochemical events that are believed to manifest in subjective pleasurable experiences. The cascade involves release of serotonin, enkephalin (an opiate-like neuropeptide), and inhibition of GABA, the brain's principal inhibitory neurotransmitter. It has been postulated that dysregulation of the reward cascade, possibly due to certain genetic variants, results in abnormal function of brain dopamine receptors, causing a global "hypodopaminergic" state. To "correct" this hypodopaminergic state, individuals affected by these genetic variants impulsively seek pleasure from high-risk activities, alcohol, or narcotics, and pursue reward-seeking drives, including gambling or multiple sex partners, in a compulsive manner. The hypodopaminergic hypothesis has broadened addiction medicine to include the concept of **process addictions,** which are compulsive, often self-destructive behaviors that result in feelings of pleasure or reward (Blum et al., 2000). Neurobiological models explain the subjective experience of craving in relation to rapid changes in brain levels of dopamine or endorphins resulting in intense feelings of dysphoria and subsequent drug-seeking behavior (Wise, 1988).

◆ The Integrative Assessment of Alcohol or Drug Abuse

Overview of Conventional Approaches Used to Assess Alcohol or Drug Abuse

The *DSM-IV* classifies symptoms related to the use of alcohol, nicotine, and illicit substances into four general categories of disorders: dependence, abuse, intoxication, and withdrawal.

Criteria for **dependence** include the development of tolerance with chronic use, a physiological syndrome of withdrawal when the substance is abruptly discontinued, a pattern of drug-seeking behavior, and (sometimes) compulsive use of the substance. The *DSM-IV* definition of substance dependence stipulates that an individual must experience significant distress in relationship to "a maladaptive pattern" of substance use, and that at least three of seven defined symptom patterns must be present during the same 12-month period. Depending on whether chronic abuse of the substance is associated with tolerance and withdrawal, dependence can occur with or without physiological dependence. According to the schema, polysubstance dependence occurs when an individual fulfills *DSM* criteria for dependence on three or more substances at the same time.

In contrast to dependence, **abuse** is defined with respect to the social, professional, or legal consequences of chronic use of a substance. The *DSM-IV* concept of substance abuse does not include tolerance or dependence. **Intoxication** is a characteristic physiological, psychological, or behavioral syndrome resulting from the use of a substance that is associated with maladaptive behavior, and possibly also impaired functioning that cannot be explained by a medical or psychiatric disorder. Characteristic *DSM-IV* syndromes of intoxication have been specified for alcohol, caffeine, methamphetamine, cannabis, cocaine, hallucinogens, inhalants, opioids, phencyclidine, and prescription narcotics, including sedative-hypnotic drugs.

DSM-IV criteria for **withdrawal** specify that a characteristic syndrome develops when a substance is reduced or discontinued following chronic use. Like intoxication, withdrawal is typically associated with a characteristic syndrome of physiological and psychological symptoms together with impaired social or occupational functioning. Symptoms of withdrawal cannot be sufficiently explained by an existing medical or psychiatric problem. Withdrawal syndromes are specified for alcohol, methamphetamine, cocaine, and opioids, but are not specified for cannabis, caffeine, hallucinogens, and phencyclidine. Physiological symptoms of intoxication or withdrawal can include changes in autonomic activity, including elevated heart rate, increases or decreases in blood pressure, and constriction or dilation of the pupils. Neurological symptoms of intoxication or withdrawal include loss of coordination, tremor, and possibly seizure. Erratic or violent fluctuations in mood often accompany intoxication and withdrawal. The *DSM-IV* describes several substance-induced psychiatric syndromes associated with chronic abuse, acute intoxication, or withdrawal. At the time of writing, these syndromes include delirium, dementia, amnestic disorder, psychotic disorder, mood disorder, anxiety disorder, sexual dysfunction, and sleep disorder. Even a thorough history often fails to differentiate between the psychological effects of chronic substance abuse and an independent syndrome affecting mood, cognition, anxiety, or sleep. **Craving,** the irresistible urge to use a substance, is a very subjective experience and is difficult to define in behavioral or neurobiological terms and therefore to observe or quantify in research studies. Analog scales have been developed with the goal of characterizing the relative intensity, frequency, and duration of craving (Halikas, Kuhn, Crosby, Carlson, & Crea, 1991). **Comorbidities,** or greater than chance correlations, have been found between nicotine abuse and schizophrenia, depression, and alcohol abuse (Hughes et al., 1986). For example, smoking is more common among depressed individuals, and smokers report beneficial changes in mood with smoking (Laje, et al., 2001). At least 30% of alcoholics have preexisting psychiatric disorders, and one fifth of bipolar patients abuse alcohol, especially during the manic phase of their illness (Schuckit, 1996). In the same vein, chronic marijuana users often have significant social anxiety or problems sustaining attention and report therapeutic effects of marijuana. Individuals who chronically abuse hallucinogens may appear to be schizophrenic, and in the absence of a clear history, a patient brought to a hospital emergency room because of a seizure or acute delirium may be mistakenly triaged as a case of primary seizure disorder or toxic encephalopathy if a drug screen is not performed.

Conventional Assessment Approaches of Substance Abuse, Dependence, and Intoxication Are Inherently limited

Assessment of substance abuse is complicated by the fact that individuals who abuse one substance frequently abuse others. Furthermore, substance abuse or dependence is frequently associated with psychiatric symptoms that may or may not be caused by the substance. Conventional assessment approaches for alcohol or illicit substance abuse include screening instruments and laboratory studies. All psychiatrists are taught how to use a simplified questionnaire to assess the seriousness of alcohol abuse. However, standardized questionnaires are seldom used when evaluating a patient who may be abusing an illicit substance, and an accurate assessment of an ongoing pattern of abuse or dependence relies on a thorough history and laboratory studies. A blood alcohol level (BAL) provides information about recent alcohol use and is a basis for inferring tolerance. Normal functioning at high BALs suggests a pattern of chronic abuse and high tolerance. An individual who is impaired with the same BAL has lower tolerance. Laboratory studies routinely used to assess the physiological consequences of alcohol abuse include liver enzyme studies, especially γ-glutamyltransferase (GGT), serum glutamic-oxaloacetic transaminase (SGOT), and alkaline phosphatase. Nicotine addiction can be estimated on the basis of the number of cigarettes smoked daily, the time of day when an individual first smokes, and the emergence of significant craving or withdrawal symptoms when tobacco is not available.

Assessing marijuana abuse and dependence is often problematic because many individuals are not impaired by long-term use, and the drug may be used almost daily for years, occasionally for recreational purposes, or by chronic pain patients following their physicians' instructions. The most useful gauge of marijuana abuse or dependence is the magnitude of social or occupational impairment associated with chronic use of the drug, including relationship stress and legal and financial problems. Classic symptoms of stimulant (i.e., methamphetamine and cocaine) intoxication are paranoia and agitation. A urine test is necessary to confirm stimulant abuse and rule out an acute psychotic episode or an evolving medical delirium. Hallucinogens, including lysergic acid diethylamide (LSD), psilocybin, and mescaline, produce visual or auditory hallucinations, distortions in the perception of time and space, illusions, and dissociative symptoms. Conventionally trained psychiatrists use history, a physical examination, and (sometimes) laboratory studies to differentiate hallucinogen-induced psychosis from a medical delirium or an acute psychotic episode. Laboratory assays of many hallucinogens are often impractical because they are difficult to obtain or insensitive to drug levels that may cause psychosis. LSD and other hallucinogens cause intense autonomic arousal, including elevated blood pressure and pulse. However, acutely psychotic patients frequently experience similar physiological changes. Phencyclidine hydrochloride (PCP) intoxication is characterized by nystagumus, an abnormal horizontal movement of the eyes, and, in contrast to other hallucinogens, is seldom accompanied by visual hallucinations. Acute heroin intoxication is difficult to discern. In contrast, abrupt cessation of heroin or other opiates is associated with a well-described withdrawal syndrome characterized by intense craving, heavy perspiration, generalized muscle pain, nasal discharge, insomnia, and restlessness. Heroin abuse is confirmed by a positive urine test. Depending on the level of tolerance following prolonged use of prescription benzodiazepines or barbiturates, it is often difficult to detect abuse of these drugs. Acute intoxication with prescription benzodiazepines or barbiturates is generally accompanied by confusion, lethargy, and loss of coordination. In contrast, acute withdrawal from either drug is accompanied by a characteristic syndrome including agitation, confusion, anxiety, sweating, and insomnia.

Overview of Nonconventional Approaches Used to Assess Alcohol or Drug Abuse and Dependence

At the time of writing, nonconventional approaches used to assess alcohol or drug abuse or dependence are not substantiated by strong evidence. Provisional biological assessment approaches that provide useful information for integrative treatment planning in cases of chronic alcohol abuse include serum assays of specific nutrients in addition to serum homocysteine levels. Specific abnormal auditory evoked potential (AEP) findings are associated with chronic heroin abuse, and may accurately predict future substance abuse in high-risk youth. Quantitative electroencephalography (qEEG) analysis is an emerging approach that possibly yields specific or accurate information when assessing the risk of relapsing in alcoholics and cocaine users. The vascular autonomic signal (VAS) reflex may provide clinically useful information about putative subtle energetic imbalances that can guide the practitioner in selecting the most effective conventional or nonconventional approaches for detoxification. **Table 13–1** lists provisional nonconventional approaches used to assess alcohol and substance abuse. **Table 13–2** provides an overview of approaches that possibly yield specific or accurate assessment findings.

Substantiated Approaches Used to Assess Substance Abuse or Dependence

At the time of writing, nonconventional approaches used to assess substance abuse or dependence are not strongly substantiated.

Provisional Approaches Used to Assess Substance Abuse or Dependence

Biological Assessment Approaches

◆ **Vitamin and mineral deficiencies are common in chronic alcohol abuse** Serious deficiencies of ascorbic acid, vitamin A, B vitamins, amino acids, essential fatty acids, zinc, and

Table 13–1   Assessment Approaches That Are Substantiated or That Probably Yield Specific Information about the Causes of Alcohol and Substance Abuse

	Assessment Approach	Evidence for Specific Diagnostic Information	Positive Finding Suggests Efficacy of This Treatment
Substantiated	None at time of writing		
Provisional			
Biological	Serum nutrient levels	Serum deficiencies of vitamins A and C, and many B vitamins, as well as zinc, magnesium, and essential fatty acids, are indicators of the severity of malnutrition related to alcohol abuse	Identified deficiencies should be treated with supplements. ***Note:*** Potential health benefits of supplementation are limited by continued alcohol consumption
	Serum homocysteine levels	Elevated serum homocysteine is an indicator of alcohol abuse and returns to normal soon after cessation of alcohol abuse	Folic acid, vitamin B_{12}, and SAMe may help to reduce abnormally high serum homocysteine levels
Somatic	None at time of writing		
Energy-information assessment approaches validated by Western science	AEP	Abnormal AEP findings are common in heroin addicts, and may predict increased risk of developing substance abuse problems in youth	Conventional treatments of heroin detoxification normalize AEP findings
Energy-information assessment approaches not validated by Western science	None at time of writing		

AEP, auditory event potential SAMe, S-adenosylmethionine

magnesium frequently result from malnutrition or malabsorption in chronic alcohol abuse, and potentially manifest as medical or psychiatric problems (Chapman, Prabhudesai, & Erdman, 1993; Darnton-Hill & Truswell, 1990; Merry, Abou-Saleh, & Coppen, 1982). Serum levels of folate, zinc, and magnesium are reliable clinical indicators of the severity of malnutrition, especially in patients who are actively drinking and who do not take supplements (World, Ryle, & Thomson, 1985).

◆ **Chronic alcoholics often have elevated serum homocysteine levels**   The serum homocysteine level is an indicator of available folate B_6 and B_{12}. Chronic alcohol consumption is associated with malabsorption of these essential B vitamins, interfering with the normal conversion of homocysteine to

S-adenosylmethionine (SAMe). The result is increased serum homocysteine levels and an associated increased risk of depressed mood and medical problems, including atherosclerosis and stroke (Cravo et al., 1996). The findings of two observational studies suggest that serum homocysteine levels are significantly elevated in chronic drinkers and that levels return to normal within a few weeks following cessation of alcohol use (Hultberg, Berglund, Anderson, & Frank, 1993).

Somatic Assessment Approaches

At the time of writing, there are no assessment approaches in this category.

Table 13–2   Assessment Approaches That May Yield Specific Information about the Causes of Alcohol or Drug Abuse

Category	Assessment Approach	Evidence for Specific Diagnostic Information	Comments
Biological	None at time of writing		
Somatic	None at time of writing		
Energy-information assessment approaches validated by Western science	qEEG	Abnormal qEEG findings in alcoholics and cocaine abusers may include high β (beta), increased α (alpha), and decreased θ (theta) power	qEEG brain mapping may prove useful in planning specific EEG-biofeedback protocols for relapsing alcoholics or narcotics abusers
Energy-information assessment approaches not validated by Western science	VAS reflex	Abnormal VAS reflex activity may characterize chronic alcohol or drug use	VAS analysis may provide clinically useful information for planning the most effective acupuncture and conventional detoxification protocols

EEG, electroencephalography; qEEG, quantitative electroencephalography; VAS, vascular autonomic signal

Assessment Approaches Based on Forms of Energy or Information Validated by Western Science

◆ **AEPs are markers of opiate abuse and may predict risk of developing substance abuse in youth**   P300 and P600 event-related potentials (ERPs) are electroencephalography (EEG) indicators of abnormal electrical brain activity that is commonly found in abusers of heroin and other opiates, and persists in abstinent addicts (Papageorgiou et al., 2001). Buprenorphine and other conventional pharmacological treatments used in heroin and cocaine detoxification are believed to improve cognitive functioning by reducing abnormal P300 ERPs (Kouri, Lukas, & Mendelson, 1996). The effectiveness of nonconventional detoxification treatments in normalizing P300 potentials in addicts has not yet been established. Auditory evoked potentials may predict the risk of developing substance abuse in prepubertal sons of substance-abusing fathers. In a small study ($N = 28$), boys at risk were compared with matched sons of non-substance-abusing fathers. Boys at risk for future substance abuse showed consistent changes in AEPs involving prolonged latency of alpha synchronization (Brigham, Herning, & Moss, 1995). AEP screening and referral of individuals who have abnormal AEP findings should be regarded as a proactive strategy for assessing high-risk adolescents.

Assessment Approaches Based on Forms of Energy or Information That Are Not Validated by Western Science

At the time of writing, there are no assessment approaches in this category.

Assessment Approaches in Current Use That Possibly Yield Specific Information about Causes of Alcohol or Drug Abuse

Table 13–2 outlines assessment approaches that possibly yield specific information about the causes of alcohol or drug abuse.

Biological Approaches

At the time of writing, there are no assessment approaches in this category.

Somatic Approaches

At the time of writing, there are no assessment approaches in this category.

Approaches Based on Forms of Energy or Information That Are Validated by Western Science

◆ **Abnormal qEEG findings may predict increased risk of relapsing among alcoholics or narcotics abusers**   Case reports suggest that alcoholics have abnormally high β (beta) activity (Bauer & Hesselbrock, 1993). Increased α (alpha) but decreased θ (theta) power has been reported during withdrawal in cocaine users (Alper et al., 1990). Quantitative EEG assessment of alcoholics who have difficulty remaining sober or relapsing narcotics abusers may provide useful information

for planning EEG-biofeedback or other biofeedback treatments addressing specific abnormal qEEG findings.

Assessment Approaches Based on Forms of Energy or Information That Are Not Validated by Western Science

◆ **The VAS reflex may help with treatment planning for detoxification**   Case reports suggest that the vascular autonomic signal reflex provides information that can guide the selection of conventional or nonconventional modalities most likely to be effective when managing a patient for alcohol or drug detoxification. Specific auriculotherapy protocols are believed to facilitate relaxation and attenuate the severity of withdrawal symptoms in the early stages of detoxification from alcohol, cocaine, and other substances of abuse (see section on acupuncture under Provisional Treatments). After detoxification has been completed, the VAS is sometimes used to obtain information about specific micronutrient supplements that are needed to "rebalance" the depleted energetic state of a patient. Unpublished case reports suggest that the VAS provides clinically useful information about amino acid precursors as well as specific vitamins and minerals required as cofactors for the synthesis of neurotransmitters that are depleted following chronic alcohol or drug abuse. The VAS can also provide supplemental information in addition to psychiatric history, mental status, and clinical experience regarding the sequential choice of medications (personal communication, J. Ackerman, M.D., June 2005).

◆ The Integrative Treatment of Alcohol and Drug Abuse and Dependence

Overview of Contemporary Western Treatments of Alcohol and Drug Abuse and Dependence

Conventional Western medical approaches to alcohol and drug abuse and dependence include pharmacological, psychotherapeutic, and psychosocial treatments (Finney & Moos, 2002; O'Brian & McKay, 2002). The treatment of alcohol, nicotine, and drug dependence generally involves detoxification followed by intensive group support. Abrupt discontinuation of alcohol following prolonged heavy consumption can result in a life-threatening syndrome called delirium tremens, which is typically managed on an inpatient basis. More gradual withdrawal from alcohol is safely managed on an outpatient basis using benzodiazepines, thiamine, and folate, preferably in the context of directed psychotherapy or a support group. Antianxiety agents are frequently used to manage physiological symptoms of withdrawal. Disulfiram (Antabuse) continues to be widely used to prevent alcohol relapse following abstinence, but it is probably not effective for this purpose (Hughes & Cook, 1997). Naltrexone is an opioid antagonist that is used conventionally to reduce alcohol or narcotic craving. Findings of a recent systematic review suggest that naltrexone is probably an effective short-term treatment of alcohol abuse, but further studies are needed to determine the most appropriate duration of treatment (Srisurapanont & Jarusuraisin, 2005). Acamprosate (Campral) is a recently introduced drug that promotes abstinence following alcohol withdrawal by modulating the imbalance between the glutamate and GABA neurotransmitter systems that occurs with chronic alcohol abuse. Combining acamprosate with naltrexone may be more effective in maintaining abstinence than either drug alone (Scott, Figgitt, Keam, & Waugh, 2005). Nicotine patches and nicotine gum are used to lessen withdrawal symptoms as smoking is gradually reduced. Psychosis and agitation frequently accompany acute stimulant (cocaine and methamphetamine) intoxication, and are treated with benzodiazepines or antipsychotics. Acidification of the urine is sometimes used in the emergency management of severe stimulant intoxication. Antidepressants and 12-step support groups are conventional treatments of depressed mood, fatigue, and social isolation that typically follow withdrawal from stimulants. Conventional pharmacological and psychological approaches aimed at reducing craving of alcohol, cocaine, and other drugs have a limited record of success (Crosby, Halikas, & Carlson, 1991; Powell et al., 1990). These include narcotic antagonists, dopamine antagonists, opioid-agonists or antagonists, antidepressants, and anticonvulsants, as well as a specialized kind of cognitive-behavioral therapy based on exposure and desensitization to the substance of abuse. Selective serotonin reuptake inhibitors (SSRIs) and other antidepressants are used to treat depressed mood, a common problem following prolonged alcohol abuse. Alcohol detoxification is managed symptomatically. Typical symptoms of opiate withdrawal, including irritability, nausea, aching joints, and sweating, are treated symptomatically. Opiate substitution based on daily methadone maintenance therapy is both an effective and cost-effective treatment approach for recovering heroin addicts. A newer longer acting opiate, levo-alpha-acetyl-methadol (LAAM), is used in some centers and has the advantage of twice weekly dosing. Buprenorphine, a partial opiate agonist, is coming into broader use to reduce craving and use of cocaine and heroin. Withdrawal from benzodiazepines following prolonged heavy use sometimes requires inpatient medical management to minimize the risk of seizures or potentially life-threatening cardiovascular complications. Withdrawal from benzodiazepines following more moderate or less prolonged use can be safely done on an outpatient basis by gradually tapering the daily dose, preferably in the context of regular supportive psychotherapy or a support group.

Social and existential well-being is related to improved overall mental health and is inversely correlated with the risk of developing alcohol abuse or dependence (Tsuang, Williams, Simpson, & Lyons, 2002). Individuals who belong to an organized religious group or follow a spiritual discipline are less likely to have problems with substance abuse or dependence, including alcohol, tobacco, and narcotics (Gorsuch, 1995). Low-income urban teenagers for whom religion is an important part of daily life are much less likely to abuse alcohol or drugs compared with nonreligious youth in stressful urban environments. Group and individual psychosocial treatments that incorporate spiritual themes are widely used following detoxification. The most effective psychosocial treatments include cognitive or behavioral interventions aimed at preventing relapse or developing stress management skills. Social skills training, brief motivational counseling, Alcoholics Anonymous (AA) and other 12-step programs, and community reinforcement are among the most effective psychosocial interventions. A religiously neutral framework of spiritual values is a central component of 12-step programs for abstinent alcoholics and substance abusers. An important component of conventional psychiatric training is the role of spiritually oriented 12-step support groups for encouraging abstinence, including and AA and Narcotics Anonymous. The success rate of AA has been ascribed largely to spiritual themes developed during meetings including self-acceptance, forgiveness, humility, and acknowledging a higher power (Kurtz, 1989). A special symposium of the 2004 annual meeting of the American Psychiatric Association reviewed recent studies showing the effectiveness of AA and other 12-step approaches in reducing relapse rates, the therapeutic benefits of AA for dual diagnosis patients, and the integration of AA group therapy and individual psychotherapy. In spite of the many successes of this model of recovery, AA and other 12-step groups are limited by their appeal to predominantly white single, middle-class males (Bean, 1975).

Conventional Treatment Approaches Are Limited in Effectiveness

Controlled studies and patient surveys suggest that most existing conventional pharmacological and psychosocial treatments of alcohol and drug abuse or dependence are sometimes effective in helping individuals to discontinue a substance or maintain abstinence. Conventional cognitive-behavioral therapy and psychosocial approaches to relapse prevention are not very effective (Bottlender, 2006). One year after discontinuing the use of alcohol or any substance of abuse, approximately one third of patients continue to abuse the same substance at the previous level, one third use the same or another substance but in a more controlled way, and roughly one third remain abstinent (McLellan, Metzger, Alterman, Cornish, & Urschel, 1992). Following the 1-year mark, abstinence rates continue to decline. At the time of writing, there are no effective conventional treatments of cocaine addiction, and recovering alcoholics engaged in 12-step programs continue to experience high relapse rates. Naltrexone and other opiate blockers haven proven ineffective in reducing the rate of heroin addiction (Fram, Marmo, & Holden, 1989). In the 1970s and 1980s, an eclectic therapeutic community at the Palo Alto (California) Veterans Administration Hospital achieved considerable success with heroin addicts using a combined psychoanalytic and Gestalt approach that directly addressed borderline and narcissistic personality traits that are common in this population (Zarcone, 1980). Only one third of recovering alcoholics who attend regular AA meetings remain sober for more than 1 year (Emrick, 1987). Less effective approaches include aversion therapy, confrontation, educational films, and general psychotherapy (Holder, Longabaugh, Miller, & Rubonis,, 1991). Guidelines have been developed for an optimal healing environment for the treatment of substance abuse in response to concerns about the limited effectiveness of conventional approaches (Wesa & Culliton, 2004). This concept incorporates conventional treatments in the context of a holistic environment that includes emerging nonconventional treatments and emphasizes the role of spirituality in recovery.

Overview of Nonconventional Treatments of Alcohol and Drug

Substantiated and Provisional Treatments

At the time of writing, there are no well-substantiated nonconventional biological treatments of alcohol abuse or dependence. However, there is consistent positive evidence that the application of weak electrical currents to the brain significantly reduces symptoms of alcohol and opiate withdrawal while improving associated symptoms of anxiety. Provisional research evidence suggests that reducing caffeine and refined sugar in the diet while increasing omega-3 consumption is associated with reduced relapse rates in abstinent alcoholics. Supplementation with amino acids may help to ameliorate many symptoms of alcohol abuse. There is evidence that taurine reduces alcohol withdrawal symptoms, SAMe reduces alcohol intake, and L-tryptophan reduces alcohol craving. Acetyl-L-carnitine (ALC) may improve cognitive functioning in abstinent alcoholics. Gamma-hydroxybutyric acid (GHBA) probably reduces craving in alcoholics. Certain vitamins are also probably beneficial treatments of symptoms associated with alcohol abuse. Antioxidant vitamins taken before heavy drinking may reduce the severity of hangover symptoms, and nicotinic acid may reduce the risk of developing dependence in chronic drinkers. Alcoholics who take magnesium and zinc supplements may mitigate the long-term neuropsychological consequences of chronic alcohol abuse. Provisional evidence suggests that the regular practice of relaxation techniques reduces withdrawal symptoms following discontinuation of benzodiazepines. The regular practice of yoga, meditation, or mindfulness training probably improves general functioning in alcoholics and may reduce the rate of relapse in abstinent alcoholics and addicts. EEG biofeedback using an alpha-theta training protocol probably reduces the rate of relapse in abstinent alcoholics. Some acupuncture protocols may reduce symptoms of withdrawal after chronic alcohol or cocaine abuse is discontinued.

Possibly Effective Nonconventional Treatments

Limited research findings and anecdotal reports suggest that certain herbs traditionally used in Chinese medicine and Ayurveda are beneficial treatments of symptoms of alcohol and drug abuse and dependence. Three herbs are used in Chinese medicine to reduce alcohol craving, reduce alcohol absorption through the gut, or lessen symptoms of withdrawal. Kudzu (*Radix puerariae*) is a traditionally used treatment of alcohol abuse and dependence in Chinese medicine. Animal studies suggest that the extract of this plant significantly reduces alcohol craving. Another herb used in Chinese medicine, danshen, or red sage (*Salvia miltiorrhiza*), reduces absorption of alcohol through the stomach and may reduce alcohol craving. *Aralia elata* is a component of a compound Chinese herbal formula traditionally used to prevent or lessen alcohol intoxication. Ibogaine is extracted from the root of an African shrub, and may significantly reduce alcohol consumption in rats genetically engineered to crave alcohol. *Cannibis indica* is an herbal used in Ayurvedic medicine that may provide an effective treatment for delirium tremens. Preliminary findings from animal studies suggest that a natural product called polyenyl phosphatidyl choline (PPC) reduces liver damage associated with chronic alcohol abuse. Ashwagondha, ginseng, and other natural products may reduce the severity of withdrawal from opiates, and reduce tolerance to cocaine, methamphetamine, and morphine. Valerian extract may reduce the severity of benzodiazepine withdrawal. Preliminary findings suggest that a proprietary Ayurvedic herbal formula called Mentat reduces the risk of relapse in abstinent alcoholics and may also reduce the severity of benzodiazepine withdrawal. The findings of one human trial suggest that

hyperbaric oxygenation is an effective treatment of acute opiate overdose. Virtual reality graded exposure therapy (VRGET) is emerging as a potentially effective nondrug therapy for reducing nicotine and cocaine craving. Regular exposure to dim morning light (250 lux) may reduce the risk of relapse in abstinent alcoholics. Finally, there is preliminary evidence that regular qigong practice may reduce the severity of withdrawal in heroin addicts.

Table 13–3 outlines nonconventional treatments of alcohol or drug abuse that are or may be effective.

Substantiated Treatments of Substance Abuse and Dependence

At the time of writing, nonconventional biological, somatic, mind–body, and energy treatments of alcohol and substance abuse and dependence have not been well substantiated.

Treatments Based on Forms of Energy or Information Validated by Western Science

◆ **CES and TES reduce symptoms of alcohol and opiate (but not nicotine) withdrawal**   Transcranial electrical stimulation (TES) is widely used in Germany for the management of withdrawal symptoms. Cranioelectrotherapy stimulation (CES) has been approved by the U.S. Food and Drug Administration (FDA) as a treatment of pain syndromes and anxiety. Both approaches involve the application of weak electrical current to specific points on the scalp or ears at regular intervals during acute withdrawal from opiates, alcohol, or nicotine. CES typically uses a single frequency setting, 100 Hz. In contrast, TES treatments use multiple pulse frequencies and waveforms to mitigate symptoms of detoxification depending on the particular substance of abuse and the stage of withdrawal that is being managed. The putative mechanism of action is stimulation of release of endogenous brain opioid peptides, including endorphins and enkephalins, and is probably similar to the biological mechanism underlying electroacupuncture (Auriacombe & Tignol, 1995). The discrepancy between largely positive outcomes from studies of CES or TES and frequent negative findings on electroacupuncture in detoxification may be partly attributable to the use of suboptimal current or frequency settings in electroacupuncture protocols evaluated to date. In contrast to conventional pharmacological approaches, microcurrent stimulation offers the important advantage of avoiding the use of other potentially addictive narcotics when managing symptoms of opiate withdrawal.

In a 7-year prospective study of CES in the treatment of alcohol, drug, and nicotine addiction, acute and chronic withdrawal symptoms were diminished, normal sleep patterns were restored more rapidly, and more patients remained addiction-free following regular CES treatments compared with conventional psychopharmacological management. CES-treated patients had significantly fewer anxiety symptoms and higher quality of life measures compared with patients who received conventional drug treatments (Patterson, Firth, & Gardiner, 1984). Regular CES treatments compare favorably with psychotherapy combined with relaxation training and biofeedback in reducing anxiety in patients abusing any substance (Overcash & Siebenthall, 1989). Findings of a sham-controlled study on 60 inpatient alcohol or polysubstance abusers suggest that daily 30-minute CES treatments significantly improve

Table 13–3 Nonconventional Treatments of Alcohol or Drug Abuse That Are Effective or Probably Effective

	Treatment Approach	Evidence for Modality or Integrative Approaches	Comments (Including Safety Issues or Contraindications)
Substantiated			
Biological	None at time of writing		
Somatic or mind–body	None at time of writing		
Validated energy-information approaches	CES and TES	Regular CES or TES treatments reduce symptoms of alcohol or opiate withdrawal but not nicotine withdrawal; both approaches reduce anxiety and improve cognitive functioning in alcoholics or drug addicts	CES and TES offer the important benefit of avoiding use of potentially addictive narcotics when managing withdrawal from alcohol or drugs; optimum therapeutic effects are achieved when specific treatment protocols are employed
Nonvalidated energy-information approaches	None at time of writing		
Provisional			
Biological	Dietary changes	Alcoholics who improve their diets, including reduced intake of refined sugar and caffeine and increased intake of omega-3 fatty acids and protein, probably have an increased chance for maintaining sobriety	Chronic alcohol abuse results in a general state of malnutrition and related medical and psychiatric problems
	Amino acid supplementation	Taurine may reduce alcohol withdrawal symptoms; SAMe may reduce alcohol intake; ALC may enhance cognitive performance in abstinent alcoholics; L-tryptophan may reduce alcohol craving	Alcoholics may have a general brain serotonin deficit. Supplementation with amino acids that increase brain serotonin levels may have beneficial effects
	Vitamin supplementation	Chronic alcoholics are generally deficient in B vitamins. Thiamine may reduce alcohol craving. Nicotinic acid may reduce the risk of alcohol dependence in chronic drinkers. Taking antioxidant vitamins soon before drinking may reduce the severity of hangover symptoms	*Note:* Individuals who chronically abuse alcohol should always be encouraged to find ways to reduce drinking behavior. All drinkers should be encouraged to take antioxidant vitamins
	Magnesium and zinc	Supplementation with magnesium and zinc in chronic alcoholics may improve global neuropsychological functioning and protect the brain against free radical damage	*Note:* Heavy drinkers should be encouraged to take magnesium and zinc supplements
	GHB	Frequent high doses of GHB (25 mg/kg up to 6 times daily) in chronic alcoholics may reduce craving and lessen withdrawal symptoms	*Caution:* Acute GHB overdose can result in profound mental status changes, respiratory depression, and death. A withdrawal syndrome occurs after prolonged use. Vertigo is a common transient adverse effect
Somatic and mind–body approaches	Exercise	Regular aerobic exercise or strength training in abstinent alcoholics may improve general emotional well-being	*Caution:* All patients should consult their primary care physician before starting a rigorous exercise program
	Mindfulness training, meditation, and spiritually focused support groups	Abstinent alcoholics and addicts who engage in a regular mindfulness practice or meditation probably have a reduced risk of relapse. Spiritually focused support groups probably reduce relapse risk	*Note:* Transcendental meditation may be more effective at reducing the risk of relapse than other meditation styles
Validated energy-information approaches	None at time of writing		
Nonvalidated energy-information approaches	Acupuncture and electroacupuncture	Some points and protocols are probably more effective than others in reducing withdrawal symptoms from alcohol or cocaine	*Note:* Inconsistent research findings probably reflect varying skill levels and different acupuncture protocols

ALC, acetyl-L-carnitine; CES, cranioelectrotherapy stimulation; GHB, γ-hydroxybutryic acid; SAMe, S-adenosylmethionine; TES, transcranial neuro-electric stimulation cognitive functioning and reduce measures of stress and anxiety in this population (Schmitt, Capo, & Boyd, 1986). Cocaine abusers undergoing medically supervised withdrawal in an inpatient setting reported positive changes in mood, anxiety, and cognitive functioning following 1 to 3 weeks of daily CES treatments, and these changes were superior to improvements observed in a matched control group (Smith & Tyson, 1991). Because of growing interest in this technique, a Cochrane protocol was proposed in 2004 to facilitate rigorous examination of efficacy claims of transcranial neuroelectric stimulation in the management of opiate withdrawal symptoms (Auriacombe, Pascale, & Notz, 2004).

Chronic alcoholics report improved cognitive functioning and perform better on standardized intelligence tests following 3 weeks of daily CES treatments (Smith, 1982). In a 4-week double-blind study, 20 depressed alcoholics were randomized to receive 20 CES treatments at 70 to 80 Hz, 4 to 7 mA, versus sham treatments. Patients who received CES treatments experienced significantly reduced anxiety by the end of the study. No adverse effects were reported. This finding suggests that CES might provide an effective nonpharmacological alternative treatment of anxiety in alcoholics while avoiding the risks of cross-tolerance and dependence associated with benzodiazepines (Krupitsky, Burakov, Karandashova, 1991). In contrast to documented therapeutic benefits in the management of withdrawal from alcohol or opiates, CES apparently does not facilitate smoking cessation or reduce nicotine withdrawal symptoms. A 5-day sham-controlled study randomized 51 smokers who were motivated to stop smoking to daily CES (30 μA, 2 msec, 10 Hz pulsed signal) versus sham CES (Pickworth, Fant, Butschky, Goffman, & Henningfield, 1998). At the end of the study, there were no significant differences between the CES and sham-CES groups in daily cigarettes smoked, smoking urges, or nicotine withdrawal symptoms. It is possible that a longer study using the same protocol might have yielded different results.

Treatments Based on Forms of Energy or Information Not Validated by Western Science

At the time of writing, there are no substantiated treatments in this category.

Provisional Treatments of Substance Abuse and Dependence

Biological Treatments

◆ **Dietary changes improve general physical and mental health in alcoholics and significantly reduce relapse risk** A significant percentage of chronic alcoholics are malnourished. The severity of malnutrition corresponds to the duration of malabsorption of essential nutrients through the mucosa of the stomach and small intestines, which significantly reduces blood levels of thiamine, folate, vitamin B_6, and important minerals (Gloria et al., 1997). Malnutrition contributes significantly to both the medical and psychiatric consequences of chronic alcohol abuse. Hypoglycemia, a consequence of toxic effects of alcohol on the liver, can manifest as confusion, anxiety, and impaired cognitive functioning. Refined carbohydrates should be avoided, and complex carbohydrates and quality food sources of protein should be encouraged. Coldwater fish or other sources of

omega-3 fatty acids should be encouraged. Alcoholics who improve their general nutrition probably have a better chance of maintaining sobriety compared with those who do not. Eighty-one percent of alcoholics who stayed on a caffeine-free, low-refined sugar diet high in wheat germ and fruit remained abstinent at 6 months (Guenther, 1983).

◆ **Amino acids and AA precursors help in the management of alcohol abuse, intoxication, and withdrawal** Amino acids are often deficient in alcoholics because of chronic malnutrition and malabsorption. Research studies have investigated the benefits of amino acid supplementation for management of alcohol craving, intoxication, and withdrawal. Animal studies suggest that taurine lowers the level of acetaldehyde, a toxic metabolite of alcohol that can interfere with normal mental functioning, by activating the enzyme that breaks down this molecule (Watanabe, Hobara, & Nagashima, 1985). Human trials have also yielded promising findings. In a double-blind, controlled trial, 60 patients hospitalized for acute alcohol withdrawal were randomized to receive taurine supplementation 1 g 3 times daily versus placebo for 1 week. Significantly fewer severe withdrawal symptoms, including delirium and hallucinations, were observed in the taurine group (Ikeda, 1977).

S-adenosylmethionine in the liver is depleted by chronic alcohol abuse. SAMe at 400 to 800 mg/day restores depleted liver SAMe levels and may reduce liver damage in individuals who chronically abuse alcohol (Lieber, 1997, 2000a,b). Abnormally low levels of SAMe are probably related to increased rates of depressed mood in alcoholics. SAMe may therefore be a logical choice when treating depressed mood complicated by chronic alcohol abuse (Agricola, Dalla Verde, & Urani, 1994). The antidepressant effects of SAMe supplementation may reduce alcohol intake (Cibin et al., 1988).

In a double-blind, placebo-controlled study, abstinent alcoholics treated with acetyl-L-carnitine at 2 g/day for 3 months performed better on tests of memory, reasoning, and language compared with a matched control group (Tempesta et al., 1990). Tyrosine may be a useful adjunctive treatment in cocaine abuse (Tutton & Crayton, 1993). Abnormally low serum levels of L-tryptophan are correlated with low serotonin in a subset of alcoholics who are at increased risk of developing early-onset alcoholism associated with antisocial behavior (Virkkunen & Linnoila, 1993). Animal research suggests that L-tryptophan may reduce alcohol craving in humans (Baskina & Lapin, 1982). Taking L-tryptophan before drinking may reduce the severity of cognitive impairment associated with alcohol use (Westrick, Shapiro, Nathan, & Brick, 1988). Supplementation with 5-hydroxytryptophan (5-HTP), a serotonin precursor, has demonstrated that many alcoholics have a serotonergic deficit (Lee & Meltzer, 1991).

◆ **B vitamins and antioxidant vitamins may have several beneficial effects in alcoholics, including decreased craving, increased alcohol clearance from the blood, and reduced severity of hangovers** Chronic alcoholics are typically deficient in thiamine, folate, and vitamins B_6 and B_{12} because of toxic effects of alcohol on the mucosal lining of the stomach and small intestine. The conventional treatment of Wernicke's encephalopathy, a condition of acute confusion and delirium sometimes seen in chronic heavy alcohol abuse, is parenteral thiamine followed by oral thiamine supplementation at 500 mg/day. Animal studies suggest that low serum thiamine levels are associated with increased alcohol craving (Zimatkin & Zimatkina, 1996). There is evidence that niacin in the form of nicotinamide (1.25 g) taken with a meal before drinking may protect the liver against the acute toxic effects of alcohol in individuals who have relapsed or are unable to abstain (Volpi et al., 1997). Niacin in the form of nicotinic acid may reduce the risk of developing alcohol dependence by interfering with the synthesis of a morphine-like substance that is formed when a metabolite of alcohol, acetaldehyde, condenses with dopamine (Davis & Walsh, 1970). For individuals who are unable to stop drinking, taking antioxidant vitamins close to the time of alcohol consumption may reduce or prevent hangover symptoms by neutralizing metabolites of alcohol that cause oxidative damage to the body and brain (Altura & Altura, 1999; Marotta et al., 2001). Taking vitamin C (2 g) 1 hour before alcohol consumption increases the rate at which alcohol is cleared from the blood, possibly reducing acute toxic effects on the liver (Chen, Boyce, & Hsu, 1990).

◆ **Magnesium and zinc supplementation may improve neuropsychological deficits in chronic alcoholics** Magnesium supplementation at 500 to 1500 mg/day may improve neuropsychological deficits associated with chronic alcohol abuse by improving cerebral blood flow, which is often diminished in alcoholics (Thomson, Pratt, Jeyasingham, & Shaw, 1988). Deficiencies in zinc, copper, manganese, and iron are common in alcoholics and worsen with continued heavy drinking. The diffuse nerve cell damage associated with chronic alcohol use is probably caused by low serum zinc levels, which indirectly promote increased formation of damaging free radicals (Menzano & Carlen, 1994). Supplementation with both magnesium and zinc is a reasonable maintenance treatment when there is ongoing alcohol abuse.

◆ **GHBA may reduce symptoms of alcohol craving and withdrawal** Gamma- hydroxybutryic acid is a natural constituent of the brain that serves as an important regulator of energy metabolism in the central nervous system and is especially concentrated in the hypothalamus. The chemical structure of GHBA is close to that of γ-hydroxybutryic acid, the brain's principal inhibitory neurotransmitter. A case report suggests that alcoholics who self-medicate with GHBA are able to reduce alcohol intake (Glisson & Norton, 2002). Frequent oral doses (25 mg/kg up to 6 times daily) of GHBA significantly reduce alcohol craving in chronic alcoholics (Addolorato et al., 1998; Gallimberti, Ferri, Ferrara, Fadda, & Gessa, 1992). In a 1-year open study (*N* = 35), severe alcoholics who had failed conventional treatments received GHBA (25 to 100 mg/kg/day; (Maremmani, Lamanna, & Tagliamonte, 2001). Sixty percent completed the study, and 40% were nonresponders. Eleven percent of those who completed the study achieved complete abstinence, and 14% reduced their intake of alcohol. Patients who took more frequent doses of GHBA (up to 6 times daily) were more likely to remain abstinent. The findings of this open study require confirmation by a double-blind, controlled trial. In one study newly abstinent alcoholics randomized to oral GHBA at 50 mg/kg experienced rapid improvement in withdrawal symptoms, including nausea, restlessness, tremor, anxiety, and depressed mood (Gallimberti et al., 1989). However, other controlled studies report negative or equivocal findings (Nimmerrichter, Walter, Gutierrez-Lobos, & Lesch, 2002; Zvosec & Smith, 2003). At doses recommended for the treatment of alcohol craving and withdrawal, a commonly reported adverse effect is transient vertigo. Recently

GHBA has become a popular recreational drug and dietary supplement. Acute overdose can result in altered mental status, respiratory depression, and death. Withdrawal from GHBA results in a syndrome that is similar to benzodiazepine withdrawal (Mason & Kerns, 2002).

Somatic and Mind–Body Approaches

◆ **Regular exercise improves mood and general well-being in recovering alcoholics** Alcoholics frequently experience depressed mood, which may trigger drinking. Findings of open trials suggest that regular exercise improves emotional well-being in abstinent alcoholics (Frankel & Murphy, 1974). In one study alcoholics hospitalized for medical monitoring during acute detoxification who followed a daily aerobic exercise program reported significant improvements in general emotional well-being (Palmer, Vacc, & Epstein, 1988). Abstinent alcoholics enrolled in outpatient recovery programs also report improved mood with regular strength training or aerobic exercise (Palmer, Palmer, Michiels, & Thigpen, 1995).

◆ **Mindfulness training and meditation probably reduce relapse risk** Mindfulness training and meditation are standard offerings in relapse prevention programs. The consistent practice of mindfulness or meditation probably reduces the risk of relapse (Breslin, Curtis, Zack, Martin, McMain, & Shelley, 2002). Transcendental meditation may be especially effective in reducing the rate of relapse in abstinent alcoholics (Alexander, Robinson, & Rainforth, 1994; Taub, Steiner, Weingarten, & Walton, 1994). Mindfulness training and spirituality are important parts of 12-step programs for relapse prevention in alcohol, tobacco, and narcotic abuse; however, a specific religious viewpoint is not endorsed. Substance abusers who successfully avoid relapse while participating in a 12-step program frequently experience increases in spirituality (Mathew, Georgi, Wilson, & Mathew, 1996). Twelve-step programs that emphasize a particular religious or spiritual philosophy may be more effective compared with "spiritually neutral" programs (Muffler, Langrod, & Larson, 1991). Recovering alcoholics should be encouraged to pursue a religious or spiritual practice consistent with their beliefs and to consider attending a spiritually focused support group.

Treatments Based on Forms of Energy or Information That Are Validated by Western Science

At the time of writing, there are no treatment approaches in this category.

Treatments Based on Forms of Energy or Information That Are Not Validated by Western Science

◆ **Acupuncture may be an effective treatment for managing nicotine withdrawal and cocaine craving but not alcohol withdrawal or smoking cessation** The effectiveness of acupuncture as a treatment for improving the duration of abstinence from alcohol, cocaine, and other drugs cannot be ascribed to a placebo effect (Brewington, Smith, & Lipton, 1994). Anecdotal reports and the findings of animal studies suggest that acupuncture treatments result in release of endogenous opioid peptides (Cheng, Pomeranz, & Yu, 1980; Clement-Jones, McLoughlin,

Lowry, Besser, Rees, & Wen, 1979; Ng, Douthitt, Thoa, & Albert, 1975). Human clinical trials suggest that stimulating specific acupuncture points on the ears, hands, and the back of the neck may reduce alcohol craving and decrease withdrawal symptoms in alcoholics. However, alcoholics treated with acupuncture generally continue to experience craving and relapse soon after treatment is discontinued (Konefal, Duncan, & Clemence, 1994; Richard, Montoya, Nelson, & Spence, 1995).

Research findings on acupuncture for relapse prevention in alcohol abuse are inconsistent, possibly reflecting differences in the selection of acupuncture points, treatment protocol used (i.e., conventional vs. electroacupuncture), frequency of treatments, duration of total treatment, and relative skill or specialized training of practitioners. In one sham-controlled study, alcoholics reported significant reductions in withdrawal symptoms within hours of the initial treatment and no withdrawal symptoms within 72 hours of the second acupuncture treatment (Yankovskis, Beldava, & Livina, 2000). Positve findings of two controlled trials provide evidence for correlations between specific acupuncture protocols and significantly reduced alcohol craving and reduced relapse rates in recovering alcoholics (Bullock, Culliton, & Olander, 1989; Bullock, Umen, Culliton, & Olander, 1987). However, another controlled study did not find significant differences in craving or relapse rates between an acupuncture protocol traditionally used to treat addiction, sham transdermal stimulation on random points, and a "wait-listed" group (Worner, Zeller, Schwartz, Zwas, & Lyon, 1992).

Acupuncture is widely used to facilitate smoking cessation and lessen the symptoms of nicotine withdrawal, although findings of most controlled trials on smoking have been negative or equivocal. Early open trials of acupuncture for smoking cessation yielded impressive results (Fuller, 1982). In a sham-controlled trial, 76 nicotine-dependent patients were randomized to receive an accepted protocol of electroacupuncture versus a sham procedure (White, Resch, & Ernst, 1998). There were no significant differences in withdrawal symptoms between the groups by the end of the 2-week treatment period. In view of numerous case reports of beneficial effects of acupuncture for nicotine withdrawal, the researchers commented that the optimal acupuncture technique may not have been correctly applied or repeated a sufficient number of times to yield a therapeutic effect. In a large 4-week sham-controlled study ($N = 238$), high school students who smoked were randomized to weekly auricular acupuncture treatments based on a protocol for reducing smoking versus another protocol (Kang, Shin, Kim & Youn, 2005). Only one student had stopped smoking by the end of the study, and there were no significant differences in the intensity of the desire to smoke between the two groups. However, students treated with the smoking cessation protocol had significantly reduced the daily number of cigarettes smoked. These findings are consistent with a Cochrane systematic review and meta-analysis of 22 sham-controlled studies on the efficacy of acupuncture for smoking cessation involving more than 2000 patients, which concluded that therapeutic acupuncture protocols and sham acupuncture yield equivalent outcomes. The meta-analysis included sham-controlled studies on conventional acupuncture, acupressure, electroacupuncture, and laser acupuncture (White, Rampes, & Ernst, 2004). An earlier meta-analysis also found no evidence supporting the use of acupuncture as a treatment of smoking cessation (White, Resch, & Ernst, 1999). These findings suggest the need for longer sham-controlled

studies to determine both the optimum frequency and the duration of acupuncture treatments for smoking cessation. It is of interest to contrast the inconsistent findings from electroacupuncture with consistent positive findings reported for Western-style treatments that use weak electrical current to reduce craving and mitigate withdrawal symptoms (see discussion of CES and TES above).

Controlled trials, a Cochrane systematic review, and a separate independent review suggest that both conventional acupuncture and electroacupuncture are equally ineffective in reducing symptoms of nicotine withdrawal and controlling cocaine addiction (D'Alberto, 2004;). Cocaine abusers frequently experience significant calming and reduced craving even after one or two acupuncture treatments, and this effect is reportedly sustained with repeated treatments. A large study examining three separate auricular acupuncture protocols for relapse prevention in individuals abusing cocaine and other narcotics concluded that all three protocols reduced the rate of drug use over time, suggesting that acupuncture reduces drug craving in general (Konefal, Duncan, & Clemence, 1995). An 8-week randomized, controlled study compared acupuncture with two conventional drugs and a placebo in 32 cocaine addicts on methadone maintenance therapy. Although one half of enrolled subjects dropped out, almost 90% of those who completed the study achieved abstinence by 8 weeks (Margolin, Avants, chang, & Posten, 1993). Patients who were able to achieve abstinence reported diminished craving and significantly improved mood.

Table 13–4 outlines possibly effective treatments of alcohol and drug abuse and dependence.

Biological Treatments

◆ **Some traditionally used herbs may reduce alcohol craving, lessen alcohol consumption, and reduce symptoms of withdrawal**   Several herbs are used in Chinese medicine to diminish alcohol craving, lessen alcohol absorption through the gut, or reduce symptoms of withdrawal (Colombo et al., 1998). Kudzu (*Radix puerariae*) has been used as a treatment of alcohol abuse and dependence in Chinese medicine for almost 2000 years. Animal studies suggest that kudzu extract significantly reduces alcohol craving (Keung & Vallee, 1993). The mechanism of action responsible for reduced alcohol craving is probably related to high plant concentrations of two isoflavones: daidzein and daidzin. *Salvia miltiorrhiza* is a widely used herb in Chinese medicine that may reduce absorption of alcohol through the stomach. Animal studies suggest that *S. miltiorrhiza* reduces alcohol-seeking behavior in rats genetically engineered to prefer alcohol. Blood alcohol levels were reduced by 60% in rats that had been pretreated with *S. miltiorrhiza*. *Aralia elata* is a component of a compound Chinese herbal formula traditionally used to prevent or mitigate alcohol intoxication. Animal studies suggest that *A. elata* is a potent inhibitor of alcohol absorption (Yoshikawa, Murakami, Harada, Murakami, Yamahara, & Matsuda, 1996). Ibogaine is a naturally occurring alkaloid extracted from the root of an African shrub (*Tabernanthe iboga*). Preparations of the herb have been used as a stimulant in traditional African culture for centuries. Animal studies suggest that ibogaine and its primary metabolite, noribogaine, significantly reduce alcohol consumption in rats genetically engineered to prefer alcohol. *Cannibis indica*, an important Ayurvedic medicinal

Table 13–4 Possibly Effective Treatments of Alcohol and Drug Abuse and Dependence

Category	Treatment Approach	Evidence for Claimed Treatment Effect	Comments
Biological	*Radix puerariae, Salvia miltiorrhiza, Aralia elata, Tabernanthe iboga,* and *Cannibis indica*	These traditionally used herbs may reduce alcohol craving, lessen alcohol consumption, and reduce symptoms of withdrawal	*Note:* To date there are no human clinical trials supporting the use of these herbals for the management of alcohol craving or withdrawal
	Ashwagondha, Panax ginseng, Aristeguietia discolor, and *Cervus elaphus*	Ashwagondha and other traditionally used herbs and natural products may reduce tolerance and decrease the severity of withdrawal from opiates, cocaine, and methamphetamine	*Note:* Human clinical trials do not support use of these herbals for the management of withdrawal from narcotics
	Valeriana officinalis and Mentat	Valerian extract normalizes sleep following benzodiazepine withdrawal.\n\nValerian extract and Mentat may lessen the severity of benzodiazepine withdrawal	*Note:* To date human trials on Mentat in benzodiazepine withdrawal have not been done
	Melatonin	Melatonin 2 mg in controlled release form may facilitate discontinuation of benzodiazepines following prolonged use for insomnia	*Note:* Chronic insomniacs are at significant risk for developing benzodiazepine dependence
	PPC	PPC taken before drinking may reduce liver damage by interfering with induction of liver enzymes	*Note:* Alcoholics should always be encouraged to reduce or discontinue alcohol use
	Fatty acids	Supplementation with omega-3 and omega-6 fatty acids may reduce the severity of alcohol withdrawal	*Note:* Omega-3 (but not omega-6) fatty acids are probably an effective adjunctive treatment for depressed mood and other psychiatric symptoms
	HBO	HBO treatment of opium-induced coma may reduce the severity of metabolic brain damage and lower the rate of neuropsychological deficits following recovery	*Note:* HBO may emerge as a standard treatment of opium-induced coma
Somatic and mind–body	Relaxation	Regular relaxation may reduce the severity of withdrawal symptoms following prolonged benzodiazepine use	Patients who are trying to discontinue conventional sedatives should be encouraged to use relaxation
	Yoga	Regular yoga practice may reduce stress and improve overall functioning in alcoholics and may lessen the risk of relapse in drug addicts	*Caution:* Patients should consult their primary care physician before starting a strenuous yoga routine
Energy-information approaches validated by Western science	Biofeedback	Some EMG, thermal, and EEG-biofeedback protocols may reduce alcohol relapse but not cocaine relapse	EEG biofeedback using alpha-theta training may induce a relaxed, calm state that reduces the urge to drink
	VRGET	VRGET may be an effective approach for extinguishing craving in nicotine or cocaine dependence	Preliminary findings of the first human clinical trial on nicotine craving are promising
	Dim morning light	Regular exposure to dim morning light (250 lux) may reduce the risk of relapse in abstinent alcoholics who have seasonal mood changes	*Note:* Increased abstinence may result from improved mood
Energy-information approaches not validated by Western science	Qigong	Regular qigong treatments may reduce the severity of withdrawal in heroin addicts	*Note:* Individuals interested in qigong should be encouraged to find a skilled instructor or therapist

EEG, electroencephalography; EMG, electromyography; HBO, hyperbaric oxygenation; PPC, polyenylphosphatidylcholine; VRGET, virtual reality graded exposure therapy

herb, may be an effective treatment for delirium tremens. Case reports from as early as the mid-19th century suggest that *C. indica* provides rapid relief from symptoms of delirium tremens when administered orally in sequential doses over a 24-hour period (Godfrey, 1996). The findings of an open trial suggest that Mentat, a proprietary Ayurvedic compound herbal formula, may reduce the risk of relapse in abstinent alcoholics (Trivedi, 1999).

◆ **Ashwagondha, ginseng, and other natural products may reduce the severity of withdrawal from opiates, and reduce tolerance to cocaine, methamphetamine, and morphine** Ashwagondha (*Withania somnifera*) is an important herb in traditional Ayurvedic medicine. Anecdotal reports and findings of animal studies suggest that Ashwagondha lessens the severity of withdrawal from morphine. Mice pretreated with Ashwagondha for 10 days did not develop tolerance to the analgesic effects of morphine, suggesting that Ashwagondha may have similar beneficial effects in human heroin addicts (Kulkarni & Ninan, 1997; Ramarao et al., 1995).

Ginseng (*Panax ginseng*) is widely used in both Chinese medicine and Western herbal medicine. Animal studies suggest that ginseng may reduce tolerance and dependence associated with the long-term abuse of cocaine, methamphetamine, or morphine (Huong, Matsumoto, Yamasaki, Duc, Nham, & Watanabe, 1997; Kim, Jang, & Lee, 1990; Kim, Kang, Seong, Nam, & Oh, 1995). Repeated use of cocaine or methamphetamine results in chronically depleted dopamine. The mechanism of action responsible for reduced tolerance observed with ginseng may involve inhibition of narcotic-induced depletion of dopamine in the brain (Oh, Kim, & Wagner, 1997).

Animal studies suggest that glycosides derived from *A. discolor*, a Peruvian medicinal plant, significantly reduce withdrawal symptoms in morphine-dependent individuals (Capasso, Saturnino, Simone, & Aquino, 2000). Velvet antler (*Cervus elaphus*) extract is a natural product added to many Chinese herbal formulas. Animal studies suggest that the water extract of velvet antler significantly reduces tolerance to morphine-induced analgesia (Kim, Lim, & Park, 1999). A putative mechanism of action is related to the high content of keratin, which contains large amounts of cysteine. Cysteine is known to promote synthesis of glutathione, the body's most important antioxidant.

◆ **Valerian extract and Mentat may reduce the severity of benzodiazepine withdrawal** Valerian (*Valeriana officinalis*) extract may lessen withdrawal symptoms and facilitate return to a normal sleep pattern following prolonged use of benzodiazepines. The findings of animal studies show that valerian in doses of 12 mg/kg attenuates withdrawal symptoms in diazepam-dependent rats (Andreatini & Leite, 1994). Findings of a small double-blind, placebo-controlled trial suggest that valerian extract reduces the frequency of middle awakenings in insomniacs who have discontinued benzodiazepines after several years of use (Poyares, Guilleminault, Ohayon, & Tufik, 2002). Individuals taking valerian extract reported significant improvements in the subjective quality of sleep and mildly reduced anxiety compared with the placebo group. These findings suggest that valerian extract may be an effective approach to the management of insomnia and anxiety symptoms during withdrawal from benzodiazepines. The Ayurvedic compound herbal formula Mentat has been found to reverse effects of acute benzodiazepine withdrawal in dependent mice, and may provide similar benefits in humans (Kulkarni & Sharma, 1994; Kulkarni & Verma, 1992).

◆ **Melatonin may help patients discontinue benzodiazepines following prolonged use** Melatonin may facilitate discontinuation of benzodiazepines when there is dependence following chronic use. In a 12-week single-blind, placebo-controlled study, patients receiving controlled release melatonin 2 mg/night were more likely to discontinue benzodiazepines compared with patients taking a placebo (Garfinkel, Zisapel, Wainstein, & Laudon, 1999). Patients taking melatonin reported significantly greater improvements in subjective sleep quality compared with the placebo group. Most patients who continued to take controlled-release melatonin at night remained off benzodiazepines 6 months after the end of the study. In view of these findings, patients who are attempting to taper and discontinue benzodiazepines following prolonged use for insomnia should be encouraged to take a nightly 2 mg dose of controlled release melatonin.

◆ **PPC may reduce liver damage in chronic alcohol abuse** Polyenylphosphatidylcholine is a natural product that is believed to reduce induction of P450 liver enzymes associated with alcohol intake. Animal studies suggest that PPC reduces liver damage when taken before alcohol consumption (Aleynik, Leo, Aleynik, & Lieber, 1999; Lieber, 1997). In some western European countries commercial products containing PPC are currently used before drinking to protect the liver from damage.

◆ **Supplementation with fatty acids may reduce the severity of alcohol withdrawal, and improve mood and overall cognitive performance** Chronic alcohol use causes depletion of omega-3 fatty acids and related molecules in nerve cell membranes, which, in turn, may predispose alcoholics to depressed mood and other psychiatric symptoms (Hibbeln & Salem, 1995). In a small double-blind, placebo-controlled trial supplementation with omega-6 fatty acids in the form of evening primrose oil, reduced the severity of withdrawal from alcohol, normalized liver enzymes, and significantly improved cognitive performance (Glen, MacDonell, & McKenzie, 1984).

◆ **Hyperbaric oxygenation may be an effective treatment of acute opiate overdose** Research evidence suggests that hyperbaric oxygenation (HBO) will emerge as an important future treatment of coma in cases of acute opium overdose. A large double-blind study randomized 136 patients with acute opium overdose or opium addiction to HBO (100% oxygen for 40 minutes up to 2 atmospheres) versus conventional pharmacological treatment (Epifanova, Romaseno, Koukchina, & Epifanov, 1999). At the time of treatment, all patients in acute opium overdose were in coma and had sustained hypoxic brain damage. Benefits of HBO therapy included a significant reduction in coma duration and a reduced incidence of chronic neuropsychological deficits following recovery. These findings suggest that HBO reduces the severity of metabolic brain injury following acute opium overdose.

Somatic and Mind–Body Approaches

◆ **Regular relaxation may facilitate benzodiazepine withdrawal** Practicing relaxation on a regular basis improves the quality of sleep and reduces withdrawal symptoms in patients who discontinue conventional sedative-hypnotic medications following chronic use. In one open study, 40 patients were randomized to receive relaxation training versus no training and instructed to gradually reduce their conventional sedative at bedtime (Lichstein, Peterson, Riedel, Means, Epperson, & Aguillard, 1999). All patients were able to reduce their doses of conventional drugs by 80%, and those who practiced daily relaxation reported improved quality of sleep and fewer withdrawal symptoms. I often recommend a consistent program of relaxation before sleep to patients who are motivated to discontinue use of conventional sedative-hypnotic medications. I have observed that most patients who use simple relaxation approaches, including deep breathing and guided imagery, are encouraged by improvements in anxiety and overall quality of sleep while trying to taper conventional sedative-hypnotics.

◆ **Regular yoga practice may lessen the risk of relapse in alcoholics and drug addicts**   The findings of open studies suggest that the regular practice of yoga reduces stress and improves overall functioning in alcoholics and drug addicts (Vedamurthachar, 2002). A regular yoga practice in conjunction with conventional treatments of alcohol abuse or narcotic addiction may lessen the rate of relapse and improve overall functioning (Shaffer, LaSalvia, & Stein, 1997). Many alcoholics and addicts are in poor physical condition and should be advised to consult their primary care physician before starting a routine of strenuous physical activity including yoga.

Treatments Based on Forms of Energy or Information That Are Validated by Western Science

◆ **Biofeedback training probably reduces the risk of relapse in abstinent alcoholics**   Limited research findings suggest that specific protocols in electromyography (EMG), thermal biofeedback (Sharp, Hurford, Allison, Sparks, & Cameron, 1997), and EEG-biofeedback training reduce relapse rates in abstinent alcoholics (Peniston & Kulkosky, 1989, 1990). In EEG-biofeedback training, the patient learns how to self-induce brain states corresponding to deep relaxation. Case studies suggest that EEG biofeedback using an alpha-theta brainwave protocol reduces the rate of relapse in alcoholics (Schneider et al., 1993), but not in cocaine abusers (Richard et al., 1995).

◆ **VRGET may extinguish craving in patients who are dependent on nicotine or cocaine**   The use of virtual environments to increase drug or alcohol craving is an important emerging approach in cognitive-behavioral therapy based on exposure and response prevention. After nicotine or cocaine craving is stimulated in a virtual environment, the therapist works with the patient to desensitize him or her to repeated exposure, thereby reducing craving. The goal of therapy is to use repeated VRGET sessions to extinguish nicotine (or other drug) craving in response to real-life situations that often trigger craving.

In a pilot study of VR cue reactivity (VRCR) for nicotine addiction, 13 nicotine-dependent adults who were not taking anticraving medication were enrolled in a VRCR protocol (Bordnick et al., 2004). All subjects were alternately ex-posed to VR smoking cues and VR neutral cues via the virtual reality nicotine cue reactivity assessment system (VR-NCRAS) (Bordnick & Graap, 2004). Virtual smoking cues stimulated nicotine craving, resulting in increased subjective experiences of craving compared to VR neutral cues (Bordnick et al., 2004). A second replication study with 10 nicotine dependent adults, supported the above results demonstrating increases in craving for VR nicotine cues versus VR neutral cues (Bordnick, Graap, Copp, Brooks, & Ferrer, 2005). In addition, increases in heart rate and GSR upon exposure to VR nicotine cues (Bordnick et. al., 2005) were observed. Building upon these initial studies, a randomized controlled trial using a VR skills training approach to teach coping skills and relapse prevention techniques for smoking cessation is currently in progress under the direction of Dr. Bordnick (personal communication, 5-12-06, Dr. Bordnick, University of Georgia). VR environments designed to study cue reactivity and assess alcohol or marijuana craving are being tested.

These new systems include smell, with the goal of creating VR scenarios that mimic real life situations to study drug-seeking behavior. Using this paradigm, researchers hope to achieve more ecologically valid VR cues in future cue reactivity and relapse prevention studies in order to find more effective ways to treat alcohol or drug abusers to environments that typically stimulate drug-using behavior. Most virtual environments are still under development and are not yet available for clinical use.

◆ **Exposure to dim morning light may reduce the risk of relapse in abstinent alcoholics**   Findings of a small double-blind study suggest that exposure to dim light (i.e., at 250 lux, an intensity simulating dawn) in the early morning improves depressed mood in abstinent alcoholics who also have seasonal affective disorder (Avery, Bolte, & Reis, 1998). Depressed mood is a significant risk factor in alcohol relapse. Confirmation of the mood-elevating effects of simulated dawn may result in a practical nonpharmacological approach to relapse prevention in abstinent alcoholics who experience seasonal mood changes.

Treatments Based on Forms of Energy or Information Not Validated by Western Science

◆ **Qigong practice may reduce the severity of withdrawal in heroin addicts**   Findings of sham-controlled trials suggest that external qigong treatments reduce the severity of withdrawal symptoms in heroin addicts (Li, Chen, & Mo, 2002). Animal studies suggest that external qigong applied to morphine-dependent mice lessens the behavioral symptoms of withdrawal following pharmacological blockade of morphine at the level of brain receptors (Zhixian, Chen, Wenwei, & Li, 2003). Regular qigong treatments may provide a useful adjunct to conventional pharmacological and behavioral management of detoxification and withdrawal from heroin and other opiates. The unskillful practice of qigong can potentially result in agitation or psychosis. Addicts who are interested in qigong should work with a skilled qigong instructor or medical qigong therapist.

◆ The Integrative Management Algorithm for Substance Abuse and Dependence

Figure 13–1 is the integrative management step-by-step approach to evaluation and treatment of substance abuse and dependence. Note that specific assessment and treatment approaches are representative examples of reasonable choices. Moderate symptoms often respond to exercise, dietary modification, mind–body practices, and energy-information therapies. When managing severe symptoms, emphasize biological therapies. Encourage exercise and other lifestyle changes in motivated patients. Consider conventional, nonconventional, and integrative approaches that have not been tried.

See evidence tables and text for complete reviews of evidence-based options.

Before implementing any treatment plan, always check evidence tables and Web site updates at www.thieme.com/mentalhealth for specific assessment and treatment protocols, and obtain patient informed consent.

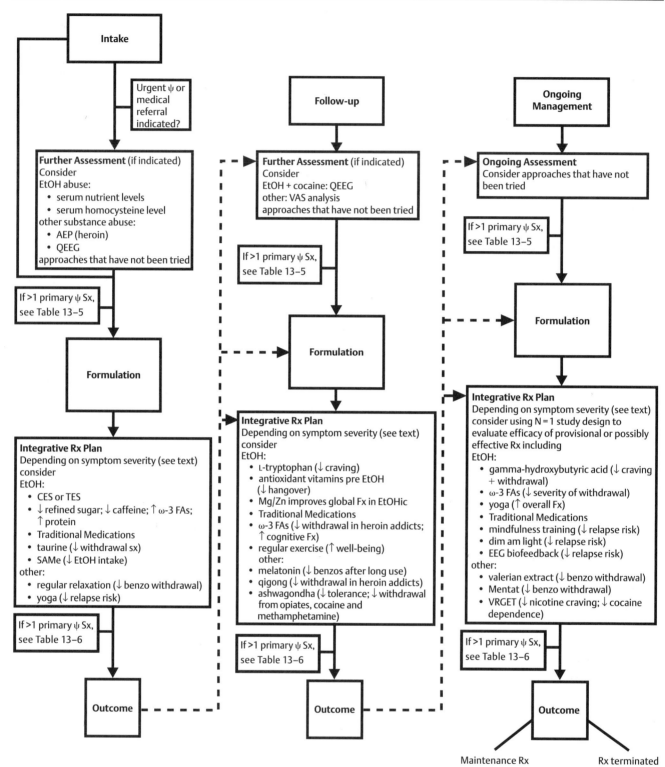

Figure 13–1 Integrative management step-by-step approach for evaluation and treatment of substance abuse and dependence. Note that specific assessment and treatment approaches are representative examples of reasonable choices. Moderate symptoms often respond to exercise, dietary modification, mind–body practices, and energy-information therapies. Fx, functioning; Rx, treatment; Sx, symptoms

◆ Integrated Approaches to Consider When Two or More Core Symptoms Are Present

Table 13–5 shows the assessment approaches to consider using when substance abuse or dependence is the focus of clinical attention and one or more other symptoms are being assessed concurrently.

Table 13–6 outlines the treatment approaches to consider using when substance abuse or dependence is the focus of clinical attention and one or more other symptoms are being treated concurrently.

Table 13–5 Assessment Approaches to Substance Abuse or Dependence When Other Symptoms Are Being Assessed Concurrently

Other Symptoms Being Assessed Concurrently	Assessment Approach	Comments
Depressed mood	Serologic studies	The magnitude of serum deficiencies of vitamins A and C, many B vitamins, zinc, magnesium, and essential fatty acids is an indicator of the severity of malnutrition related to alcohol abuse.
		Low serum folate levels predict nonresponse to conventional and nonconventional treatments of depressed mood
	qEEG brain mapping	Characteristic abnormal qEEG findings in alcoholics and cocaine abusers may include high β, increased α, and decreased θ power.
		Specific qEEG findings predict differential response rates of depressed mood to both conventional and nonconventional treatments
	Analysis of the VAS	Limited evidence suggests that abnormal VAS reflex activity characterizes chronic alcohol or drug use.
		There is also preliminary evidence that analysis of the VAS may provide useful information when evaluating depressed mood.
Mania and cyclic mood changes	Serologic studies	Low trace lithium levels (i.e., from low nutritional intake) are common in acutely manic patients.
		Limited evidence suggests that pretreatment serum GABA levels predict improved response of mania and cyclic mood changes to divalproex (Depakote) but not other mood stabilizers
	qEEG brain mapping	Limited evidence suggests that pretreatment qEEG in acutely manic or cycling patients (showing left-sided abnormalities) predicts improved response to conventional treatments
	Analysis of the VAS	Limited evidence suggests that analysis of the VAS provides useful information when evaluating energetic factors related to mania
Anxiety	Serologic studies	Deficiencies of vitamins B6, C, and E and niacin are sometimes associated with generalized anxiety.
		Limited evidence suggests that total serum cholesterol is elevated in chronically anxious patients
	qEEG brain mapping	Emerging evidence suggests that specific qEEG changes correspond to disparate anxiety syndromes
Psychosis	Serologic studies	Limited evidence suggests that abnormally low serum and RBC folate levels correlate with increased risk of schizophrenia and other psychotic syndromes.
		Limited evidence suggests that high pretreatment serum HVA levels predict improved response to lower doses of conventional antipsychotics in acutely manic patients with psychotic symptoms
	qEEG brain mapping	Limited evidence suggests that specific qEEG findings may correlate with disparate syndromes of chronic psychosis
Cognitive impairment	Serologic studies	Abnormally low levels of zinc and magnesium may correlate with the risk of developing Alzheimer's disease; however' findings are inconsistent
	qEEG brain mapping	Limited evidence suggests that qEEG brain mapping provides useful information when planning specific EEG-biofeedback protocols for relapsing alcoholics or narcotics abusers
Disturbance of sleep or wakefulness	Serologic studies	Deficiencies in vitamins C, E, B_{12}, and folic acid are correlated with increased daytime sleepiness and insomnia.
		Abnormally low serum levels of magnesium and zinc are often associated with increased daytime sleepiness
	Chinese pulse diagnosis	Limited evidence suggests that Chinese pulse diagnosis provides clinically useful information about energetic imbalances that manifest as daytime sleepiness or nighttime wakefulness

EEG, electroencephalography; GABA, γ-aminobutyric acid; HVA, homovanillic acid; qEEG, quantitative electroencephalography; RBC, red blood cell (count); VAS, vascular autonomic signal

Table 13–6 Treatment Approaches to Substance Abuse or Dependence When Other Symptoms Are Being Treated Concurrently

Other Symptoms Being Treated Concurrently	Treatment Approach	Comments
Depressed mood	Dietary changes	Alcoholics who improve their diets, including reduced intake of refined sugar and caffeine and increased intake of omega-3 fatty acids and protein, probably have an increased chance for maintaining sobriety.
		Limited evidence suggests that restricting caffeine and refined sugar and increasing consumption of fatty fish and whole foods rich in B vitamins improve depressed mood and reduce the risk of becoming depressed
	Vitamins and minerals	Limited evidence suggests that thiamine reduces alcohol craving, nicotinic acid reduces the risk of alcohol dependence in chronic drinkers, and taking antioxidant vitamins soon before drinking reduces the severity of hangover symptoms. Limited evidence suggests that supplementation of chronic alcoholics with magnesium and zinc improves global neuropsychological functioning and protects the brain against free radical damage.
		Folate 0.5 to 1 mg/day augments the effects of conventional antidepressants and SAMe
	Amino acid supplementation	Taurine may reduce alcohol withdrawal symptoms; SAMe may reduce alcohol intake; ALC may enhance cognitive performance in abstinent alcoholics; L-tryptophan may reduce alcohol craving.
		Note: Alcoholics may have a general brain serotonin deficit. Supplementation with amino acids that increase brain serotonin levels may have beneficial effects.
		5-HTP 300 mg/day is probably as effective as conventional antidepressants for moderate depressed mood.
		Note: Some cases of treatment-refractory depression improve when 5-HTP 300 to 600 mg/day is combined with carbidopa or conventional antidepressants.
		L-tryptophan 2 g augments fluoxetine 20 mg and improves sleep quality in depressed individuals.
		L-tryptophan 1 to 2 g combined with bright light therapy is more effective than either approach alone in seasonal depressed mood.
		Limited evidence suggests that L-tryptophan 1 to 2 g is equivalent to imipramine 150 mg and other conventional antidepressants
	Omega-3 fatty acids	Limited evidence suggests that supplementation with omega-3 and omega-6 fatty acids reduces the severity of alcohol withdrawal.
		Note: Omega-3 (but not omega-6) fatty acids are probably an effective adjunctive treatment for depressed mood and other psychiatric symptoms.
		Limited evidence suggests that combining omega-3 fatty acids (especially EPA) 1 to 2 g/day with conventional antidepressants improves response and may accelerate response rate.
		Limited evidence suggests that EPA alone is an effective treatment of severe depressed mood
	Somatic approaches	Limited evidence suggests that regular aerobic exercise or strength training in abstinent alcoholics improves general emotional well-being.
		Caution: All patients should consult with their primary care physician before starting a rigorous exercise program
	Mindfulness training	Abstinent alcoholics and addicts who engage in a regular mindfulness practice or meditation probably have a reduced risk of relapse.
		Spiritually focused support groups probably reduce relapse risk.
		Note: Transcendental meditation may be more effective at reducing the risk of relapse compared with other meditation styles.
		Mindfulness training is probably as effective as cognitive therapy in moderate depressed mood.
		Limited evidence suggests that regular yoga (breathing or postures) practice is as effective as conventional antidepressants in severe depressed mood.
		Combining mindfulness training or guided imagery with conventional antidepressants is more effective than conventional treatments alone
	Acupuncture	Some acupuncture points and protocols are probably more effective than others in reducing symptoms of alcohol or cocaine withdrawal.
		Limited evidence suggests that conventional acupuncture is effective against severe depressed mood.
		Limited evidence suggests that electroacupuncture alone is as effective as electroacupuncture combined with amitriptyline or other conventional antidepressants.

Table 13–6 Treatment Approaches to Substance Abuse or Dependence When Other Symptoms Are Being Treated Concurrently *(Continued)*

Other Symptoms Being Treated Concurrently	Treatment Approach	Comments
		Limited evidence suggests that computer-controlled electroacupuncture using high-frequency currents is more effective than conventional or standard electroacupuncture
	Ayurvedic herbals	Limited evidence suggests that Ashwagondha and other traditionally used herbs and natural products reduces tolerance and decrease the severity of withdrawal from opiates, cocaine, and methamphetamine.
		Note: Human clinical trials do not support use of these herbals for the management of withdrawal from narcotics.
		Several Ayurvedic herbs and compound herbal formulas are probably beneficial for depression.
		Note: Patients taking Ayurvedic herbs should be supervised by an Ayurvedic physician
	Somatic and mind–body approaches	Limited evidence suggests that regular aerobic exercise or strength training in abstinent alcoholics improves general emotional well-being.
		Regular exercise at least 30 minutes 3 times a week is probably as effective as conventional antidepressants, St. John's wort, and cognitive therapy for moderate depressed mood.
		Exercising under bright light is more effective against depression than exercise or bright light alone
	Microcurrent electrical stimulation (CES and TES)	Regular CES or TES treatments reduce symptoms of alcohol or opiate withdrawal but not nicotine withdrawal.
		Note: Both approaches reduce anxiety and improve cognitive functioning in alcoholics or drug addicts.
		Note: Optimum therapeutic effects are achieved when specific treatment protocols are employed.
		Limited evidence suggests that daily 40 minute CES treatments is beneficial in some cases of depressed mood
	Biofeedback	Limited evidence suggests that some EMG, thermal, and EEG biofeedback protocols reduces alcohol relapse but not cocaine relapse.
		Limited evidence suggests that EEG-biofeedback training using alpha-theta training induces a relaxed, calm state that reduces the urge to drink.
		Limited evidence suggests that combined EEG-HRV biofeedback (energy cardiology) training improves depressed mood
	Light exposure	Limited evidence suggests that regular exposure to dim morning light (250 lux) may reduce the risk of relapse in abstinent alcoholics with seasonal mood changes.
		Limited evidence suggests that increased abstinence results from improved mood.
		Limited evidence suggests that regular bright light exposure (10,000 lux for 30 to 40 minutes/day) improves depressed mood and has more rapid onset than conventional antidepressants.
		Limited evidence suggests that regular exposure to dim red or blue light is as effective as bright light exposure in seasonal depression.
		Limited evidence suggests that dim green light 2 hours before exposure to natural light accelerates response to conventional antidepressants
	Qigong	Limited evidence suggests that regular qigong treatments reduce the severity of withdrawal in heroin addicts.
		Regular qigong practice results in generally improved emotional well-being
Mania and cyclic mood changes	Vitamins and minerals	Limited evidence suggests that folic acid 200 μg/day augments the effects of lithium in mania and that monthly B_{12} injections reduce the risk of recurring manic episodes.
		Limited evidence suggests that magnesium supplementation 40 mEq/day is an effective treatment of rapid cycling episodes, and that potassium 20 mEq bid reduces lithium-induced tremor and improves compliance
	Omega-3 fatty acids	Limited evidence suggests that EPA 1 to 2 g/day in combination with conventional mood stabilizers reduces the severity and frequency of manic episodes.
		Note: At the time of writing, there is one case report of EPA-induced hypomania

(Continued)

Table 13–6 Treatment Approaches to Substance Abuse or Dependence When Other Symptoms Are Being Treated Concurrently (Continued)

Other Symptoms Being Treated Concurrently	Treatment Approach	Comments
	Mind–body approaches	Limited evidence suggests that certain yogic breathing practices and postures reduce the severity of mania or hypomania
	Mindfulness training	Limited evidence suggests that certain meditation practices promote calmness and are beneficial in mania or hypomania
Anxiety	Dietary modifications	Limited evidence suggests that avoiding refined sugar and caffeine and increasing protein and foods containing tryptophan reduce symptoms of generalized anxiety and panic
	Somatic approaches	Regular aerobic or strengthening exercise reduces generalized anxiety symptoms, and there is limited evidence that exercise may also reduce the frequency and severity of panic attacks
Psychosis	Dietary changes	Limited evidence suggests that chronically psychotic patients with higher intake of unsaturated fats, reduced gluten, and improved glucose regulation may experience milder symptoms
	Vitamins	Combining niacin (in the form of nicotinamide 3–8 g), folate (in the form of methylfolate 15 mg), or thiamine (500 mg tid) with conventional antipsychotics may improve outcomes.
		Note: Flushing and discomfort are associated with large doses of niacin and reportedly diminished when niacin is taken in the form of niacinamide
	Omega-3 fatty acids	Limited evidence suggests that EPA (1–4 g) alone or in combination with conventional antipsychotics (and especially clozapine) improves outcomes. Beneficial effects of omega-3 essential fatty acids may be more robust in the early-acute phase of the illness.
	Ayurvedic herbs	Limited evidence suggests that Brahmyadiyoga 8 to 12 g is as effective as conventional antipsychotics; Mentat may reduce severity of negative psychotic symptoms
	Somatic and mind–body approaches	Limited evidence suggests that a sensory stimulation technique known as the Wilbarger method improves sensory integration in schizophrenics
	Spiritually oriented group therapy and mindfulness training	Combining spiritually oriented group therapy with yogic breathing practice and conventional medications improves global functioning in stable chronically psychotic patients.
		Caution: Patients who are delusional or have other acute psychotic symptoms should be discouraged from participating in spiritual or religious practices.
		Limited evidence suggests that patients who have well-controlled psychotic symptoms benefit from social support in organized religious activity.
		Caution: Patients who are actively psychotic should be advised to avoid intense religious or spiritual activity
Cognitive impairment	Dietary changes	Moderate wine consumption, reduced saturated fats, and reduced total caloric intake are correlated with reduced risk of developing Alzheimer's disease
	Vitamins and minerals	Limited evidence suggests that diets high in fish or other sources of omega-3 fatty acids and low in omega-6 fatty acids are associated with a reduced risk of developing dementia.
		Limited evidence suggests that high niacin intake from food or supplements significantly reduces the risk of developing dementia and decreases the rate of cognitive decline in healthy elderly individuals
	Ayurvedic herbs	Limited evidence suggests that Ashwagondha 50 mg/kg improves short- and long-term memory and executive functioning in cognitively impaired individuals.
		Note: Individuals who use Ayurvedic herbs should do so only under the supervision of an Ayurvedic physician
	Somatic approaches	Limited evidence suggests that 4 to 8 weekly Snoezelen sessions reduces apathy and psychomotor agitation while enhancing language in demented individuals.
		Limited evidence suggests that regular massage therapy reduces agitated behavior in demented nursing home patients.
		Wander gardens permit demented or post-stroke patients to enjoy nature-related activities and reportedly improve baseline functioning in the early stages of dementia

Table 13–6   Treatment Approaches to Substance Abuse or Dependence When Other Symptoms Are Being Treated Concurrently *(Continued)*

Other Symptoms Being Treated Concurrently	Treatment Approach	Comments
	Microcurrent electrical stimulation	Two forms of microcurrent electrical stimulation—TENS and CES—resulted in improvements in word recall, face recognition, and motivation in demented individuals.
		Note: The beneficial effects of weak electrical stimulation are not sustained several weeks after treatment ends
	Light exposure	Limited evidence suggests that regular bright light (10,000 lux) exposure improves sleep, reduces "sundowning," reduces agitation and other inappropriate behaviors, and delays the time of peak agitation in Alzheimer's patients
	Biofeedback	EEG and HRV biofeedback training may enhance cognitive performance in healthy adults.
		EEG biofeedback may accelerate recovery following stroke or traumatic brain injury
	Qigong	Limited evidence suggests that regular qigong practice or external qigong treatments normalize EEG slowing and reverse cerebral atrophy associated with dementia.
		Note: Controlled studies of qigong in dementia have not been done, but case reports suggest dramatic beneficial effects
Disturbance of sleep or wakefulness	Dietary changes	Alcohol use at bedtime causes rebound insomnia.
		Caffeine in beverages or medications causes insomnia; caffeine withdrawal causes daytime sleepiness and fatigue.
		Limited evidence suggests that refined sugar snacks at night cause rebound hypoglycemia and disturbed sleep
	Vitamin, mineral, and amino acid supplementation	Supplementation with folate, thiamine, iron, zinc, and magnesium in deficient individuals reduces daytime sleepiness and improves nighttime sleep.
		5-HTP and L-tryptophan probably reduce symptoms of mild or situational insomnia.
		5-HTP increases sleep duration in obstructive sleep apnea and narcolepsy.
		Combining L-tryptophan 2 g with a conventional antidepressant probably enhances antidepressant response and improves sleep quality
	Ayurvedic herbs	Limited evidence suggests that Ashwagondha and an Ayurvedic compound herbal formula are effective treatments of chronic primary insomnia
	Somatic approaches	Many somatic and mind–body practices, including progressive muscle relaxation, massage, meditation, and guided imagery, are as effective as conventional sedative-hypnotics for mild to moderate insomnia.
		Regular physical exercise increases the quality and duration of sleep in the elderly.
		Limited evidence suggests that regular daily practice of Tibetan yoga improves sleep quality and reduces the need for conventional hypnotics
	Light exposure	Regular carefully timed bright light exposure resynchronizes phase-advanced or phase-delayed sleep to the patient's time zone
	Microcurrent electrical stimulation	CES is probably beneficial in some cases of chronic insomnia.
		Patients who reported improved sleep following CES treatment exhibited increased "delta sleep" that continued months after treatments ended
	Biofeedback	Some EEG-biofeedback protocols, especially SMR (alpha-theta training), are effective treatments of chronic insomnia
	Acupuncture	Some acupuncture and auriculotherapy protocols probably reduce the severity of sleep disturbances, including insomnia related to a mental or emotional problem

ALC, acetyl-L-carnitine; CES, cranioelectrotherapy stimulation; EEG, electroencephalography; EMG, electromyography; EPA, ecosapentanoic acid; 5-HTP, 5-hydroxytryptophan; HRV, heart rate variability; SAMe, S-adenosylmethionine; SMR, sensori-motor rhythm; TES, transcranial neuroelectric stimulation

Case Vignette

History and Initial Presentation

As a child, Nick had only known about what people *don't* have. He had only seen how relationships *don't* work. His mother took Nick and his two older brothers to live in the projects of Detroit soon after his father was murdered in a gang war. Alcohol was available almost from the time he could talk. Nick was barely 12 when his cousin introduced him to marijuana one bright summer morning. Two years later, he free-based for the first time in a dirty alley behind his middle school, but what worked best to "calm him down" was a fifth of rum. Nick remembers the rum giving him a warm, safe feeling when he was hungry. At age 15 he was detained overnight in juvenile hall for shoplifting. A 2-year run of petty theft charges and weekend detentions was followed by his first felony arrest at age 17. By that point, Nick had been out of school and on the street for almost a year. He was sentenced to 3 months in juvenile hall followed by 100 hours of community service, including mandatory weekly attendance at a teen Narcotics Anonymous (NA) group. He was acutely detoxed with benzodiazepines and transferred to the main detention area. After the detox ended, there were daily required groups. Nick recalls looking forward to meals, and he began to see himself in a new way through individual therapy sessions and support groups. He began to realize that anxiety had been a long-standing problem. For the first time in years he started to feel hopeful about the future after learning about opportunities to finish high school or try vocational training. In the safety of therapy sessions, he learned how to express his fears and feelings of "being this lost kid that didn't belong anywhere." After his detox, Nick continued to take lorazepam (Ativan) for 2 weeks to manage residual withdrawal symptoms. He was started on paroxetine (Paxil) for generalized anxiety. After 3 months, Nick was released to a group home for repeat juvenile offenders. He continued in weekly individual therapy sessions, and was required to attend daily NA meetings at the home. A referral to Dr. Wechsler, a community psychiatrist, was scheduled 2 weeks following his release date.

Assessment, Formulation, and Treatment Plan

Dr. Wechsler began the interview by asking Nick about the group home, his appetite, and the quality of food there. At first Nick didn't feel comfortable telling Dr. Wechsler about the cravings, but he finally disclosed that the Ativan made them less intense. Dr. Wechsler asked him about the vocational training program he had started. Nick had an aptitude for electronics and computer repair work, and he had started

a training program earlier that week. He denied anxious or depressed mood, and there were no adverse effects to Paxil. Dr. Wechsler suggested that Nick continue the Paxil for 3 months even though his anxiety had already improved significantly. She also encouraged Nick to continue paying attention to his diet and exercise, explaining that both help with depressed mood, and that a healthy diet, cutting down on fast food, refined sugar, and caffeine, probably reduces craving. Nick described his craving for cocaine as "almost too hard to hold on to," but he denied craving alcohol. Dr. Wechsler wrote a prescription for naltrexone 50 mg/day and told Nick that she would notify the residential counselor about the craving. Dr. Wechsler described the benefits of relaxation and yoga for mental health and encouraged Nick to begin a regular practice. At the end of the session, Dr. Wechsler told Nick about L-tryptophan, explaining its possible role in reducing craving. Nick agreed to call the following week with an update on his craving, and agreed to return in 1 month. When the session was over, Nick noticed that he felt reassured and relaxed.

Follow-Up

Nick reported that had gained about 4 pounds in the past month, and he was in excellent physical shape. His craving had markedly diminished with naltrexone, and there were no adverse effects. He had continued on the Paxil and tried the L-tryptophan but felt very sedated in the morning, so he had stopped taking it after only a few days. Nick had continued on a healthy diet, avoiding junk food and refined sugar, and had kept up a regular exercise program. His sleep had markedly improved, and there had been no significant anxiety symptoms. He had made progress in group therapy. Nick had joined a regular morning yoga class at the group home and was apparently enjoying it. Early morning yoga sessions included 15 minutes of meditation followed by 30 minutes of yoga postures and breathing exercises. He had experienced significantly reduced anxiety almost from the first day of yoga practice, and was now practicing yoga postures and breathing exercises twice daily. Nick had already completed three electronics projects in his vocational training program, and in the waiting room he was reading the technical manual on radio repair. Dr. Wechsler agreed that Nick was doing very well but reminded him of how far he had come in a short time, and suggested that he continue taking both the naltrexone and Paxil for at least 6 more months while remaining committed to a healthy diet, daily yoga practice, exercise, and group support meetings, and pursuing his goals in the vocational program. At the end of the session, Nick felt confident and encouraged. A routine follow-up appointment was scheduled for 2 months later.

References

Addolorato, G., Cibin, M., & Capristo, E., et al. (1998). Maintaining abstinence from alcohol with γ-hydroxybutyric acid: Research letter. *Lancet, 351*, 38.

Agricola, R., Dalla Verde, G., & Urani, R. (1994). S-adenosyl-L-methionine in the treatment of major depression complicating chronic alcoholism. *Current Therapeutic Research, 55*, 83–92.

Alexander, C. N., Robinson, P., & Rainforth, M. (1994). Treating and preventing alcohol, nicotine and drug abuse through Transcendental Meditation: A review and statistical meta-analysis. *Alcoholism Treatment Quarterly, 11* (1–2), 13–87.

Aleynik, M. K., Leo, M. A., Aleynik, S. I., & Lieber, C. S. (1999). Polyenylphosphatidylcholine opposes the increase of cytochrome P-4502E1 by ethanol and corrects its iron-induced decrease. *Alcoholism, Clinical and Experimental Research, 23*(1), 96–100.

Alper, K., Chabot, R., Kim, A., et al. (1990). Quantitative EEG correlates of crack cocaine dependence. *Psychiatry Research, 35*, 95–106.

Altura, B. M., & Altura, B. T. (1999). Association of alcohol in brain injury, headaches, and stroke with brain-tissue and serum levels of ionized magnesium: A review of recent findings and mechanisms of action. *Alcohol, 19*(2), 119–130.

Andreatini, R., & Leite. J. R. (1994). Effect of valepotriates on the behavior of rats in the elevated plus-maze during diazepam withdrawal. *European Journal of Pharmacology, 260*(2–3), 233–235.

Auriacombe, M., Pascale, F., & Notz, N. (2004). Neuroelectric stimulation for the management of opioid withdrawal (Protocol for a Cochrane Review). In *The Cochrane Library* (Issue 2). Chichester, UK: John Wiley & Sons.

Auriacombe, M., & Tignol, J. (1995). Detoxification and management of opiate dependence [in French]. *Revue du Praticien, 45*, 1383–1387.

Avery, D. H., Bolte, M. A., & Ries, R. (1998). Dawn simulation treatment of abstinent alcoholics with winter depression. *Journal of Clinical Psychiatry, 59*(1), 36–44.

Baskina, N. F., & Lapin, I. P. (1982). Changes in alcohol choice by chronically alcoholized cats as affected by tryptophan, its metabolites and preparations affecting its metabolism [in Russian]. *Farmakologiia itoksikologiia, 45*(1), 70–76.

Bauer, L., Hesselbrock, V. (1993). EEG autonomic and subjective correlates of the risk for alcoholism. *Journal of Studies on Alcohol, 54*, 577–589.

Bean, M. (1975). Alcoholics Anonymous: AA. *Psychiatric Annals, 5*(2), 3–64.

Blum, K., Braverman, E. R., Holder, J. M., Lubar, J. F., Monastra, V. J., Miller, D., et al. (2000).Reward deficiency syndrome: A biogenetic model for the diagnosis and treatment of impulsive, addictive, and compulsive behaviors. *Journal of Psychoactive Drugs, 32*(Suppl. i–iv), 1–112.

Bordnick, P. S., & Graap, K. (2004). Virtual reality nicotine cue reactivity assessment system (VR-NCRAS) (1.0) (Version 1.0) [PC]. Decatur, GA: Virtually Better, Inc.

Bordnick, P. S., Graap, K. M., Copp, H. L., Brooks, J., & Ferrer, M. (2005). Virtual reality cue reactivity assessment in cigarette smokers. *Cyberpsychology and Behavior, 8*(5), 487–492.

Bordnick, P. S., Graap, K. M., Copp, H. L., Brooks, J. S., Ferrer, M., & Logue, B. (2004). Utilizing virtual reality to standardize nicotine craving research: A pilot study. *Addictive Behaviors, 29*, 1889–1894.

Breslin, F., Curtis, Zack, Martin, McMain, & Shelley. (2002). An information-processing analysis of mindfulness: Implications for relapse prevention in the treatment of substance abuse. *Clinical Psychology: Science and Practice, 9*(3), 275–299.

Brewington, V., Smith, M., & Lipton, D. (1994). Acupuncture as a detoxification treatment: An analysis of controlled research. *Journal of Substance Abuse Treatment, 11*(4), 289–307.

Brigham, J., Herning, R. I., & Moss, H. B. (1995). Event-related potentials and alpha synchronization in preadolescent boys at risk for psychoactive substance use. *Biological Psychiatry, 37*(12), 834–846.

Bullock, M., Culliton, P., & Olander, R. (1989). Controlled trial of acupuncture for severe recidivist alcoholism. *Lancet, 1*(8652), 1435–1439.

Bullock, M., Umen, A., Culliton, P., & Olander, R. (1987). Acupuncture treatment of alcoholic recidivism: A pilot study. *Alcoholism, Clinical and Experimental Research, 11*(3), 292–295

Capasso, A., Saturnino, P., Simone, F., & Aquino, R. (2000). Flavonol glycosides from Aristeguietia discolor reduce morphine withdrawal in vitro. *Phytotherapy Research;14*(Suppl. 59), 538–540.

Bottlender, M., Kohler, J., Soyka, M. (2006). The effectiveness of psychosocial treatment approaches for alcohol dependence—a review. *Fortshcr Neurological Psychiatry, 74*(1), 19–31.

Chapman, K. M., Prabhudesai, M., & Erdman, J. W., Jr. (1993). Vitamin status of alcoholics upon admission and after two weeks of hospitalization. *Journal of the American College of Nutrition, 12*(1), 77–83.

Chen, M. F., Boyce, H. W., Jr., & Hsu, J. M. (1990). Effect of ascorbic acid on plasma alcohol clearance. *Journal of the American College of Nutrition, 9*(3), 185–189.

Cheng, R., Pomeranz, B., & Yu, G. (1980). Electroacupuncture treatment of morphine-dependent mice reduces signs of withdrawal, without showing cross-tolerance. *European Journal of Pharmacology, 68*, 477–481.

Cibin, M., Gentile, N., Ferri, M., et al. (1988). S-adenosyl-methionine (SAMe) is effective in reducing ethanol abuse in an outpatient program for alcoholics. In K. Kuriyama, A. Taka, & M. Ishii (Eds.), *Biomedical and social aspects of alcohol and alcoholism* (pp. 357–360). Amsterdam: Elsevier.

Clement-Jones, V., McLoughlin, L., Lowry, P., Besser, G., Rees, L., & Wen, H. (1979). Acupuncture in heroin addicts: Changes in met-enkephalin and B-endorphin in blood and cerebrospinal fluid. *Lancet, 2*, 380–383.

Coach, W. (1990). Benzodiazepines: An overview. In *Community epidemiology work group, epidemiologic trends in drug abuse: proceedings* (pp. 88–89). Rockville, MD: National Institute on Drug Abuse.

Colombo, G., Agabio, R., Lobina, C., Reali, R., Gessa, G., Bombardelli, E., et al. (1998). From medicinal plants promising treatments for alcoholism. *Fitoterapia, 69*(Suppl. 5), 20.

Community Epidemiology Work Group. (2005). Epidemiologic trends in drug abuse: advance report. Bethesda, Maryland: United States Department of Health and Human Services, National Institutes of Health.

Compton, W., Grant, B., Colliver, J., Glantz, M., Stinson, F. Prevalence of marijuana use disorders in the United States: 1991–1992 and 2001–2002. *JAMA,* 291, 2114–2121.

Cravo, M. L., Gloria, L. M., & Selhub, J., et al. (1996). Hyperhomocysteinemia in chronic alcoholism: Correlation with folate, vitamin B-12 and vitamin B-6 status. *American Journal of Clinical Nutrition, 63,* 220–224.

Crosby, R. D., Halikas, J.A., & Carlson, G. (1991). Pharmacotherapeutic interventions for cocaine abuse: Present practices and future directions. *Journal of Addictive Diseases, 10*(4), 13–30.

Cutrona, C. E., Cadoret, R. E., Suhr, J. A., et al. (1994). Interpersonal variables in the prediction of alcoholism among adoptees: Evidence for gene–environment interaction. *Comprehensive Psychiatry, 35,* 171–179.

D'Alberto, A. (2004). Auricular acupuncture in the treatment of cocaine/crack abuse: A review of the efficacy, the use of the National Acupuncture Detoxification Association protocol, and the selection of sham points. *Journal of Alternative and Complementary Medicine, 10*(6), 985–1000.

Darnton-Hill, I., & Truswell, A. S. (1990). Thiamin status of a sample of homeless clinic attenders in Sydney. *Medical Journal of Australia, 152*(1), 5–9.

Davis, V. E., & Walsh, M. J. (1970). Alcohol, amines, and alkaloids: A possible biochemical basis for alcohol addiction. *Science, 167,* 1005–1007.

Emrick, C. D. (1987). Alcoholics Anonymous: Affiliation processes and effectiveness as treatment. *Alcoholism, Clinical and Experimental Research, 11,* 416–423.

Epifanova, N., Romaseno, M., Koukchina, A., & Epifanov, I. (1999). Some clinico-biochemical aspects of hyperbaric oxygenation effect in the treatment of opium poisoning. *Journal of the European College of Neuropsychopharmacology, 9*(Suppl. 5), S335.

Fenichel, O. (1945). *The psychoanalytic theory of neurosis.* New York: W. W. Norton, esp. 375–386.

Finney, J., & Moos, R. (2002). Psychosocial treatments for alcohol use disorders. In P. Nathan & J. Gorman (Eds.), *A guide to treatments that work* (2nd ed., pp. 157–168). New York: Oxford University Press.

Fram, D., Marmo, J., & Holden, R. (1989). Naltrexone treatment—the problem of patient acceptance. *Journal of Substance Abuse Treatment, 6,* 119–122.

Frankel, A., & Murphy, J. (1974). Physical fitness and personality in alcoholism: Canonical analysis of measures before and after treatment. *Quarterly Journal of Studies on Alcohol, 35,* 1272–1278.

Fuller, J. (1982). Smoking withdrawal and acupuncture. *Medical Journal of Australia, 1,* 28–29.

Gallimberti, L., Canton, G., Gentile, N., et al. (1989). Gamma-hydroxybutyric acid for treatment of alcohol withdrawal syndrome. *Lancet, 2*(8666), 787–789.

Gallimberti, L., Ferri, M., Ferrara, S. D., Fadda, F., & Gessa, G. L. (1992). Gamma-hydroxybutyric acid in the treatment of alcohol dependence: A double-blind study. *Alcoholism, Clinical and Experimental Research, 16*(4), 673–676.

Garfinkel, D., Zisapel, N., Wainstein, J., & Laudon, M. (1999). Facilitation of benzodiazepine discontinuation by melatonin: A new clinical approach. *Archives of Internal Medicine, 159*(20), 2456–2460.

Glen, I., MacDonell, L., & McKenzie, J. (1984). Possible pharmacological approaches to the prevention and treatment of alcohol-related CNS impairment: Results of a double blind trial of essential fatty acids. In G. Edwards & J. Littleton (Eds.), *Pharmacological treatments for alcoholism* (pp. 331–350). London: Croom, Helm.

Glisson, J., & Norton, J. (2002). Self-medication with gamma-hydroxybutyrate to reduce alcohol intake. *Southern Medical Journal, 95*(8), 926–928.

Gloria, L., Cravo, M., Camilo, M. E., et al. (1997). Nutritional deficiencies in chronic alcoholics: Relation to dietary intake and alcohol consumption. *American Journal of Gastroenterology, 92*(3), 485–489.

Godfrey, J. (1996). Delirium tremens treated by *Cannabis indica. Eclectic Medical Journals, 2*(3), 12–13.

Golombok, S., Moodley, P., & Lader, M. (1988). Cognitive impairment in long-term benzodiazepine users. *Psychological Medicine, 18*(2), 365–374.

Gorsuch, G. (1995). Religious aspects of substance abuse and recovery. *Journal of Social Issues, 51,* 65–83.

Grant, B. F. (1997). Prevalence and correlates of alcohol use and DSM-IV alcohol dependence in the United States: Results of the National Longitudinal Alcohol Epidemiologic Survey. *Journal of Studies on Alcohol, 58,* 464–473.

Guenther, R. (1983). Role of nutritional therapy in alcoholism treatment. *International Journal of Biosocial and Medical Research, 4*(1), 5–18.

Halikas, J., Kuhn, K., Crosby, R., Carlson, G., & Crea, F. (1991). The measurement of craving in cocaine patients using the Minnesota Cocaine Craving Scale. *Comprehensive Psychiatry, 32*(1), 22–27.

Health, A. C., Whitfield, J. B., Madden, P. A., et al. (2001). Towards a molecular epidemiology of alcohol dependence: Analysing the interplay of genetic and environmental risk factors. *British Journal of Psychiatry, 178*(Suppl. 40), S33–S40

Hibbeln, J., & Salem, N. (1995). Dietary polyunsaturated fatty acids and depression: When cholesterol does not satisfy. *American Journal of Clinical Nutrition, 62,* 1–9.

Holder, H., Longabaugh, R., Miller, W., & Rubonis, A. (1991). The cost effectiveness of treatment for alcoholism: A first approximation. *Journal of Studies on Alcohol, 52,* 517–540.

Hughes, J. C., & Cook, C. C. (1997). The efficacy of disulfiram: A review of outcome studies. *Addiction, 92,* 381–395.

Hughes, J., Hatsukami, D., Mitchel, J., et al. (1986). Prevalence of smoking among psychiatric outpatients. *American Journal of Psychiatry, 143*, 993–997.

Hultberg, B., Berglund, M., Anderson, A., & Frank, A. (1993). Elevated plasma homocysteine in alcoholics. *Alcoholism, Clinical and Experimental Research, 17*(3), 687–689.

Huong, N. T., Matsumoto, K., Yamasaki, K., Duc, N. M., Nham, N. T., & Watanabe, H. (1997). Majonoside-R2, a major constituent of Vietnamese ginseng, attenuates opioid-induced antinociception. *Pharmacology, Biochemistry, and Behavior, 57*(1–2), 285–291.

Ikeda, H. (1977). Effects of taurine on alcohol withdrawal [Letter]. *Lancet, 2*, 509.

Johnson, B., & Muffler, J. (1997). Sociocultural. In J. Lowinson, P. Ruiz, R. Millman, & J. Langrod (Eds.), *Substance abuse: A comprehensive textbook* (3rd ed., pp. 107–117). Baltimore, MD: William & Wilkins.

Kandel, D., & Logan, J. (1984). Patterns of drug use from adolescence to young adulthood: 1. Period of risk for initiation, continued use and discontinuation. *American Journal of Public Health, 74*, 660–667.

Kang, H., Shin, K., Kim, K., & Youn, B. (2005). The effects of the acupuncture treatment for smoking cessation in high school student smokers. *Yonsei Medical Journal, 46*(2), 206–212.

Keung, W., & Vallee, B. (1993). Daidzein and daidzin suppress free-choice ethanol intake by Syrian golden hamsters. *Proceedings of the National Academy of Sciences of the United States of America, 90*, 10008–10012.

Kim, H., Jang, C., & Lee, M. (1990). Antinarcotic effects of the standardized ginseng extract G115 on morphine. *Planta Medica, 56*, 158–163.

Kim, H., Kang, J., Seong, Y. H., Nam, K. Y., & Oh, K. W. (1995). Blockade of ginseng total saponin of the development of cocaine induced reversed tolerance and dopamine receptor supersensitivity in mice. *Pharmacology, Biochemistry, and Behavior, 50*, 23–27.

Kim, H. S., Lim, H. K., & Park, W. K. (1999). Antinarcotic effects of the velvet antler water extract on morphine in mice. *Journal of Ethnopharmacology, 66*, 41–49.

Konefal, J., Duncan, R., & Clemence, C. (1994). The impact of an acupuncture treatment program to an existing Metro-Dade County outpatient substance abuse treatment facility. *Journal of Addictive Diseases, 13*(3), 71–99.

Konefal, J., Duncan, R., & Clemence, C. (1995). Comparison of three levels of auricular acupuncture in an outpatient substance abuse treatment program. *Alternative Medicine Journal, 2*, 5.

Kouri, E. M., Lukas, S. E., & Mendelson, J. H. (1996). P300 assessment of opiate and cocaine users: Effects of detoxification and buprenorphine treatment. *Biological Psychiatry, 40*(7), 617–628.

Krupitsky, E., Burakov, G., & Karandashova, J. (1991). The administration of transcranial electric treatment for affective disturbances therapy in alcoholic patients. *Drug and Alcohol Dependence, 27*, 1–6.

Kulkarni, S. K., & Ninan, I. (1997). Inhibition of morphine tolerance and dependence by *Withania somnifera* in mice. *Journal of Ethnopharmacology, 57*(3), 213–217.

Kulkarni, S., & Sharma, A. (1994). Reversal of diazepam withdrawal induced hyperactivity in mice by BR 16-A (Mentat), a herbal preparation. *Indian Journal of Experimental Biology, 32*(12), 886–888.

Kulkarni, S., & Verma, A. (1992). Prevention of development of tolerance and dependence to opiate in mice by BR-16A (Mentat), a herbal psychotropic preparation. *Indian Journal of Experimental Biology, 30*(10), 885–888.

Kurtz, E. (1989, June 9). *Alcoholics Anonymous and spirituality*. Workshop presented by Green Oaks Psychiatric Hospital, Dallas, TX.

Laje, R. P., Berman, J. A., & Glassman, A.H. (2001). Depression and nicotine: preclinical and clinical evidence for common mechanisms. *Current Psychiatry Report, 3*(6), 470–474.

Lee, M. A., & Meltzer, H. Y. (1991). Neuroendocrine responses to serotonergic agents in alcoholics. *Biological Psychiatry, 30*(10), 1017–1030.

Li, M., Chen, K., & Mo, Z. (2002). Detoxification with qigong therapy for heroin addicts. *Alternative Therapies in Health and Medicine, 8*, 50–59.

Lichstein, K. L., Peterson, B. A., Riedel, B. W., Means, M. K., Epperson, M. T., & Aguillard, R. N. (1999). Relaxation to assist sleep medication withdrawal. *Behavior Modification, 23*(3), 379–402.

Lieber, C. S. (1997). Role of oxidative stress and antioxidant therapy in alcoholic and nonalcoholic liver diseases. *Advances in Pharmacology, 38*, 601–628.

Lieber, C. S. (2000a). Alcohol: Its metabolism and interaction with nutrients. *Annual Review of Nutrition, 20*, 395–430.

Lieber, C. S. (2000b). Alcoholic liver disease: New insights in pathogenesis lead to new treatments. *Journal of Hepatology, 32*(1), 113–128.

Maremmani, I., Lamanna, F., & Tagliamonte, A. (2001). Long-term therapy using GHB (sodium gamma hydroxybutyrate) for treatment-resistant chronic alcoholics. *Journal of Psychoactive Drugs, 33*(2), 135–142.

Margolin, A., Avants, K., Chang, P., & Kosten, T. (1993). Acupuncture for the treatment of cocaine dependence in methadone-maintained patients. *American Journal on Addictions, 2*(3), 194–201.

Marotta, F., Safran, P., Tajiri, H., Princess, G., Anzulovic, H., Ideo, G. M., et al. (2001). Improvement of hemorrheological abnormalities in alcoholics by an oral antioxidant. *Hepatogastroenterology, 48*(38), 511–517.

Mason, P., & Kerns, W. (2002). Gamma hydroxybutyric acid (GHB) intoxication. *Academic Emergency Medicine, 9*(7), 730–739.

Mathew, R., Georgi, J., Wilson, W., & Mathew, V. (1996). A retrospective study of the concept of spirituality as understood by recovering individuals. *Journal of Substance Abuse Treatment, 13*, 67–73.

McLellan, A., Metzger, D., Alterman, A., Cornish, J., & Urschel, H. (1992). How effective is substance abuse treatment—compared to what? In C. O'Brien & J. Jaffe (Eds.), *Advances in understanding the addictive states*. New York: Raven Press.

Menzano, E., & Carlen, P. (1994). Zinc deficiency and corticosteroids in the pathogenesis of alcoholic brain dysfunction—a review. *Alcoholism, Clinical and Experimental Research, 18*(4), 895–901.

Merikangas, K. R., & Swendsen, J. D. (1997). Genetic epidemiology of psychiatric disorders. *Epidemiologic Reviews, 19*, 144–155.

Merry, J., Abou-Saleh, M., & Coppen, A. (1982). Alcoholism, depression and plasma folate [Letter]. *British Journal of Psychiatry, 141*, 103–104.

Muffler, J., Langrod, J., & Larson, D. (1991). There is a balm in Gilead: Religion and substance abuse treatment. In J. H. Lowinson, P. Ruiz, R. Milman, & J. Langrod (Eds.), *Substance abuse: A comprehensive textbook* (2nd ed., pp. 584–595). Baltimore, MD: Williams & Wilkins.

Myers, J., Weissman, M., Tischler, G., Holzer, C., Leaf, P., Orvaschel, H., et al. (1984). Six month prevalence of psychiatric disorders in three communities, 1980–1982. *Archives of General Psychiatry, 41*, 959–967.

National Narcotics Intelligence Consumers Committee. (1990). The NNICC report. *Marijuana Digest, 3*, 3.

Ng, L., Douthitt, T., Thoa, N., & Albert. C. (1975). Modification of morphine-withdrawal syndrome in rats following transauricular stimulation: An experimental paradigm for auricular acupuncture. *Biological Psychiatry, 10*, 575–580.

Nimmerrichter, A., Walter, H., Gutierrez-Lobos, K., & Lesch, O. (2002). Double-blind controlled trial of gamma-hydroxybutyrate and clomethiazole in the treatment of alcohol withdrawal. *Alcohol and Alcoholism, 37*(1), 67–73.

O'Brian, C., & McKay, J. Pharmacological treatments for substance use disorders. In P. Nathan & J. Gorman (Eds.), *A guide to treatments that work* (2nd ed., pp. 125–156). New York: Oxford University Press.

Office of Applied Studies. (1995). *Preliminary estimates from the 1994 National Household Survey on Drug Abuse*. Rockville, MD: Substance Abuse and Mental Health Services Administration.

Oh, K. W., Kim, H. S., & Wagner, G. C. (1997). Ginseng total saponin inhibits the dopaminergic depletions induced by methamphetamine [Letter] *Planta Medica, 63*, 80–81.

Overcash, S., & Siebenthall, A. (1989). The effects of cranial electrotherapy stimulation and multisensory cognitive therapy on the personality and anxiety levels of substance abuse patients. *American Journal of Electromedicine, 6*(2), 105–111.

Palmer, J., Palmer, L., Michiels, K., & Thigpen, B. (1995). Effects of type of exercise on depression in recovering substance abusers. *Perceptual and Motor Skills, 80*, 523–530.

Palmer, J., Vacc, N., & Epstein, J. (1988). Adult inpatient alcoholics: Physical exercise as a treatment intervention. *Journal of Studies on Alcohol, 49*, 418–421.

Papageorgiou, C., Liappas, I., Asvestas, P., Vasios, C., Matsopoulos, G. K., Nikolaou, C., et al. (2001). Abnormal P600 in heroin addicts with prolonged abstinence elicited during a working memory test. *Neuroreport, 12*(8), 1773–1778.

Patterson, M., Firth, J., & Gardiner, R. (1984). Treatment of drug, alcohol and nicotine addiction by neuroelectric therapy: Analysis of results over 7 years. *Journal of Bioelectricity, 3*(1–2), 193–221.

Peniston, E. G., & Kulkosky, P. J. (1989). Alpha-theta brainwave training and beta-endorphin levels in alcoholics. *Alcoholism, Clinical and Experimental Research, 13*, 271–279.

Peniston, E. G., & Kulkosky, P. J. (1990). Alcoholic personality and alpha-theta brainwave training. *Medical Psychotherapy, 3*, 37–55.

Pickworth, W. B., Fant, R. V., Butschky, M. F., Goffman, A. L., & Henningfield, J. E. (1998). Evaluation of cranial electrostimulation therapy on short-term smoking cessation [Comment]. *Biological Psychiatry, 43*(6), 468–469.

Powell, J., Gray, J., Bradley, B., et al. (1990). Effects of exposure to drug-related cues in detoxified opiate addicts: A theoretical review and some new data. *Addictive Behaviors, 15*(4), 339–354.

Poyares, D. R., Guilleminault, C., Ohayon, M. M., & Tufik, S. (2002). Can valerian improve the sleep of insomniacs after benzodiazepine withdrawal? *Progress in Neuropsychopharmacology and Biological Psychiatry, 26*(3), 539–545.

Prescott, C. A., & Kendler, K. S. (1999). Genetic and environmental contributions to alcohol abuse and dependence in a population-based sample of male twins. *American Journal of Psychiatry, 156*, 34–40.

Ramarao, P., Rao, K. T., Srivastava, R. S., et al. (1995). Effects of glycowithanolides from *Withania somnifera* on morphine-induced inhibition of intestinal motility and tolerance to analgesia in mice. *Phytotherapy Research, 9*(1), 66–68.

Rice, D. P., Kelman, S., & Miller, L. S. (1991). Estimates of economic costs of alcohol and drug abuse and mental illness, 1985 and 1988. *Public Health Reports, 106,* 280–292.

Richard, A. J., Montoya, I. D., Nelson, R., & Spence, R. T. (1995). Effectiveness of adjunct therapies in crack cocaine treatment. *Journal of Substance Abuse Treatment, 12*(6), 401–413.

Schmitt, R., Capo, T., & Boyd, E. (1986). Cranial electrotherapy stimulation as a treatment for anxiety in chemically dependent persons. *Alcoholism, Clinical and Experimental Research, 10*(2), 158–160.

Schneider, F., Elbert, T., Heimann, H., Welker, A., Stetter, F., Mattes, R., et al. (1993). Self-regulation of slow cortical potentials in psychiatric patients: Alcohol dependency. *Biofeedback and Self-Regulation, 18*(1), 23–32.

Schuckit, M. (1996). *Drug and alcohol abuse. A clinical guide to diagnosis and treatment* (4th ed.). New York: Plenum Medical Book Co.

Scott, L., Figgitt, D., Keam, S., & Waugh, J. (2005). Acamprosate: A review of its use in the maintenance of abstinence in patients with alcohol dependence. *CNS Drugs, 19*(5), 445–464.

Shaffer, H. J., LaSalvia, T. A., & Stein, J. P. (1997). Comparing Hatha yoga with dynamic group psychotherapy for enhancing methadone maintenance treatment: A randomized clinical trial. *Alternative Therapies in Health and Medicine, 3*(4), 57–66.

Sharp, C., Hurford. D. P., Allison, J., Sparks, R., & Cameron, B. P. (1997). Facilitation of internal locus of control in adolescent alcoholics through a brief biofeedback-assisted autogenic relaxation training procedure. *Journal of Substance Abuse Treatment, 14*(1), 55–60.

Smith, R. B. (1982). Confirming evidence of an effective treatment for brain dysfunction in alcoholic patients. *Journal of Nervous and Mental Disease, 170*(5), 275–278.

Smith, R., & Tyson, R. (1991). The use of transcranial electrical stimulation in the treatment of cocaine and/or polysubstance abuse.

Smoking rates climb among American teenagers. (1995, July 17). *News and Information Service,* (University of Michigan).

Srisurapanont, M., & Jarusuraisin, N. (2005). Naltrexone for the treatment of alcoholism: A meta-analysis of randomized controlled trials. *International Journal of Neuropsychopharmacology, 8*(2), 267–280.

Taub, E., Steiner, S., Weingarten, E., & Walton, K. (1994). Effectiveness of broad spectrum approaches to relapse prevention in severe alcoholism: A long-term randomized, controlled-trial of transcendental meditation, EMG biofeedback, and electronic neurotherapy. *Alcoholism Treatment Quarterly, 11,* 187–220.

Tempesta, E., Troncon, R., Janiri, L., et al. (1990). Role of acetyl-L-carnitine in the treatment of cognitive deficit in chronic alcoholism. *International Journal of Clinical Pharmacology Research, 10*(1–2), 101–107.

Thomson, A. D., Pratt, O. E., Jeyasingham, M., & Shaw, G. K. (1988). Alcohol and brain damage. *Human Toxicology, 7*(5), 455–463.

Trivedi, B. T. (1999). A clinical trial on Mentat. *Probe, 4*(38), 226.

Tsuang, M., Williams, W., Simpson, J., & Lyons, M. (2002). Pilot study of spirituality and mental health in twins. *American Journal of Psychiatry, 159*(3), 486–488.

Tutton, C. S., & Crayton, J. W. (1993). Current pharmacotherapies for cocaine abuse: A review. *Journal of Addictive Diseases, 12*(2), 109–127.

U.S. Department of Health and Human Services. (1990). *Seventh annual report to the U.S. Congress on Alcohol and Health from the Secretary of Health and Human Services.* Rockville, MD: National Institute on Alcohol Abuse and Alcoholism, 1990.

U.S. Department of Health and Human Services. (1991). *Drug abuse and drug abuse research: The third triennial report to Congress from the Secretary, Department of Health and Human Services.* Rockville, MD: U.S. Department of Health and Human Services.

Vedamurthachar, A. (2002). *Biological effects of Sudarshan Kriya on alcoholics.* Unpublished doctoral dissertation. Mangalore University, Bangalore, India, National Institute of Mental Health and Neurosciences.

Virkkunen, M., & Linnoila, M. (1993). Brain serotonin, type II alcoholism and impulsive violence. *Journal of Studies on Alcohol 11*(Suppl.), 163–169.

Volpi, E., Lucidi, P., Cruciani, G., et al. (1997). Nicotinamide counteracts alcohol-induced impairment of hepatic protein metabolism in humans. *Journal of Nutrition, 127*(2), 2199–2204.

Watanabe, A., Hobara, N., & Nagashima, H. (1985). Lowering of liver acetaldehyde but not ethanol concentrations by pretreatment with taurine in ethanol-loaded rats. *Experientia, 41*(11), 1421–1422.

Weller, R. A., & Halikas, J. A. (1980). Objective criteria for the diagnosis of marijuana abuse. *Journal of Nervous and Mental Disease, 168,* 98–103.

Wesa, K. M., & Culliton P. (2004). Recommendations and guidelines regarding the preferred research protocol for investigating the impact of an optimal healing environment on patients with substance abuse. *Journal of Alternative and Complementary Medicine, 10*(Suppl. 1), S193–S199.

Westrick, E. R., Shapiro, A. P., Nathan, P. E., & Brick, J. (1988). Dietary tryptophan reverses alcohol-induced impairment of facial recognition but not verbal recall. *Alcoholism, Clinical and Experimental Research, 12*(4), 531–533.

White, A. R., Rampes, H., & Ernst, E. (2004). Acupuncture for smoking cessation (Cochrane Review). In *The Cochrane Library* (Issue 2). Chichester, UK: John Wiley & Sons.

White, A., Resch, K., & Ernst, E. (1998). Randomized trial of acupuncture for nicotine withdrawal symptoms. *Archives of Internal Medicine, 158,* 2251–2255.

White, A. R., Resch, K. L., & Ernst, E. (1999). A meta-analysis of acupuncture techniques for smoking cessation. *Tobacco Control, 8,* 393–397.

Wieder, H., & Kaplan, E. H. (1969). Drug use in adolescents: Psychodynamic meaning and pharmacogenic effect. *Psychoanalytic Study of the Child, 24,* 399–431.

Wise, R. (1988). The neurobiology of craving: Implications for the understanding and treatment of addiction. *Journal of Abnormal Psychology, 97*(2), 118–132.

World, M. J., Ryle, P. R., & Thomson, A. D. (1985). Alcoholic malnutrition and the small intestine. *Alcohol and Alcoholism, 20*(2), 89–124.

Worner, T., Zeller, B., Schwartz, H., Zwas, F., & Lyon D. (1992). Acupuncture fails to improve treatment outcomes in alcoholics. *Drug and Alcohol Dependence, 30,* 169–173.

Yankovskis, G., Beldava, I., & Livina, B. (2000). Osteoreflectory treatment of alcohol abstinence syndrome and craving for alcohol in patients with alcoholism. *Acupuncture and Electro-Therapeutics Research, 25*(1), 9–16.

Yoshikawa, M., Murakami, T., Harada, E., Murakami, N., Yamahara, J., & Matsuda, H. (1996). Bioactive saponins and glycosides: 6. Elatosides A and B, potent inhibitors of ethanol absorption, from the bark of *Aralia elata* SEEM (Araliaceae): The structure-requirement in oleanolic acid glucuronide-saponins on the inhibitory activity. *Chemical and Pharmaceutical Bulletin (Tokyo), 44*(10), 1915–1922.

Zarcone, V. (1980). An eclectic therapeutic community for the treatment of addiction. *International Journal of the Addictions, 15*(4), 515–527.

Zhixian, M., Chen, K., Wenwei, O., & Li, M. (2003). Benefits of External Qigong Therapy on morphine-abstinent mice and rats. *Journal of Alternative and Complementary Medicine, 9*(6), 827–835.

Zimatkin, S. M., & Zimatkina, T. I. (1996). Thiamine deficiency as predisposition to, and consequence of, increased alcohol consumption. *Alcohol and Alcoholism, 31,* 421–427.

Zvosec, D., & Smith, S. (2003). Unsupported "efficacy" claims of gamma hydroxybutyrate (GHB). *Academic Emergency Medicine, 10*(1), 95–96.

14

Integrative Management of Disturbances of Sleep and Wakefulness

This chapter focuses on the integrative treatment of disturbances of sleep and wakefulness, specifically daytime sleepiness and nighttime wakefulness. Following a brief overview of the medical and psychiatric causes of disturbances of sleep and wakefulness; conventional biomedical approaches used to assess and treat these problems are described. The balance of the chapter reviews the evidence for non-conventional and integrative assessment and treatment approaches including biological, mind–body and energy-information modalities.

◆ Background

Disturbances of Sleep and Wakefulness Affect All Segments of the Population

Disturbed sleep and excessive daytime sleepiness are very frequent complaints. Approximately one third of the population is affected by disturbed sleep, including difficulty falling asleep, early awakening, and interrupted sleep, and

~5% meet the criteria for a sleep disorder established by the *Diagnostic and Statistical Manual of Mental Disorders* (4th ed., *DSM-IV*; Ford & Kamerow, 1989; Ohayon, 2002b). Many patients who report chronic insomnia also experience daytime fatigue that may impair their work performance. However, chronic fatigue is not always associated with insomnia, and it is not the focus of this discussion. Disturbed sleep is an especially important problem among the elderly and people afflicted with mental illnesses. Almost 60% of individuals who seek mental health care report chronic problems with insomnia or daytime sleepiness (Sweetwood et al., 1980). Seventy-five percent of outpatients seen at sleep clinics meet *DSM-IV* criteria for at least one psychiatric disorder (Buysse et al., 1994). Insomnia is caused by medical and psychiatric problems that directly or indirectly interfere with normal sleep. About 15% of children and 1% of the adult population report episodes of sleepwalking at some point during their lifetime. Twenty percent of children and ~10% of adults experience recurrent nightmares. In Western countries one half of all cases of insomnia are probably related to psychological factors, including anxiety, depressed mood, chronic stress, and substance abuse. Pain syndromes, sleep apnea, neurological diseases, endocrinological imbalances, and circadian rhythm problems are common physiological causes of insomnia.

Difficulties maintaining daytime wakefulness fall into two basic categories: feelings of excessive sleepiness and excessive time spent sleeping. Epidemiologic data suggest that roughly 10% of men and 20% of women experience excessive daytime sleepiness without actually falling asleep, and a significant percentage of these report impaired occupational functioning (Hara, Lopes, & Lima-Costa, 2004). These rates are probably higher among the unemployed and low-income groups. Excessive daytime sleepiness interferes with work performance and significantly increases the risk of motor vehicle accidents and workplace accidents (Lyznicki et al., 1998; Rogers, Phan, Kennaway, & Dawson, 2003). About 4% of adults complain of excessive sleep time, which is probably more common in women. At some point in their lifetimes, ~16% of adults will probably experience subjective distress because of excessive time spent sleeping and associated impairments in social or occupational functioning (Breslau et al., 1996; Ford & Kamerow, 1989).

Disturbances of Sleep and Wakefulness Are Highly Subjective, Difficult to Characterize, and Underreported

Abnormalities of sleep and wakefulness are understood in relationship to agreed-on "normal" patterns of sleep and wakefulness. A wide range of normal sleep and wakefulness experiences at different ages and in different cultures, and the vagueness of terminology used to describe subjective qualities of different states of consciousness makes it difficult to define and quantify symptoms of abnormal sleep and wakefulness. The *DSM-IV* defines five primary sleep disorders, or *dyssomnias*, as persisting disturbances in the amount, quality, or timing of sleep. *Primary hypersomnia* is described as "excessive sleepiness for at least 1 month that

cannot be accounted for by an inadequate amount of sleep." Four other *DSM-IV* primary sleep disorders are

◆ *Primary insomnia*—a pattern of difficulty initiating or maintaining sleep or nonrestorative sleep that persists for at least 1 month

◆ *Breathing-related sleep disorder*—a disruption of sleep that causes excessive daytime sleepiness or insomnia and is related to a sleep-related breathing condition

◆ *Circadian rhythm sleep disorder*—a persistent and recurrent pattern of sleep disruption leads to excessive sleepiness or insomnia due to a mismatch between the individual's sleep–wake schedule and his or her own circadian rhythm

◆ *Narcolepsy*—a pattern of irresistible sleep attacks that occur daily for at least 3 months that is accompanied by cataplexy, hallucinations, at sleep onset or waking, and sleep paralysis

Disturbances of sleep or wakefulness caused by disruptions in the body's normal circadian rhythms are commonplace in developed countries because of steadily increasing jet travel and the widespread practice of shift work. Circadian rhythm disturbances often result in clinically significant insomnia and excessive daytime sleepiness. Narcolepsy is a severe disorder of wakefulness characterized by sudden onset sleep attacks, sleep-onset hallucinations, sleep paralysis, and *cataplexy*—the sudden loss of muscle tone precipitated by intense emotions. In contrast to dyssomnias, *parasomnias* are defined in relation to abnormal events that take place during sleep, including nightmares, sleep terrors, and sleepwalking. *Rapid eye movement (REM) sleep behavior disorder* is a rare parasomnia in which nightmares during REM sleep are accompanied by purposeful movements (i.e., the normal paralysis of voluntary muscles during sleep is lost), sometimes resulting in harm to the patient or his or her partner. In addition to these two major categories of sleep disorders, the *DSM-IV* establishes criteria for insomnia or hypersomnia (i.e., excessive daytime sleepiness) related to a psychiatric disorder when a pattern of disturbed sleep or wakefulness persists for at least 1 month and can be attributed to a major psychiatric disorder. Two other *DSM-IV* sleep disorders are sleep disorder due to a general medical condition and substance-induced sleep disorder. It is important to note that other widely used classification systems employ different criteria to define abnormal patterns of sleep and wakefulness. For example, the American Academy of Sleep Medicine defines *excessive sleepiness* in very subjective terms: "a complaint of difficulty in maintaining desired wakefulness or a complaint of an excessive amount of sleep" (American Sleep Disorders Association, 1997). Defining abnormal patterns of sleep and wakefulness in different ways has practical clinical consequences because disparate diagnostic criteria lead to different clinical assessment and treatment approaches, which translate into significant differences in outcomes (De Valck & Cluydts, 2003).

Complaints of excessive daytime sleepiness and disturbed sleep are highly underreported (Ancoli-Israel & Roth, 1999). Whereas some individuals view persisting problems falling asleep or intermittent nighttime awakenings as normal, others interpret the same pattern as abnormal or impairing and seek medical attention. Subjective differences also separate individuals who experience daytime somnolence. Epidemiologic studies show that many people who cope with severe insomnia or daytime somnolence for many years often interpret these symptoms as "tiredness," and subsequently underreport them as debilitating symptoms (Dement, Hall, & Walsh, 2003). Many individuals who report disrupted sleep also report daytime somnolence or fatigue, but not all individuals who complain of chronic fatigue have problems sleeping or difficulties staying awake in the daytime. Many individuals who have difficulty falling asleep or staying asleep have a history of a medical problem, substance abuse, or a psychiatric disorder that was diagnosed after their sleep disturbance. Patients with complicated medical or psychiatric histories frequently report changing symptoms of insomnia or daytime sleepiness, and it is often impossible to establish a discrete cause of their symptoms. To add to these complications, what is considered "normal" sleep continues to change throughout the life span, and healthy elderly individuals commonly report reduced nighttime sleep, fragmented sleep, and increased daytime napping. Thus normal sleep and wakefulness among the elderly is probably quite different than normal sleep in young or middle-aged people.

◆ The Integrative Assessment of Daytime Sleepiness and Nighttime Wakefulness

Disturbances in Sleep or Wakefulness Are Often Associated with Medical and Psychiatric Problems

Many neurotransmitters contribute to normal sleep and wakefulness. Gamma-aminobutyric acid (GABA) inhibits release of serotonin, norepinephrine, and other neurotransmitters that maintain wakefulness and is considered the most important regulator of sleep. Brain levels of norepinephrine increase with normal aging, possibly explaining the observed increased incidence of sleep fragmentation in the elderly. Hypocretin is a recently discovered neurotransmitter that probably plays a central role in maintaining normal wakefulness (Siegel, 2004). Individuals who have narcolepsy have severe losses of hypocretin-secreting neurons (Thannickal et al., 2000). Both GABA and hypocretin are synthesized and released from the hypothalamus, the part of the brain that regulates sleep and wake cycles in relation to the body's circadian rhythms. In a normal sleep cycle, REM sleep alternates with non-REM sleep in ~90-minute intervals throughout the night. REM and non-REM sleep periods are associated with characteristic electroencephalography (EEG) activity. Non-REM sleep normally predominates in the first hours of sleep, whereas REM sleep accounts for most of the final hours of sleep.

Changes in an individual's normal pattern of nighttime sleep or daytime wakefulness are often caused by medication side effects, substance abuse, and medical problems that directly or indirectly affect sleep-regulating neurotransmitters. Heart disease, diabetes, chronic pain syndromes, and respiratory illnesses are often associated with excessive daytime sleepiness or nighttime wakefulness (Katz & McHorney, 1998). Disturbances in sleep or wakefulness occur more often in the elderly and medically ill compared with younger or healthy individuals, and are frequently associated with depressed mood, chronic anxiety, and Alzheimer's disease and other neurodegenerative diseases (Foley, Ancoli-Israel, Britz, & Walsh, 2004; McCurry et al., 1999). Elderly patients who report severe insomnia experience more rapid cognitive decline compared with individuals with normal sleep (Cricco, Simonsick, & Foley, 2001). The complex relationships between disturbed sleep and depressed mood or other psychiatric symptom patterns have not been clearly elucidated, but they may involve dysregulation of the hypothalamic-pituitary-adrenal (HPA) axis affecting both mood and wakefulness (Richardson & Roth, 2001). Disturbed sleep is so commonly associated with depressed mood that it is a diagnostic criterion of major depressive disorder in the *DSM-IV*. Approximately 90% of depressed patients and 70% of anxious patients complain of chronic insomnia (Anderson, Noyes, Crowe, & Noyes, 1984; McCall et al., 2000), and almost half of individuals who report chronic insomnia fulfill *DSM-IV* criteria for at least one psychiatric disorder (Ford & Kamerow, 1989). There is also a strong correlation between substance abuse and disturbances of wakefulness and sleep. Half of alcoholics report persisting insomnia (Brower, 2003). Many prescription drugs deleteriously affect sleep or wakefulness. Most pharmacologic treatments used in conventional mental health care adversely affect sleep or wakefulness (Obermeyer & Benca, 1996). For example, psychostimulant drugs such as methylphenidate (Ritalin) and so-called activating antidepressants such as buproprion (Wellbutrin) and venlafaxine (Effexor) often result in disrupted sleep; other antidepressants, including many selective serotonin reuptake inhibitors (SSRIs), cause daytime somnolence.

Overview of Conventional Approaches Used to Assess Daytime Sleepiness and Nighttime Wakefulness

The conventional practitioner's central goal is to determine the environmental, medical, or psychiatric causes of disturbed sleep or wakefulness. A primary disorder of sleep or wakefulness is diagnosed only when a persisting pattern of insomnia or daytime sleepiness cannot be adequately explained by a known medical or psychiatric disorder, substance abuse, or the effects of a medication. Because of the known relationships between insomnia and daytime sleepiness and psychiatric and medical problems, a thorough history, including a history of alcohol and substance abuse, should always be the starting place when evaluating both complaints. All medications and supplements should be carefully documented, including exact doses and dosing schedules. The Mini-Mental State Examination (MMSE) provides useful clinical information when there is evidence of impaired cognitive functioning.

Standardized instruments used to assess daytime sleepiness include the Stanford Sleepiness Scale and the Multiple Sleep Latency Test (MSLT). In the self-administered Stanford Sleepiness Scale, the individual estimates his or her sleepiness at different times of the day. In the MSLT, the patient is asked to estimate the time required to fall asleep (i.e., *sleep latency*) at five specified times during the course of the day. The MSLT probably yields more reliable information about symptoms of daytime sleepiness than the Stanford

Table 14–1 Nonconventional Assessment Approaches That Are Substantiated or Probably Yield Specific Diagnostic Information about the Causes of Daytime Sleepiness or Nighttime Wakefulness

	Assessment Approach	Evidence for Specific Diagnostic Information	Positive Finding Suggests Efficacy of This Treatment
Substantiated	None at time of writing		
Provisional			
Biological	Serum levels of several vitamins and minerals	Deficiencies in vitamins C, E, B$_{12}$, and folic acid are correlated with increased daytime sleepiness and insomnia.	Supplementation with vitamins and minerals that are deficient sometimes results in reduced daytime sleepiness and nighttime wakefulness
		Abnormally low serum levels of magnesium and zinc are often associated with increased daytime sleepiness	
Somatic	None at time of writing		
Energy-information assessment approaches validated by Western science	None at time of writing		
Energy-information assessment approaches not (yet) validated by Western science	None at time of writing		

Sleepiness Scale (Doghramji, 2004). Instruments used to assess insomnia include the Pittsburgh Sleep Quality Index and the Hamilton Rating Scale for Depression (HAM-D), which contains several questions about sleep. A sleep log is probably the most practical assessment tool when evaluating patients who complain of either insomnia or daytime sleepiness. The patient is instructed to designate times of falling asleep, waking up in the middle of the night, final waking, and daytime naps, in addition to amounts and times of caffeine, nicotine, or alcohol use and the timing and doses of prescribed medications. On the basis of findings in the clinical interview and the mental state exam, the therapist advises the patient about cognitive and behavioral approaches that address factors that probably contribute to problems of sleep or wakefulness. Polysomnography using EEG to measure brain wave activity during sleep is the gold standard for evaluating insomnia and abnormal behaviors during sleep, but EEG studies are seldom ordered because this technology is expensive, often impractical, and frequently unavailable (Haponik, 1992).

Overview of Nonconventional Approaches Used to Assess Excessive Daytime Sleepiness and Nighttime Wakefulness

At the time of writing, nonconventional methods used to assess disturbances in normal wakefulness or sleep have not been substantiated by compelling evidence. Provisional assessment approaches include checking serum levels of vitamins C, E, and B$_{12}$, which are frequently deficient in patients who report excessive daytime sleepiness and insomnia. Abnormally low serum levels of zinc and magnesium are frequently associated with increased daytime sleepiness. Several possibly useful diagnostic tests of the causes of daytime sleepiness and nighttime wakefulness are emerging. Limited data suggest that abnormal serum levels of two cytokines, interleukin-6

(IL-6) and tumor necrosis factor (TNF), may be causally related to changes in sleep and wakefulness. Food sensitivities and chronic or reactive hypoglycemia may explain some cases of excessive daytime sleepiness. Finally, the use of Chinese medical pulse diagnosis may help elucidate energetic imbalances associated with daytime sleepiness or nighttime wakefulness and lead to the most appropriate energetic treatments of these symptom patterns. **Tables 14–1** and **14–2**, respectively, list provisional and possibly specific nonconventional approaches used to assess daytime sleepiness or nighttime wakefulness.

Substantiated Approaches Used to Assess Daytime Sleepiness or Nighttime Wakefulness

At the time of writing, there are no well-substantiated nonconventional assessment approaches of daytime sleepiness or nighttime wakefulness.

Provisional Approaches Used to Assess Daytime Sleepiness or Nighttime Wakefulness

Biological Approaches

◆ **Deficiency states of certain vitamins and minerals result in fatigue or insomnia** Abnormally low serum levels of vitamins C and E and some B vitamins, including thiamine, pantothenic acid, folic acid, and B$_{12}$, may result in increased daytime sleepiness and fatigue (Cheraskin, Ringsdorf, & Medford, 1976; Smidt, Cremin, Grivetti, & Clifford, 1991; Tahiliani & Beinlich, 1991). Deficiencies in iron, folic acid, and B$_{12}$ cause anemia and associated fatigue (Higgins, 1995; Kuleshova & Riabova, 1989). Depressed mood, which is commonly associated with insomnia and daytime somnolence, is also a frequent concomitant of folic acid deficiency. Low serum magnesium is

Table 14–2 Nonconventional Assessment Approaches That May Yield Specific Diagnostic Information about Causes of Daytime Sleepiness or Nighttime Wakefulness

Category	Assessment Approach	Evidence for Specific Diagnostic Information	Comments
Biological	Serum levels of norepinephrine, IL-6, and TNF. Check for food allergies. Check for hypoglycemia	Abnormally high nighttime serum norepinephrine levels and abnormaly low nighttime serum IL-6 and TNF levels may be associated with increased rates of chronic insomnia. Abnormally high daytime serum levels of IL-6 and TNF may be associated with excessive daytime sleepiness. Sensitivities to dairy and wheat products may result in increased daytime sleepiness. Hypoglycemia may result in increased daytime sleepiness	***Note:*** The serum norepinephrine level may not be useful in the elderly, as levels increase with normal aging. ***Note:*** It is not clear whether changes in IL-6 and TNF are causes of insomnia and excessive sleepiness or markers of immunological processes that are indirectly related to these problems. Test for food allergies in chronically sleepy individuals who are otherwise healthy. Check fasting glucose and glucose tolerance test in chronically tired individuals who are otherwise healthy
Somatic	None at time of writing		
Energy-information assessment approaches validated by Western science	None at time of writing		
Energy-information assessment approaches not validated by Western science	Chinese medical diagnosis	Chinese pulse diagnosis may provide clinically useful information about energetic imbalances that manifest as daytime sleepiness or nighttime wakefulness	Specific pulse diagnosis findings are useful in planning Chinese medical treatments that address energetic imbalances associated with reduced daytime sleepiness or nighttime wakefulness

IL, interleukin; TNF, tumor necrosis factor

often associated with anxiety, daytime fatigue, increased difficulty falling asleep, and night terrors, as well as restless legs syndrome and other automatisms of sleep (Durlach et al., 1994; Popoviciu et al., 1990, 1993). A deficiency in zinc is often associated with easy fatigability or increased daytime sleepiness (Bakan, 1990). It is prudent to check serum levels of folic acid and B_{12} in patients who do not take these vitamin supplements and complain of persisting insomnia or daytime sleepiness.

Somatic Approaches

At the time of writing, there are no assessment approaches in this category.

Approaches Based on Forms of Energy or Information That Are Validated by Western Science

At the time of writing, there are no assessment approaches in this category.

Approaches Based on Forms of Energy or Information That Are Not Validated by Western Science

At the time of writing, there are no assessment approaches in this category.

Assessment Approaches That Possibly Yield Specific Diagnostic Information about Causes of Daytime Sleepiness or Nighttime Wakefulness

Biological Approaches

◆ **Chronic insomnia may be correlated with changes in immune functioning and increased risk of cardiovascular death** Young or middle-aged patients who experience chronic insomnia may have increased serum levels of norepinephrine at night, decreased immune functioning, and increased risk of cardiovascular death. As noted above, nighttime serum norepinephrine normally increases with aging. In one small double-blind study, diminished quality of sleep was correlated with elevated nighttime norepinephrine levels (Irwin, Clark, Kennedy, Christian Gillian, & Ziegler, 2003). Preliminary findings suggest that chronic insomnia is related to abnormal secretion patterns of two important cytokines, IL-6 and TNF, that regulate the body's immune functioning. High levels of these naturally circulating cytokines characterize normal sleep and induce excessive daytime fatigue and sleepiness when they occur during the daytime. Conversely, low cytokine levels normally occur during the day and are associated with increased wakefulness when present at night. Chronic insomniacs have abnormally high daytime and low nighttime serum levels of both IL-6 and TNF (Vgontzas et al., 2002). These findings may help to explain difficulties falling asleep at night and problems remaining awake during the day reported by chronic insomniacs.

◆ **Food allergies and reactive hypoglycemia probably account for many cases of increased daytime sleepiness** Food allergies, including sensitivities to dairy and wheat products, probably contribute to many cases of daytime sleepiness in individuals who follow healthy diets (Kondo et al., 1992). Testing for food allergies may be useful when excessive daytime sleepiness persists in spite of an apparently healthy diet and otherwise good physical and mental health.

◆ **Hypoglycemia is often associated with increased daytime sleepiness** Hypoglycemia is frequently associated with easy fatigability, anxiety, and difficulty concentrating. In a large observational study, two thirds of patients with hypoglycemia reported significant daytime sleepiness (Salzer 1966). The fasting blood glucose level and the glucose tolerance test are important conventional tests for verifying hypoglycemia.

Somatic Approaches

At the time of writing, there are no assessment approaches in this category.

Approaches Based on Forms of Energy or Information That Are Validated by Western Science

At the time of writing, there are no assessment approaches in this category.

Approaches Based on Forms of Energy or Information That Are Not Validated by Western Science

◆ **Chinese medical diagnosis may provide clinically useful information about energetic imbalances underlying daytime sleepiness or nighttime wakefulness** Chinese medical diagnosis, including a thorough history and examination of the tongue and pulses, reveals the energetic pattern associated with complaints of insomnia or daytime somnolence (Flaws & Lake, 2001). Different energetic imbalances, including specific excesses and deficiencies in yin or yang, manifest as insomnia or daytime sleepiness. The identified energetic pattern determines the most appropriate acupuncture or herbal treatment.

◆ The Integrative Treatment of Daytime Sleepiness and Nighttime Wakefulness

Overview of Conventional Treatments of Daytime Sleepiness and Nighttime Wakefulness

Conventionally trained physicians use both pharmacologic and nonpharmacologic approaches to prevent or treat daytime somnolence and nighttime wakefulness. Cognitive-behavioral interventions are often effective for the management of insomnia, but they are infrequently recommended compared with sedative-hypnotic drugs (Morin, Culbert, & Schwartz, 1994). *Sleep hygiene* is an important part of conventional management. Effective sleep hygiene includes restricting time spent in bed, going to bed only when sleepy, getting out of bed when unable to sleep, reducing noise or light in the sleep environment, getting up at the same time every morning, and avoiding daytime naps. Moderately severe cases of insomnia often respond well to improved sleep hygiene. Relaxation before bedtime, including progressive muscle relaxation, meditation, and listening to music, is an effective intervention for many sleep problems but is often not recommended by conventionally trained physicians.

The conventional management of situational or chronic insomnia generally relies on prescription benzodiazepines or other sedative-hypnotic drugs. Two more recently introduced drugs, zolpidem (Ambien) and zaleplon (Sonata), act on benzodiazepine receptors but are not true benzodiazepines. These short-acting agents do not have the same potential for abuse and dependence that has made long-term use of benzodiazepines problematic in chronic insomniacs.

The conventional management of excessive daytime sleepiness or fatigue often includes psychostimulants, including methylphenidate (Ritalin) and dextroamphetamine (Dexedrin). Psychostimulants are the established conventional treatments of narcolepsy, although only limited research findings support their use (Fry, 1998; Mitler, Jaudukovic, & Erman, 1993). Modafinil (Provigil) is a recently introduced drug that enhances wakefulness but is not considered a stimulant. The efficacy of modafinil for excessive daytime sleepiness associated with narcolepsy and obstructive sleep apnea has been established by large multicenter clinical trials. Recent research on sodium oxybate (γ-hydroxybutyrate) has yielded promising results in the management of cataplexy and excessive daytime sleepiness associated with narcolepsy (Scharf et al., 1985; U.S. Xyrem Multicenter Study Group, 2004).

Conventional Treatments Are Limited by Poor Efficacy and Unresolved Safety Problems

Recent surveys suggest that prescription benzodiazepines are used to manage 80 to 90% of all complaints of insomnia in Western countries (Mant, de Burgh, Mattick, Donnelly, & Hall, 1996; Straand & Rokstad, 1997). This practice has led to the overprescribing or inappropriate prescribing of potentially addictive sedative-hypnotics (Dollman et al., 2003). Over 40% of all patients who are hospitalized for any reason are prescribed benzodiazepines for management of sleep or anxiety, and many continue to use these drugs long after being discharged (Zisselman, Rovner, Kelly & Woods, 1994). Morning drowsiness, dizziness, and headache are common adverse effects of benzodiazepines. Inappropriate long-term use or high doses of benzodiazepines frequently result in confusion, daytime somnolence, and short-term memory impairment (Mant et al., 1995). Benzodiazepine use in the elderly is especially problematic because of the significantly increased risk of serious fall injuries associated with their use in this population (Herings et al., 1995).

Conventional antidepressants are widely used to treat insomnia; however, few controlled clinical trials have evaluated their efficacy or safety for this application (Walsh & Schweitzer, 1999). Many antidepressants, including doxepin (Siniquan), trazodone (Desyrel), and mirtazapine (Remeron), are moderately sedating, and their use in the management of insomnia has steadily increased since the mid-1980s (Walsh &

Schweitzer, 1999). However, research findings suggest that antidepressants used to treat insomnia cause serious adverse effects more often compared with benzodiazepines, including elevated liver enzymes, dry mouth, nausea, weight gain, orthostatic hypotension, daytime sleepiness, and dizziness (Hajak et al., 2001; Riemann et al., 2002).

Diphenhydramine, an antihistamine, is frequently prescribed for insomnia because of its sedating side effects. In recent years certain atypical antipsychotics that have sedating side effect profiles have come into increasing use for the management of insomnia in the absence of approval from the U.S. Food and Drug Administration (FDA) for this clinical application, and in spite of the absence of findings from controlled trials supporting the efficacy and safety of these drugs for the treatment of insomnia. Atypical agents frequently prescribed for insomnia include quetiapine (Seroquel) and olanzapine (Zyprexa).

In many cases the conventional pharmacologic management of insomnia is inappropriate or potentially unsafe because of a nondisclosed history of alcohol abuse or prescription drug dependence, concurrent use of medications that interact with sedative-hypnotics, or the existence of medical conditions that make the use of benzodiazepines unsafe (Morin et al., 1992). The effectiveness of insomnia treatments is difficult to evaluate because of the absence of rating scales that are able to show correlations between subjective complaints of insomnia or excessive daytime sleepiness and objective measures of sleep. Meta-analyses of conventional treatment approaches suggest that conventional drugs are probably more effective in the acute management of insomnia, whereas cognitive-behavioral approaches are more effective over the long term (Holbrook, Crowther, Lotter, Cheng, & King, 2000; Morin, Colecchi, Stone, Sood, & Brink, 1999).

Overview of Nonconventional Treatments of Daytime Sleepiness and Nighttime Wakefulness

Many nonconventional treatments of insomnia or daytime somnolence have been substantiated by strong research evidence and extensive clinical use. Dietary modifications, including reduced alcohol and daytime caffeine consumption, improve both symptom patterns. Depending on dosing, preparation, and timing, melatonin improves the quality and duration of sleep in both chronic insomnia and circadian rhythm sleep disturbances. Valerian extract is often as effective as conventional sedative-hypnotics while avoiding the risk of dependence. Somatic and mind–body approaches, including exercise, progressive muscle relaxation, guided imagery, and meditation, are as effective as conventional drugs for the management of mild to moderate insomnia. Carefully timed bright light exposure is an effective treatment of insomnia caused by circadian rhythm disturbances. EEG-biofeedback protocols based on alpha-theta training effectively reduce the severity of insomnia. Provisional nonconventional biological treatments of insomnia include a traditional Japanese herbal called Yoku-kan-san-ka-chimpi-hange, L-tryptophan, and 5-hydroxytryptophan (5-HTP). Some cranioelectrotherapy stimulation (CES) and EEG-biofeedback protocols are probably beneficial in cases of chronic insomnia. Certain acupuncture protocols probably reduce the severity of chronic insomnia.

Limited or inconsistent research findings suggest that the following biological treatments may be beneficial in some cases of insomnia or excessive daytime sleepiness: certain vitamins and minerals, melatonin, *Ginkgo biloba, St.* John's wort (*Hypericum perforatum*), an Ayurvedic herbal formula, ginseng (many species), Ashwagondha, yohimbine, indolepyruvic acid (IPA), and dehydroepiandrosterone (DHEA). Passive body heating may reduce symptoms of insomnia, and training in lucid dreaming induction may be beneficial when a disturbance in sleep is caused by recurring nightmares. Possibly effective treatments of insomnia based on forms of energy which are validated by current Western science include timed bright light exposure, low energy emission therapy (LEET), impulse magnetic field therapy, and white noise. **Table 14–3** lists substantiated and provisional treatments of insomnia and excessive daytime sleepiness. **Table 14–4** lists treatments that are possibly effective.

Table 14–3 Nonconventional Treatments of Daytime Sleepiness or Nighttime Wakefulness That Are Substantiated or Probably Effective

	Substantiated Treatment Approach	Evidence for Modality or Integrative Approaches That Include it	Comments (Including Safety Issues or Contraindications)
Biological	Dietary changes	Alcohol use at bedtime causes rebound insomnia.	Advise patients who complain of chronic insomnia or daytime sleepiness to reduce or eliminate refined sugar snacks and drinking alcohol at bedtime, and to reduce daytime caffeine consumption
		Caffeine in beverages or medications causes insomnia; caffeine withdrawal causes daytime sleepiness and fatigue.	
		Refined sugar snacks at night cause rebound hypoglycemia and disturbed sleep	
	Melatonin	Melatonin at doses between 0.3 and 3.0 mg improves sleep quality and duration in chronic insomnia.	*Note:* The best preparation of melatonin depends on the nature of the sleep disturbance.
		Melatonin 0.5 mg resynchronizes the sleep–wake cycle in circadian rhythm sleep disturbances	Melatonin may be safely combined with benzodiazepines to reduce middle awakening and reduce the risk of falling in elderly patients

Table 14–3 Nonconventional Treatments of Daytime Sleepiness or Nighttime Wakefulness That Are Substantiated or Probably Effective *(Continued)*

	Substantiated Treatment Approach	Evidence for Modality or Integrative Approaches That Include it	Comments (Including Safety Issues or Contraindications)
	Valerian	Valerian 600 mg at bedtime is probably as effective as benzodiazepines in the management of chronic insomnia, and facilitates discontinuation of benzodiazepines (i.e., used for insomnia) following prolonged use	Chronic use of valerian extract does not result in dependence, and daytime psychomotor slowing does not occur. **Caution:** Pregnant or nursing women should not use valerian extract
Somatic or mind–body	Somatic and mind–body practices	Many somatic and mind–body practices, including progressive muscle relaxation, massage, meditation, and guided imagery, are as effective as conventional sedative-hypnotics for mild to moderate insomnia. Using a somatic or mind–body approach together with a sedative-hypnotic is more effective than either approach alone	**Note:** Somatic and mind–body practices require more time to work but over the long term are less expensive and more cost-effective compared with conventional drugs. **Caution:** Sedentary and physically impaired patients, as well as patients with heart or lung disease, should consult a physician before beginning to exercise
	Exercise	Regular physical exercise increases the quality and duration of sleep in the elderly	
Validated energy-information approaches	Bright light exposure	Regular carefully timed bright light exposure resynchronizes phase-advanced or phase-delayed sleep to the patient's time zone	**Important:** When recommending light exposure therapy, always provide detailed instructions, review important safety information, and provide the name of a reputable manufacturer
	EEG biofeedback	Some EEG biofeedback protocols, especially SMR (alpha-theta training), are effective treatments of chronic insomnia	EEG biofeedback compares favorably with progressive muscle relaxation in the management of chronic insomnia
Nonvalidated energy-information approaches	None at time of writing		
Provisional			
Biological	5-HTP and L-tryptophan	5-HTP and L-tryptophan probably reduce symptoms of mild or situational insomnia. 5-HTP increases sleep duration in obstructive sleep apnea and narcolepsy. Combining L-tryptophan 2 g with a conventional antidepressant probably enhances antidepressant response and improves sleep quality	**Note:** L-tryptophan does not reduce the frequency of sleep attacks or improve the subjective quality of sleep in narcolepsy
	Yoku-kan-san-ka-chimpi-hange	Yoku-kan-san-ka-chimpi-hange, a widely used treatment of insomnia in traditional Japanese medicine (Kampo), probably increases overall quality and duration of sleep in chronic insomniacs	**Note:** The sleep-inducing mechanism of action of Yoku-kan-san-ka-chimpi-hange probably does not involve GABA
Somatic or mind–body	None at time of writing		
Validated energy-information approaches	CES	CES is probably beneficial in some cases of chronic insomnia. Patients who reported improved sleep following CES treatment exhibited increased "delta sleep" that continued months after treatments ended	**Note:** Reported disparities in research outcomes are probably related to customized equipment, the use of different protocols, the severity of symptoms treated, and the timing and duration of treatment
Nonvalidated energy-information approaches	Acupuncture and auriculotherapy	Some acupuncture and auriculotherapy protocols probably reduce the severity of sleep disturbances, including insomnia related to a mental health problem	**Note:** A long history of clinical use and consistent positive anecdotal evidence support the use of some acupuncture and auriculotherapy protocols for insomnia

CES, cranioelectrotherapy stimulation; EEG, electroencephalography; 5-HTP, 5-hydroxytryptophan; GABA, γ-aminobutyric acid; SMR, sensorimotor rhythm

Table 14–4   Possibly Effective Treatments of Daytime Sleepiness or Nighttime Wakefulness

Category	Treatment Approach	Evidence for Claimed Treatment Effect	Comments
Biological	Vitamins and minerals	Supplementation with folate, thiamine, iron, zinc, and magnesium in deficient individuals may reduce daytime sleepiness and improve nighttime sleep	*Note:* Most findings pertaining to vitamins and minerals come from open trials or observational studies
	Melatonin	Melatonin 2 mg (controlled release) may facilitate discontinuation of benzodiazepines following prolonged use and improve subjective sleep quality.	*Note:* Combining melatonin with a benzodiazepine taper at bedtime may be an effective strategy for transitioning patients off benzodiazepines following prolonged use
		Melatonin 9 to 12 mg may reduce symptoms of REM sleep behavior disorder	
	Ginkgo biloba	*Ginkgo biloba* 240 mg/day used in combination with a conventional antidepressant may improve the quality of sleep and reduce the frequency of middle awakenings in depressed patients	*Note:* The mechanism of action associated with enhanced non-REM sleep may be related to reduced levels of CRH. Other research findings (see Chapter 8) suggest that *G. biloba* improves depressed mood, possibly via the same mechanism
	St. John's wort (*Hypericum perforatum*)	St. John's wort may improve sleep quality in depressed patients who respond to treatment	*Note:* Like many conventional antidepressants, improved sleep quality may be a significant therapeutic effect of St. John's wort
	Ashwagondha (*Withania somnifera*), Ayurvedic herbal formula	Ashwagondha and an Ayurvedic compound herbal formula may be effective treatments of chronic primary insomnia	*Caution:* Half of patients reported adverse gastrointestinal effects. One ingredient (*Rauwolfia serpentina*) is known to cause or worsen depressed mood, and depressed patients should be advised to *not* use this formula
			Note: No human trials to date on Ashwagondha, but strong anecdotal support for use in insomnia
	Ginseng (many species)	Standardized ginseng preparations may enhance daytime wakefulness and reduce symptoms of insomnia	*Note:* Limited research findings suggest good efficacy using a wide range of doses. A conservative strategy is to begin with a low dose and increase the dose gradually while monitoring for changes in wakefulness or insomnia
	Yohimbine	Yohimbine 8 mg/day may be an effective treatment of daytime sleepiness in narcolepsy	*Caution:* Adverse effects of yohimbine include diarrhea, insomnia, gastrointestinal upset, and flushing
	IPA	IPA 200 to 300 mg may improve symptoms of mild or situational insomnia	*Note:* Adverse effects of IPA at these doses have not been reported including morning grogginess
	DHEA	DHEA 500 mg may increase REM sleep, and may be beneficial in sleep disturbances associated with diminished REM sleep.	*Note:* Women with a history of estrogen-receptor-positive breast cancer should avoid DHEA
		DHEA may be effective in some cases when insomnia and depressed mood occur together	
Somatic and mind–body	Passive body heating	Total passive body heating, especially taking a hot bath, soon before bedtime may improve overall sleep quality and reduce the frequency of middle awakenings	*Note:* Assuming the absence of serious physical impairments, all patients who complain of chronic insomnia should be encouraged to take a hot bath or use other means for passive body heating soon before bedtime
	Lucid dreaming	Developing skill at lucid dreaming may permit patients who have recurring nightmares to control their dreams and improve the quality of sleep	*Note:* Lucid dreaming training is used as a treatment of post-traumatic stress (see Chapter 10)
	Tibetan yoga	Regular daily practice of Tibetan yoga may improve sleep quality, and may also reduce the need for conventional hypnotics	*Note:* Improved sleep quality was not associated with reduced anxiety or depressed mood

Table 14–4 Possibly Effective Treatments of Daytime Sleepiness or Nighttime Wakefulness *(Continued)*

Category	Treatment Approach	Evidence for Claimed Treatment Effect	Comments
Energy-information approaches validated by Western science	Bright light exposure	Bright light exposure may improve sleep quality in some cases of insomnia that are not related to circadian rhythm disturbances	*Note:* Timed bright light exposure is an established treatment of circadian phase sleep disturbances; however, no controlled studies were identified in a systematic review
	LEET	LEET 15 minutes/night may improve overall sleep quality in chronic insomnia	*Note:* LEET is currently unavailable in the United States but may be a promising future approach to chronic insomnia
	Impulse magnetic field therapy	70% of chronic insomniacs randomized to nightly impulse magnetic field therapy reported significant improvements in sleep over a 2-week period	*Note:* No adverse effects of impulse magnetic field therapy were reported in the only controlled study done to date
	White noise	Nighttime exposure to white noise may be beneficial	*Note:* Adverse effects to white noise during sleep have not been reported
Energy-information approaches not validated by Western science	None at time of writing		

CRH, corticotrophin-releasing hormone; DHEA, dehydroepiandrosterone; IPA, indole-3-pyruvic acid; LEET, low energy emission therapy; REM, rapid eye movement

Substantiated Treatments of Daytime Sleepiness and Nighttime Wakefulness

Biological Treatments

◆ **Dietary changes can sometimes improve daytime wakefulness and nighttime sleep**   In general, consumption of alcohol and caffeine is associated with a relatively greater risk of insomnia. Drinking soon before bedtime often results in initial grogginess followed by rebound insomnia (Shinba, Murashima, & Yamamoto, 1994). Individuals who use caffeine-containing medications have greater difficulty falling asleep compared with those who do not (Brown et al., 1995). A common symptom of caffeine withdrawal is daytime sleepiness (Hughes et al., 1991). Chronic fatigue or sleepiness typically accompanies hypoglycemia (Salzer, 1966). A large epidemiological study concluded that reactive hypoglycemia during sleep caused by late-night snacking is probably a significant risk factor in many cases of insomnia (Mogi et al., 1996). Daytime snacks with high refined sugar content typically lead to initially increased energy followed by reactive hypoglycemia and increased fatigue or sleepiness (Thayer, 1987). Reducing dietary intake of refined sugar and taking frequent small meals are usually an effective approach to hypoglycemia.

◆ **Melatonin is an effective treatment of chronic insomnia and circadian rhythm sleep disturbances**   Melatonin is a validated treatment of both chronic insomnia in patients with low serum melatonin levels and jet lag when five or more time zones have been crossed. Sustained-release preparations are most effective for improving the duration of sleep, whereas patients who have trouble falling asleep (*prolonged sleep latency*) respond best to immediate-release forms of melatonin. A meta-analysis of 17 double-blind, controlled studies involving a total of 284 patients concluded that exogenous melatonin decreases the time required to fall asleep (*sleep onset latency*), and increases total sleep duration (Brzezinski et al., 2005). Doses that replace normal physiological levels (0.3 mg) in insomnia patients with low serum melatonin levels improve restful sleep in the middle part of the sleep cycle. In contrast, higher pharmacologic doses (3.0 mg) improve sleep quality but are sometimes associated with hypothermia, elevated daytime melatonin levels, and residual grogginess (Zhdanova, Wurtman, Regan, Taylor, Shi, & Leclair, 2001). Adding controlled-release melatonin 2 mg to the patient's existing regimen of benzodiazepines significantly improves sleep time, sleep continuity, and sleep latency in elderly patients with low serum melatonin levels (Garfinkel, Laudon, & Zisapel, 1997). Patients who do not have chronic insomnia but have low serum melatonin levels do not report changes in sleep with melatonin. In view of the high risk of falling among elderly insomniacs when they get up in the middle of the night, it is reasonable to augment or replace existing conventional hypnotic treatments with melatonin in this population, with the goal of reducing the number of middle awakenings. Bright light exposure can be effectively combined with melatonin in the management of circadian rhythm sleep disturbances (see discussion below). Double-blind studies demonstrate consistent improvements in sleep quality and duration, and reduced sleep latency in chronic insomniacs who take melatonin at doses between 0.3 and 3 mg (Kayumov et al., 2001).

Melatonin is beneficial in resynchronizing the sleep–wake cycle back to a rhythm that is normal with respect to a particular time zone. A Cochrane systematic review of 10 double-blind, placebo-controlled studies concluded that melatonin was effective in jet lag at doses of 0.5 to 5.0 mg when taken close to bedtime in the country of destination (Herxheimer & Petrie, 2004). The overall efficacy of melatonin was relatively less for westward flights and relatively greater when more time zones were crossed. In cases of *phase advance*, in which a patient is rising early and going to sleep early with respect to his or her time zone, melatonin 0.5 mg can be used to incrementally delay the sleep phase if taken during middle awakenings and at the time of rising in the early morning. In cases of *phase delay, in which a patient goes to sleep late and awakens late*, melatonin 0.5 mg should be taken ~7 hours after sleep onset to incrementally advance the individual to a normal sleep–wake schedule.

Melatonin has been used to treat insomnia in schizophrenics (Shamir et al., 2000) and agitated manic patients (Bersani & Garavini, 2000) with moderate success. Daytime use of melatonin should be avoided (except when treating a sleep disturbance caused by circadian phase advance—see discussion above) because of potentially impairing decrements in cognition and job performance, including reduced response time and slowed problem solving (Rogers, Dorrian, & Dinges, 1998). Uncommon mild side effects of melatonin include headache and itching.

◆ **Valerian (*Valeriana officinalis*) is an effective and safe treatment of chronic insomnia** Valerian has been an important medicinal plant in many traditional systems of medicine for more than a thousand years. A systematic review of double-blind studies of valerian extract for insomnia concluded that a 600 to 900 mg dose at bedtime improves the subjective quality of sleep with few side effects (Krystal & Ressler, 2001). The mechanism of action has not yet been established, but it may involve inhibition of GABA reuptake or binding to serotonin receptors by valepotriates, important active constituents of the herb. At doses that are therapeutic, valerian extract is sedating, and research does not support the daytime use of the herb as a treatment of anxiety (Kohnen & Oswald, 1988). In contrast to benzodiazepines, valerian preparations do not entail a risk of addiction, and there are no reports of daytime psychomotor slowing following use (Schultz, Hubner, & Ploch, 1997). In a large multicenter 6-week study, valerian extract 600 mg/day had comparable efficacy to oxazepam (Serax) 10 mg, a benzodiazepine, in the management of chronic insomnia (Ziegler, Ploch, Miettinen-Baumann, & Collet, 2002). Chronic insomniacs who take valerian extract following discontinuation of benzodiazepines report improved quality of sleep and fewer awakenings (Poyares, Guilleminault, Ohayon, & Tufik, 2002). Findings from a pilot study suggest that an effective integrative approach to stress-induced insomnia is a combined regimen of daytime kava 120 mg and nighttime valerian 600 mg (Wheatley, 2001). Combining these two herbals avoids the risk of dependence with prolonged benzodiazepine use in chronically stressed individuals. Because of its potentiating effect on GABA, valerian should not be combined with benzodiazepines or alcohol. There are rare reports of elevated liver enzymes (Shepherd, 1993). Valepotriates contained in valerian may be mutagenic, and the herb should be avoided in pregnant or nursing women.

Somatic and Mind–Body Approaches

◆ **Somatic and mind–body approaches are beneficial for mild to moderate insomnia** Many somatic and mind–body techniques have been investigated in controlled trials of insomnia, including progressive muscle relaxation, massage, meditation, desensitization, guided imagery, autogenic training, and hypnosis. Progressive muscle relaxation and sustained deep breathing are especially effective at reducing the time needed to fall asleep (i.e., sleep latency) in chronic insomniacs. The regular use of audiocassettes at bedtime guides individuals who have difficulty falling asleep through relaxing images while also causing sleep-promoting mental fatigue. I have found that patients who have trouble falling asleep because of anxiety or work stress frequently benefit from listening to a relaxing imagery tape starting 30 minutes before their regular bedtime. Individuals who have difficulty falling asleep because of somatic complaints respond better to progressive muscle relaxation, and those who stay awake because of chronic worrying are more likely to sleep better with imagery (Titlebaum, 1998). Effective relaxation approaches probably work by increasing parasympathetic activity and decreasing overall sympathetic activity, thus increasing the threshold for arousal during sleep. Cognitive approaches for relaxation, including meditation and guided imagery, are probably more effective than somatic approaches such as progressive muscle relaxation for the management of mild or situational insomnia, but these approaches are of little benefit in cases of severe insomnia (National Institutes of Health Technology Assessment Panel, 1996). Fibromyalgia patients report significant increases in the duration of sleep and reduced pain with regular massage treatments (Field, Diego, Cullen, Hernandez-Reif, Sunshine, & Douglas, 2002). Insomniac patients who consistently practice a validated somatic or cognitive-behavioral technique alone or in combination with sedative-hypnotic drugs report that nonpharmacologic or combined approaches are more effective than conventional drugs alone. Furthermore, clinical improvements in insomnia are sustained longer in patients who use nonpharmacologic or combined approaches compared with conventional pharmacologic treatments alone (Morin et al., 1999). A Cochrane meta-analysis of 66 studies (including almost 2000 patients) of somatic and mind–body treatments of insomnia concluded that all interventions resulted in "reliable and durable benefits" that were superior to placebo, including improved quality of sleep and reduced sleep latency (Murtagh & Greenwood, 1995). A separate Cochrane meta-analysis concluded that although nonpharmacologic treatments of chronic insomnia are initially more expensive and require more time compared with conventional drug therapy, in the long run they are reliable, result in sustained benefits, and are more cost-effective than drugs alone (Morin et al., 1994). In view of the adverse effects and the potential for abuse with prolonged use of sedative-hypnotic drugs, especially in the elderly and in substance-abusing patients, the consistent practice of an effective somatic or mind–body approach should be strongly encouraged in all patients who complain of insomnia.

◆ **Regular exercise in the elderly probably enhances the quality and duration of sleep** Physical exercise is widely recommended by both conventionally trained and alternative medical practitioners as an approach to reduce stress and improve the quality of sleep. A Cochrane systematic review of studies on the relationship between exercise and sleep in the elderly concluded that exercise probably enhances sleep and improves the overall quality of life (Montgomery & Dennis, 2004b). Both sleep duration and the quality of sleep improved significantly with regular exercise. In view of the documented risk of adverse effects associated with sedative-hypnotic drugs in the elderly, and the general benefits of exercise to health and mood, all patients complaining of chronic insomnia should be encouraged to exercise on a regular basis. Elderly patients, individuals who have been sedentary, and patients with physical impairments, heart disease, or pulmonary disorders should consult their physicians before starting an exercise program.

Treatment Approaches Based on Forms of Energy or Information That Are Validated by Western Science

◆ **Regular bright light exposure is an effective treatment for circadian rhythm sleep disturbances** Because of the relationship between bright light exposure, melatonin levels, and sleep, researchers have investigated the benefits of bright light exposure as a treatment of insomnia (Dijk, Boulos, Eastman, Lewy, Campbell, & Terman, 1995; Lewy & Sack, 1986). The entrainment of sleep–wake cycles by external bright light cues, along with the associated suppression of melatonin production by the pineal gland, is the established mechanism of action underlying the therapeutic benefits of light exposure on sleep, wakefulness, and mood (Campbell, Eastman, Terman, Lewy, Boulos, & Dijk, 1995). Controlled studies and an expert consensus report on light treatment for sleep disorders provide compelling evidence for the efficacy of bright light exposure in the management of circadian rhythm sleep problems but not for insomnia in general (Campbell et al., 1995).

There are two basic kinds of circadian rhythm sleep disturbances: phase delay and phase advance (Lewy, 1987; Lewy & Sack, 1986). In phase-delayed circadian disturbances, sleep onset and waking are shifted to times that are later than usual for an individual with respect to the time zone where he or she lives. The phase-delayed individual typically goes to sleep late and wakes up late. Phase-delayed circadian sleep disturbances are relatively common in adolescents and night-shift workers. In contrast, phase-advanced sleep disturbances are characterized by early sleep onset and early awakening relative to the time zone where the patient resides. Phase-advanced sleep disturbances are common in the elderly. The most appropriate strategy for bright light exposure is determined on the basis of the phase-advanced or phase-delayed nature of the sleep disturbance. If a patient complains of consistently going to sleep and waking up very early, he or she is probably phase advanced, and daily bright light exposure soon after waking will gradually normalize the sleep–wake cycle. In contrast, patients who complain about going to sleep and waking up too late are probably phase delayed and will respond best to daily bright light exposure in the early evening hours (i.e., relative to the time zone where they reside).

Jet lag is a clinically significant disturbance of normal sleep and wakefulness caused by a phase delay or phase advance, depending on the direction of travel. Traveling east over several time zones results in a need for a phase advance, and often responds to early morning bright light. In contrast, traveling west induces a relative phase delay and often responds to bright light exposure in the early evening hours (Boulos, Campbell, Lewy, Terman, Dijk, & Eastman, 1995; Daan & Lewy, 1984). Most protocols recommend 30 to 40 minutes of bright light exposure daily for beneficial effects in shifting circadian rhythms and changing sleep–wake cycles (Campbell et al., 1995). Beneficial effects of bright light exposure therapy are usually noticeable within a few days, and an appropriate treatment plan often resynchronizes the patient's sleep–wake cycle with his or her time zone in 2 or 3 weeks.

Correct timing of light exposure is essential for successful treatment of circadian sleep problems. In this context, it is important to note that bright light exposure between the hours of late morning and late afternoon probably has no effect on circadian rhythm phase. Melatonin taken in conjunction with bright light exposure sometimes results in more rapid normalization of the sleep–wake cycle (see discussion above).

When recommending exposure to natural sunlight for a circadian rhythm sleep disturbance, the patient should be instructed to avoid looking directly at the sun or to close the eyes while orienting to the sun. When using an artificial light source, patients should be provided with written instructions describing the timing and duration of treatment, and the names of reputable manufacturers. All patients should be cautioned to avoid using sun lamps (which emit harmful ultraviolet rays), and instructed to keep the eyes open while viewing the light fixture at an oblique (~45 degree) angle to avoid excessive eye strain.

◆ **EEG biofeedback is an effective treatment of chronic insomnia** The American Academy of Sleep Medicine has recommended EEG biofeedback for the treatment of chronic insomnia (Standards of Practice Committee of the American Academy of Sleep Medicine, 1999). In a review of nonpharmacologic treatments of insomnia, EEG biofeedback was found to be more effective than progressive muscle relaxation (Morin, Hauri, Espie, Spielman, Buysse, & Bootzin, 1998). Research findings suggest that an innovative form of EEG biofeedback that transforms the unique EEG signal of an individual who has insomnia into musical tones improves the quality and duration of sleep when listened to before bedtime. In a 2-week double-blind study, 58 patients with chronic insomnia were instructed to listen to music generated from certain EEG segments corresponding to sleep phases from their own or another's EEG recordings (Levine, 1997). All subjects enrolled in the study had been off prescription medications or alternative remedies for at least 2 weeks, and none had been diagnosed with a major psychiatric disorder. Based on a clinical questionnaire, standardized psychological tests, and EEG sleep recordings, significantly more patients who listened to their own "brain music" before sleeping experienced increased total duration of sleep, increased delta (slow wave) and fewer middle awakenings compared with individuals who listened to the "brain music" of others. Several EEG-biofeedback protocols are probably beneficial in insomnia, but a protocol that modulates α (alpha) and θ (theta) activity along the primary sensory and motor regions in the frontal and prefrontal areas of the cortex may yield the most consistently beneficial outcomes in improving the overall quality of sleep and reducing the frequency of middle awakenings (Hauri, Percy, Hellekson, Hartmann, & Russ, 1982).

Approaches Based on Forms of Energy or Information That Are Not Validated by Western Science

At the time of writing, there are no treatment approaches in this category.

Provisional Approaches

Biological Treatments

◆ **L-tryptophan and 5-HTP are beneficial and well tolerated for mild or situational insomnia** Both L-tryptophan and 5-HTP are widely used to treat depressed mood and sleep disturbances, but evidence supporting the use of these amino acids in insomnia is limited. L-tryptophan 1 g at bedtime reduces the time required to fall asleep in mild or situational insomnia, and doses up to 15 g are required in more severe cases of insomnia (Schneider-Helmert & Spinweber, 1986). L-tryptophan is generally well tolerated at doses that are beneficial for insomnia. Combining L-tryptophan 2 g with conventional antidepressants accelerates antidepressant response and improves the overall quality of sleep (Levitan, Shen, Jindal, Driver, Kennedy, & Shapiro, 2000). There have been no reports of serotonin syndrome or other serious adverse effects using this protocol.

Nighttime use of 5-HTP may improve some cases of mild to moderate insomnia and sleep disturbances related to obstructive sleep apnea (Hudgel, Gordon, & Meltzer, 1995) and narcolepsy (Autret et al., 1977). In one series, patients with narcolepsy treated with 5-HTP 600 mg at bedtime reported increased nighttime sleep but did not experience improved sleep quality or decreased narcoleptic attacks (Autret et al., 1977). Patients with obstructive sleep apnea who improved with 5-HTP (0.4 mg/kg) had higher pretreatment cortisol levels compared with controls (Hudgel et al., 1995).

◆ **A Japanese traditional herbal medicine is probably a safe and effective treatment of insomnia** Yoku-kan-san-ka-chimpi-hange is widely used to treat insomnia in traditional Japanese herbal medicine (Kampo). A double-blind, placebo-controlled study concluded that total sleep time was significantly increased, sleep latency was decreased, and the subjective quality of sleep was enhanced (Aizawa et al., 2002). There were no reports of significant adverse effects or changes in REM or other aspects of sleep polysomnography suggesting a benzodiazepine-like effect.

Somatic and Mind–Body Approaches

At the time of writing, there are no treatment approaches in this category.

Treatment Approaches Based on Forms of Energy or Information That Are Validated by Western Science

◆ **Ces is beneficial in some cases of insomnia** The use of weak electrical currents applied to the scalp or earlobes has been explored as a treatment of insomnia since the late 1960s. The technique is variously called "electrosleep" and "electroanesthesia." In Russia, electrosleep has been accepted as a mainstream medical approach for the management of insomnia for several decades (Iwanovsky et al., 1968). A meta-analysis of sham-controlled studies of cranioelectrotherapy stimulation for insomnia has not been done, and findings of published studies are inconsistent. Although some sham-controlled studies show no beneficial effects of CES in insomnia

(Coursey, Frankel, Gaarder, & Mott, 1980; Frankel, Buchbinder, & Snyder, 1973; Hearst, Cloninger, Crews, & Cadoret, 1974), others report sustained improvements in the timing of sleep onset and total sleep duration (Cartwright & Weiss, 1975; Weiss 1973). A private survey by a company that manufactures a popular CES machine found that a significant percentage of patients report improved sleep and reduced sleep latency when using a CES device made by that company (Kirsch, 2002). Patients who reported improved sleep following CES treatment exhibited increased stage IV, or delta, sleep that was sustained several months after treatments ended. Reported differences in the therapeutic benefits of CES in insomnia probably depend on differences between equipment designs, the protocol that is used, and the duration and timing of treatment.

Treatment Approaches Based on Forms of Energy or Information That Are Not Validated by Western Science

◆ **Acupuncture and auriculotherapy are probably beneficial in many cases of insomnia** Acupuncture is a widely used treatment of insomnia in countries where Chinese medicine is practiced, including United States, Canada, and most western European countries. The analgesic and sedating effects of specific acupuncture treatment protocols are probably mediated by the release of endogenous opioid peptides in the brain (Lin, 1995). Disparate acupuncture protocols are used to treat insomnia depending on the specific energetic imbalance associated with this symptom pattern. Like many nonconventional modalities, the absence of standardized acupuncture treatment protocols for insomnia has interfered with efforts to design rigorously controlled double-blind studies. A systematic review of all studies on acupuncture for insomnia published in the English language through 2002 identified few studies suitable for analysis because most studies had not used formal randomized, double-blind procedures (Sok, Erlen, & Kim, 2003). Furthermore, most studies included small numbers of patients who reported insomnia symptoms of varying duration and severity. On the basis of study findings that were able to be included in a systematic comparison, the reviewers concluded that acupuncture may be an effective intervention for the relief of insomnia (Sok et al., 2003). Consistent case report findings also support the claim that some acupuncture protocols have significant and beneficial effects in the management of insomnia (Xu, 1997).

Acupuncture is probably a beneficial treatment of insomnia associated with psychiatric symptoms, including generalized anxiety and schizophrenia. In a large case series, 500 schizophrenics reported significant improvements in sleep following acupuncture treatments (Shi & Tan, 1986). In one double-blind, controlled study (Montakab 1999), 40 patients were randomized to an acupuncture protocol traditionally used to improve sleep versus a sham protocol. All patients in the study were first diagnosed using established Chinese medical assessment methods (see discussion above) and were subsequently matched to appropriate acupuncture protocols addressing specific energetic "imbalances" associated with complaints of insomnia. Significant improvements in the subjective quality of sleep and commensurate therapeutic changes on EEG polysomnography were found in patients in the treatment group but not the sham group.

Auricular acupuncture (**auriculotherapy**) is a widely used approach in Chinese medicine in which the energetic imbalance associated with a particular symptom pattern is treated by attaching magnetic pearls to specific points on the ears. In one controlled trial, 15 elderly patients were randomized to a traditionally used protocol versus a sham treatment protocol for a 3-week period. Sleep patterns were evaluated at 1, 3, and 6 months (Suen, Wong, Leung, & Ip, 2003). Significant improvements in sleep quality and duration were reported in the treatment group throughout the treatment period but not the sham group, and these differences persisted 6 months after the study ended. Traditional acupuncture or auriculotherapy treatments of sleep complaints should always be administered by a skilled Chinese medical practitioner who has clinical experience treating sleep-related problems.

Possibly Effective Treatments of Insomnia or Daytime Sleepiness

Table 14–4 outlines the possibly effective treatments of daytime sleepiness or nighttime wakefulness.

Biological Treatments

◆ **Vitamin and mineral supplements sometimes reduce fatigue and daytime sleepiness and improve the quality of sleep** When a patient complaining of daytime sleepiness or fatigue is found to be deficient in certain vitamins or minerals, supplementation sometimes results in dramatic improvements in energy and wakefulness. Supplements are widely used in Western countries to treat complaints of daytime sleepiness or fatigue, but few controlled studies have verified their effectiveness. Findings of a small open trial suggest that folic acid 10 mg/day in folate-deficient patients significantly reduces fatigue and daytime sleepiness after 2 to 3 weeks of treatment (Botez et al., 1979). Findings of a double-blind study showed that elderly individuals who are marginally thiamine deficient respond to supplementation (10 mg/day) with improved energy, increased daytime wakefulness, and improved sleep (Smidt et al., 1991). The evidence for a fatigue-decreasing effect of vitamin B_{12} is inconsistent (Ellis & Nasser, 1973). Findings of a small open trial suggest that vitamin B_{12} 3 mg/day results in earlier sleep onset in adolescents who complain of chronic daytime sleepiness associated with a phase delay in their circadian rhythm (Ohta et al., 1991). There is limited and inconclusive evidence for vitamins C and E as treatments of daytime sleepiness and fatigue (Gerster, 1989; Heseker, Kubler, Pudel, & Westenhoffer, 1992). Iron deficiency invariably results in anemia and fatigue. Findings of controlled studies show that iron supplementation in individuals who are deficient results in significantly reduced levels of fatigue and daytime sleepiness (Ballin et al., 1992; Schultz & Freedman, 1987). Individuals who are zinc deficient report significant improvements in fatigability and daytime sleepiness with daily supplementation (Krotkiewski, Gudmundsson, Backstrom, & Mandroukas, 1982). Insomnia and anxiety are common manifestations of

magnesium deficiency. Findings of two observational studies suggest that magnesium supplementation improves overall sleep quality, and oral potassium chloride supplementation 96 mEq/day helps to consolidate fragmented sleep in individuals found to have low potassium serum levels (Davis & Ziady, 1976; Drennan, Kripke, Klemfuss, & Moore, 1991).

◆ **Melatonin may facilitate discontinuation of benzodiazepines in chronic insomniacs and reduce symptoms of REM sleep behavior disorder** Chronic insomniacs are at high risk for benzodiazepine abuse. The findings of one study suggest that controlled-release melatonin 2 mg taken at bedtime facilitates discontinuation of benzodiazepines when there is dependence following chronic use (Garfinkel, Zisapel, Wainstein, & Laudon, 1999). In this population, regular bedtime use of melatonin may result in significant improvements in subjective sleep quality. Findings from another study suggest that melatonin is an effective treatment of an unusual sleep disturbance called **REM sleep behavior disorder**, in which there is a loss of normal sleep paralysis during REM sleep and the individual physically acts out his or her dreams, potentially causing injury to the individual or his or her partner (Kunz & Bes, 1997). Conventional drug treatments of this unusual condition are associated with significant toxicities or side effects. Melatonin may be effective at bedtime doses of 9 to 12 mg, with few minor adverse effects.

◆ ***Ginkgo biloba* extract may improve insomnia related to depressed mood** *Ginkgo biloba* extract may improve sleep disturbances and the severity of cognitive impairments in depressed patients when used in combination with a conventional antidepressant. A small open study found significant improvements in the quality of sleep and the number of middle awakenings in patients taking a standardized ginkgo preparation 240 mg/day and trimipramine 200 mg compared with patients taking only the conventional antidepressant (Hemmeter et al., 2001). Sleep studies showed that non-REM sleep was especially enhanced in the group receiving ginkgo, and this beneficial effect was lost when ginkgo was discontinued. These findings suggest that ginkgo improves non-REM sleep by reducing the activity of corticotropin-releasing hormone (CRH).

◆ **St. John's wort may reduce symptoms of insomnia related to depressed mood** Improved sleep may be a significant beneficial effect when depressed patients respond to St. John's wort. After 6 weeks of therapy, elderly depressed individuals who responded to treatment with St. John's wort extract had increased slow-wave sleep and improved overall sleep quality (Holsboer-Trachsler, 2000).

◆ **Ayurvedic herbal medicines may be beneficial in chronic insomnia** Forty patients diagnosed with chronic insomnia were randomized to receive an herbal formula consisting of *Rauwolfia serpentina* root (100 mg), *Nardostachys jatamansi* root (100 mg), and *Tinospora cordifolia* (100 mg) versus placebo at bedtime for 3 weeks (Rani & Naidu, 1998). Patients taking the herbal formula slept longer and had significantly fewer middle awakenings compared with the placebo group. REM sleep was not affected, and morning drowsiness was not reported; however, half of patients taking the herbal formula experienced significant adverse gastrointestinal effects. The results of this study are promising though preliminary. Of note, *R. serpentina* may worsen depressed mood and should not be used by depressed patients. In traditional Ayurvedic medicine, Ashwagondha (*Withania somnifera*) is frequently used for its sedative-hypnotic properties in the management of insomnia, agitation, and anxiety symptoms, depending on dosing and timing of administration. However, human clinical trials on insomnia have not been conducted to date. Animal studies suggest that the extract of this herbal has moderately sedating effects and may improve the quality and duration of sleep (Das, 1994; Prabhu, Rao, & Karanth, 1990; Vaidya, 1997).

◆ **Ginseng may enhance daytime wakefulness and improve the quality of sleep** Preparations of different ginseng species are widely used as adaptogens to treat both insomnia and daytime fatigue and sleepiness. Many biologically active constituents of ginseng probably have therapeutic roles, though steroid-like molecules called ginsenosides have been studied most. These molecules mediate changes in arousal by competitively binding to brain GABA receptors (Kimura, Saunders, & Kim, 1994). Doses of 200 to 600 mg/day of standardized ginseng extract are reportedly effective and well tolerated for enhancing daytime wakefulness in patients who complain of chronic low energy and sleepiness. Findings of a randomized double-blind, controlled trial suggest that 40 mg of a standardized ginseng preparation significantly improves both daytime wakefulness and sleep quality in a population of healthy adults (Marasco, Ruiz, Villagomez, & Infante, 1996). Mild anxiety is an infrequent adverse effect at usual therapeutic doses.

◆ **Yohimbine may be an effective treatment for narcolepsy** Findings of a small open trial suggest that yohimbine at 8 mg/day may result in significantly improved control over daytime sleepiness in narcolepsy (Wooten, 1994). The putative mechanism of action involves decreased REM sleep through blockade of α-2 receptors in the brain. Seven of 8 patients in the study reported consistent beneficial effects for the duration of the 18-month trial. Adverse effects included diarrhea, insomnia, gastrointestinal upset, and flushing.

◆ **IPA may improve overall sleep quality** Results of a pilot study suggest that indole-pyruvic acid has mild hypnotic effects at doses of 200 to 300 mg and may improve the quality of sleep (Shamsi, Stanley, Yoon, & Hindmarch, 1996). All 10 patients enrolled in the study reported significant improvements in sleep, and there were no reports of morning grogginess. Pending corroboration by larger studies, IPA may provide an alternative to conventional hypnotics for mild or situational insomnia.

◆ **DHEA may be beneficial for insomnia related to REM sleep disturbances** A pilot study tested the effects of oral DHEA 500 mg on sleep polysomnography in 10 healthy young men (Friess et al., 1995). REM sleep was significantly increased during the first 2 hours of sleep, suggesting that DHEA may be beneficial for insomnia related to REM sleep disturbances. DHEA is a provisional treatment of depressed mood, and therefore may be an effective treatment of some cases where insomnia and depressed mood occur together. DHEA may increase the risk of breast cancer in women who have a history of estrogen-receptor-positive breast cancer and should be avoided in this population.

Somatic and Mind–Body Approaches

◆ **Passive body heating may improve the overall quality of sleep** Taking a hot bath before going to bed is a common approach to alleviating stress and is often recommended to patients who struggle with chronic insomnia. Limited evidence supports the putative beneficial effects of hot baths on the quality of sleep. Taking a hot bath and other approaches that result in total passive body heating probably improve insomnia by increasing slow-wave sleep at an individual's customary time of sleep onset. Slow-wave sleep is diminished with normal aging and is probably associated with the observed increased rate of insomnia in the elderly. A pilot study found that elderly women (ages 60 to 72) with chronic insomnia who took a hot bath (40 to 40.5°C) 1.5 hours before bedtime experienced significant improvements in uninterrupted sleep and had more slow-wave sleep (Dorsey et al., 1996). Assuming the absence of physical impairments or serious medical risks that may be associated with passive body heating, chronic insomniacs should be encouraged to take a hot bath or use other means to effectively achieve passive body heating before bedtime.

◆ **Lucid dreaming methods may be beneficial for sleep disturbances related to recurring nightmares** In a *lucid dream*, the dreamer is conscious while dreaming and thus aware that he or she is dreaming and not awake. Considerable research has substantiated the neurobiological basis of lucid dreaming (Gackenbach & LaBerge, 1988). Individuals who have been traumatized often experience interrupted sleep because of recurring disturbing dreams or nightmares. Many have learned how to use lucid dreams to confront and transform the content of their dreams, and in so doing are able to achieve refreshing sleep. When it does not result in severe arousal and awakening, anxiety in dreams frequently leads to the spontaneous experience of lucidity. Many individuals who have disturbed sleep related to recurring anxiety-provoking dreams develop a capacity for spontaneous lucidity. Those who do not become lucid spontaneously can become proficient lucid dreamers by practicing associative cues during the day. Special devices have also been designed to "cue" the sleeping brain during REM sleep and "remind" the dreamer that he or she is dreaming, resulting in self-awareness during dreaming. Practical strategies for improving skill at lucid dreaming are elaborated elsewhere (LaBerge & Rheingold, 1990).

Lucid dreaming methods include the use of word-association mnemonics when awake to trigger awareness of dreaming when asleep, along with machines that detect REM sleep and activate a dim flashing light or a subaudible tone to "remind" the dreamer that he or she is dreaming, thereby inducing a lucid state. Once lucidity is achieved, the dreamer can "confront" unpleasant images or experiences while still "in" the dream, which often has the effect of dissolving frightening imagery. Emerging findings suggest that anxious or traumatized patients who use this approach eventually achieve increased control over their dreams, reduce the frequency and intensity of nightmares and anxiety-inducing dream images, and report clinical improvements in daytime anxiety and the quality of sleep (see Chapter 10, Anxiety) (Brylowski & McCay, 1991). Dr. LaBerge comments: "Lucid dreaming gives us the power to banish the terror of nightmares and at the same time to strengthen our courage—if we master our fear sufficiently to recognize our most disturbing images as our own creations and face them."

◆ **Tibetan yoga may improve overall sleep quality** The findings of a small randomized trial on lymphoma patients suggest that the daily practice of a form of Tibetan yoga (Tsa lung and Trul khor), which incorporates controlled breathing, visualization, mindfulness techniques and low-impact postures, results in generally improved sleep quality, longer sleep, and fewer middle awakenings, and may also reduce the need for conventional hypnotics (Cohen et al., 2004). Significantly, improvements in anxiety, depressed mood, and fatigue were not reported by individuals who used this technique.

Treatment Approaches Based on Forms of Information or Energy That Are Validated by Western Science

◆ **Bright light exposure may be beneficial in some cases of chronic insomnia that are not related to circadian rhythm disturbances** Daytime exposure to bright light with an intensity of 10,000 lux is sometimes used as a treatment of chronic insomnia that is unrelated to circadian phase disturbances. Anecdotal reports suggest that bright light exposure is beneficial in some cases. However, a Cochrane systematic review failed to identify any randomized double-blind studies on bright light therapy for chronic primary insomnia that met rigorous inclusion criteria (Montgomery & Dennis, 2004a).

◆ **LEET may be beneficial in some cases of chronic insomnia** Low energy emission therapy employs a device that is held between the tongue and hard palate that emits low-frequency radio waves, with the goal of inducing relaxation or drowsiness. The mechanism of action is complex and probably involves radio wave–induced changes in EEG activity, and associated increased release of melatonin and GABA (Kaczmarek & Adey, 1973; Reiter, 1993). Findings of a small double-blind study suggest that regular nightly LEET treatments (15 minutes) reduce the time needed to fall asleep, and improve the duration and quality of sleep in chronic insomniacs (Pasche et al., 1996). Adverse effects or discontinuation effects have not been reported by patients who use this approach. LEET is not commercially available in the United States at present, and its use requires careful training and specialized technical knowledge. However, pending continued findings verifying its efficacy and safety, LEET can be regarded as a potentially beneficial nonconventional treatment of chronic insomnia in cases where more established conventional or nonconventional approaches prove ineffective or in patients for whom nonbiological treatments are more appropriate. Like CES and other therapies based on electromagnetic energy, LEET avoids the risks associated with chronic benzodiazepine use.

◆ **Impulse magnetic field therapy may be beneficial in some cases of insomnia** Anecdotal reports and findings of double-blind studies suggest that exposure to magnetic fields may improve insomnia. In one placebo-controlled study, 101 patients complaining of insomnia characterized by delayed sleep onset, middle awakening, or nightmares were randomized to an active treatment group versus sham treatment. The treatment group received pulsed magnetic field therapy nightly over 4 weeks. Seventy percent of patients in the treatment group experienced significant improvement or complete remission of all target symptoms in contrast to 2% of patients in the sham treatment group (Pelka, Jaenicke, & Gruenwald, 2001). No adverse outcomes were reported.

◆ **Nighttime exposure to white noise may be an effective treatment for some cases of insomnia** Nighttime exposure to a white noise background may be an effective treatment in some cases of insomnia (Lopez, Bracha, & Bracha, 2002). White noise is believed to reduce middle awakenings by increasing the threshold of perceived sounds during sleep. This approach is inexpensive, and adverse effects have not been reported.

Treatment Approaches Based on Forms of Information or Energy That Are Not Validated by Western Science

At the time of writing, there are no treatment approaches in this category.

◆ The Integrative Management Algorithm for Disturbances of Sleep and Wakefulness

Figure 14–1 is the integrative management step-by-step approach to evaluation and treatment of disturbances of sleep and wakefulness. Note that specific assessment and treatment approaches are representative examples of reasonable choices. Moderate symptoms often respond to exercise, dietary modification, mind–body practices, and energy-information therapies. When managing severe symptoms, emphasize biological therapies. Encourage exercise and other lifestyle changes in motivated patients. Consider conventional, nonconventional, and integrative approaches that have not been tried.

See evidence tables and text for complete reviews of evidence-based options.

Before implementing any treatment plan, always check evidence tables and Web site updates at www.thieme.com/mentalhealth for specific assessment and treatment protocols, and obtain patient informed consent.

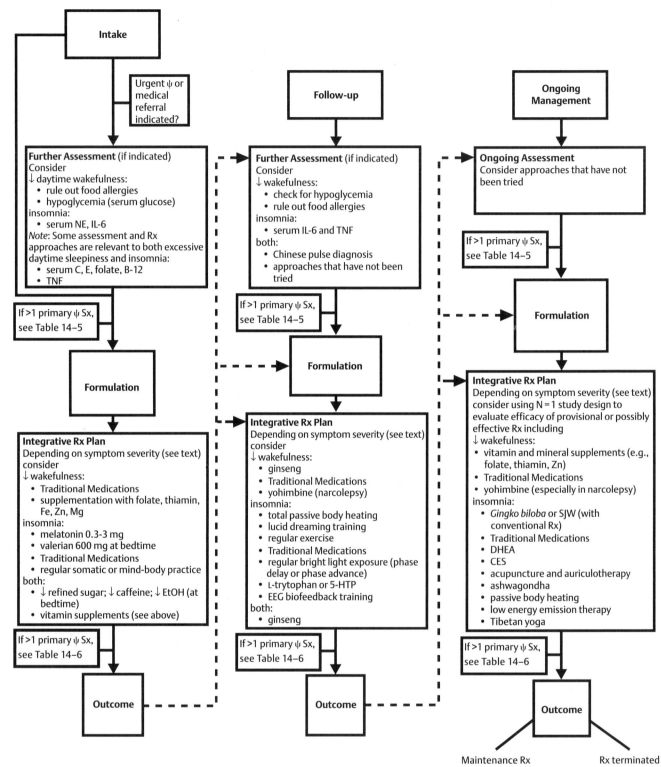

Figure 14–1 Integrative management step-by-step approach for evaluation and treatment of disturbances of sleep and wakefulness. Note that specific assessment and treatment approaches are representative examples of reasonable choices. Moderate symptoms often respond to exercise, dietary modification, mind–body practices, and energy-information therapies. Rx, treatment; Sx, symptoms

◆ Integrated Approaches to Consider When Two or More Core Symptoms Are Present

Table 14–5 shows the assessment approaches to consider using when a disturbance or nighttime sleep or daytime wakefulness is the focus of clinical attention and one or more other symptoms are being assessed concurrently.

Table 14–6 outlines the treatment approaches to consider using when a disturbance of nighttime sleep or daytime wakefulness is the focus of clinical attention and one or more other symptoms are being treated concurrently.

Table 14–5 Assessment Approaches to Disturbance of Nighttime Sleep or Daytime Wakefulness When Other Symptoms Are Being Assessed Concurrently

Other Symptom(s) Being Assessed Concurrently	Assessment Approach	Comments
Depressed mood	Serologic studies	Deficiencies in vitamins C, E, B$_{12}$, and folic acid are correlated with increased daytime sleepiness and insomnia.
		Abnormally low serum levels of magnesium and zinc are often associated with increased daytime sleepiness.
		Limited evidence suggests that abnormally high nighttime serum norepinephrine levels and abnormally low nighttime IL-6 and TNF serum levels are associated with increased rates of chronic insomnia, and that abnormally high daytime serum levels of IL-6 and TNF are associated with an increased risk of excessive daytime somnolence.
		Low serum folate levels predict nonresponse to conventional and nonconventional treatments of depressed mood
	Chinese pulse diagnosis	Limited evidence suggests that Chinese pulse diagnosis provides clinically useful information about energetic imbalances that manifest as daytime sleepiness or nighttime wakefulness.
		Recent grief, anguish, agitated depression, and hysterical depression are associated with distinctive pulse characteristics, according to TCM theory
Mania and cyclic mood changes	Serologic studies	Low trace lithium levels (i.e., from low nutritional intake) are common in acutely manic patients.
		Limited evidence suggests that pretreatment serum GABA levels predict improved response of mania and cyclic mood changes to divalproex (Depakote) but not other mood stabilizers
	qEEG brain mapping	Limited evidence suggests that pretreatment qEEG in acutely manic or cycling patients (showing left-sided abnormalities) predicts improved response to conventional treatments
	Analysis of the VAS	Limited evidence suggests that analysis of the VAS provides useful information when evaluating energetic factors related to mania
Anxiety	Serologic studies	Deficiencies of vitamins B$_6$, C, and E and niacin are sometimes associated with generalized anxiety.
		Limited evidence suggests that total serum cholesterol is elevated in chronically anxious patients
	qEEG brain mapping	Limited evidence suggests that specific qEEG changes correspond to disparate anxiety syndromes
Psychosis	Serologic studies	Limited evidence suggests that abnormally low serum and RBC folate levels correlate with increased risk of schizophrenia and other psychotic syndromes.
		Limited evidence suggests that high pretreatment serum HVA levels predict improved response to lower doses of conventional antipsychotics in acutely manic patients with psychotic symptoms
	qEEG brain mapping	Limited evidence suggests that specific qEEG findings may correlate with disparate syndromes of chronic psychosis
Cognitive impairment	Serologic studies	Limited evidence suggests that abnormally low levels of zinc and magnesium are correlated with increased risk of developing Alzheimer's disease
	qEEG brain mapping	qEEG mapping provides useful information when planning EEG-biofeedback protocols addressing cognitive impairment in general.
		Specific qEEG findings correlate with Alzheimer's; specific VEP or AER findings correlate with milder cognitive impairment
Substance abuse or dependence	Serologic studies	The magnitude of serum deficiencies of A, C, and many B vitamins, as well as zinc, magnesium, and essential fatty acids, is an indicator of the severity of malnutrition related to alcohol abuse
	Analysis of the VAS	Limited evidence suggests that abnormal VAS reflex activity characterizes chronic alcohol or drug use

AER, auditory evoked response; EEG, electroencephalography; GABA, γ-aminobutyric acid; HVA, homovanillic acid; IL, interleukin; qEEG, quantitative electroencephalography; RBC, red blood cell (count); TCM, traditional Chinese medicine; TNF, tumor necrosis factor; VAS, vascular autonomic signal; VEP, visual evoked potential

Table 14–6   Treatment Approaches to Disturbance of Nighttime Sleep or Daytime Wakefulness When Other Symptoms Are Being Treated Concurrently

Other Symptom(s) Being Treated Concurrently	Treatment Approach	Comments
Depressed	Dietary changes	Alcohol use at bedtime causes rebound insomnia.
		Caffeine in beverages or medications causes insomnia; caffeine withdrawal causes daytime sleepiness and fatigue.
		Limited evidence suggests that refined sugar snacks at night cause rebound hypoglycemia and disturbed sleep
	Vitamins and minerals	Limited evidence suggests that restricting caffeine and refined sugar and increasing consumption of fatty fish and whole foods rich in B vitamins improve depressed mood and reduce the risk of becoming depressed
	Amino acid supplementation	Supplementation with folate, thiamine, iron, zinc, and magnesium in deficient individuals reduces daytime sleepiness and improves nighttime sleep.
		Folate 0.5 to 1 mg/day augments the effects of conventional antidepressants and SAMe.
		5-HTP and L-tryptophan probably reduce symptoms of mild or situational insomnia.
		5-HTP increases sleep duration in obstructive sleep apnea and narcolepsy.
		Combining L-tryptophan 2 g with a conventional antidepressant probably enhances antidepressant response and improves sleep quality.
		5-HTP 300 mg/day is probably as effective as conventional antidepressants for moderate depressed mood.
		Note: Some cases of treatment-refractory depression improve when 5-HTP 300 to 600 mg/day is combined with carbidopa or conventional antidepressants.
		l-tryptophan 1 to 2 g combined with bright light therapy is more effective than either approach alone in seasonal depressed mood.
		Limited evidence suggests that L-tryptophan 1 to 2 g is equivalent to imipramine 150 mg and other conventional antidepressants.
		Limited evidence suggests that L-tyrosine (500–1500 mg/day) has antidepressant effects and that L-phenylalanine is beneficial in depressed patients with low serum PEA levels.
		Limited evidence suggests that ALC 1 to 3 g/day in divided doses is beneficial in elderly depressed or depressed demented patients.
		Note: Supplementation with ALC should be considered when depression is related to post-traumatic brain injury or age-related cognitive decline
	St. John's wort (*Hypericum perforatum*)	Limited evidence suggests that St. John's wort improves sleep quality in depressed patients who respond to treatment.
		Standardized St. John's wort preparations 300 mg tid is comparable in efficacy to conventional antidepressants for moderate depressed mood. There are case reports of severe depression responding to higher doses (up to 1800 mg/day)
	Ginkgo biloba	Limited evidence suggests that *Ginkgo biloba* 240 mg/day used in combination with a conventional antidepressant improves the quality of sleep and reduces the frequency of middle awakenings in depressed patients.
		G. biloba may augment conventional antidepressants in treatment-refractory patients
	Ayurvedic herbs	Limited evidence suggests that Ashwagondha and an Ayurvedic compound herbal formula are effective treatments of chronic primary insomnia.
		Several Ayurvedic herbs and compound herbal formulas are probably beneficial for depression.
		Note: Patients taking Ayurvedic herbs should be supervised by an Ayurvedic physician
	Somatic and mind–body approaches	Many somatic and mind–body practices, including progressive muscle relaxation, massage, meditation, and guided imagery, are as effective as conventional sedative-hypnotics for mild to moderate insomnia.
		Regular physical exercise increases the quality and duration of sleep in the elderly.
		Limited evidence suggests that total passive body heating, especially taking a hot bath, soon before bedtime improves overall sleep quality and reduces the frequency of middle awakenings.
		Limited evidence suggests that regular daily practice of Tibetan yoga improves sleep quality and reduces the need for conventional hypnotics.
		Regular exercise at least 30 minutes 3 times a week is probably as effective as conventional antidepressants, St. John's wort, and cognitive therapy for moderate depressed mood.

Table 14–6 Treatment Approaches to Disturbance of Nighttime Sleep or Daytime Wakefulness When Other Symptoms Are Being Treated Concurrently (Continued)

Other Symptom(s) Being Treated Concurrently	Treatment Approach	Comments
		Exercising under bright light is more effective against depression than exercise or bright light alone.
		Mindfulness training is probably as effective as cognitive therapy in moderate depressed mood.
		Combining mindfulness training or guided imagery with conventional antidepressants is more effective than conventional treatments alone.
		Limited evidence suggests that regular yoga (breathing or postures) practice is as effective as conventional antidepressants in severe depressed mood
	Light exposure	Regular carefully timed bright light exposure resynchronizes phase-advanced or phase-delayed sleep to the patient's time zone.
		Limited evidence suggests that regular bright light exposure (10,000 lux for 30–40 minutes/day) improves depressed mood and has more rapid onset than conventional antidepressants.
		Limited evidence suggests that regular exposure to dim red or blue light is as effective as bright light exposure in seasonal depression.
		Limited evidence suggests that dim green light 2 hours before exposure to natural light accelerates response to conventional antidepressants
	Microcurrent electrical stimulation (CES and TES)	CES is probably beneficial in some cases of chronic insomnia.
		Patients who reported improved sleep following CES treatment exhibited increased "delta sleep" that continued months after treatments ended.
		Limited evidence suggests that daily 40-minute CES treatments is beneficial in some cases of depressed mood
	Biofeedback	Some EEG-biofeedback protocols, especially SMR (alpha-theta training), are effective treatments of chronic insomnia.
		Limited evidence suggests that combined EEG-HRV biofeedback (energy cardiology) training improves depressed mood
	Acupuncture	Some acupuncture and auriculotherapy protocols probably reduce the severity of sleep disturbances, including insomnia related to a mental or emotional problem.
		Limited evidence suggests that conventional acupuncture is effective against severe depressed mood.
		Limited evidence suggests that electroacupuncture alone is as effective as electroacupuncture combined with amitriptyline or other conventional antidepressants.
		Limited evidence suggests that computer-controlled electroacupuncture using high-frequency currents is more effective than conventional or standard electroacupuncture
Mania and cyclic mood changes	Vitamins and minerals	Limited evidence suggests that folic acid 200 μg/day augments the effects of lithium in mania and that monthly B$_{12}$ injections reduce the risk of recurring manic episodes.
		Limited evidence suggests that magnesium supplementation 40 mEq/day is an effective treatment of rapid cycling episodes, and that potassium 20 mEq bid reduces lithium-induced tremor and improves compliance
	Mind–body approaches	Limited evidence suggests that certain yogic breathing practices and postures reduce the severity of mania or hypomania
	Mindfulness training	Limited evidence suggests that certain meditation practices promote calmness and are beneficial in mania or hypomania
Anxiety	Dietary modifications	Limited evidence suggests that avoiding refined sugar and caffeine and increasing protein and foods containing tryptophan reduce symptoms of generalized anxiety and panic
	Vitamins and minerals	Limited evidence suggests that phosphorus reduces the frequency of panic attacks, and that magnesium 100 to 200 mg reduces symptoms of generalized anxiety
	Ayurvedic herbs	Ashwagondha is an Ayurvedic herbal used to treat anxiety and chronic stress
	Somatic approaches	Regular aerobic or strengthening exercise reduces generalized anxiety symptoms, and there is limited evidence that exercise may also reduce the frequency and severity of panic attacks
	Microcurrent electrical stimulation	Limited evidence suggests that microcurrent stimulation of the paraspinal regions reduces the severity of PTSD symptoms

(Continued)

Table 14–6 Treatment Approaches to Disturbance of Nighttime Sleep or Daytime Wakefulness When Other Symptoms Are Being Treated Concurrently (Continued)

Other Symptom(s) Being Treated Concurrently	Treatment Approach	Comments
Psychosis	Dietary changes	Limited evidence suggests that chronically psychotic patients with higher intake of unsaturated fats, reduced gluten, and improved glucose regulation may experience milder symptoms
	Vitamins	Combining niacin (in the form of nicotinomide 3–8 g), folate (in the form of methylfolate 15 mg), or thiamine (500 mg tid) with conventional antipsychotics may improve outcomes.
		Note: Flushing and discomfort are associated with large doses of niacin and reportedly diminished when niacin is taken in the form of niacinamide
	Ginkgo biloba	Combining *Ginkgo biloba* (360 mg/day) with a conventional antipsychotic may be more effective for both positive and negative symptoms compared with conventional treatments alone
	Ayurvedic herbs	Limited evidence suggests that Brahmyadiyoga 8 to 12 g is as effective as conventional antipsychotics; Mentat may reduce severity of negative psychotic symptoms
	Acupuncture	Daily 15-minute laser acupuncture treatments of the yamen point may reduce psychotic symptoms in schizophrenics
	Somatic and mind–body approaches	Limited evidence suggests that a sensory stimulation technique known as the Wilbarger method improves sensory integration in schizophrenics
	Spiritually oriented group therapy and mindfulness training	Combining spiritually oriented group therapy with yogic breathing practice and conventional medications improves global functioning in stable chronically psychotic patients.
		Caution: Patients who are delusional or have other acute psychotic symptoms should be discouraged from participating in spiritual or religious practices.
		Limited evidence suggests that patients who have well-controlled psychotic symptoms benefit from social support in organized religious activity.
		Caution: Patients who are actively psychotic should be advised to avoid intense religious or spiritual activity
Cognitive impairment	Dietary changes	Moderate wine consumption, reduced saturated fats, and reduced total caloric intake are correlated with reduced risk of developing Alzheimer's disease.
		Limited evidence suggests that diets high in fish or other sources of omega-3 fatty acids and low in omega-6 fatty acids are associated with a reduced risk of developing dementia
	Vitamins and minerals	Limited evidence suggests that high niacin intake from food or supplements significantly reduces the risk of developing dementia and decreases the rate of cognitive decline in healthy elderly individuals
	Ayurvedic herbs	Limited evidence suggests that Ashwagondha 50 mg/kg improves short- and long-term memory and executive functioning in cognitively impaired individuals.
		Note: Individuals who use Ayurvedic herbs should do so only under the supervision of an Ayurvedic physician
	Somatic approaches	Limited evidence suggests that 4 to 8 weekly Snoezelen sessions reduces apathy and psychomotor agitation while enhancing language in demented individuals.
		Limited evidence suggests that regular massage therapy reduces agitated behavior in demented nursing home patients.
		Wander gardens allow demented or post-stroke patients to enjoy nature-related activities and reportedly improve baseline functioning in the early stages of dementia
	Microcurrent electrical stimulation	Two forms of microcurrent electrical stimulation—TENS and CES—resulted in improvements in word recall, face recognition, and motivation in demented individuals.
		Note: The beneficial effects of weak electrical stimulation are not sustained several weeks after treatment ends
	Light exposure	Limited evidence suggests that regular bright light (10,000 lux) exposure improves sleep, reduces "sundowning," reduces agitation and other inappropriate behaviors, and delays the time of peak agitation in Alzheimer's patients
	Biofeedback	EEG- and HR- biofeedback training may enhance cognitive performance in healthy adults.
		EEG biofeedback may accelerate recovery following stroke or traumatic brain injury
Substance abuse or dependence	Dietary changes	Alcoholics who improve their diets, including reduced intake of refined sugar and caffeine and increased intake of omega-3 fatty acids and protein, probably have an increased chance for maintaining sobriety
	Vitamins and minerals	Limited evidence suggests that thiamine reduces alcohol craving, nicotinic acid reduces the risk of alcohol dependence in chronic drinkers, and taking antioxidant vitamins soon before drinking reduces the severity of hangover symptoms

Table 14–6 Treatment Approaches to Disturbance of Nighttime Sleep or Daytime Wakefulness When Other Symptoms Are Being Treated Concurrently *(Continued)*

Other Symptom(s) Being Treated Concurrently	Treatment Approach	Comments
	Amino acid supplementation	Limited evidence suggests that supplementation of chronic alcoholics with magnesium and zinc improves global neuropsychological functioning and protects the brain against free radical damage.
		Taurine may reduce alcohol withdrawal symptoms; SAMe may reduce alcohol intake; ALC may enhance cognitive performance in abstinent alcoholics; L-tryptophan may reduce alcohol craving.
		Note: Alcoholics may have a general brain serotonin deficit
	Ayurvedic herbs	Limited evidence suggests that Ashwagondha and other traditionally used herbs and natural products reduces tolerance and decrease the severity of withdrawal from opiates, cocaine, and methamphetamine.
		Note: Human clinical trials do not support use of these herbals for the management of withdrawal from narcotics
	Somatic approaches	Limited evidence suggests that regular aerobic exercise or strength training in abstinent alcoholics improves general emotional well-being.
		Caution: All patients should consult with their primary care physician before starting a rigorous exercise program
	Mindfulness training and meditation	Abstinent alcoholics and addicts who engage in a regular mindfulness practice or meditation probably have a reduced risk of relapse.
		Spiritually focused support groups probably reduce relapse risk.
		Note: Transcendental meditation may be more effective at reducing the risk of relapse compared with other meditation styles
	Light exposure	Limited evidence suggests that regular exposure to dim morning light (250 lux) may reduce the risk of relapse in abstinent alcoholics with seasonal mood changes.
		Limited evidence suggests that increased abstinence results from improved mood
	Microcurrent electrical stimulation	Regular CES or TES treatments reduce symptoms of alcohol or opiate withdrawal but not nicotine withdrawal.
		Note: Both approaches reduce anxiety and improve cognitive functioning in alcoholics or drug addicts.
		Note: Optimum therapeutic effects are achieved when specific treatment protocols are employed
	Biofeedback	Limited evidence suggests that some EMG, thermal, and EEG-biofeedback protocols reduce alcohol relapse but not cocaine relapse.
		Limited evidence suggests that EEG-biofeedback training using alpha-theta training induces a relaxed, calm state that reduces the urge to drink
	Acupuncture	Some acupuncture points and protocols are probably more effective than others in reducing symptoms of alcohol or cocaine withdrawal

ALC, acetyl-L-carnitine; CES, cranioelectrotherapy stimulation; EEG; electroencephalography; EMG, electromyography; 5-HTP, 5-hydroxytryptophan; HRV, heart rate variability; PEA, phenylethylamine; PTSD, post-traumatic stress disorder; SAMe, S-adenosylmethionine; SMR, sensorimotor rhythm; TES, transcranial neuroelectric stimulation

Case Vignettes

History and Initial Presentation

Julie, a registered nurse, had been on the evening shift for 5 years before she realized that her general health was declining. Before being placed on the night shift, Julie had an irregular schedule for 2 years; prior to that, she had worked days in the intensive care unit (ICU). Although she had enjoyed the intensity of the ICU, the pace had been too intense, and there had been no time to raise her children. At the age of 32 Julie had chosen to "explore quieter options" in her nursing career. She accepted an evening position in the community hospital.

Julie was often abruptly awakened at 5:30 A.M., when her husband woke up to get ready for his commute to Silicon Valley, where he worked as an engineer. Mornings had gotten much easier in the past few years. Both of her children now slept through the night. After dropping the kids off at day care, Julie usually felt awake for a few hours and enjoyed going to a café for an espresso. The rest of her morning was spent running errands and straightening up around the house. Julie's efforts to take a nap before picking up the kids at 1:30 P.M. had been frustrated because of street noises and the phone ringing. After fetching the kids from school, she would usually sip on a diet soda to stay awake until her spouse arrived home around 7:00 P.M. Julie would then climb back into her car and drive the 2 miles up the winding highway to the hospital to start her next shift.

On busy nights Julie often felt herself tense and unable to focus, and sometimes there wasn't enough time to eat. During those shifts she used caffeinated coffee and soft drinks to keep going. Julie realized that she was making mistakes, sometimes not charting all the medications she had administered, sometimes forgetting to transcribe verbal orders. As she became more exhausted, she felt herself becoming more anxious. When the supervising nurse met with her for her 6-month review, Julie began to cry and felt an enormous sense of relief as she was told about her deficiencies. Terri had been nursing supervisor for the night shift for 6 years, and although demanding, she was also understanding and empathic. Terri wrote down the name and phone number of a local psychiatrist and suggested that Julie take a week off "to get some help."

Assessment, Formulation, and Treatment Plan

By the time Julie showed up at Dr. Ziegler's door, she had not worked for at least 5 days and had been sleeping ~10 hours every night. She continued to wake up in the middle of the night, sometimes two or three times. She felt drowsy much of the day, and had been drinking ~3 cups of caffeinated coffee on average. She felt almost constantly jittery and had not had a healthy meal in days. Julie described the daily anxiety, the mind–jarring fatigue, the problems getting a full night's sleep, and "playing musical parents" with her spouse, as well as her worries about "losing my mental edge." In the intake interview, Dr. Ziegler confirmed that Julie had no serious medical problems, did not have a history of manic episodes or severe depressive episodes, wasn't abusing alcohol or drugs, and had not experienced anxiety until a few months ago. He asked Julie about stress management, and she told him there had never been time to work on her stress. Dr. Ziegler described several relaxation approaches, including progressive muscle relaxation and guided imagery. He commented on the value of quiet music and recommended taking a hot bath before going to sleep. Dr. Ziegler advised Julie to stop drinking coffee in the morning and recommended putting on dark sunglasses when driving the kids to school, then returning home and sleeping again. He commented on the benefits of exercise, suggested dark shades for the bedroom windows, and briefly described

the therapeutic uses of bright light exposure and melatonin. He suggested avoiding refined sugar snacks while working and encouraged Julie to take a vitamin supplement including a good quality B complex. He briefly mentioned that Julie's circadian rhythms were out of phase and then commented on napping, suggesting that all naps should be short and restricted to the early afternoon hours before beginning the next night shift. Dr. Ziegler then described rebound insomnia from excessive evening caffeine consumption, and advised Julie to forgo caffeinated beverages after ~3:00 P.M. He advised her to take a controlled-release form of melatonin before going to bed. At the end of the session, Dr. Ziegler asked Julie if evening shift work was really necessary and invited her to consider ongoing psychotherapy to examine possible psychological issues that may have led to her decision to work in a way that was consistently resulting in severe stress and exhaustion.

Follow-up

Four weeks later, Dr. Ziegler hardly recognized Julie in the waiting room. Her eyes seemed brighter, and she appeared visibly younger. She had already started psychotherapy and had reviewed possible self-defeating aspects of some personal and professional choices. Julie had met with the nurse supervisor a few days after the initial session, and they had come to a mutual understanding. Julie was well regarded for her skill, but her colleagues realized that the evening shift was too difficult to maintain, given her parenting responsibilities and the guarantee of disrupted sleep for years to come. They had agreed that Julie would return to her previous position as a float nurse, with the goal of finding a day shift in a unit that was less stressful than the ICU. Since the date of that meeting, Julie had continued to follow Dr. Ziegler's advice about exercise, sleep hygiene, relaxation, and vitamins. She had initially used bright light and melatonin but had let go of these techniques a few weeks later after her sleep had normalized.

References

Aizawa, R., Kanbayashi, T., Saito, Y., Ogawa, Y., Sugiyama, T., Kitajima, et al. (2002). Effects of Yoku-kan-san-ka-chimpi-hange on the sleep of normal healthy adult subjects. *Psychiatry and Clinical Neurosciences, 56*(3), 303–304.

American Sleep Disorders Association. (1997). *International Classification of Sleep Disorders: Diagnostic and coding manual* (Rev.). Rochester, MN: Author.

Ancoli-Israel, S. (1999). Roth T characteristics of insomnia in the United States: Results of the 1991 National Sleep Foundation Survey. *Sleep, 22*(Suppl. 2), S347–S353.

Anderson, D., Noyes, R., Crowe, R., & Noyes, R., Jr. (1984). A comparison of panic disorder and generalized anxiety disorder. *American Journal of Psychiatry, 141*(4), 572–575.

Autret, A., Minz, M., Beillevaire, T., et al. (1977). Clinical and polygraphic effects of d, l-HTP on narcolepsy-cataplexy. *Biomedicine, 27*(5), 200–203.

Bakan, P. (1990). Confusion, lethargy and leukonychia. *Journal of Orthomolecular Medicine, 5*(4), 198–202.

Ballin, A., Berar, M., Rubinstein, U., et al. (1992). Iron state in female adolescents. *American Journal of Diseases of Children, 146*(7), 803–805.

Bersani, G., & Garavini, A. (2000). Melatonin add-on in manic patients with treatment resistant insomnia. *Progress in Neuro-Psychopharmacology and Biological Psychiatry, 24*, 185–191.

Botez, M., Botez, T., Leveille, J., et al. (1979). Neuropsychological correlates of folic acid deficiency: Facts and hypotheses. In M. I. Botex & E. H. Reynolds (Eds.), *Folic acid in neurology, psychiatry and internal medicine* (pp. 435–461). New York: Raven Press.

Boulos, Z., Campbell, S., Lewy, A., Terman, M., Dijk, D., & Eastman, C. (1995). Light treatment for sleep disorders: Consensus report. 7. Jet lag. *Journal of Biological Rhythms, 10*(2), 167–176.

Breslau, N., Roth, T., Rosenthal, L., et al. (1996). Sleep disturbances and psychiatric disorders: A longitudinal epidemiological study of young adults. *Biological Psychiatry, 39*, 411–418.

Brower, K. (2003). Insomnia, alcoholism and relapse. *Sleep Medicine Reviews, 7*(6), 523–539.

Brown, S., Salive, M., Pahor, M., et al. (1995). Occult caffeine as a source of sleep problems in an older population. *Journal of the American Geriatric Society, 43*(8), 860–864.

Brylowski, A., & McKay, D. (1991, April 26–27). *Lucid dreaming as a treatment for nightmares in posttraumatic stress of Vietnam combat veterans.* Presented at the Southern Association for Research in Psychiatry meeting, Tampa, FL.

Brzezinski, A., Vangel, M., Wurtman, R., Norrie, G., Zhdanova, I., & Ben-Shushan, A. (2005). Effects of exogenous melatonin on sleep: A meta-analysis. *Sleep Medicine Reviews, 9*, 41–50.

Buysse, D., Reynolds, C., Hauri, P., et al. (1994). Diagnostic concordance for DSM-IV sleep disorders: A report from the APA/NIMH DSM-IV field trial. *American Journal of Psychiatry, 151*(9), 1351–1360.

Campbell, S., Eastman, C., Terman, M., Lewy, A., Boulos, Z., & Dijk, D. (1995). Light treatment for sleep disorders: Consensus report. 1. Chronology of seminal studies in humans. *Journal of Biological Rhythms, 10*(2), 105–109.

Cartwright, R., & Weiss, M. (1975). The effects of electro-sleep on insomnia revisited. *Journal of Nervous and Mental Disease, 161*(2), 134–137.

Cheraskin, E., Ringsdorf, W., & Medford, F. (1976). Daily vitamin C consumption and fatigability. *Journal of the American Geriatric Society, 24*(3), 136–137.

Cohen, L., Warneke, C., Fouladi, R., et al. (2004). Psychological adjustment and sleep quality in a randomized trial of the effects of a Tibetan yoga intervention in patients with lymphoma. *Cancer, 100,* 2253–2260.

Coursey, R. D., Frankel, B. L., Gaarder, K. R., & Mott, D. E. (1980). A comparison of relaxation techniques with electrosleep therapy for chronic sleep-onset insomnia: A sleep-EEG study. *Biofeedback and Self-Regulation, 5*(1), 57–73.

Cricco, M., Simonsick, E., & Foley, D. (2001). The impact of insomnia on cognitive functioning in older adults. *Journal of the American Geriatric Society, 49*(9), 1185–1189.

Daan, S., & Lewy, A. J. (1984). Scheduled exposure to daylight: A potential strategy to reduce "jet lag" following transmeridian flight. *Psychopharmacology Bulletin, 20*(3), 566–568.

Das, S. N. (1994). Some pharmacological studies on Zeetress. *Indian Journal of Indigenous Medicine, 10*(2), 49–52.

Davis, W., & Ziady, F. (1976). Presented at the Second International Symposium on Magnesium, Montreal.

Dement, W., Hall. J., & Walsh, J. (2003). Tiredness versus sleepiness: Semantics or a target for public education? *Sleep, 26,* 485–486.

De Valck, E., & Cluydts, R. (2003). Sleepiness as a state-trait phenomenon, comprising both a sleep drive and a wake drive. *Medical Hypotheses, 60,* 509–512.

Dijk, D., Boulos, Z., Eastman, C., Lewy, A., Campbell S, & Terman, M. (1995). Light treatment for sleep disorders: Consensus report. 2. Basic properties of circadian physiology and sleep regulation. *Journal of Biological Rhythms, 10*(2), 113–125.

Doghramji, K. (2004). Assessment of excessive sleepiness and insomnia as they relate to circadian rhythm sleep disorders. *Journal of Clinical Psychiatry, 65*(Suppl. 16), 17–22.

Dollman, W., Le Blanc, V., & Roughhead, E. (2003). Managing insomnia in the elderly—what prevents us using non-drug options. *Journal of Clinical Pharmacy and Therapeutics, 28*(6), 485–491.

Dorsey, C. M., Lukas, S. E., Teicher, M. H., Harper, D., Winkelman, J. W., Cunningham, S. L., et al. (1996). Effects of passive body heating on the sleep of older female insomniacs. *Journal of Geriatric Psychiatry and Neurology, 9*(2), 83–90.

Drennan, M., Kripke, D., Klemfuss, H., & Moore, J. (1991). Potassium affects actigraph-identified sleep. *Sleep, 14*(4), 357–360.

Durlach, J., Durlach, V., Bac, P., et al. (1994). Magnesium and therapeutics. *Magnesium Research, 7*(3–4), 313–328.

Ellis, F., & Nasser, S. (1973). A pilot study of vitamin B12 in the treatment of tiredness. *British Journal of Nutrition, 30,* 277–283.

Field, T., Diego, M., Cullen, C., Hernandez-Reif, M., Sunshine, W., & Douglas, S. (2002). Fibromyalgia pain and substance P decrease and sleep improves after massage therapy. *Journal of Clinical Rheumatology, 8*(2), 72–76.

Flaws, B., & Lake, J. (2001). Insomnia. In *Chinese medical psychiatry: A textbook and clinical manual* (pp. 181–194). Boulder, CO: Blue Poppy Press.

Foley, D., Ancoli-Israel, S., Britz, P., & Walsh, J. (2004). Sleep disturbances and chronic disease in older adults: Results of the 2003 National Sleep Foundation Sleep in America survey. *Journal of Psychosomatic Research, 56*(5), 497–502.

Ford, D., & Kamerow, D. (1989). Epidemiologic study of sleep disturbance and psychiatric disorders: An opportunity for prevention. *Journal of the American Medical Association, 262*(11), 1479–1484.

Frankel, B., Buchbinder, R., & Snyder, F. (1973). Ineffectiveness of electrosleep in chronic primary insomnia. *Archives of General Psychiatry, 29,* 563–568.

Friess, E., Trachsel, L., Guldner, J., et al. (1995). DHEA administration increases rapid eye movement sleep and EEG power in the sigma frequency range. *American Journal of Physiology, 268*(1, pt. 1), E107–E113.

Fry, J. (1998). Treatment modalities for narcolepsy. *Neurology, 50*(Suppl. 1), S43–S48.

Gackenbach, J., & LaBerge, S. (Eds.). (1988). *Conscious mind, sleeping brain: Perspectives on lucid dreaming.* New York: Plenum Press.

Garfinkel, D., Laudon, M., & Zisapel, N. (1997). Improvement of sleep quality by controlled-release melatonin in benzodiazepine-treated elderly insomniacs. *Archives of Gerontology and Geriatrics, 24*(2), 223–231.

Garfinkel, D., Zisapel, N., Wainstein, J., & Laudon M. (1999). Facilitation of benzodiazepine discontinuation by melatonin: A new clinical approach. *Archives of Internal Medicine, 159*(20), 2456–2460.

Gerster, H. (1989). The role of vitamin C in athletic performance. *Journal of the American College of Nutrition, 8*(6), 636–643.

Hajak, G., Rodenbeck, A., Voderholzer, U., et al. (2001). Doxepin in the treatment of primary insomnia: A placebo-controlled, double-blind, polysomnographic study. *Journal of Clinical Psychiatry, 62,* 453–463.

Haponik, E. (1992). Sleep disturbances of older persons: Physicians' attitudes. *Sleep, 15*(2), 168–172.

Hara, C., Lopes, R., & Lima-Costa, M. (2004). Prevalence of excessive daytime sleepiness and associated factors in a Brazilian community: The Bambui study. *Sleep Medicine, 5,* 31–36.

Hauri, P. J., Percy, L., Hellekson, C., Hartmann, E., & Russ, D. (1982). The treatment of psychophysiologic insomnia with biofeedback: A replication study. *Biofeedback and Self-Regulation, 7*(2), 223–235.

Hearst, E., Cloninger, R., Crews, E., & Cadoret, R. (1974). Electrosleep therapy: A double-blind trial. *Archives of General Psychiatry, 30,* 463–466.

Hemmeter, U., Annen, B., Bischof, R., Bruderlin, U. Hatzinger, M., Rose, U., et al. (2001). Polysomnographic effects of adjuvant ginkgo biloba therapy in patients with major depression medicated with trimipramine. *Pharmacopsychiatry, 34*(2), 50–59.

Herings, R., Stricker, B., de Boer, A., et al. (1995). Benzodiazepines and the risk of falling leading to femur fractures: Dosage more important than elimination half-life. *Archives of Internal Medicine, 155*(16), 1801–1807.

Herxheimer, A., & Petrie, K. J. (2004). Melatonin for the prevention and treatment of jet lag (Cochrane Review). In *The Cochrane Library* (Issue 2). Chichester, UK: John Wiley & Sons.

Heseker, H., Kubler, W., Pudel, V., & Westenhoffer, J. (1992). Psychological disorders as early symptoms of a mild-moderate vitamin deficiency. *Annals of the New York Academy of Sciences, 669,* 352–357.

Higgins, C. (1995). Deficiency testing for iron, vitamin B-12 and folate. *Nursing Times, 91*(22), 38–39.

Holbrook, A. M., Crowther, R., Lotter, A., Cheng, C., & King, D. (2000). Meta-analysis of benzodiazepine use in the treatment of insomnia. *Canadian Medical Association Journal, 162*(2), 225–233.

Holsboer-Trachsler, E. (2000). Phytotherapeutics and sleep. *Schweizerische Rundschau fur Medizin Praxis, 89*(51–52), 2178–2182.

Hudgel, D. W., Gordon, E. A., & Meltzer, H. Y. (1995). Abnormal serotonergic stimulation of cortisol production in obstructive sleep apnea. *American Journal of Respiratory and Critical Care Medicine, 152*(1), 186–192.

Hughes, J. R., Higgins, S. T., Bickel, W. K., et al. (1991). Caffeine self-administration, withdrawal, and adverse effects among coffee drinkers. *Archives of General Psychiatry, 48,* 611–617.

Irwin, M., Clark, C., Kennedy, B., Christian Gillin, J., & Ziegler, M. (2003). Nocturnal catecholamines and immune function in insomniacs, depressed patients, and control subjects. *Brain, Behavior, and Immunity, 17*(5), 365–372.

Iwanovsky, A., & Dodge, C. H. (1968). Electrosleep and elecroanesthesia: Theory and clinical experience. *Foreign Science Bulletin, 4*(2), 1–64.

Kaczmarek, L., & Adey, W. (1973). The efflux of Ca and gamma-amino butyric acid from cat cerebral cortex. *Brain Research, 63,* 331–342.

Katz, D., & McHorney, C. (1998). Clinical correlates of insomnia in patients with chronic illness. *Archives of Internal Medicine, 158*(10), 1099–1107.

Kayumov, L., Brown, G., Jindal, R., et al. (2001). A randomized, double-blind, placebo-controlled crossover study of the effect of exogenous melatonin on delayed sleep phase syndrome. *Psychosomatic Medicine, 63,* 40–48.

Kimura, T., Saunders, P., & Kim, H. (1994). Interactions of ginsenosides with ligand-bindings of GABA-A, and GABA-B receptors. *General Pharmacology, 25,* 193–199

Kirsch, D. (2002). *The science behind cranial electrotherapy stimulation* (2nd ed.). Edmonton, Alberta, Canada: Medical Scope Publishing.

Kohnen, R., & Oswald, W. D. (1988). The effects of valerian, propanolol, and their combination on activation, performance, and mood of healthy volunteers under social stress conditions. *Pharmacopsychiatry, 21,* 447–448.

Kondo, N., Shinoda, S., Agata, H., et al. (1992). Lymphocyte responses to food antigens in food sensitive patients with allergic tension-fatigue syndrome. *Biotherapy, 5*(4), 281–284.

Krotkiewski, M., Gudmundsson, M., Backstrom, P., & Mandroukas, K. (1982). Zinc and muscle strength and endurance. *Acta Physiologica Scandinavica, 116*(3), 309–311.

Krystal, A. D., & Ressler, I. (2001). The use of valerian in neuropsychiatry. *CNS Spectrums, 6,* 841–847.

Kuleshova, E. A., & Riabova, N. V. (1989). Effect of iron deficiency of the body on the work capacity of women engaged in mental work. [in Russian]. *Terapevticheski arkhiv, 61*(1), 92–95.

Kunz, D., & Bes, F. (1997). Melatonin effects in a patient with severe REM sleep behavior disorder: Case report and theoretical considerations. *Neuropsychobiology, 36,* 211–214.

LaBerge, S., & Rheingold, H. (1990). *Exploring the world of lucid dreaming: A workbook of dream exploration and discovery that will help you put the ideas in Lucid Dreaming into practice.* New York: Ballantine Books.

Levine, Y. A. (1997). Music of the brain. In *Treatment of Insomnia Patients (Double Blind Research).* The Eighth International Rappaport Symposium and the Annual Meeting of the Israel Sleep Research Society held at the Sleep Disorders Centre, I. M.Sechenov Moscow Medical Academy, 83.

Levitan, R. D., Shen, J. H., Jindal, R., Driver, H. S., Kennedy, S. H., & Shapiro, C. M. (2000). Preliminary randomized double-blind placebo-controlled trial of tryptophan combined with fluoxetine to treat major depressive disorder: Antidepressant and hypnotic effects. *Journal of Psychiatry and Neuroscience, 15*(4), 337–346.

Lewy, A., Sack, R., & Singer, C. (1985).Treating phase typedchronobiologic sleep and mood disorders with appropriately timed bright artificial light. *Psychopharmacology Bulletin, 21*(3), 368–372.

Lewy, A., & Sack, R. (1986). Light therapy and psychiatry. *Proceedings of the Society for Experimental Biology and Medicine, 183,* 11–18.

Lin, Y. (1995). Acupuncture treatment for insomnia and acupuncture analgesia. *Psychiatry and Clinical Neurosciences, 49,* 119–120.

Lopez, H. H., Bracha, A. S., & Bracha, H. S. (2002). Evidence based complementary intervention for insomnia. *Hawaii Medical Journal, 61*(9), 192, 213.

Lyznicki, J., Doege, T., Davis, R., et al. (1998). Sleepiness, driving and motor vehicle crashes. *Journal of the American Medical Association, 279,* 1908–1913.

Mant, A., de Burgh, S., Mattick, R. P., Donnelly, N., & Hall, W. (1996). Insomnia in general practice: Results from the NSW General Practice Survey 1991–1992. *Australian Family Physician, 25*(Suppl. 1), S15–S18.

Mant, A., Mattick, R., de Burgh, S., et al. (1995). Benzodiazepine prescribing in general practice: Dispelling some myths. *Family Practice, 12*(1), 37–43.

Marasco, A., Ruiz, R., Villagomez, A., & Infante, C. (1996). Double-blind study of a multivitamin complex supplemented with ginseng extract. *Drugs Under Experimental and Clinical Research, 22,* 323–329.

McCall, W., Reboussin, B., & Cohen, W. (2000). Subjective measurement of insomnia and quality of life in depressed inpatients. *Journal of Sleep Research, 9*(1), 43–48.

McCurry, S. M., Logsdon, R. G., Teri, L., et al. (1999). Characteristics of sleep disturbance in community-dwelling Alzheimer's disease patients. *Journal of Geriatric Psychiatry and Neurology, 12*(2), 53–59.

Mitler, M., Jaudukovic, & Erman. M. (1993). Treatment of narcolepsy with methamphetamine. *Sleep, 16,* 306–317.

Mogi, T., Wada, Y., Hirosawa, I., et al. (1996). Epidemiological study on hypoglycemia endemic to female nurses and other workers. *Industrial Health, 34*(4), 335–346.

Montakab, H. (1999). Acupuncture and insomnia [in German]. *Forsch Komplementarmed* (Suppl. 1), 29–31.

Montgomery, P., & Dennis, J. (2004a). Bright light therapy for sleep problems in adults aged 60+ (Cochrane Review). In *The Cochrane Library* (Issue 2). Chichester, UK: John Wiley & Sons.

Montgomery, P., & Dennis, J. (2004b). Physical exercise for sleep problems in adults aged 60+ (Cochrane Review). In *The Cochrane Library* (Issue 2). Chichester, UK: John Wiley & Sons.

Morin, C. M., Colecchi, C., Stone, J., Sood, R., & Brink, D. (1999). Behavioral and pharmacological therapies for late-life insomnia: A randomized controlled trial [Comment]. *Journal of the American Medical Association, 281*(11), 991–999.

Morin, C., Culbert, J., & Schwartz, M. (1994). Nonpharmacological interventions for insomnia: A meta-analysis of treatment efficacy. *American Journal of Psychiatry, 151,* 1172–1180.

Morin, C., Gaulier, B., Barry, T., et al. (1992). Patients' acceptance of psychological and pharmacological therapies for insomnia. *Sleep, 15,* 302–305.

Morin, C. M., Hauri, P. J., Espie, C. A., Spielman, A. J., Buysse, D. J., & Bootzin, R. R. (1998). Nonpharmacologic treatment of chronic insomnia: An American Academy of Sleep Medicine Review. *Neuroscience and Behavioral Physiology, 22*(8), 1134–1156.

Murtagh, D. R., & Greenwood, K. M. (1995). Identifying effective psychological treatments for insomnia: A meta-analysis. *Journal of Consulting and Clinical Psychology, 63*(1), 79–89.

National Institutes of Health, Technology Assessment Panel. (1996). Integration of behavioral and relaxation approaches into the treatment of chronic pain and insomnia. *Journal of the American Medical Association, 276,* 313–318.

Obermeyer, W., & Benca, R. (1996). Effects of drugs on sleep. *Neurologic Clinics, 14*(4), 827–840.

Ohayon, M., Priest, R., Zulley, J., et al. (2002a). Prevalence ofnarcolepsy symptomatology and diagnosis in the European general population. *Neurology, 58*(12), 1826–1833.

Ohayon, M. (2002b). Epidemiology of insomnia: What we know and what we still need to learn. *Sleep Medicine Reviews, 6,* 97–111.

Ohayon, M., Priest, R., Zulley, J., Smirne, S., & Paiva, T. (2002). Prevalence of narcolepsy symptomatology and diagnosis in the European general population. *Neurology, 58,* 1826–1833.

Ohta, T., Ando, K., Iwata. T., et al. (1991). Treatment of persistent sleep–wake schedule disorders in adolescents with methylcobalamin (vitamin B$_{12}$). *Sleep, 14*(5), 414–418.

Pasche, B., Erman, M., Hayduk, R., et al. (1996). Effects of low energy emission therapy in chronic psychophysiological insomnia. *Sleep, 19,* 327–336.

Pelka, R. B., Jaenicke, C., & Gruenwald, J. (2001). Impulse magnetic-field therapy for insomnia: A double-blind, placebo-controlled study. *Advances in Therapy, 18*(4), 174–180.

Popoviciu, L., Asgian, B., Delast-Popoviciu, D., et al. (1993). Clinical, EEG, electromyographic and polysomnographic studies in restless legs syndrome caused by magnesium deficiency. *Romanian Journal of Neurology and Psychiatry, 31*(1), 55–61.

Popoviciu, L., Delast-Popoviciu, D., Delast-Popoviciu R, et al. (1990). Parasomnias (non-epileptic nocturnal episodic manifestations) in patients with magnesium deficiency. *Romanian Journal of Neurology and Psychiatry, 28*(1), 19–24.

Poyares, D. R., Guilleminault, C., Ohayon, M. M., & Tufik, S. (2002). Can valerian improve the sleep of insomniacs after benzodiazepine withdrawal? *Progress in Neuro-Psychopharmacology and Biological Psychiatry, 26*(3), 539–545.

Prabhu, M. Y., Rao, A., & Karanth, K. S. (1990). Neuropharmacological activity of Withania somnifera. *Fitoterapia, 61*(3), 237–240.

Rani, P, & Naidu, M. (1998). Subjective and polysomnographic evaluation of a herbal preparation in insomnia. *Phytomedicine, 5,* 253–257.

Reiter, R. J. (1993). Electromagnetic fields and melatonin production. *Biomedicine and Pharmacotherapy, 47,* 439–444.

Richardson, G., & Roth, T. (2001). Future directions in the management of insomnia. *Journal of Clinical Psychiatry, 62*(Suppl. 10), 39–45.

Riemann, D., Volderholzer, U., Cohrs, S., et al. (2002). Trimipramine in primary insomnia: Results of a polysomnographic double-blind controlled study. *Pharmacopsychiatry, 35,* 165–174.

Rogers, N., Dorrian, T., & Dinges, D. (2003). Sleep, waking and neurobehavioral performance. *Frontiers in Bioscience, 8,* S1056–S1067.

Rogers, N. L., Phan, O., Kennaway, D. J., & Dawson, D. (1998). Effect of daytime oral melatonin administration on neurobehavioral performance in humans. *Journal of Pineal Research, 25*(1), 47–53.

Salzer, H.M. (1966). Relative hypoglycemia as a cause of neuropsychiatric illness. *Journal of the National Medical Association,58*(1), 12–17.

Scharf, M., Brown, D., Woods, M., et al. (1985). The effects and effectiveness of gamma-hydroxybutyrate in patients with narcolepsy. *Journal of Clinical Psychiatry, 46,* 222–225.

Schneider-Helmert, D., & Spinweber, C. (1986). Evaluation of L-tryptophan for treatment of insomnia: A review. *Psychopharmacology (Berlin), 89*(1), 1–7.

Schultz, B., & Freedman, M. (1987). Iron deficiency in the elderly. *Baillière's Clinical Haematology, 1*(2), 291–313.

Schultz, V., Hubner, W. D., & Ploch, M. (1997). Clinical trials with phytopsychopharmacological agents. *Phytomedicine, 4,* 379–387.

Shamir, E., Laudon, M., Barak, Y., et al. (2000). Melatonin improves sleep quality of patients with chronic schizophrenia. *Journal of Clinical Psychiatry, 61,* 373–377.

Shamsi, Z., Stanley, N., Yoon, J., & Hindmarch, I. (1996). Effects of three doses of 3-indole pyruvic acid on subjective and objective measures of sleep and early morning performance. *Human Psychopharmacology, 11*(3), 235–239.

Shepherd, C. (1993). Sleep disorders: Liver damage warning with insomnia remedy. *British Medical Journal, 306,* 1477

Shi, Z. X., & Tan, M.Z. (1986). An analysis of the therapeutic effect of acupuncture in 500 cases of schizophrenia. *Journal of Traditional Chinese Medicine, 6*(2), 99–104.

Shinba, T., Murashima, Y., & Yamamoto, K. (1994). Alcohol consumption and insomnia in a sample of Japanese alcoholics. *Addiction, 89*(5), 587–592.

Siegel, J. (2004). The neurotransmitters of sleep. *Journal of Clinical Psychiatry, 65*(Suppl. 16), 4–7.

Smidt, L., Cremin, F., Grivetti, L. &, Clifford, A. (1991). Influence of thiamin supplementation on the health and general well-being of an elderly Irish population with marginal thiamin deficiency. *Journal of Gerontology, 46*(1), M16–M22.

Sok, S. R., Erlen, J. A., & Kim, K. B. (2003). Effects of acupuncture therapy on insomnia. *Journal of Advanced Nursing, 44*(4), 375–384.

Standards of Practice Committee of the American Academy of Sleep Medicine. (1999). An American Academy of Sleep Medicine report: Practice parameters for the nonpharmacologic treatment of chronic insomnia. *Sleep, 22*(8), 1134–1156.

Straand, J., & Rokstad, K. (1997). General practitioners' prescribing patterns of benzodiazepine hypnotics: Are elderly patients at particular risk from over prescribing? A report from the More & Romsdal Prescription study. *Scandinavian Journal of Primary Health Care, 15*(1), 16–21.

Suen, L. K., Wong, T. K., Leung, A. W., & Ip, W. C. (2003). The long-term effects of auricular therapy using magnetic pearls on elderly with insomnia. *Complementary Therapies in Medicine, 11*(2), 85–92.

Sweetwood, H., Grant, I., Kripke, D., et al. (1980). Sleep disorder over time: Psychiatric correlates among males. *British Journal of Psychiatry, 136,* 456–462.

Tahiliani, A., & Beinlich, C. (1991). Pantothenic acid in health and disease. *Vitamins and Hormones, 46,* 165–228.

Thannickal, T., Moore, R., Nienhuis, R., et al. (2000). Reduced number of hypocretin neurons in human narcolepsy. *Neuron, 27,* 469–474.

Thayer, R. (1987). Energy, tiredness, and tension effects of a sugar snack versus moderate exercise. *Journal of Personality and Social Psychology, 52*(1), 119–125.

Titlebaum, H. M. (1998). Relaxation. *Alternative Health Practitioner, 4*(2), 123–146.

U.S. Xyrem Multicenter Study Group. (2004). Sodium oxybate demonstrates long-term efficacy for the treatment of cataplexy in patients with narcolepsy. *Sleep Medicine, 5,* 119–123.

Vaidya, A. D. (1997). The status and scope of Indian medicinal plants acting on central nervous system. *Indian Journal of Pharmacology, 29*(5), S340–S343.

Vgontzas, A. N., Zoumakis, M., Papanicolaou, D. A., et al. (2002). Chronic insomnia is associated with a shift of interleukin-6 and tumor necrosis factor secretion from nighttime to daytime. *Metabolism, 51*(7), 887–892.

Walsh, J., & Schweitzer, P. (1999). Ten-year trends in the pharmacological treatment of insomnia. *Sleep, 22*(3), 371–375.

Weiss, M. (1973). The treatment of insomnia through use of electrosleep: An EEG study. *Journal of Nervous and Mental Disease, 157*(2), 108–120.

Wheatley, D. (2001). Stress-induced insomnia treated with kava and valerian: Singly and in combination. *Human Psychopharmacology, 16*(4), 353–356.

Wooten, V. (1994). Effectiveness of yohimbine in treating narcolepsy. *Southern Medical Journal, 87,* 1065–1066.

Xu, G. (1997). [Forty-five cases of insomnia treated by acupuncture]. *Shanghai Journal of Acupuncture and Moxibustion, 16,* 6–10.

Zhdanova, I. V., Wurtman, R. J., Regan, M. M., Taylor, J. A., Shi, J. P., & Leclair, O. U. (2001). Melatonin treatment for age-related insomnia. *Journal of Clinical Endocrinology and Metabolism, 86*(10), 4727–4730.

Ziegler, G., Ploch, M., Miettinen-Baumann, A., & Collet, W. (2002). Efficacy and tolerability of valerian extract LI 156 compared with oxazepam in the treatment of non-organic insomnia: A randomized, double-blind, comparative clinical study. *European Journal of Medical Research, 7*(11), 480–486.

Zisselman, M., Rovner, B., Kelly, K., & Woods, C. (1994). Benzodiazepine utilization in a university hospital. *American Journal of Medical Quality, 9*(3), 138–141.

Appendix A

Assessment and Treatment Approaches by Core Symptom and Level of Evidence

◆ **Assessment Approaches**, 329
   Substantiated (in current use and effective)
   Provisional assessment approaches
   Possibly specific assessment approaches/all symptoms
◆ **Treatment Approaches**, 332
   Substantiated treatments (in current use and effective)
   Provisional treatments/all symptoms
   Possibly effective treatments/all symptoms

◆ Assessment Approaches

Substantiated (in Current Use and Effective)

Approaches listed in **Table A–1** are characterized by the following:

1. Systematic review findings are compelling or strongly support claims that a particular assessment modality provides accurate information about the causes or meanings of a symptom pattern, OR
2. Three or more rigorously conducted cohort studies support claims of outcomes of the modality with respect to a specified symptom pattern.
3. The modality is in current use for the assessment of a specified symptom pattern, AND
4. The use of the modality with respect to a specified symptom pattern is endorsed by a relevant professional association.

Provisional Assessment Approaches

Provisional (in Current Use and Probably Effective)

Approaches listed in **Table A–2** are characterized by the following:

1. Systematic review findings are highly suggestive but not compelling, or have not been conducted because of insufficient numbers of studies or uneven quality of completed studies; OR
2. Three or more rigorously conducted double-blind, randomized controlled trials (cohort studies for assessment approaches) yield findings that are suggestive but not compelling; AND
3. The approach is in current use for the assessment of a specified symptom pattern.
4. The use of the modality with respect to a specified symptom pattern may be endorsed by a relevant professional association.

Table A–1   Substantiated Assessment Approaches

Symptom	Approach	Comment
Depression	Serum levels of certain vitamins	Low serum folate predicts nonresponse to conventional and nonconventional treatments.
		Low vitamin B_{12} and E levels often found in depressed patients
	Serum triglyceride and cholesterol levels	Low total serum triglycerides and cholesterol levels correlate with more severe depressed mood and higher risk of suicide
	qEEG brain mapping and AEP	Increased alpha (α) or theta (θ) power, decreased interhemispheric coherence in unipolar depression.
		Reduced α and increased beta (β) power in bipolar depression.
		High AEP predicts improved response to SSRIs.
		Negative prefrontal cordance predicts improved response to SSRIs and homeopathic treatments
Mania and cyclic mood changes	None at time of writing	
Anxiety	None at time of writing	
Psychosis	None at time of writing	
Dementia and cognitive impairment	qEEG and neurometric brain mapping	qEEG mapping shows correlations between cognitive impairment related to dementia or stroke (CVA) and diminished activity in the alpha and beta ranges; neurometric brain mapping compares qEEG findings with normative age-matched brain activity
Alcohol and substance abuse	None at time of writing	
Disturbances of nighttime sleep and daytime wakefulness	None at time of writing	

AEP, auditory evoked potential; CVA, cerebrovascular accident; qEEG, quantitative electroencephalography; SSRI, selective serotonin reuptake inhibitor

Table A–2   Provisional Assessment Approaches

Symptom	Approach	Comment
Depression	RBC fatty acids	Low RBC omega-3 fatty acids are correlated with more severe depressed mood
	qEEG brain mapping	Low RBC n-3 fatty acids are correlated with more severe depressed mood
Mania and cyclic mood changes	RBC folate level	Abnormally low RBC folate levels (but normal serum folate levels) are common in bipolar patients
	qEEG brain mapping	Left-sided qEEG abnormalities in acute mania may correlate with improved response to conventional treatments
Anxiety	qEEG and HRV analysis	Specific qEEG changes may correspond to disparate anxiety symptoms
		In patients diagnosed with obsessive-compulsive disorder, increased α power predicts response to SSRIs, and increased θ power predicts nonresponse to SSRIs
Psychosis	RBC fatty acid levels	Consistently low RBC levels of two fatty acids (arachidonic acid and DHA) suggests low brain levels in schizophrenia
	Serum DHEA levels	Abnormally low serum DHEA may correlate with increased risk of schizophrenia
	Niacin challenge test	Schizophrenics exhibit a reduced flushing response to niacin
	Serum estradiol levels (in women)	Abnormally low serum estradiol levels in women may correspond to increased risk of developing psychosis
	Serum and RBC folate levels	Abnormal low serum and RBC folate levels may correlate with increased risk of schizophrenia and other psychotic syndromes
	qEEG brain mapping	Specific qEEG findings may correlate with disparate symptom patterns
Dementia and cognitive impairment	Serum zinc and magnesium levels	Abnormally low levels of zinc and magnesium may correlate with the risk of developing Alzheimer's disease; however, findings are inconsistent
	qEEG and VEP or AEP	Specific qEEG findings correlate with Alzheimer's disease; specific VEP or AEP findings correlate with milder cognitive impairment
	VR testing	VR testing environments will permit earlier and more accurate assessment of moderate and severe cognitive impairment

Table A–2 Provisional Assessment Approaches *(Continued)*

Symptom	Approach	Comment
Alcohol and substance abuse	Serum nutrient levels	The magnitude of serum deficiencies of vitamins A and C and many B vitamins, as well as zinc, magnesium, and essential fatty acids, is an indicator of the severity of malnutrition related to alcohol abuse
	Serum homocysteine levels	Elevated serum homocysteine is an indicator of chronic alcohol abuse and returns to normal levels soon after cessation of alcohol abuse
	AEP	Abnormal AEP findings are common in heroin addicts and may predict increased risk of developing substance abuse problems in youth
Disturbances of nighttime sleep and daytime wakefulness	Serum levels of several vitamins and minerals	Deficiencies in folic acid and vitamins B$_{12}$, C, and E are correlated with increased daytime sleepiness and insomnia.
		Abnormally low serum levels of magnesium and zinc are often associated with increased daytime sleepiness

AEP, auditory evoked potential; DHA, docosahexaenoic acid; DHEA, dehydroepiandrosterone; HRV, heart rate variability; qEEG, quantitative electroencephalography; RBC, red blood cell (count); SSRI, selective serotonin reuptake inhibitor; VR, virtual reality

Possibly Specific Assessment Approaches/All Symptoms

Possibly Effective (in Current Use and Possibly Effective)

Approaches listed in **Table A–3** are characterized by the following:

1. Research findings or anecdotal reports are limited or inconsistent AND
2. There are insufficient quality studies on which to base a systematic review or meta-analysis.
3. The modality is currently used but remains controversial and may be endorsed by a relevant professional association.

Table A–3 Possibly Specific Assessment Approaches

Symptom	Approach	Comment
Depression	Dexamethasone suppression test	Serum cortisol levels are suppressed following dexamethasone in severely depressed women but not in men
	Urinary PEA and PAA	PEA and PAA levels may be consistently low in bipolar depressed mood
	Chinese medical pulse diagnosis and VAS reflex	Low PEA (or PAA) suggests dietary amino acid deficiency or metabolic problem
	Homeopathic constitutional assessment	A specific energetic pattern obtained using pulse diagnosis or VAS may suggest the most effective energetic or conventional treatment for depressed mood
	Applied kinesiology	Constitutional analysis may permit identification of most effective homeopathic remedies.
		Findings on applied kinesiology testing suggest certain kinds of energetic treatments
Mania and cyclic mood changes	Serum lithium level	Supplementation with trace lithium in the diet may reduce the risk of acute mania in predisposed individuals
	Serum GABA level	Manic patients with low pretreatment serum GABA levels should be preferentially started on divalproex (Depakote)
	CNS *N*-acetylaspartate	A possible beneficial role of supplementation remains unclear
	MRS	MRS is not indicated as a routine screening approach for at-risk children
	Serum HVA	Check serum HVA level to estimate effective dose range when treating an acute manic episode to achieve optimum antipsychotic dosing strategy and minimize risk of adverse effects
	VAS analysis	Measuring the VAS reflex is an easy and inexpensive method that can be used adjunctively in integrative treatment planning
Anxiety	Total serum cholesterol	Total serum cholesterol may be elevated in chronically anxious patients
	Serum vitamin levels	Deficiencies of niacin and vitamins B6, C, and E may be associated with generalized anxiety
	Serum mineral levels	Deficiencies of magnesium, selenium, and phosphorus may be associated with chronic anxiety
	Urinary glutamate level	High urinary glutamate levels may correlate with general anxiety
	Constitutional assessment	Constitutional assessment findings may guide selection of effective homeopathic remedies in anxious patients

Table A–3 Possibly Specific Assessment Approaches *(Continued)*

Symptom	Approach	Comment
	EDST	EDST may provide a way to measure energetic changes following Healing Touch or conventional treatments of anxiety
Psychosis	Serum phospholipase A$_2$	Supplementation with omega-3 fatty acids may compensate for the acquired trait of abnormally high phospholipase A$_2$ levels
	Serum HVA levels	Abnormally high serum HVA levels may predict lower effective doses of first-generation antipsychotics
	Brain glutamate levels	Dietary modifications addressing abnormal brain glutamate activity may ameliorate psychotic symptoms
	VAS	The VAS reflex may provide clinically useful information for identifying treatments and doses that will be effective in previously nonresponsive patients
Dementia and cognitive impairment	Serum levels of vitamins and trace elements	Chronic malnutrition caused by malabsorption of essential dietary factors may increase the risk of developing Alzheimer's disease or mild cognitive impairment
	Serum DHA levels	Abnormally low serum DHA levels may correlate with increased risk of developing Alzheimer's disease
Alcohol and substance abuse	qEEG	qEEG brain mapping may prove useful in planning specific EEG-biofeedback protocols for relapsing alcoholics or narcotics abusers
	VAS reflex	VAS analysis may provide clinically useful information about most effective acupuncture and conventional detoxification protocols
Disturbances of nighttime sleep and daytime wakefulness	Serum levels of norepinephrine, IL-6, and TNF	Abnormally high nighttime serum norepinephrine levels and abnormally low nighttime serum IL-6 and TNF levels may be associated with increased rates of chronic insomnia.
		Abnormally high daytime serum levels of IL-6 and TNF may be associated with increased risk of excessive daytime sleepiness
	Check for food allergies	Sensitivities to dairy and wheat products may result in increased daytime sleepiness
	Check for hypoglycemia	Hypoglycemia may result in increased daytime sleepiness

CNS, central nervous system; DHA, docosahexaenoic acid; EDST, electrodermal skin testing; EEG, electroencephalography; GABA, γ-aminobutyric acid; HVA, homovanillic acid; IL, interleukin; MRS, magnetic resonance spectroscopy; PAA, phenylacetic acid; PEA, phenylethylamine; qEEG, quantitative electroencephalography; TNF, tumor necrosis factor; VAS, vascular autonomic signal

◆ Treatment Approaches

Substantiated Treatments (in Current Use and Effective)

Approaches listed in **Table A–4** are characterized by the following:

1. Systematic review findings are compelling or strongly support claims that a particular treatment approach results in consistent positive outcomes with respect to a specified symptom pattern; OR

2. Three or more rigorously conducted double-blind, randomized controlled trials support claims of outcomes of the modality with respect to a specified symptom pattern.

3. The modality is in current use for the treatment of a specified symptom pattern, AND

4. The use of the modality with respect to a specified symptom pattern is endorsed by a relevant professional association.

Table A–4 Substantiated Treatment Approaches

Symptom	Approach	Comment
Depression	St. John's wort	Standardized St. John's wort preparations 300 mg tid comparable to conventional antidepressants for moderate depressed mood.
		Case reports of severe depression responding to higher doses (up to 1800 mg/day)
	SAMe	SAMe 400 to 1600 mg/day has comparable efficacy to conventional antidepressants.
		SAMe has synergistic beneficial effects when combined with folate (1 mg), vitamin B$_{12}$ (800 μg), or conventional antidepressants.
		SAMe accelerates response, improves outcomes, and may lower effective doses of conventional antidepressants.
		Case reports of response in treatment-refractory patients
	Vitamins (including folate and vitamins B$_6$, B$_{12}$, C, D, and E)	Folate 0.5 to 1 mg/day augments the effects of conventional antidepressants, and SAMe patients with normal vitamin B$_{12}$ serum levels respond better to conventional antidepressants than patients who are B$_{12}$ deficient.
		Large doses of vitamin D 100,000 IU may be more effective than bright light therapy in seasonal depressed mood

Table A–4 Substantiated Treatment Approaches (*Continued*)

Symptom	Approach	Comment
	Omega-3 fatty acids	Combining omega-3 fatty acids (especially EPA) 1 to 2 g/day with conventional antidepressants improves response and may accelerate response rate.
		Case reports of EPA effective in severe depressed mood
	Exercise	Regular exercise at least 30 minutes 3 times a week is as effective as conventional antidepressants, St. John's wort, and cognitive therapy for moderate depressed mood.
		Exercising under bright light is more effective than exercise or bright light alone
	Bright light exposure	Regular bright light exposure (10,000 lux for 30—40 minutes/day) improves depressed mood and may have more rapid onset than conventional antidepressants. Bright artificial and natural light are equally effective.
		Benefits are greater when there is a seasonal pattern.
		Safe conventional treatment of depression in pregnant women.
		Exposure to bright light when exercising is more effective than either approach alone
Mania and cyclic mood changes	None at time of writing	
Anxiety	Kava (*Piper methysticum*)	Kava 70 to 240 mg/day is probably as effective as conventional drugs for generalized anxiety.
		Caution: Rare cases of liver failure are probably related to contamination.
		Caution: Avoid concurrent use of benzodiazepines
	L-theanine	L-theanine 50 to 200 mg/day is effective for moderate anxiety, 800 mg/day in divided doses for more severe anxiety
	Relaxation and guided imagery	Relaxation is as effective as conventional treatments of moderate generalized anxiety.
		Guided imagery is beneficial for generalized anxiety, panic, and traumatic memories.
		Caution: Panic attacks have been reported during relaxation exercises in predisposed patients
	Yoga	Regular yoga practice is beneficial for many anxiety symptoms and may permit reductions in conventional medications
	Meditation and mindfulness-based stress reduction	Regular meditation or mindfulness training reduces symptoms of generalized anxiety.
		Mindfulness training reduces the severity of physical symptoms associated with chronic anxiety, including irritable bowel syndrome
	VRGET	VRGET is as effective as conventional exposure therapies for specific phobias, social phobia, and panic disorder.
		Caution: Psychotic patients, patients with seizure disorders or other neurologic disorders, and substance-abusing patients should be advised against using VRGET
	Videoconferencing	Videoconferencing permits establishment of a therapeutic alliance and is as effective as face-to-face CBT for many anxiety symptoms, including agoraphobia and panic attacks
	Biofeedback	EEG, EMG, GSR, and thermal biofeedback are effective treatments of generalized anxiety and may permit dose reductions of conventional drugs.
		Combined GSR biofeedback and relaxation is more effective than either approach alone
	Microcurrent electrical stimulation (CES)	Microcurrent electrical stimulation (CES) has comparable efficacy to conventional drug treatments of generalized anxiety and phobias and may permit dose reductions of conventional drugs
Psychosis	None at time of writing	
Dementia and cognitive impairment	Dietary modification	Moderate wine consumption, reduced saturated fats, and reduced total caloric intake are correlated with reduced risk of developing Alzheimer's disease
	Ginkgo biloba	Standardized extracts of *G. biloba* 120 to 600 mg/day improve memory and cognitive performance in mild to moderate Alzheimer's disease, vascular dementia, and post-stroke patients and may slow cognitive decline in severe dementia.
		Combining *G. biloba* with ginseng enhances cognitive performance in nonimpaired healthy adults
		Possibly enhanced effect when combined with piracetam or CDP-choline.
		Caution: G. biloba is contraindicated in patients taking anticoagulants.
		Cases of serotonin syndrome have been reported when combined with SSRIs
	Huperzine-A (*Huperzia serrata*)	Huperzine-A 200 to 400 μg may have beneficial effects in age-related memory loss and Alzheimer's disease that are comparable to conventional cholinesterase inhibitors

(Continued)

Table A–4   Substantiated Treatment Approaches *(Continued)*

Symptom	Approach	Comment
	CDP-choline	CDP-choline enhances the rate of cognitive recovery following stroke and may be beneficial in traumatic brain-injured patients.
		Note: CDP-choline may not improve attention, but it does improve global functioning and memory
	Phosphatidylserine	Phosphatidylserine (300 mg/day) is beneficial for age-related cognitive decline and Alzheimer's disease.
		Caution: Bovine brain-derived phoshatidylserine is probably more effective than the soy-derived product, but there is growing concern over acquiring a slow virus from infected brain tissue
	Idebenone	Idebenone 360 mg may be more effective than conventional cholinesterase inhibitors in the treatment of mild to moderate Alzheimer's disease. Post-stroke recovery may be enhanced by combining idebenone with vinpocetine.
		Note: Use of idebenone in post-stroke patients is based on animal studies and must be confirmed by human clinical trials before being recommended
	Exercise	Regular physical exercise in healthy elderly individuals significantly reduces the risk of all categories of dementia.
		Note: Exercise is probably not an effective intervention after the onset of dementia.
		Caution: Individuals who have been sedentary or who have a chronic pain syndrome or a major medical illness should be evaluated by a physician before starting a rigorous exercise program
Alcohol and substance abuse	CES and TES	Regular CES or TES treatments reduce symptoms of alcohol or opiate withdrawal but not nicotine withdrawal; both approaches reduce anxiety and improve cognitive functioning in alcoholics and drug addicts.
		Note: Optimum therapeutic effects are achieved when specific treatment protocols are employed
Disturbances of nighttime sleep and daytime wakefulness	Dietary changes	Alcohol use at bedtime causes rebound insomnia.
		Caffeine in beverages or medications causes insomnia; caffeine withdrawal causes daytime sleepiness and fatigue.
		Refined sugar snacks at night cause rebound hypoglycemia and disturbed sleep
	Melatonin	Melatonin at doses between 0.3 and 3 mg improves sleep quality and duration in chronic insomnia.
		Melatonin 0.5 mg resynchronizes the sleep–wake cycle in circadian rhythm sleep disturbances.
		Note: The best preparation of melatonin depends on the nature of the sleep disturbance.
		Melatonin may be safely combined with benzodiazepines to reduce middle awakening and reduce fall risk in elderly patients
	Valerian (*Valeriana officinalis*)	Valerian 600 mg at bedtime is probably as effective as benzodiazepines in the management of chronic insomnia and facilitates discontinuation of benzodiazepines (i.e., used for insomnia) following prolonged use.
		Caution: Pregnant or nursing women should not use valerian extract
	Somatic and mind–body practices	Many somatic and mind–body practices, including progressive muscle relaxation, massage, meditation, and guided imagery, are as effective as conventional sedative-hypnotics for mild to moderate insomnia.
		Using a somatic or mind–body approach together with a sedative-hypnotic is more effective than either approach alone.
		Note: Somatic and mind–body practices require more time to work but over the long term are less expensive and more cost-effective compared with conventional drugs
	Exercise	Regular physical exercise increases the quality and duration of sleep in the elderly.
		Caution: Sedentary, physically impaired patients, or patients with heart or lung disease should consult with a physician before beginning to exercise
	Bright light exposure	Regular carefully timed bright light exposure resynchronizes phase-advanced or phase-delayed sleep to the patient's time zone.
		Important: When recommending light exposure therapy, always provide detailed instructions, review important safety information, and provide the name of a reputable manufacturer
	EEG biofeedback	Some EEG-biofeedback protocols, especially SMR (alpha-theta training), are effective treatments of chronic insomnia

CBT, cognitive-behavioral therapy; CDP, cytidine diphosphate; CES, cranioelectrotherapy stimulation; EEG, electroencephalography; EMG, electromyography; EPA, ecosapentanoic acid; GSR, galvanic skin response; IU, international unit; SAMe, S-adenosylmethionine; SMR, TK; SSRI, selective serotonin reuptake inhibitor; TES, transcanial neuroelectric stimulation; VRGET, virtual reality graded exposure therapy

Provisional Treatments/All Symptoms

Provisional Treatments (in Current Use and Probably Effective)

Approaches listed in **Table A–5** are characterized by the following:

1. Systematic review findings are highly suggestive but not compelling, or have not been conducted because of insufficient numbers of studies or uneven quality of completed studies; OR

2. Three or more rigorously conducted, double-blind, randomized controlled trials yield findings that are suggestive but not compelling; AND

3. The approach is in current use for the treatment of a specified symptom pattern. The use of the modality with respect to a specified symptom pattern may be endorsed by a relevant professional association.

Table A–5 Provisional Treatment Approaches

Symptom	Approach	Comment
Depression	Dietary modifications	Restricting caffeine and refined sugar and increasing consumption of fatty fish and whole foods rich in B vitamins may improve depressed mood or reduce the risk of becoming depressed
	Ayurvedic herbs	Several Ayurvedic herbs and compound herbal formulas are probably beneficial.
		Note: Patients taking Ayurvedic herbs should be supervised by an Ayurvedic physician
	5-HTP	5-HTP 300 mg/day is probably as effective as conventional antidepressants for moderate depressed mood.
		Note: Some cases of treatment-refractory depression improve when 5-HTP 300 to 600 mg/day is combined with carbidopa or conventional antidepressants
	L-tryptophan	L-tryptophan 1 to 2 g may be equivalent to imipramine 150 mg and other conventional antidepressants.
		L-tryptophan 2 g augments fluoxetine 20 mg and improves sleep quality in depressed individuals.
		L-tryptophan 1 to 2 g combined with bright light therapy is more effective than either approach alone in seasonal depressed mood
	ALC	ALC 1 to 3 g/day in divided doses may be beneficial in elderly depressed or depressed demented patients.
		ALC should be considered when depression is related to post-traumatic brain injury or age-related cognitive decline
	Inositol	Inositol 12 to 20 g/day may be beneficial in both unipolar and bipolar depressed mood.
		Inositol may have synergistic effects when combined with conventional mood stabilizers
	DHEA	DHEA 90 to 450 mg/day in mild to moderate depressed mood.
		DHEA has synergistic effects when combined with conventional antidepressants and may be an effective monotherapy for moderate depressed mood.
		DHEA may be beneficial when depressed mood occurs together with anxiety, psychosis, or cognitive impairment
	Cortisol-lowering agents	Cortisol-lowering agents, including ketoconazole, aminoglutethimide, and metyrapone, may be beneficial.
		Note: Cortisol-lowering agents are probably ineffective and should be avoided when depression occurs together with psychosis
	Total or partial sleep deprivation	One night of total sleep deprivation followed by sleep phase advance is effective in severe depressed mood. Partial sleep deprivation improves moderate depressed mood.
		Partial sleep deprivation combined with maintenance lithium therapy and morning bright light exposure may be more effective than either approach alone in bipolar depression.
		Combining periodic partial sleep deprivation with a conventional antidepressant in severely depressed patients is probably more effective than either approach alone
	Mindfulness training and yoga	Mindfulness training is probably as effective as cognitive therapy in moderate depressed mood.
		Regular yoga (breathing or postures) practice may be as effective as conventional antidepressants in severe depressed mood.
		Combining mindfulness training or guided imagery with conventional antidepressants is more effective than conventional treatments alone
	High-density negative ions	Regular daily exposure to high-density negative ions is probably an effective treatment of seasonal depressed mood.
		Antidepressant effects of exposure to high-density negative ions and bright light may be equivalent
	Dim green, blue, or red light	Regular exposure to dim red or blue light may be as effective as bright light exposure in seasonal depression.
		Dim green light 2 hours before exposure to natural light may accelerate response to conventional antidepressants

(Continued)

Table A–5   Provisional Treatment Approaches *(Continued)*

Symptom	Approach	Comment
	Music or binaural sound	Attentive listening to music probably improves moderately depressed mood.
		Combining music with guided imagery is more beneficial than either approach alone.
		Listening to binaural sounds in the beta frequency range (16–24 Hz) may improve depressed mood
	EEG biofeedback and HRV biofeedback	Combined EEG-HRV biofeedback (energy cardiology) training may improve depressed mood
	Acupuncture, electroacupuncture, and computer-controlled electroacupuncture	Conventional acupuncture may be effective against severe depressed mood.
		Electroacupuncture alone may be as effective as electroacupuncture combined with amitriptyline or other conventional antidepressants.
		Computer-controlled electroacupuncture using high-frequency currents may be more effective than conventional or standard electroacupuncture
	Homeopathic preparations	Homeopathic remedies may be beneficial in some cases of depressed mood depending on constitutional findings
	Spirituality and religious beliefs	Spirituality and religious beliefs are associated with reduced risk of depressed mood.
		Regular support groups with spiritual-religious themes reduce the severity of depressed mood and increase emotional well-being
	Healing Touch and Therapeutic Touch	Regular HT or TT treatments may reduce the severity of depressed mood and bereavement
	Qigong	Regular qigong practice results in generally improved emotional well-being
Mania and cyclic mood changes	EMPowerPlus	EMPowerPlus may be an effective adjunctive or stand-alone treatment of depressive and manic symptoms in patients diagnosed with bipolar disorder.
		Some bipolar patients were able to reduce conventional medications by one half when taking EMPowerPlus.
		Some bipolar patients remain stable off all conventional medications when taking EMPowerPlus
	Acute tyrosine depletion	A branched-chain amino acid drink that excludes tyrosine may be an effective treatment in some cases of acute mania.
		Note: Specialized preparations of branched-chain amino acids should be administered under medical supervision
	L-tryptophan	L-tryptophan may reduce the frequency of depressive mood swings and reduce the severity of mania in bipolar patients.
		L-tryptophan 3 g tid added to lithium may improve symptoms of mania more than lithium alone.
		Caution: Dietary restriction of L-tryptophan can precipitate depressed mood in bipolar patients
	Omega-3 fatty acids	EPA 1 to 2 g/day in combination with conventional mood stabilizers may reduce the severity and frequency of manic episodes.
		Note: There is one case report of EPA-induced hypomania
	Choline and phosphatidylcholine	Adding choline (2–7 g/day) to therapeutic doses of lithium may improve response in rapid-cycling episodes
		Adding phosphatidylcholine (15–30 g/day) improves both depression and mania in bipolar patients
	Folic acid 200 μg/day	Folic acid 200 μg/day may augment the effects of lithium in mania
	Trace lithium supplementation	Lithium in trace amounts (50 μg with meals) may reduce the frequency and severity of both depressive and manic symptoms.
		Note: There are no contraindications to the use of lithium in trace amounts
	Magnesium supplementation	Magnesium supplementation 40 mEq/day may be an effective treatment of rapid cycling episodes
Anxiety	Dietary changes	Avoiding refined sugar and caffeine, increasing protein and foods containing tryptophan may reduce symptoms of generalized anxiety or panic
	Ayurvedic herbs	Ayurvedic herbs, including *Bacopa monniera*, *Centella asiatica*, and a compound herbal formula, Geriforte, reduce symptoms of generalized anxiety
	L-tryptophan and 5-HTP	L-tryptophan 2 to 3g/day or 5-HTP 25 to 100 mg up to 3 times a day is probably an effective treatment of generalized anxiety.
		5-HTP may prevent panic attacks.
		Caution: When combining 5-HTP and a conventional medication, the risk of serotonin syndrome can be minimized by starting 5-HTP at low doses (e.g., 25 mg/day) and gradually increasing the dose while monitoring for adverse effects including insomnia and nervousness
	Inositol	Inositol (up to 20 g/day) is probably an effective treatment of panic attacks and may reduce symptoms of agoraphobia, obsessions, and compulsions

Table A–5   Provisional Treatment Approaches *(Continued)*

Symptom	Approach	Comment
	Exercise	Regular aerobic or strengthening exercise reduces generalized anxiety symptoms and may reduce frequency and severity of panic attacks.
		Caution: Patients with heart disease, chronic pain syndromes, or other serious medical illnesses should always consult with their physician before starting an exercise program
	Massage	Regular massage reduces the severity of chronic moderate anxiety.
		Note: Individuals with chronic pain syndromes should consult with their physician before receiving massage therapy
	Music and binaural sound	Regular listening to soothing music or certain binaural sounds can significantly reduce generalized anxiety.
		Note: The experience of music or binaural sound is more effective when there are no distractions. Anxious patients should be encouraged to become absorbed in music or binaural sounds on a regular basis
	HRV-biofeedback training	Biofeedback training using HRV probably reduces symptoms of generalized anxiety
	Acupuncture and electroacupuncture	Some acupuncture and electroacupuncture protocols probably reduce symptoms of generalized anxiety
		Note: Rare adverse effects of acupuncture include bruising, fatigue, and fainting. Very rare cases of pneumothorax have been reported
	Reiki	Regular Reiki treatments may be beneficial for anxiety related to pain or depressed mood.
		Note: Both contact and noncontact Reiki may reduce anxiety symptoms
Psychosis	Brahmyadiyoga and Mentat	Brahmyadiyoga 8 to -12 g may be as effective as conventional antipsychotics; Mentat may reduce severity of negative psychotic symptoms
	Korean compound herbal formulas	Many Korean traditional herbal formulas may be beneficial in psychosis.
		Note: Few human trials have been done on Korean herbal formulas, and safety issues have not been clearly defined
	EEPA, an omega-3 fatty acid	EPA (1–4 g) alone or in combination with conventional antipsychotics (and especially clozapine) may improve outcomes. Beneficial effects may be more robust in the early acute phase of the illness.
	Estrogen supplementation	Estrogen replacement therapy may be an effective treatment for postpartum psychosis. Adding estrogen to conventional antipsychotics may improve outcomes.
		Caution: Estrogen supplementation may increase risk of breast cancer or heart disease in susceptible women
	Niacin, folate, and thiamine	Combining niacin (in the form of nicotinomide 3–8 g), folate (in the form of methylfolate 15 mg), or thiamine (500 mg tid) with conventional antipsychotics may improve outcomes.
		Note: Flushing and discomfort are associated with large doses of niacin and reportedly diminished when niacin is taken in the form of niacinamide
	Glycine	Combining glycine 60 g with a conventional antipsychotic may improve both positive and negative symptoms.
		Glycine supplementation may improve mood and overall cognitive functioning in chronic psychotics.
		Caution: Case reports suggest that therapeutic doses of glycine may precipitate acute psychosis
	Spiritually oriented group therapy	Combining spiritually oriented group therapy with yogic breathing practice and conventional medications improves global functioning in stable chronically psychotic patients.
		Caution: Patients who are delusional or have other acute psychotic symptoms should be discouraged from participating in spiritual or religious practices
	Religious or spiritual involvement	Patients who have well-controlled psychotic symptoms may benefit from social support in organized religious activity.
		Caution: Patients who are actively psychotic should be advised to avoid intense religious or spiritual activity
	Qigong	Patients who have well-controlled psychotic symptoms may benefit from the regular practice of certain qigong exercises.
		Caution: Patients who have a history of psychosis should practice qigong only under the supervision of a qualified instructor
Dementia and cognitive impairment	Dietary modifications	Diets high in fish or other sources of omega-3 fatty acids and low in omega-6 fatty acids may be associated with reduced risk of dementia.
		Note: Epidemiologic data on relationships between specific foods and the risk of developing dementia are inconsistent

(Continued)

Table A–5 Provisional Treatment Approaches *(Continued)*

Symptom	Approach	Comment
	Ginkgo biloba	*G. biloba* extract (1.9 mL/day) may improve the efficiency and speed of information processing in healthy elderly individuals.
		G. biloba may slow progression to mild cognitive impairment.
		Caution: *G. biloba* should be avoided in patients taking aspirin or anticoagulant drugs
	Kami-untan-to (KUT)	KUT, a compound herbal formula, stimulates production of nerve growth factor and the synthetic enzyme for acetylcholine and may slow the rate of progression of Alzheimer's disease.
		Note: One open study used KUT combined with vitamin E and a nonsteroidal anti-inflammatory drug, making it difficult to attribute cognitive-enhancing effects to KUT alone
	Golden root (*Rhodiola rosea*)	*R. rosea* 500 mg/day improves memory and performance in healthy adults and may accelerate recovery of normal cognitive functioning following head injury.
		Neuroprotective effects may be enhanced by piracetam, ginkgo, or ginseng
		Caution: *R. rosea* may induce mania in bipolar patients and should be avoided in this population
	Choto-san	Choto-san, a compound herbal formula, affects dopamine and serotonin receptors and has strong antioxidant properties. Choto-san improves global functioning and improves cognition in vascular dementia.
		Note: There is evidence that Choto-san reduces symptoms of psychosis in demented individuals
	ALC	ALC 1500 to 3000 mg may be beneficial for mild cognitive decline and Alzheimer's disease.
		ALC may improve cognitive performance in healthy adults, and in depressed individuals and abstinent alcoholics. Neuroprotective effects of ALC may be enhanced when combined with CoQ10, alpha lipoic acid, or omega-3 fatty acids.
		Note: Initial beneficial cognitive effects in dementia may not be sustained beyond 1 year with continuous treatment
	B vitamins (folate, B_{12}, and thiamine)	Daily folate, vitamin B_{12}, or thiamine supplementation may be beneficial in some cases of age-related cognitive decline and Alzheimer's disease.
		Folate 50 mg/day may improve mood and cognition in depressed demented individuals.
		Note: The evidence for vitamin B_{12} is limited and largely anecdotal. A systematic review did not find strong evidence for folate or B_{12} in dementia or other forms of severe cognitive impairment
	Vitamins C and E	Daily combined use of vitamin C (at least 500 mg) and vitamin E (at least 400 IU) may significantly reduce the risk of developing Alzheimer's disease.
		Note: There is probably little protective benefit from taking either vitamin C or vitamin E alone.
		A systematic review did not find strong evidence for a beneficial effect of vitamin E in dementia.
		Caution: High doses of vitamin E may increase the risk of stroke in at-risk patients
	DHEA and testosterone	DHEA 25 to 50 mg/day may improve mental performance in healthy adults, and 200 mg/day may improve cognitive functioning in vascular dementia Testosterone 75 mg may slow the rate of progression of Alzheimer's disease.
		Note: There is no evidence for a cognitive-enhancing effect of DHEA in Alzheimer's disease
		Caution: DHEA can cause insomnia or agitation and should be taken in the morning; testosterone replacement can increase the risk of prostate cancer
	Essential oils	Essential oils of lavender and lemon balm applied to the face and arms (but not as aromatherapy) have beneficial calming effects on agitation in demented patients.
		Caution: Essential oils can cause skin allergies and phototoxic reactions. Lavender oil increases the sedating effects of conventional sedatives.
		Pregnant women should not apply essential oils to the skin because of systemic absorption and potentially toxic effects on the fetus
	Snoezelen, a multimodal sensory stimulation therapy	Four to 8 weekly Snoezelen sessions may reduce apathy and psychomotor agitation while enhancing language in demented individuals
	Transcranial electrical nerve stimulation (TENS) and CES	TENS and CES treatments resulted in improvements in word recall, face recognition, and motivation in demented individuals
		Note: The beneficial effects of weak electrical stimulation are not sustained several weeks after treatment ends
	Music therapy and binaural sound	Regular music therapy probably enhances global functioning in demented individuals, reduces agitation and wandering, enhances social interaction, improves depressed mood, increases cooperative behavior, and increases baseline cognitive functioning. Binaural sounds in the beta frequency range may enhance cognitive functioning in healthy adults.
		Note: Most studies on music in dementia are small, and findings are limited by the absence of quantitative outcomes measures, randomization, and blinding

Table A–5 Provisional Treatment Approaches *(Continued)*

Symptom	Approach	Comment
	Healing Touch and Therapeutic Touch	Regular HT or TT treatments may reduce agitation, improve global functioning, improve sleep schedule, and enhance compliance with nursing home routines.
		Patients who receive regular HT treatments may require lower doses of medications for agitated behavior.
		Note: Findings of HT and TT as treatments of agitation in dementia are limited by study design flaws, including lack of blinding, small size, and the absence of control groups receiving sham treatments in most studies
Alcohol and substance abuse and dependence	Dietary changes	Alcoholics who improve their diets, including reduced intake of refined sugar and caffeine and increased intake of omega-3 fatty acids and protein, probably have an increased chance for maintaining sobriety
	Amino acid supplementation	Taurine may reduce alcohol withdrawal symptoms; SAMe may reduce alcohol intake; ALC may enhance cognitive performance in abstinent alcoholics; L-tryptophan may reduce alcohol craving.
		Note: Alcoholics may have a general brain serotonin deficit. Supplementation with amino acids that increase brain serotonin levels may have beneficial effects
	Vitamin supplementation	Chronic alcoholics are generally deficient in B vitamins. Thiamine may reduce alcohol craving. Nicotinic acid may reduce the risk of alcohol dependence in chronic drinkers. Taking antioxidant vitamins soon before drinking may reduce the severity of hangover symptoms
	Magnesium and zinc	Supplementation of chronic alcoholics with magnesium and zinc may improve global neuropsychological functioning and protect the brain against free radical damage
	GHBA	Frequent high doses of GHBA (25 mg/kg up to 6 times daily) in chronic alcoholics may reduce craving and lessen withdrawal symptoms.
		Caution: Acute GHBA overdose can result in profound mental status changes, respiratory depression, and death. A withdrawal syndrome occurs after prolonged use. Vertigo is a common transient adverse effect
	Exercise	Regular aerobic exercise or strength training in abstinent alcoholics may improve general emotional well-being
		Caution: All patients should consult with their primary care physician before starting a rigorous exercise program
	Mindfulness training, meditation, and spiritually focused support groups	Abstinent alcoholics and addicts who engage in a regular mindfulness practice or meditation probably have a reduced risk of relapse.
		Spiritually focused support groups probably reduce relapse risk.
		Note: Transcendental meditation may be more effective at reducing the risk of relapse compared with other meditation styles
	Acupuncture and electroacupuncture	Some points and protocols are probably more effective than others in reducing symptoms of alcohol or cocaine withdrawal.
		Note: Inconsistent research findings on acupuncture for alcohol and drug abuse probably reflect varying skill levels and protocols
Disturbances of nighttime sleep and daytime wakefulness	5-HTP and L-tryptophan	5-HTP and L-tryptophan probably reduce symptoms of mild or situational insomnia.
		5-HTP increases sleep duration in obstructive sleep apnea and narcolepsy.
		Combining L-tryptophan 2 g with a conventional antidepressant probably enhances antidepressant response and improves sleep quality
	Yoku-kan-san-ka-chimpi-hange	Yoku-kan-san-ka-chimpi-hange, a widely used treatment of insomnia in traditional Japanese medicine (Kampo), probably increases overall quality and duration of sleep in chronic insomniacs
	CES	CES is probably beneficial in some cases of chronic insomnia.
		Patients who reported improved sleep following CES treatment exhibited increased delta sleep that continued months after treatments ended.
		Note: Reported disparities in research outcomes are probably related to customized equipment, the use of different protocols, the severity of symptoms treated, and the timing and duration of treatment
	Acupuncture and auriculotherapy	Some acupuncture and auriculotherapy protocols probably reduce the severity of sleep disturbances, including insomnia related to a mental or emotional problem

ALC, acetyl-L-carnitine; CES, cranioelectrotherapy stimulation; CoQ10, coenzyme Q$_{10}$; DHEA, dehydroepiandrosterone; EEG, electroencephalography; EPA, ecosapentanoic acid; 5-HTP, 5-hydroxytryptophan; GHBA, γ-hydroxybutyric acid; HRV, heart rate variability; HT, Healing Touch; IU, international units; SAMe, *S*-adenosylmethionine; TT Therapeutic Touch

Possibly Effective Treatments/All Symptoms

Possibly Effective (in Current Use and Possibly Effective)

Approaches listed in **Table A–6** are characterized by the following:

1. Fewer than three studies or poorly designed studies have been done to determine whether a particular treatment modality results in consistent positive outcomes with respect to a specified symptom pattern,

2. Research findings or anecdotal reports are limited or inconsistent,

3. There are insufficient quality studies on which to base a systematic review or meta-analysis, AND

4. The modality is in current use but remains controversial and may be endorsed by a relevant professional association.

Table A–6   Possibly Effective Treatment Aproaches

Symptom	Treatment	Comment
Depression	*Rhodiola rosea* (golden root)	*R. rosea* may augment conventional antidepressants
	Ginkgo biloba	*G. biloba* may provide a safe alternative to conventional augmentation strategies.
		Caution: *G. biloba* should not be taken with warfarin or other drugs that affect bleeding time
	L-tyrosine	L-tyrosine 500 to 1500 mg may have antidepressant effects.
		Caution: Large doses of L-tyrosine may promote growth of malignancies
	L-phenylalanine	L-phenylalanine may be beneficial in depressed patients with low serum PEA levels.
		Note: Targeted amino acid therapy uses specific combinations of amino acids to treat identified neurotransmitter deficiencies (see discussion in text)
	Mineral supplements	Supplementation with selenium or rubidium may be effective when these elements are deficient in the diet
		Note: Supplementation with selenium or rubidium may be effective when these elements are deficient in the diet
	Massage	Regular massage therapy probably improves general emotional well-being and is beneficial in pre-menstrual or postpartum depression
	High-density negative ions	High-density negative ions may be as effective as bright light exposure in patients who experience seasonal depressed mood.
		Note: Low-density negative ions are probably ineffective
	CES	Daily 40-minute CES treatments may be beneficial in some cases of depression.
		Note: CES may reduce alcohol or substance abuse in depressed alcoholics or addicts
	Reiki	Regular Reiki treatments may be beneficial for depressed patients
	Prayer and distant healing intention	Individuals who pray and those prayed for may benefit from shared beliefs.
		Note: There is no current evidence that intercessory prayer has beneficial effects on depressed mood
Mania	St. John's wort (*Hypericum perforatum*)	St. John's wort may be an effective treatment of SAD.
		Combining St. John's wort with bright light exposure may be more effective in SAD than either approach alone.
		Caution: Patients should use St. John's wort under medical supervision. St. John's wort interacts with many conventional drugs, including protease inhibitors, oral contraceptives, and warfarin
	Rauwolfia serpentina	*R. serpentina* may be beneficial in mania that does not respond to conventional mood stabilizers.
		R. serpentina may augment the mood-stabilizing effects of lithium.
		Note: *R. serpentina* may be safely combined with lithium but should be used only under the supervision of a trained Ayurvedic practitioner
	Vitamin B$_{12}$ supplementation	Monthly B$_{12}$ injections may reduce the risk of recurring manic episodes.
		Check serum level before giving B$_{12}$ injections (patients who are not deficient will probably not benefit)
	Potassium supplementation	Potassium 20 mEq bid may reduce lithium-induced tremor and improve compliance.
		Caution: Patients who have cardiac arrhythmias or take antiarrhythmic drugs should consult with their physicians before taking potassium
	Meditation and mindfulness training	Certain meditation practices promote calmness and may be beneficial in mania or hypomania.
		Caution: Rare cases of hypomania have been reported following meditation. Bipolar patients should avoid "activating" meditation practices
	Yoga	Certain yogic breathing practices and postures probably promote calmness in general and may be beneficial in mania or hypomania.
		Caution: Bipolar patients should avoid yoga practices that are stimulating

Table A–6   Possibly Effective Treatment Aproaches *(Continued)*

Symptom	Treatment	Comment
Anxiety	Passionflower (*Passiflora incarnata*)	Passionflower extract may have anxiety-reducing effects comparable to benzodiazepines
	Ashwagondha (*Withania somnifera*)	Ashwagondha is an Ayurvedic herbal used to treat anxiety and chronic stress. *Note:* Individuals who use Ayurvedic herbs should do so only under the supervision of an Ayurvedic physician
	Lavender and rosemary essential oils	When used as aromatherapy or applied to the skin during massage, lavender and rosemary essential oils may reduce generalized anxiety
	D-cycloserine	D-cycloserine 500 mg facilitates the effectiveness of VRGET in acrophobia
	Bach flower remedies	Certain Bach flower remedies may reduce test anxiety
	DHEA	DHEA 100 mg/day may reduce anxiety symptoms in psychotic patients. *Note:* Combining DHEA with conventional medications may reduce the severity of anxiety associated with depressed mood or psychosis
	Vitamins (including thiamine, B6, B12, niacinamide, C and E)	Two forms of niacin, nicotinamide and niacinamide, may have calming effects. Niacinamide 1 to 3 g/day may reduce anxiety caused by hypoglycemia
	Minerals (phosphorus, magnesium, and selenium)	Phosphorus may reduce the frequency of panic attacks. Magnesium 100 to 200 mg may reduce symptoms of generalized anxiety
	Animal-facilitated psychotherapy	Animal-facilitated psychotherapy may improve general emotional well-being and reduce symptoms of generalized anxiety
	Lucid dreaming	Training in lucid dreaming induction may reduce the severity of PTSD symptoms
	Paraspinal electrical stimulation	Paraspinal electrical stimulation may be a viable alternative for PTSD patients who have not responded to other treatments
	Healing Touch and Therapeutic Touch	HT and TT may reduce symptoms of generalized anxiety and anxiety related to pain or trauma *Note:* Sham-controlled studies suggest nonspecific beneficial effect versus placebo effect
	Qigong and Tai Chi	The regular practice of qigong and Tai Chi may reduce symptoms of generalized anxiety. *Note:* Tai Chi was more effective than progressive muscle relaxation in PTSD combat veterans *Caution:* Psychotic individuals or patients diagnosed with severe personality disorders should practice qigong only under the supervision of a skilled instructor
	Homeopathic remedies	Case reports suggest that certain homeopathic remedies are beneficial in cases of social phobia, PTSD, panic attacks, and OCD, but two double-blind studies showed no beneficial effects
	Thought field therapy (TFT) and Emotional Freedom Techniques (EFT)	TFT and EFT claim to reduce anxiety by rebalancing energy in the meridians. Both approaches are widely used to treat different anxiety syndromes. *Note:* Sham-controlled studies suggest that observed benefits of EFT are achieved by desensitization and distraction
	Somatoemotional release and craniosacral therapy	Case reports and one study suggest beneficial effects in trauma survivors *Note:* The only study on somatoemotional release and craniosacral therapy in PTSD is small and methodologically flawed
	Religious attitudes and affiliation	Individuals who have strong religious beliefs or religious affiliations may be more resilient when facing stressful circumstances
	Intercessory prayer	Praying at a distance may be associated with a reduction in symptoms of pain and anxiety. *Note:* Beneficial effects of intercessory prayer on anxiety and emotional well-being may be due to group suggestion
Psychosis	Dietary changes, including decreased intake of saturated fats and increased intake of omega-3 fatty acids, reduced gluten, and improved glucose regulation	Chronically psychotic patients with higher intake of unsaturated fats, reduced gluten, and improved glucose regulation may experience milder symptoms
	Ginkgo biloba	Combining *G. biloba* (360 mg/day) with a conventional antipsychotic may be more effective for both positive and negative symptoms compared with conventional treatments alone. *Note:* Combining *G. biloba* with a conventional antipsychotic may reduce adverse neurological effects

Table A–6 Possibly Effective Treatment Aproaches (Continued)

Symptom	Treatment	Comment
	DHEA	Combining DHEA 100 mg with a conventional antipsychotic may reduce the severity of negative symptoms and improve depressed mood and anxiety.
		Caution: DHEA can be activating and should be taken in the morning. Patients with a history or BPH or prostate cancer should consult their physician before taking DHEA
	Mineral supplements	Manganese, selenium, or zinc supplementation may improve psychotic symptoms in some cases.
		Note: The evidence for beneficial effects of mineral supplementation in schizophrenia is limited and inconsistent
	Evening primrose (*Oenothera biennis*) oil	Putative mechanism of action involves restoring deficient prostaglandins with essential fatty acids. May improve psychotic symptoms in some cases
		Note: Few double-blind studies and inconsistent findings
	Yoga	Regular practice of certain yogic breathing routines and postures may reduce severity of psychotic symptoms in some cases.
		Caution: Certain yogic breathing practices can cause agitation and transient worsening of psychotic symptoms. Chronically psychotic patients should practice yoga only under the guidance of a qualified instructor.
	Wilbarger intervention	The Wilbarger method is a sensory stimulation technique involving frequent passive stretching and touching of the body. Preliminary findings suggest improved sensory integration in schizophrenics.
		Note: Beneficial effects of this technique may be related to frequent human contact
	Laser acupuncture	Daily 15-minute laser acupuncture treatments of the yamen point may reduce psychotic symptoms in schizophrenics
Cognitive impairment	Vinpocetine	Vinpocetine 30 to 60 mg/day may be beneficial in both Alzheimer's disease and vascular dementia.
		Note: Only a few small human trials on vinpocetine in dementia have been done, and findings are inconsistent
	Ashwagondha (*Withania somnifera*)	Ashwagondha 50 mg/kg may improve short and long-term memory and executive functioning in cognitively impaired individuals.
		Note: Few human trials on Ashwagondha have been published
	Ginseng (*Panax ginseng*)	Ginseng may enhance memory and overall cognitive performance in healthy adults.
		Note: Some negative trials with ginseng, and at least one reported case of mania induction
	Lemon balm (*Melissa officinalis*) and common sage (*Salvia officinalis*)	Extracts of lemon balm and common sage (60 drops/day) may slow the rate of decline in Alzheimer's disease
	Dronabinol	Dronabinol may reduce agitated behavior, improve global functioning, and enhance mental status in Alzheimer's disease
	Dehydroevodiamine (DHED), Qian Jin Yi Fang, Trasina, Mentat, and lobeline	DHED may be more effective than cholinesterase inhibitors in Alzheimer's disease.
		A Chinese compound herbal formula called Qian Jin Yi Fang reportedly reduces symptoms of dementia.
		Two proprietary Ayurvedic compound herbal formulas, Trasina and Mentat, may be beneficial in Alzheimer's disease and age-related cognitive impairment.
		Lobeline is a promising memory-enhancing agent.
		Note: Human clinical trials data for these herbals are extremely limited or entirely absent
	Niacin	Findings of a single study suggest that high niacin intake from food or supplements may significantly reduce the risk of developing dementia and decrease the rate of cognitive decline in healthy elderly individuals.
		Note: Only epidemiologic studies have been done on niacin and dementia.
		Confirmation of a protective effect of niacin will require a large controlled trial
	Centrophenoxine (CPH), phosphatidyl choline, and lecithin	CPH may improve global functioning and cognitive performance in Alzheimer's disease. Benefits of CPH are possibly enhanced when combined with vitamins. Phosphatidyl choline and lecithin are probably ineffective.
		Note: Beneficial findings for CPH in dementia are still preliminary
	Piracetam	Piracetam alone may be ineffective, but piracetam (up to 4800 mg/day) in combination with vinpocetine or CDP-choline may improve cognitive performance in mild to moderate dementia. Piracetam in combination with ginkgo may improve overall cognitive performance in dyslexic individuals.
		Note: Few human trials, and findings of a Cochrane review on piracetam in dementia were equivocal

Table A–6   Possibly Effective Treatment Aproaches (Continued)

Symptom	Treatment	Comment
	Nicergoline	Nicergoline may be beneficial in cognitive decline caused by various underlying pathologies, including vascular dementia and Alzheimer's disease.
		Note: A systematic review of 14 double-blind studies found only "some evidence" of efficacy
	Alpha lipoic acid (ALA)	Animal studies suggest that ALA may enhance recovery following stroke. Human case reports suggest that ALA may accelerate return of cognitive function after traumatic brain injury.
		Note: Findings on ALA in dementia are largely from case studies, and a 2004 Cochrane review identified no controlled trials
	Estrogen and proges-terone replacement in women	Case reports suggest efficacy; however, meta-analyses fail to show that hormonal replacement with estrogen/progesterone slows progression of dementia in postmenopausal women diagnosed with Alzheimer's disease or prevents cognitive decline in healthy postmenopausal women.
		Caution: Estrogen replacement therapy is associated with increased risk of breast cancer, heart disease, and stroke
	SAMe	SAMe (up to 3200 mg/day) may improve post-stroke survival and enhance return to baseline cognitive functioning.
		SAMe (150 mg/day) may accelerate return of normal cognitive functioning following traumatic brain injury.
		Note: Findings of small studies on SAMe in Alzheimer's disease are inconsistent.
		Caution: SAMe at high doses may cause agitation, and there are rare reports of hypomania in bipolar patients
	Picamilon	Picamilon (50 mg 3 times/day) may reduce cognitive impairments related to cerebrovascular disease and accelerate recovery following traumatic brain injury.
		Note: Few human trials have been done on picamilon in dementia or traumatic brain injury
	Pyritinol	Pyritinol (600 mg/day) may have general beneficial effects on cognitive functioning following traumatic brain injury.
		Note: Few studies on pyritinol, and inconsistent findings
	Melatonin	Melatonin 3 mg at bedtime may improve alertness and wakefulness while reducing agitation in Alzheimer's patients
	Massage	Regular massage therapy may reduce agitated behavior in demented nursing home patients.
		Note: Anecdotal reports and open studies provide the only evidence for calming effects of massage in dementia
	Wander garden	Wander gardens permit demented or post-stroke patients to enjoy nature-related activities and reportedly improve baseline functioning in the early stages of dementia
	Bright light exposure	Regular bright light (10,000 lux) exposure may improve sleep, reduce "sundowning," reduce agitation and other inappropriate behaviors, and delay the time of peak agitation in Alzheimer's patients
	EEG and HRV biofeedback	EEG- and HRV-biofeedback training may enhance cognitive performance in healthy adults.
		EEG biofeedback may accelerate recovery following stroke or traumatic brain injury.
		Caution: Certain EEG-biofeedback protocols can cause seizures and should be avoided in patients who have epilepsy
	Qigong	Regular qigong practice or external qigong treatments may normalize EEG slowing and reverse cerebral atrophy associated with dementia.
		Note: Controlled studies of qigong in dementia have not been done, but case reports suggest dramatic beneficial effects
Alcohol/drugs	*Radix puerariae, Salvia miltiorrhiza, Aralia elata, Tabernanthe iboga,* and *Cannibis indica*	These traditionally used herbs may reduce alcohol craving, lessen alcohol consumption, and reduce symptoms of withdrawal.
		Note: To date there are no human clinical trials supporting the use of these herbals for the management of alcohol craving or withdrawal
	Ashwagondha, Panax ginseng, Aristeguietia discolor, and *Cervus elaphus*	Ashwagondha and other traditionally used herbs and natural products may reduce tolerance and decrease the severity of withdrawal from opiates, cocaine, and methamphetamine.
		Note: Human clinical trials do not (yet) support use of these herbals for the management of withdrawal from narcotics
	Valeriana officinalis and *Mentat*	Valerian extract normalizes sleep following benzodiazepine withdrawal.
		Valerian extract and Mentat may lessen the severity of benzodiazepine withdrawal
	Melatonin	Melatonin 2 mg in controlled-release form may facilitate discontinuation of benzodiazepines following prolonged use for insomnia

(Continued)

Table A–6   Possibly Effective Treatment Aproaches *(Continued)*

Symptom	Treatment	Comment
	PPC	PPC taken before drinking may reduce liver damage by interfering with induction of liver enzymes.
		Note: Alcoholics should always be encouraged to reduce or discontinue alcohol use
	Fatty acids	Supplementation with omega-3 and omega-6 fatty acids may reduce the severity of alcohol withdrawal.
		Note: Omega-3 (but not omega-6) fatty acids are probably an effective adjunctive treatment for depressed mood and other psychiatric symptoms
	HBO	HBO treatment of opium-induced coma may reduce the severity of metabolic brain damage and lower the rate of neuropsychological deficits following recovery.
		Note: HBO may emerge as a standard treatment of opium-induced coma
	Relaxation	Regular relaxation may reduce the severity of withdrawal symptoms following prolonged benzodiazepine use
	Yoga	Regular yoga practice may reduce stress and improve overall functioning in alcoholics and may lessen the risk of relapse in drug addicts.
		Caution: Patients should consult with their primary care physician before starting a strenuous yoga routine
	Biofeedback	Some EMG-thermal, and EEG-biofeedback protocols may reduce alcohol relapse but not cocaine relapse.
		EEG biofeedback using alpha-theta training may induce a relaxed, calm state that reduces the urge to drink
	VRGET	VRGET may be an effective approach for extinguishing craving in nicotine or cocaine dependence
	Dim morning light	Regular exposure to dim morning light (250 lux) may reduce the risk of relapse in abstinent alcoholics with seasonal mood changes.
		Increased abstinence may result from improved mood
	Qigong	Regular qigong treatments may reduce the severity of withdrawal in heroin addicts
Insomnia/ sleepiness	Vitamins and minerals	Supplementation with folate, thiamine, iron, zinc, and magnesium in deficient individuals may reduce daytime sleepiness and improve nighttime sleep.
		Note: Most findings pertaining to vitamins and minerals and sleep come from open trials or observational studies
	Melatonin	Melatonin 2 mg (controlled release) may facilitate discontinuation of benzodiazepines following prolonged use and improve subjective sleep quality.
		Melatonin 9 to 12 mg may reduce symptoms of REM sleep behavior disorder.
		Note: Combining melatonin with a benzodiazepine taper at bedtime may be an effective strategy for transitioning patients off benzodiazepines following prolonged use
	Ginkgo biloba	*G. biloba* 240 mg/day used in combination with a conventional antidepressant may improve the quality of sleep and reduce the frequency of middle awakenings in depressed patients
	St. John's wort (*Hypericum perforatum*)	St. John's wort may improve sleep quality in depressed patients who respond to treatment
	Ashwagondha (*Withania somnifera*) Ayurvedic herbal formula	Ashwagondha and an Ayurvedic compound herbal formula may be effective treatments of chronic primary insomnia
	Ginseng (many species)	Standardized ginseng preparations may enhance daytime wakefulness and reduce symptoms of insomnia.
		Note: Limited research findings suggest good efficacy using a wide range of doses. A conservative strategy is to begin with a low dose and increase the dose gradually while monitoring for changes in wakefulness or insomnia
	Yohimbine	Yohimbine 8 mg/day may be an effective treatment of daytime sleepiness in narcolepsy
	IPA	IPA 200 to 300 mg may improve symptoms of mild or situational insomnia
	DHEA	DHEA 500 mg may increase REM sleep and may be beneficial in sleep disturbances associated with diminished REM sleep.
		DHEA may be effective in some cases when insomnia and depressed mood occur together.
		Note: Women with a history of estrogen-receptor-positive breast cancer should avoid DHEA
	Passive body heating	Total passive body heating, especially taking a hot bath, soon before bedtime may improve overall sleep quality and reduce the frequency of middle awakenings
	Lucid dreaming	Developing skill at lucid dreaming may permit patients who have recurring nightmares to control their dreams and improve the quality of sleep

Table A–6   Possibly Effective Treatment Aproaches *(Continued)*

Symptom	Treatment	Comment
	Tibetan yoga	Regular daily practice of Tibetan yoga may improve sleep quality and may also reduce the need for conventional hypnotics
	Bright light exposure	Bright light exposure may improve sleep quality in some cases of insomnia not related to circadian rhythm disturbances.
		Note: Timed bright light exposure is an established treatment for circadian phase sleep disturbances; however, no controlled studies were identified in a systematic review
	LEET Impulse magnetic field therapy	LEET 15 minutes/night may improve overall sleep quality in chronic insomnia.
		Note: LEET is currently unavailable in the United States but may be a promising future approach to chronic insomnia.
		Seventy percent of chronic insomniacs randomized to nightly impulse magnetic field therapy reported significant improvements in sleep over a 2-week period
	White noise	Nighttime exposure to white noise may be beneficial in some cases of insomnia

ALC, acetyl-L-carnitine; BPH, benign prostatic hypertrophy; CDP, cytidine diphosphate; CES, cranioelectrotherapy stimulation; DHEA, dehydroepiandrosterone; EEG, electroencephalography; EMG, electromyography; 5-HTP, 5-hydroxytryptophan; HBO, hyperbaric oxygenation; HRV, heart rate variability; HT, Healing Touch; IPA, indole-pyruvic acid; LEET, low energy emission therapy; OCD, obsessive-compulsive disorder; PEA, phenylethylamine; PPC, polyenylphosphatidylcholine; PTSD, post-traumatic stress disorder; REM, rapid eye movement; SAD, seasonal affective disorder; SAMe, *S*-adenosylmethionine; TT, Therapeutic Touch; VRGET, virtual reality graded exposure therapy

Appendix B

Internet Resources on Conventional and Nonconventional Mental Health Care

- ◆ Glossaries of Terms Used in Mental Health and Nonconventional Medicine, 346
- ◆ Clinical Practice Guidelines for the Conventional Treatment of Mental Health Problems, 346
- ◆ General Resources on Nonconventional Medicine, 347
- ◆ Resources for Monitoring Research in Conventional and Nonconventional Treatments, 348
- ◆ Evaluating Natural Products and Selecting Brands, 349
- ◆ Identifying Qualified Practitioners of Nonconventional Therapies, 349
- ◆ Biological Therapies, 350
- ◆ Somatic and Mind–Body Approaches, 350
- ◆ Therapies Based on Forms of Energy-Information Validated by Current Western Science, 351
- ◆ Approaches Based on Forms of Energy-Information Not Validated by Current Western Science, 351
- ◆ Miscellaneous Resources, 352

This appendix includes only Web-based resources, on the assumption that the majority of readers have access to the Internet and use it to obtain medical information. For readers who do not use the Internet, extensive references of published journal articles, monographs, and books follow each chapter. For those who are just starting to use the Internet to identify reliable information on nonconventional approaches in medicine or mental health care, I strongly recommend *Complementary Therapies on the Internet*, by Beckner and Berman (Churchill-Livingstone, 2003). The authors are at the Center for Integrative Medicine, University of Maryland School of Medicine, where they manage the part of the Cochrane Collaboration on nonconventional medicine. Their book is an excellent introduction to effective Internet search strategies in nonconventional medicine.

◆ Glossaries of Terms Used in Mental Health and Nonconventional Medicine

Interactive Glossary of Mental Health and Disability Terms   This site provides a list of frequently used health, mental health, and disability terms that are defined in clear and simple everyday language.

Alternative Medicine Terms   This site provides a comprehensive list of terms, modalities, and specific brands of nonconventional medical products and includes hypertext links to relevant phytochemical and ethnobotanical databases.

◆ Clinical Practice Guidelines for the Conventional Treatment of Mental Health Problems

www.library.nhs.uk/mentalhealth   This is the site of the National Electronic Library for Health of the United Kingdom's National Health Service. It is intended to provide comprehensive information on the range of conventional treatments for mental health problems. There is no fee. There are links to patient resources. The site includes guidelines and treatment appraisals, Cochrane systematic reviews, and a compendium of best practice articles (including clinical evidence chapters and World Health Organization guidelines for mental health in primary care).

http://www.guideline.gov/   This very useful site contains summaries of, and links to, over 50 different sets of practice guidelines covering a range of mental health diagnoses and issues.

www.psychguides.com   This site offers practical clinical recommendations for the conventional treatment of common mental health problems based on expert consensus. The *Expert Consensus Guidelines* present practical clinical recommendations based on a survey of expert opinions. The guidelines are based on both research and clinical expertise. Although the guidelines are comprehensive, they emphasize medications over psychotherapy and other conventional treatments.

http://www.psych.org/psych_pract/treatg/pg/prac_guide.cfm
This site is sponsored by the American Psychiatric Association and includes full text of many (but not all) of the practice guidelines developed by this organization. Topics include Psychiatric Evaluation of Adults, Bipolar Disorder, Major Depressive Disorder in Adults, Eating Disorders, Substance Use Disorders (Alcohol, Cocaine, Opioids), Alzheimer's Disease and Other Dementias of Late Life, Schizophrenia, and Nicotine Dependence.

http://www.mhmr.state.tx.us/centraloffice/medicaldirector/TMAP toc.html Sponsored by the Texas Department of Mental Health and Mental Retardation, this site offers detailed treatment recommendations (the Texas Medication Algorithm Project, or TMAP) for each of three major disorders (schizophrenia, bipolar disorder; and major depressive disorder).

http://www.asam.org/publ/withdrawal.htm This site consists of a meta-analysis and evidence-based practice guideline developed by the American Society of Addiction Medicine, Committee on Practice Guidelines, Working Group on Pharmacological Management of Alcohol Withdrawal.

http://www.state.sc.us/dmh/clinical/port.htm This is the site of an article published in *Schizophrenia Bulletin* that offers a comprehensive set of guidelines for the conventional biomedical treatment of schizophrenia. Development of these Patient Outcomes Research Team (PORT) guidelines was funded by the National Institute of Mental Health. Eighteen of the recommendations address antipsychotic agents and other conventional drug treatments. The remaining 12 recommendations address other conventional treatments of schizophrenia, including electroconvulsive therapy, psychological interventions, family interventions, vocational rehabilitation, and intensive case management.

◆ General Resources on Nonconventional Medicine

http://www.pitt.edu/~cbw/database.html This is the Alternative Medicine Homepage, a project coordinated by the staff of the Falk Library of Health Sciences, University of Pittsburgh, Pennsylvania. The site provides extensive links to reviewed Web sites on professional associations, centers of excellence where nonconventional medical care is available, and databases on many nonconventional treatments. The site includes links to professional e-bulletin boards and e-journals in many areas of nonconventional medicine.

National Center for Complementary and Alternative Medicine (NCCAM) NCCAM is one of the 27 institutes and centers that make up the National Institutes of Health (NIH). The NIH is one of eight agencies under the Public Health Service (PHS) in the Department of Health and Human Services (DHHS). NCCAM is dedicated to exploring complementary and alternative healing practices in the context of rigorous science, training complementary and alternative medicine (CAM) researchers, and disseminating authoritative information to the public and professionals. The NCCAM citation index contains over 200,000 citations of studies on all areas of nonconventional medicine indexed in the National Library of Medicine beginning in 1966. The four primary focus areas are research, career development, outreach, and integration of nonconventional and conventional approaches.

PubMed NCCAM and the National Library of Medicine (NLM) have partnered to create a subset of the National Library of Medicine's PubMed. A literature search from this Web site will automatically be limited to the subset of PubMed pertaining to nonconventional medicine. PubMed provides access to citations from the MEDLINE database and additional life science journals. It also includes links to many full-text articles at journal Web sites and other related Web resources.

CRISP—a Database of Biomedical Research Funded by the National Institutes of Health CRISP (Computer Retrieval of Information on Scientific Projects) is a searchable database of federally funded biomedical research projects conducted at universities, hospitals, and other research institutions, including research in many areas of nonconventional medicine. The database is maintained by the Office of Extramural Research at NIH and includes projects funded by the institute, Substance Abuse and Mental Health Services (SAMHSA), U.S. Food and Drug Administration (FDA), Agency for Health Care Research and Quality (AHRQ), and other federal agencies. The site can be used to search for scientific concepts and emerging trends and techniques or to identify specific projects and/or investigators.

Natural Standard, the Authority on Integrative Medicine is an excellent resource covering the range of nonconventional modalities. *Natural Standard* is an international research collaboration that aggregates and synthesizes data on nonconventional therapies. The goal of this collaboration is to provide objective, reliable information that aids clinicians, patients, and health care institutions in making more informed and safer therapeutic decisions.

Embase This Web site is a gateway to biomedical and pharmacological information pertaining to both conventional and nonconventional treatments. The site includes but is not limited to MedLine entries. Approximately 2,000 records are added daily, and 600,000 articles are added annually. It includes many search tools quick to facilitate rapid identification of relevant clinical or research information, and the user can generate table-of-content alerts to keep up-to-date with significant emerging findings.

Complementary and Alternative Medicine (CAM) includes five databases on nonconventional and integrative medicine that cover herbal medicines and supplements, clinical information on integrative approaches, patient education information, a database on herb–drug and supplement–drug interactions, and referenced monographs on herbal medicinals.

The FACTs-Home is the Web site for the Friends of Alternative and Complementary Therapies Society. The goal of this society of healers and patients is to create "a repository of health information that is factual, accessible, credible and ethical." Information included in the Web site comes from different traditions of medicine and different cultures. FACT is an Associate Member of the Canadian Health Network.

Trip Database Plus The TRIP (Turning Research into Practice) database started in 1997 as a small search engine with a focus on evidence-based medicine. The goal of the TRIP database is to allow health professionals to easily find the highest-quality material available on the Web on a range of conventional and nonconventional medical practices. Typically 300 to 400 new articles are added monthly. The content of the TRIP database is separated into a number of categories: evidence-based medicine, guidelines, query answering, medical images, e-textbooks, patient information leaflets, and peer-reviewed journals.

Alt HealthWatch   provides a gateway to full-text searches of over 100 serials on all major nonconventional medical approaches. The list is maintained by EBSCO Publishing. EBSCO is a leading provider of popular secondary databases such as MLA International Bibliography, CINAHL, and PsycINFO. Extensive use of linking enables users to access full text information from virtually all library holdings.

www.rosenthal.hs.columbia.edu   includes a link to the directory of databases on CAM of the Richard and Hinda Rosenthal Center for Complementary and Alternative Medicine includes extensive links to reviewed databases on a range of non-conventional modalities. The site is a powerful gateway to numerous online databases covering six major areas: biomedical bibliographic information; complementary and alternative medicine; medical, pharmaceutical, or scientific data; traditional medicine systems; therapy- or modality-specific; and clinical trials and research projects. Brief information on each linked site is included, together with type of literature covered and whether the site is fee-based access or free.

Osher Institute, Harvard Medical School, Division for Research and Education in Complementary and Integrative Medicine   The mission of the Harvard Osher Center and the Web site is to facilitate interdisciplinary and interinstitutional faculty collaboration for purposes of research evaluation of complementary and integrative medical therapies, delivery of educational programs to the medical community and the public, and investigation of the design of sustainable models of complementary and integrative care delivery in an academic setting.

UCSF-Osher Center for Integrative Medicine   The mission of the University of California, San Francisco, Osher Center for Integrative Medicine is to search for the most effective treatments for patients by combining both conventional and alternative approaches that address all aspects of health and wellness—biological, psychological, social and spiritual. The center is working to transform health care by conducting rigorous research on the medical outcomes of complementary and alternative healing practices; educating medical students, health professionals, and the public about these practices; and creating new models of clinical care.

Research Council for Complementary Medicine (RCCM)   The RCCM was founded in 1983 by practitioners and researchers from both orthodox and nonconventional systems of medicine. Their goal is to develop the evidence base for nonconventional medicine in order to provide both practitioners and patients with information about the effectiveness of individual therapies and the treatment of specific conditions. The School of Integrated Health at the University of Westminster hosts the Web site.

Focus on Alternative and Complementary Therapies (FACT) *FACT* is a quarterly review journal that aims to present the evidence on complementary and alternative medicine in an analytical and impartial manner. With increasing interest and growing research into nonconventional medicine, there are dozens of specific complementary medicine journals and thousands of general medical journals that present articles and research findings in this area. Realizing that it is impossible to scan all pertinent publications, *FACT* systematically searches the world literature to uncover key articles

in CAM research. The most important factual papers found worldwide are summarized and then critically appraised in *FACT*. They are followed by an expert commentary written by a member of *FACT*'s international editorial board and include a reply from the author of the original paper. All *FACT* summaries and commentaries are evidence-based, reporting clinical trials, systematic reviews, or meta-analyses and compiling, interpreting, and disseminating the up-to-date evidence for or against complementary medicine.

The Cochrane Library   This Web site provides a gateway to *The Cochrane Library*, and the Cochrane Field on Complementary and Alternative Medicine. The Cochrane CAM Field is coordinated by an international group of individuals dedicated to creating systematic reviews of randomized clinical trials in diverse areas of nonconventional medicine, including acupuncture, massage, chiropractic, herbal medicine, homeopathy, and mind–body therapy. The Cochrane CAM Field was founded in 1996 and is coordinated by the University of Maryland Center for Integrative Medicine.

www.bl.uk/collections/health/amed.html   Allied and Complementary Medicine Database (AMED), produced by the Medical Information Centre of the British Library, has over 100,000 references, including 400 biomedical journals.

Bandolier—Evidence-based Thinking about Healthcare Bandolier is an independent journal about evidence-based health care written by Oxford University scientists. The journal first appeared in February 1994. It is directed at both health care professionals and patients. The e-journal provides information about evidence of effectiveness in bullet format based on critical analysis of systematic reviews, meta-analyses, and single randomized, controlled trials drawn from the Cochrane Library and PubMed. The electronic version of *Bandolier* now has over one million visitors each month from all over the world. Many visitors are health care professionals; however, *Bandolier* is also a source of useful information for patients.

bmj.com Collected Resources: Complementary Medicine   This site provides a searchable database of articles published in the *British Medical Journal* pertaining to complementary and alternative medicine. It is indexed and cross-referenced.

◆ Resources for Monitoring Research in Conventional and Nonconventional Treatments

NCCAM Grantee Publications Database   This database provides citations of publications by NCCAM grantees. It covers the results of NCCAM-funded research. Publications are regularly added to this database. Specific citations can be found by the principal investigator's last name, title of article, journal name, grant mechanism, or grant number. Searches can also be done by key word or phrase contained in the title of the article.

www.clinicaltrials.gov   This site includes mostly government-sponsored studies and is the most comprehensive clinical trials directory on the Internet. It provides regularly updated information about federally funded and some privately supported human clinical trials that are currently in progress, and includes studies on nonconventional modalities. Data include the purpose of the study, who may participate, locations, and phone numbers for more details.

Oregon Center for Complementary and Alternative Medicine in Neurological Disorders (ORCCAMIND) ORCCAMIND is a center without walls committed to research on nonconventional treatments of neurological disorders. The center was created in 1999 through funding from NCCAM. Initial studies have examined treatment approaches using antioxidants, yoga, acupuncture, and chiropractic manipulation.

www.centerwatch.com This site is an excellent resource for identifying studies sponsored by the pharmaceutical industry or private institutions. The site lists more than 41,000 active industry and government-sponsored clinical trials, as well as new drug therapies in research and those recently approved by the FDA. Patients interested in participating in clinical research can make inquiries about specific ongoing trials.

◆ Evaluating Natural Products and Selecting Brands

www.naturaldatabase.com (subscription fee) This Web site is a valuable resource for both practitioners and patients. The Natural Medicines Comprehensive Database was released in September 1999 and is updated daily. The mission of the research and editorial team at Therapeutic Research Center is to critically evaluate the literature to produce an objective, evidence-based resource designed for health care professionals. This database provides a comprehensive listing of brand name natural product ingredients, and the ingredients of brand name products are linked to a monograph on the particular ingredient. Clinically relevant information is in a user-friendly format. Thousands of new references are added each year, and new interactions and safety concerns are added as soon as they are recognized. Effectiveness ratings are raised or lowered based on emerging research findings. There is an interface that permits identification of potential interactions between a specified natural product, other natural products, and conventional drugs. A new database and Web site have recently been created specifically for patients with the goal of providing patient-friendly wording on natural medicines. Sections of the patient database can be printed for patients during sessions.

www.factsandcomparisons.com (subscription) Facts and Comparisons is an established information service on new drug research that has been in existence for over 5 decades. Its mission is to compile unbiased, essential, and appropriate drug information. Thousands of articles, drug package inserts, lectures, and other relevant data are culled and edited year-round by a professional panel of pharmacists, physicians, and nurses to provide the most current drug information. The company annually publishes an updated version of Drug Facts and Comparisons and many other information services as printed reports.

http://www.consumerlab.com (subscription fee) Consumer-Lab.com (CL) provides independent test results and information to help consumers and health care professionals evaluate health, wellness, and nutrition products. It publishes results on its Web site and in published form in an annually updated book, *ConsumerLab.com's Guide to Buying Vitamins and Supplements*, and in technical reports covering a range of supplements. ConsumerLab is a certification company and enables companies of all sizes to have their products voluntarily tested for potential inclusion in its list of Approved Quality products and bear its seal of approval. In the past 5 years, CL has tested more than 1200 products. Products tested and rated include herbal products, vitamins and minerals, other natural product supplements, sports and energy products, functional foods, foods and beverages, and personal hygiene products.

http://www.nnfa.org The National Nutritional Foods Association (NNFA) was founded in 1936. Its mission is to promote the values and shared interests of retailers and suppliers in the natural nutritional foods and products industry, to safeguard retailers and suppliers of foods and natural products, and to create standards and procedures for self-regulation aimed at improving the quality and safety of natural foods, products, services, and labeling information.

http://www.usp.org The United States Pharmacopeia (USP) is the official public standards-setting authority for all prescription and over-the-counter medicines, dietary supplements, and other health care products manufactured and sold in the United States. USP is an independent, science-based public health organization. It sets standards for the quality of these products and works with health care providers to help them reach the standards. USP's standards are recognized and used in many other countries. Prescription and over-the-counter medicines available in the United States must, by federal law, meet USP's public standards, where such standards exist. USP disseminates its standards to pharmaceutical manufacturers, pharmacists, and other users through publications, official USP Reference Standards materials, and courses. USP also conducts verification programs for dietary supplement ingredients and products. These programs involve independent testing and review to verify ingredient and product integrity, purity, and potency for manufacturers who choose to participate.

http://www.nsf.org NSF International is a not-for-profit, nongovernmental organization, devoted to standards development, product certification, education, and risk management for public health and safety that has been in existence over 60 years and provides services for manufacturers in 80 countries. It provides third-party conformity assessment services. NSF has earned the Collaborating Center designation by the World Health Organization for Food and Water Safety and Indoor Environment.

◆ Identifying Qualified Practitioners of Nonconventional Therapies

http://www.pitt.edu/~cbw/prac.html This is a section of the Alternative Medicine Homepage (see above) that contains links to directories of practitioners in many areas of nonconventional medicine, including Chinese medicine, naturopathy, homeopathy, and mind–body practices. The site can be used to help identify qualified nonconventional practitioners when referring patients.

The ByRegion Network The site lists registered practitioners by practice area and geographic region. It is a useful tool for identifying practitioners who use a range of nonconventional approaches.

http://www.naturopathic.org The official Web site of the American Association of Naturopathic Physicians includes a search engine for identifying naturopathic physicians by specified geographic location or city.

http://www.holisticmedicine.org   The official Web site for the American Holistic Medicine Association (AHMA), the major organization for physicians who practice holistic medicine, includes a search engine for identifying AHMA members when looking for appropriate referrals in your area.

Note that appropriate referrals to nonconventional practitioners can also be identified through many Web sites included in the following sections.

◆ Biological Therapies

Bastyr University Library Resources Using CAM Medline   offers a user-friendly gateway to medical subject hierarchy (MEsH) terms in Medline that facilitate effective searches on a range of nonconventional biological therapies, including herbs and other natural products used as medicine, foods, aromatherapy, and many others.

Office of Dietary Supplements IBIDS Database   (subscription fee) The International Bibliographic Information on Dietary Supplements (IBIDS) database is the official Web site of the Office of Dietary Supplements, National Institutes of Health. The IBIDS database provides access to bibliographic citations and abstracts from published international and scientific literature on a range of dietary supplements. Users can search the full IBIDS database, a subset of Consumer Citations Only or Peer Reviewed Citations Only.

Phytochemical and Ethnobotanical Databases   This site is the homepage of Dr. Jim Duke, noted ethnobotanist, and the Agricultural Research Service of the U.S. Department of Agriculture. It is a valuable clinical resource that includes links to many phytochemical and ethnobotanical and nutritional databases and is intended primarily for researchers. The site includes an online dictionary of ethnobotany.

Phytotherapies.org   (free service for registered users) Although this site is the product of an herbal company based in Australia, it is a valuable resource for herbal practitioners and conventionally trained medical practitioners interested in learning more about herbal medicine. The site is updated weekly and includes editorial content, articles, and an extensive searchable and hyperlinked herbal database that includes monographs on current herbal therapeutics. Online inquiries can be submitted to experienced herbalists.

The Institute for Functional Medicine   (IFM) (subscription fee) The mission of the IFM is to improve patient outcomes through prevention, early assessment, and comprehensive management of complex, chronic disease by developing the functional medicine knowledge base as a bridge between research and clinical practice; teaching physicians and other health care providers the basic science and clinical applications of functional medicine; and working with policy makers, practitioners, educators, researchers, and the public to disseminate the functional medicine knowledge base more widely.

Herbal Medicine Internet Resources—the Alternative Medicine Homepage   This is part of the Alternative Medicine Homepage (see above), and is valuable gateway to the official Web sites of numerous professional associations concerned with all aspects of herbal medicine.

HerbMed   This Website is an interactive, electronic herbal database and provides hyperlinked access to the scientific data underlying the use of herbs for a range of medical and mental health problems. It is an evidence-based information resource about herbal medicines provided by the Alternative Medicine Foundation, Inc., a nonprofit organization. A limited free version of the database contains information on 75 common herbs, and a fee-based professional version, HerbMedPro, uses hyperlinks to cross-reference an extensive bibliographic collection on all aspects of herbal medicine. The databases are updated on a regular basis. Subscribers can request searches on specific herbs or particular clinical applications. The Web site is linked to numerous medical, scientific, and health-related Web sites, including the National Library of Medicine, MEDLINEPlus, and TEK*PAD, a project of the American Association for the Advancement of Medicine and the U.S. Patent and Trademarks Office.

Herb Research Foundation—Herbs and Herbal Medicine for Health   (subscription fee) This site includes expert compilations on specific herbals that contain carefully selected articles, studies, and/or discussions by experts that are available as downloads or in print form. The work of the Herb Research Foundation is based on its dedicated holdings of more than 300,000 scientific articles on thousands of herbs.

American Botanical Council—Herbal Medicine   (subscription fee) Established in 1988, the American Botanical Council (ABC) is the leading independent, nonprofit, international member-based organization providing education using science-based and traditional information to promote the responsible use of herbal medicine. The site includes databases on safety, use conditions for specific herbals, and searchable monographs depending on the level of membership.

NAPRALERT Database Summary Sheet   (subscription fee) The NAPRALERT File (NAtural PRoducts ALERT) contains bibliographic and factual data on natural products, including information on the pharmacology, biological activity, taxonomic distribution, chemistry of plant, microbial, and animal (including marine) extracts, as well as ethnomedicine use records. In addition, the database has information on the chemistry and pharmacology of secondary metabolites that are derived from natural sources and that have known structure. NAPRALERT contains records from 1650 to the present; however, roughly half of the content comes from systematic literature reviews from 1975 to the present. NAPRALERT is a valuable information research tool for practitioners interested in the history and basic science of natural product–derived medicines.

International Journal of Aromatherapy   This site is the home of the *International Journal of Aromatherapy*, which covers the uses of aromatherapy for mental, emotional, or physical complaints. Subjects include the use of natural, aromatic plant oils and essential oils and massage and touch therapy.

◆ Somatic and Mind–Body Approaches

Federation MBS   This is the Web site of the Federation of Massage, Body Work and Somatic Practice Organizations, a nonprofit membership organization in the massage, bodywork, and somatic practice field. The site is a gateway to other Websites of organizations related to different somatic approaches, including massage, Rolfing, Feldenkrais, and the Alexander technique.

TRI Homepage The Touch Research Institute is dedicated to studying the effects of touch therapy. TR has researched the effects of massage therapy at all stages of life, from newborns to senior citizens. The site includes summaries of studies conducted through TRI as well as abstracts of studies on Tai Chi, yoga, and acupuncture.

Manual Healing Internet Resources—the Alternative Medicine Homepage This part of the Alternative Medicine Homepage (see above) provides valuable links to official Web sites of numerous professional associations concerned with a broad range of somatic therapies.

Journal of Bodywork and Movement Therapies The site provides access to the electronic version of *Journal of Bodywork and Movement Therapies,* which covers therapeutic advances using bodywork, including the Alexander technique, chiropractic, cranial therapy, dance, Feldenkrais, massage therapy, osteopathy, Shiatsu and Tuina massage, Tai Chi, qigong, and yoga.

Mind Body Control—the Alternative Medicine Homepage This part of the Alternative Medicine Homepage (see above) acts as a valuable gateway to numerous Web sites pertaining to a range of mind–body practices. Note that this site also includes links to many Websites on somatic approaches and therapies based on subtle energy.

AMTA Foundation Research Database This is the Web site of the Massage Therapy Foundation and the Massage Therapy Research Database. The mission of the foundation is to chart an agenda for research on health benefits of massage therapy. The initial version of the database was compiled in 2000 and is updated quarterly. There are currently more than 4,700 citations of articles and books about massage therapy. Citations are reviewed by a committee of massage therapists, physicians, and researchers. There is no subscription fee, and the database is available only through the foundation's Web site.

◆ Therapies Based on Forms of Energy-Information Validated by Current Western Science

American Music Therapy Association The mission of the American Music Therapy Association is to advance public awareness of the benefits of music therapy and increase access to quality music therapy services in a rapidly changing world.

The Biofeedback Network provides extensive links to societies and research groups that study various applications of biofeedback.

Scientific Articles and Citations incorporates the research library for Applied Neuroscience Inc. and contains research articles on clinical applications of quantitative electroencephalography (qEEG) and EEG biofeedback in mental health care.

www.ambientintelligence.org/ This Web site is an excellent and comprehensive resource for research and Web-based tools for virtual reality therapy. The site provides summaries of books and research papers on virtual reality–based therapy and includes links to the leading research centers. It provides free downloads of development tools and programs to facilitate learning about clinical uses of virtual reality technologies.

VR Therapy—the Future of Mental Health Treatment This site is an excellent resource for mental health practitioners who are considering using virtual reality (VR) exposure therapy. The aim of the VR Therapy Project is the promotion of information and use of VR over the Internet. The mission of the site developers is to offer an accessible global knowledge base on emerging clinical applications of virtual reality.

◆ Approaches Based on Forms of Energy-Information Not Validated by Current Western Science

The Samueli Institute This is the Web site of the Rockfeller-Samueli Center for Research in Mind-Body Energy, established in 2002. The goals of the program are to promote and support scientifically credible research on spiritual and energy healing. The purpose of the program is to test the impact of healing energy on patients and to explore mechanisms of healing energy in the laboratory. Development of objective and clinically relevant measures is a key focus of the program. These measurements include patients' quality of life, changes in health, effects on brain function, cell and gene changes, and the overall risks, benefits, and costs associated with delivery of spiritual and energy healing practices in health care.

Wellcome Centre—Asia's Medical Systems and Traditions This site provides extensive links to other Web sites on traditional Asian systems of medicine, including Chinese medicine, Ayurveda, and Tibetan medicine. Wellcome Centre members edit the Wellcome series, publishing fine editions of classical texts in their own language. This Web site aims to introduce key areas in history of Asian medicine and focuses on current work in the field.

Acubriefs.com—a Comprehensive Acupuncture Research Resource Acubriefs was established by a grant from the Medical Acupuncture Research Foundation (MARF) and is supported through foundation grants. Its mission is to create a comprehensive online database of English languages references on acupuncture. The site plans to eventually incorporate non-English references depending on funding.

British Acupuncture Council (BAcC) represents professional acupuncturists who have extensive training in acupuncture and the biomedical sciences. The Acupuncture Research Resource Centre has produced a valuable set of briefing papers reviewing the evidence of effectiveness of acupuncture in the treatment of specific medical and mental health conditions, including addiction and substance abuse, anxiety and depression, stroke, menopause, and migraine. The briefing papers are available as free downloads in PDF format.

Welcome to TCM Online This resource is a gateway to over 20 online databases on Chinese medicine, most of which are in Chinese but some of which are in English. Databases cover Chinese herbal medicine, Tibetan medicine, clinical indications for Chinese medical treatments, services available in thousands of Chinese hospitals, and newspaper articles on Chinese medicine (i.e., in China). This Web site is a valuable research tool for individuals interested in the practice of Chinese medicine and Tibetan medicine in Asian countries.

Welcome to Acudetox   This is the official Web site of the National Acupuncture Detoxification Association (NADA). The mission of the site is to promote improved understanding of the principles of both Chinese medicine and chemical dependency. The site includes NADA protocols that have been carefully developed and extensively tested. More than 500 clinical sites in the United States, Europe, Australia, and the Caribbean currently utilize these protocols for the management of detoxification in alcohol and drug abuse. The protocols are promoted through public education about acupuncture as a recovery tool, training and certification of professionals in use of the techniques, consultation with local organizations in setting up treatment sites, and the distribution of NADA-approved literature, audiotapes, and videotapes.

IAAM   is the Web site for the International Association for Auricular Medicine, whose mission is to provide an international nonbiased forum for developing the science and practice of auricular acupuncture, based on the teachings of Paul Nogier. The association provides a forum for medical practitioners, dentists, physical therapists, acupuncturists, and mental health practitioners who have a particular interest in auricular therapy and auricular medicine. Several chat rooms are available to facilitate discussion on various aspects of auricular therapy in order to contribute to the research knowledge and clinical applications of auricular therapy.

INDEX   is the Web site of Emory University's Center on Complementary and Alternative Medicine in Neurodegenerative Diseases, whose mission is to rigorously study promising nonconventional interventions that preserve or enhance function and quality of life among individuals with neurodegenerative disorders. The center was started in 2000 under a 5-year National Institutes of Health grant. Ongoing pilot studies include the investigation of nonconventional treatments of insomnia in patients with Parkinson's disease, the investigation of qigong and Tai Chi on movement symptoms in Parkinson's disease, the putative role of sex hormone therapy as neuroprotective agents in transgenic mice with Huntington's disease, and the investigation of the effects of neuromuscular massage therapy in Parkinson's disease.

Welcome to www.hom-inform.org   (no fee) This Web site is the home of the British Homeopathic Library, an information service dedicated to the research and practice of homeopathy. Library services include a database of over 25,000 article and book references on homeopathy, and access to Hom-Inform, a search and query service on homeopathy. Both services are available free of charge.

www.hpus.com   This is the official Web site of the Homeopathic Pharmacopoeia of the United States. It has been in continuous publication since 1897 and includes information on homeopathic remedies that are regulated by the FDA and listed in the Homeopathic Pharmacopoeia of the United States. A series of loose-leaf binders providing comprehensive information about FDA-endorsed homeopathic remedies is available for purchase through the site.

Healing Touch International Home Page   The mission of Healing Touch International is to disseminate information about Healing Touch while supporting member practitioners. The site is a gateway to three large professional organizations of Healing Touch practitioners: Healing Touch International, the Colorado Center for Healing Touch, and Healing Touch International Foundation. The site for Healing Touch International includes an extensive bibliography of studies on Healing Touch in all areas of medicine and descriptions of ongoing research.

ISSSEEM,   the International Society for the Study of Subtle Energies and Energy Medicine, was established to explore the application of subtle energies to the experience of consciousness, healing, and human potential and is designed as a bridging organization for scientists, clinicians, therapists, healers, and laypeople. ISSSEEM encourages open-minded exploration of phenomena associated with the practice of energy healing. The site includes abstracts and contents of the *Subtle Energies and Energy Medicine Journal.* Links to conferences on subtle energy healing, shamanic healing, and consciousness research are provided.

Center for Spirituality and Healing   Established in 1995 at the University of Minnesota, the Center for Spirituality and Healing has the goal of integrating biomedical, complementary, cross-cultural, and spiritual care. The center provides interdisciplinary education, clinical care, and outreach while integrating evidence-based research to renew, enhance, and transform health care practice, health sciences education, and clinical care.

Also see   the TRI Homepage and the *Journal of Bodywork and Movement Therapies* (under Somatic and Mind–Body Approaches).

◆ Miscellaneous Resources

www.APACAM.org   is the dedicated Web site of the Caucus on Complementary, Alternative and Integrative Approaches in Mental Health Care of the American Psychiatric Association. There is no subscription fee, but you must be a psychiatrist to be a full member of the caucus. The site is evolving rapidly and includes online forums that are useful for networking with other psychiatrists regarding a range of nonconventional treatments. The site includes a library and links to related sites reviewed by caucus members.

IHSM   The Institute for Healing in Society and Medicine (IHSM) is dedicated to catalyzing the transformation of medicine from the inside out by reconnecting individual health care providers with the richness of their own inner lives, their authentic professional mission, and the sacred roots of medicine. By promoting increased awareness in the lives of health care providers, IHSM strives to restore the primary focus of medicine in healing, enhance the quality of the doctor–patient relationship, increase the delivery of effective, low-cost preventive therapies based on patient self-care, and provide an impetus to adopt new educational and research models for better health care delivery. IHSM conducts research on patient care and health care provider education and uses findings to develop educational, training, and retreat opportunities for health care providers.

Index